MEDICAL SURGICAL NURSING
Made Easy

MEDICAL SURGICAL NURSING
Made Easy

Seenidurai Paulraj
MSc (Nursing) MPhil (Nursing) PhD (Nursing)
MA (Political Science) MS (Psychotherapy and Counseling)

Chief Health Consultant
Sarva Shiksha Abhiyan
Department of School Education
Vijayawada, Andhra Pradesh, India

Ex-Member
UG and PG Board of Studies for Nursing
Rajiv Gandhi University of Health Sciences
Bengaluru, Karnataka, India

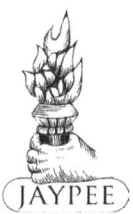

JAYPEE BROTHERS MEDICAL PUBLISHERS
The Health Sciences Publisher
New Delhi | London

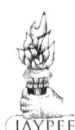 **Jaypee Brothers Medical Publishers (P) Ltd**

Headquarters
Jaypee Brothers Medical Publishers (P) Ltd
EMCA House, 23/23-B
Ansari Road, Daryaganj
New Delhi 110 002, India
Landline: +91-11-23272143, +91-11-23272703
+91-11-23282021, +91-11-23245672
Email: jaypee@jaypeebrothers.com

Corporate Office
Jaypee Brothers Medical Publishers (P) Ltd
4838/24, Ansari Road, Daryaganj
New Delhi 110 002, India
Phone: +91-11-43574357
Fax: +91-11-43574314
Email: jaypee@jaypeebrothers.com

Overseas Office
J.P. Medical Ltd
83 Victoria Street, London
SW1H 0HW (UK)
Phone: +44 20 3170 8910
Fax: +44 (0)20 3008 6180
Email: info@jpmedpub.com

Website: www.jaypeebrothers.com
Website: www.jaypeedigital.com

© 2022, Jaypee Brothers Medical Publishers

The views and opinions expressed in this book are solely those of the original contributor(s)/author(s) and do not necessarily represent those of editor(s) of the book.

All rights reserved. No part of this publication may be reproduced, stored or transmitted in any form or by any means, electronic, mechanical, photocopying, recording or otherwise, without the prior permission in writing of the publishers.

All brand names and product names used in this book are trade names, service marks, trademarks or registered trademarks of their respective owners. The publisher is not associated with any product or vendor mentioned in this book.

Medical knowledge and practice change constantly. This book is designed to provide accurate, authoritative information about the subject matter in question. However, readers are advised to check the most current information available on procedures included and check information from the manufacturer of each product to be administered, to verify the recommended dose, formula, method and duration of administration, adverse effects and contraindications. It is the responsibility of the practitioner to take all appropriate safety precautions. Neither the publisher nor the author(s)/editor(s) assume any liability for any injury and/or damage to persons or property arising from or related to use of material in this book.

This book is sold on the understanding that the publisher is not engaged in providing professional medical services. If such advice or services are required, the services of a competent medical professional should be sought.

Every effort has been made where necessary to contact holders of copyright to obtain permission to reproduce copyright material. If any have been inadvertently overlooked, the publisher will be pleased to make the necessary arrangements at the first opportunity.

Inquiries for bulk sales may be solicited at: jaypee@jaypeebrothers.com

Medical Surgical Nursing Made Easy

First Edition: **2022**
ISBN: 978-93-90595-80-8

Dedicated to
My beloved Parents
Mr M Seenidurai and Mrs Esther Seenidurai

who were the role models, guide and friend to me in all through my life endeavors and also supported me a lot at times of my professional and personal downfall and for giving their valuable suggestions and support in a constant manner for my upliftment in life.

I just wanted to say thank you for all the sacrifices you have made, all the support you have given me, all the guidance you gave when I needed it most and moulding me into the person I have become today

Contributors

Anand M MSc (N)
Principal
Chinai College of Nursing
Bengaluru, Karnataka, India

Asha P Nair MSc (N) MPhil (N)
Registered Nurse
Government Medical College
SAT Hospital
Thiruvananthapuram, Kerala, India

Auxilia PD MSc (N)
Professor in Nursing
St John's College of Nursing
Bengaluru, Karnataka, India

Gopalakrishnan N BSc (N) CHCWM
Registered Nurse
Government General Hospital
Puducherry, India

Hemavati G MSc (N) PhD (N)
Professor
Medical Surgical Nursing
Postgraduate College of Nursing
Bhilai, Chhattisgarh, India

Jihi Melba J MSc (N)
Professor in Nursing
Al Shifa College of Nursing
Malappuram, Kerala, India

Priyanka Gurrala MSc (N)
Assistant Professor
Nightingale College of Nursing
Bengaluru, Karnataka, India

Punithamani G MSc (N)
Principal
St Mary's College of Nursing
Chitradurga, Karnataka, India

Ramesh C MSc (N) PhD (N)
Lecturer
Department of Medical Surgical Nursing
Manipal College of Nursing
Manipal, Karnataka, India

Ramya Satheesh MSc (N)
Clinical Instructor
Kuwait Cancer Control Center
Kuwait

Sudhakar Dayalan MSc (N) PhD (N)
Principal
RL College of Nursing
Gwalior, Madhya Pradesh, India

Suresh S MSc (N)
Registered Nurse
Perambur Headquarters Railway Hospital
Chennai, Tamil Nadu, India

Preface

We welcome our readers to the new book *Medical Surgical Nursing Made Easy*. In planning this book, a firm commitment has been made in assuring a thorough and complete text. Latest concepts and newer classifications have been highlighted in it to keep the students abreast with recent advances. A lot of information has been packed in the form of easy flowcharts. Almost all the chapters are adorned with figures related to the content. The art and science of medical surgical nursing have progressed considerably in recent times and every effort has been made to keep pace with the advancement in it. This book has been arranged in 14 chapters and every chapter provides latest information. I hope this book will be a complete one in its own field. Yet I have always tried to make this book handy. The future of the nursing promises dynamic changes and continual challenges. Nurses of tomorrow need a broad knowledge base from which to provide care. This textbook is designed for beginning students in all types of professional nursing programmes. I am indebted to the many educators and students who have shared their thoughts, visions and ideas with me and I credit each of them as valuable collaborators for this book. I hope that I have provided a comprehensive and enduring guide and reference for nurses to pursue excellence in nursing care. Nursing care is structured by the activities planned and carried out through clinical reasoning and uses multiple thinking strategies when applying the nursing process. So friends happy reading/understanding and all the best.

Seenidurai Paulraj

Acknowledgments

The writing of this book began with the idea of providing nurses with a resource that would allow them to have enough information on medical surgical nursing at their fingertips. Providing a resource that contains all information in one location makes the book a very valuable resource.

This book would not have been possible without the help of many wonderful friends and colleagues. I wish to extend a heartfelt thanks to all those who supported this journey of writing the book.

I will be failing badly if I do not mention the encouragement which I received from my wife (Ms Jerene Paulraj), sister (Ms Prema Charles) and brother (Mr Moses Jayaraj) in writing the book which has been a unique experience. I am grateful to M/s Jaypee Brothers Medical Publishers (P) Ltd, New Delhi, India for doing a commendable job.

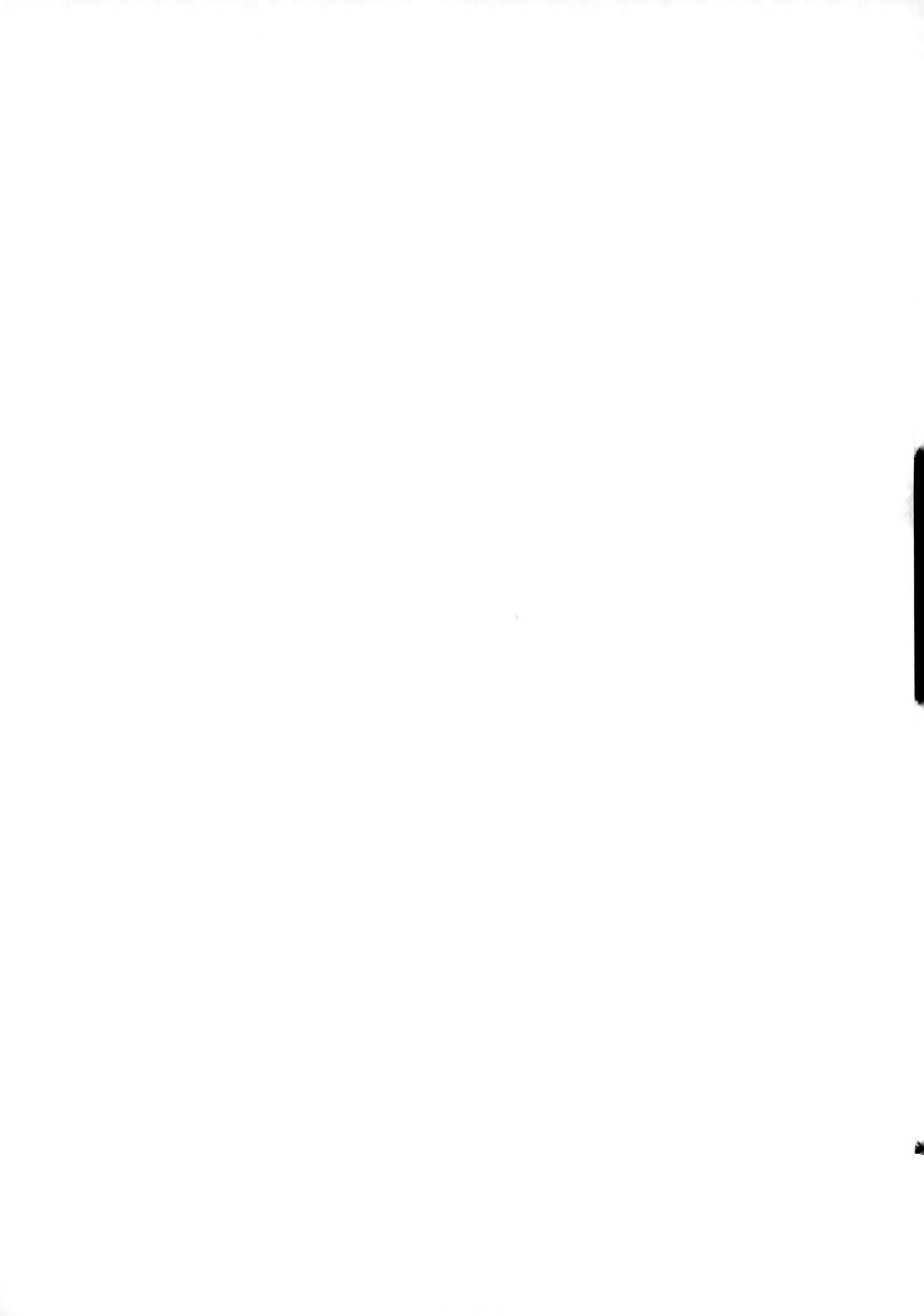

Contents

1. **Disorders of Nervous System** 1

   Alzheimer's Disease *1*
   Amyotrophic Lateral Sclerosis (Lou Gehrig's Disease) *3*
   Bell's Palsy *5*
   Brain Abscess *6*
   Cerebral Infarction *7*
   Coma *9*
   Decompression Sickness *12*
   Delirium *15*
   Dementia *16*
   Encephalitis *18*
   Epilepsy or Seizure *19*
   Floppy Infant Syndrome (Hypotonia) *22*
   Gilles de la Tourette Syndrome *24*
   Guillain-Barre Syndrome *26*
   Headache *28*
   Herniated Disc *30*
   Huntington's Disease *32*
   Hydrocephalus *34*
   Increased Intracranial Pressure *36*
   Kennedy's Disease *38*
   Meningitis *39*
   Moebius Syndrome *42*
   Multiple Sclerosis *43*
   Myasthenia Gravis (Goldflam Disease) *45*
   Myoglobinuria *47*
   Neurosarcoidosis *49*
   Paraneoplastic Syndromes *50*
   Parkinson's Disease *53*
   Prion Disease *55*
   Spinal Cord Injury *57*
   Stroke (Cerebrovascular Accident) *59*
   Susac's Syndrome *62*
   Syncope (Sudden Fainting) *63*

Syringomyelia *65*
Thoracic Outlet Syndrome *67*
Transient Ischemic Attack (Mini-Stroke) *69*
Traumatic Brain Injury *71*

2. Disorders of Endocrine 75

Addison's Disease *75*
Cushing's Syndrome *77*
Diabetes Insipidus *78*
Diabetes Mellitus *80*
Diabetic Ketoacidosis *83*
Hyperaldosteronism *85*
Hyperosmolar Hyperglycemic Nonketotic Syndrome *87*
Hyperparathyroidism *89*
Hyperpituitarism *91*
Hyperthyroidism *92*
Hypoglycemia *94*
Hypoparathyroidism *96*
Hypopituitarism (Simmond's Disease) *98*
Hypothyroidism (Myxedema) *100*
Syndrome of Inappropriate Anti-diuretic Hormone Secretion *102*

3. Disorders of Eye 105

Age-related Macular Degeneration *105*
Blepharitis *107*
Cataract *108*
Chalazion *110*
Conjunctivitis *112*
Correctable Refractive Errors *114*
Diabetic Retinopathy *117*
Eye Trauma *119*
Glaucoma *120*
Hordeolum (Stye) *123*
Keratitis *124*
Retinal Detachment *126*
Strabismus (Squint Eyes) (Crossed Eyes) *127*
Visual Impairment (Blindness) *129*

4. Disorders of Ear, Nose and Throat 132

Acute Pharyngitis (Sore Throat) *132*
Cerumen Impaction (Earwax) *134*
Deviated Nasal Septum *135*

Epistaxis *137*
Hearing Loss *139*
Labyrinthitis *141*
Mastoiditis *143*
Meniere's Disease (Endolymphatic Hydrops) *145*
Nasal Polyps *147*
Otitis Media *149*
Otosclerosis *151*
Peritonsillar Abscess (Quinsy) *153*
Rhinitis *155*
Sinusitis *157*
Tonsillitis *159*

5. Disorders of Gastrointestinal System 161
Amoebic Dysentery (Amoebiasis) *161*
Anal Fissure *162*
Anal Fistula *164*
Appendicitis *166*
Bacillary Dysentery or Shigellosis *167*
Cholecystitis *168*
Cholelithiasis *170*
Constipation (Dyschezia) *172*
Crohn's Disease *174*
Deficiency Diseases *176*
Diarrhea *180*
Gastritis *181*
Gastroesophageal Reflux Disease with Esophagitis *183*
Hemorrhoids *185*
Hepatic Encephalopathy *186*
Hepatitis *188*
Hernia *189*
Intestinal Obstruction *192*
Liver Abscess *193*
Liver Cirrhosis *195*
Malabsorption Syndrome *197*
Pancreatitis *199*
Parasitic Infestations *201*
Peptic Ulcer Disease *203*
Peritonitis *205*
Pharyngitis *207*
Ulcerative Colitis *208*

6. Disorders of Respiratory System 211

Atelectasis 211
Bronchial Asthma 213
Bronchiectasis 215
Bronchitis 216
Chest Trauma 218
Chronic Obstructive Pulmonary Disease 220
Cor Pulmonale 222
Cystic Fibrosis (Cystic Lungs) 224
Hypoxia 225
Lung Abscess 228
Pleural Effusion 230
Pleurisy (Pleuritis or Pleurodynia) 231
Pneumonia 233
Pneumothorax 235
Pulmonary Embolism 237
Pulmonary Hypertension 240
Pulmonary Tuberculosis 242
Respiratory Failure 244
Sarcoidosis 246
Tracheal Obstruction 248

7. Disorders of Cardiac System 250

Angina Pectoris 250
Aortic Aneurysm 252
Atherosclerosis 254
Cardiac Arrest 257
Cardiac Dysrhythmias 259
Cardiomyopathy 262
Congestive Cardiac Failure 265
Coronary Artery Disease (Ischemic Heart Disease) 268
Endocarditis 271
Hypertension (Silent Killer) 273
Hypotension 275
Myocardial Infarction 277
Myocarditis 279
Pericarditis 281
Rheumatic Fever 283
Valvular Heart Disease 285

8. Disorders of Vascular System 291

Acute Blood Loss 291
Anemia 293

Hemochromatosis *298*
Hemophilia (The Royal Disease) *299*
Raynaud's Phenomenon *301*
Thromboangiitis Obliterans (Buerger's Disease) *303*
Varicose Veins *305*
Venous Thrombosis *307*
Von Willebrand Disease *308*

9. Disorders of Renal System 311

Acute Kidney Injury (Acute Renal Failure) *311*
Chronic Kidney Disease (End-stage Renal Disease) *314*
Cystitis *316*
Glomerulonephritis *318*
Nephrosclerosis *320*
Nephrotic Syndrome *322*
Polycystic Kidney Disease *324*
Pyelonephritis *325*
Renal Calculi (Kidney Stones) *327*
Uremic Encephalopathy *329*
Urethral Strictures *331*
Urethritis *332*
Urinary Incontinence *334*
Urinary Tract Infection *336*

10. Disorders of Reproductive System 338

Male Reproductive System **338**

Benign Prostatic Hyperplasia *338*
Cryptorchidism (Undescended Testes) *340*
Epididymitis *341*
Erectile Dysfunction (Impotence) *343*
Male Infertility *345*
Prostatitis *347*
Varicocele *349*

Female Reproductive System **350**

Abortion *350*
Bartholin's Abscess *352*
Dysmenorrhea *354*
Ectopic Pregnancy *356*
Endometritis *357*
Female Infertility *359*
Fibroid Uterus *361*
Pelvic Inflammatory Disease *362*
Polycystic Ovary Disease (Stein-Leventhal Syndrome) *364*

Toxic Shock Syndrome *367*
Uterine Prolapse *369*

11. Disorders of Skin 371

Acne Vulgaris *371*
Athlete's Foot (Tinea Pedis) *373*
Burns *374*
Candidiasis *378*
Cellulitis *379*
Dermatitis (Eczema) *381*
Impetigo *383*
Onychomycosis (Fungal Nail Infection) *384*
Psoriasis *385*
Tinea Corporis (Ringworm of the Body) *387*
Scabies *388*
Shingles *390*

12. Disorders of Musculoskeletal System 392

Acute Low Back Pain *392*
Ankylosing Spondylitis *394*
Carpal Tunnel Syndrome *395*
Fracture *397*
Gout *401*
Herniated Lumbar Disk *402*
Muscular Dystrophy *404*
Myositis Ossificans (Heterotopic Ossification) *406*
Osteoarthritis *408*
Osteomalacia *409*
Osteomyelitis *411*
Osteoporosis *413*
Paget's Disease *414*
Rheumatoid Arthritis *416*
Sprain *418*
Strain *420*
Systemic Lupus Erythematosus *421*

13. Communicable Diseases 424

Acquired Immunodeficiency Syndrome *424*
Chikungunya *426*
Chickenpox *428*
Chlamydia (Silent Infection) *429*
Cholera *430*
Dengue Fever *432*

Diphtheria *434*
Ebola Virus Disease *435*
Filariasis *437*
Gonorrhea *439*
Influenza *440*
Japanese Encephalitis (JE) *442*
Kala-Azar (Visceral Leishmaniasis) *444*
Leprosy (Hansen's Disease) *445*
Leptospirosis *448*
Malaria *450*
Measles (Rubeola) *452*
Mumps (Epidemic Parotitis) *454*
Pertussis (Whooping Cough) *455*
Plague *457*
Poliomyelitis *459*
Rubella (German Measles or Three-day Measles) *461*
Severe Acute Respiratory Syndrome *462*
Smallpox *464*
Swine Flu *466*
Syphilis *468*
Tetanus (Lockjaw) *470*
Typhoid (Enteric Fever) *471*
Yellow Fever *473*
Zika Virus Disease *475*

14. Oncology-related Disorders 477

Etiology *478*
Risk Factors *478*
Pathophysiology *478*
Types of Cancer *479*
Stages of Cancer *479*
Clinical Features *480*
Complications *480*
Prevention of Cancer *497*
Management *497*

Index *501*

CHAPTER 1

Disorders of Nervous System

CHAPTER OUTLINE

- Alzheimer's disease
- Amyotrophic lateral sclerosis
- Bell's palsy
- Brain abscess
- Cerebral infarction
- Coma
- Decompression sickness
- Delirium
- Dementia
- Encephalitis
- Epilepsy or seizure
- Floppy infant syndrome
- Gilles de la Tourette syndrome
- Guillain-Barre syndrome
- Headache
- Herniated disc
- Huntington's disease
- Hydrocephalus
- Increased intracranial pressure
- Kennedy's disease
- Meningitis
- Moebius syndrome
- Multiple sclerosis
- Myasthenia gravis
- Myoglobinuria
- Neurosarcoidosis
- Paraneoplastic syndromes
- Parkinson's disease
- Prion disease
- Spinal cord injury
- Stroke
- Susac's syndrome
- Syncope
- Syringomyelia
- Thoracic outlet syndrome
- Transient ischemic attack
- Traumatic brain injury

ALZHEIMER'S DISEASE

Definition

Alzheimer's disease is a chronic, progressive, degenerative disease of the brain which interferes with memory, thinking, affect, and judgment.

Etiology

- Idiopathic
- Viral or bacterial infections
- Autoimmune dysfunction
- Genetic abnormalities
- Down's syndrome.

Risk Factors

- Advancing age
- Overproduction of Amyloid-beta
- Heredity
- Sex
- Mild cognitive impairment
- Lifestyle modification.

2. Disorders of Nervous System

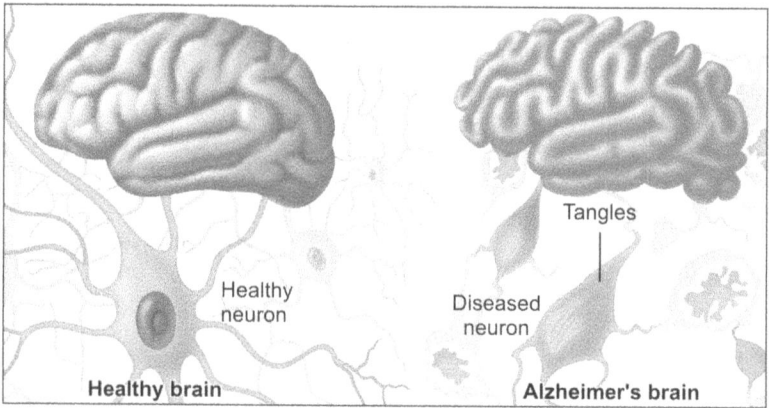

Fig. 1.1: Shows the comparison of a healthy brain and a brain with Azheimer's.

Types
There are three types of Alzheimer's disease as follows:
1. *Mild Alzheimer's disease:*
   - Getting lost of oneself
   - Trouble in handling money and paying bills
   - Repeating questions
   - Taking much time than before to complete normal daily tasks
   - Poor judgment:
     - Losing things or misplacing them in odd places
     - Mood and personality changes
2. *Moderate Alzheimer's disease:*
   - Increased memory loss and confusion
   - Problems of recognizing family members and friends
   - Inability to learn new things
   - Difficulty in carrying out tasks that involve multiple steps
   - Problems of coping with new situations
   - Delusions and paranoia
   - Impulsive behavior
3. *Severe Alzheimer's disease:*
   - Inability to recognize oneself or family
   - Inability to communicate
   - Weight loss
   - Seizures
   - Skin infections
   - Difficulty in swallowing
   - Groaning, moaning, or grunting,
   - Increased sleep duration
   - Lack of bowel and bladder control.

Pathophysiology

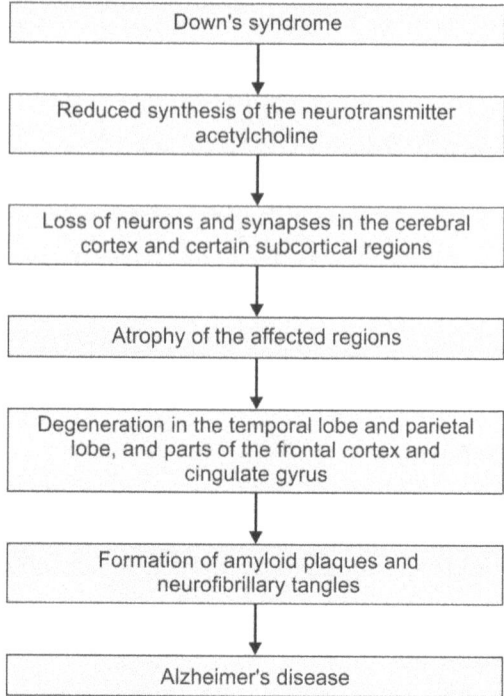

Clinical Features
- Memory loss that affects job skills
- Difficulty in performing familiar tasks
- Problems with language

- Disorientation to time and place
- Poor or decreased judgment
- Problems with abstract thinking
- Misplacing things
- Changes in mood or behavior
- Changes in personality
- Loss of initiative.

Complications

- Wandering tendency
- Getting lost
- Falls and combative behavior leading to injuries and fractures
- Infections
- Pneumonia.

Diagnostic Tests

- History
- Physical examination
- Magnetic resonance imaging
- Positron emission tomography
- Single photon emission computed tomography
- Urine testing
- Histopathological examination
- Neuropsychological testing
- Electrocardiogram
- Blood tests
- Thyroid function test.

Management

Medical

- **Acetylcholinesterase inhibitors:** It reduces the rate at which acetylcholine is broken down, thereby increasing the concentration of acetylcholine in the brain and combating the loss of acetylcholine caused by the death of cholinergic neurons. For example, donepezil, galantamine, rivastigmine, etc.
- **N-Methyl D-Aspartate (NMDA) receptor antagonist:** It acts on the glutamatergic system by blocking NMDA receptors and inhibiting their overstimulation by glutamate. For example, Memantine.
- **Selective serotonin reuptake inhibitors:** It helps in improving cognitive ability. For example, sertraline, fluvoxamine, citalopram, fluoxetine, etc.
- **Neuroleptics:** It helps to reduce aggression and improves cognitive behavior. For example, haloperidol, loxapine, risperidone, olanzapine, etc.
- **Antioxidants:** It slows down progression of the disease by preventing nerve cell damage by destroying toxic free radicals. For example, vitamin-C, vitamin-A, selegiline, etc.

Nursing

- Maintain patient's usual routines as much as possible
- Communicate clearly to the patient
- Reduce stressors such as fatigue, overstimulation or pain
- Involve family members in care
- Keep them active-physically, mentally and socially.

AMYOTROPHIC LATERAL SCLEROSIS (LOU GEHRIG'S DISEASE)

Definition

It is a progressive neurodegenerative disease that attacks the nerve cells (neurons) in the brain and the spinal cord that control voluntary muscles.

Etiology

- Gene mutation
- Chemical imbalance
- Disorganized immune response
- Protein mishandling.

Risk Factors

- Heredity
- People between the age 40 to 60 years
- Men
- Smoking
- Lead exposure
- People in military service.

4. Disorders of Nervous System

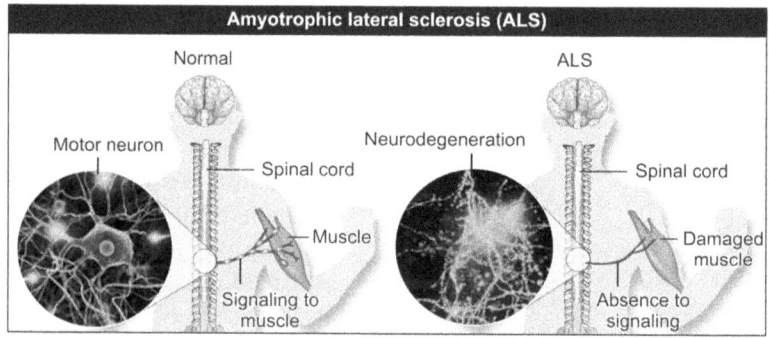

Fig. 1.2: Shows the comparison of a normal brain and amyotrophic lateral sclerosis (ALS).

Pathophysiology

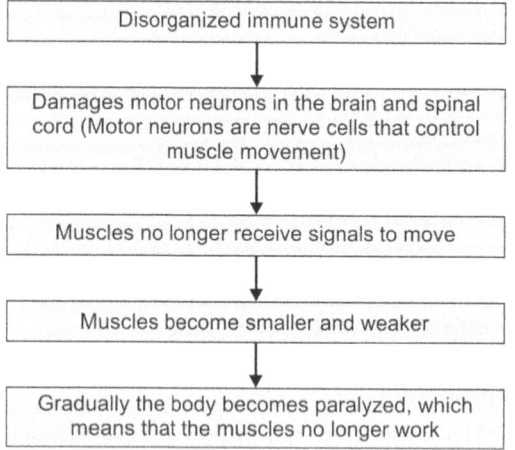

Clinical Features

Initial Symptoms

- Twitching
- Cramping
- Weakness in the legs and arms
- Difficulty speaking, chewing or swallowing.

Late Symptoms

- Weight loss
- Fatigue
- Exaggerated reflexes
- Decreased coordination.

Complications

- Respiratory problems
- Muscle twitches
- Muscle tightness
- Eating problems
- Speaking problems
- Dementia.

Diagnostic Tests

- History
- Physical examination
- Electromyography—to detect electrical activity in muscles
- Nerve conduction study (NCS)—to measure electrical energy by assessing the nerve's ability to send a signal
- Magnetic resonance imaging
- Spinal tap (lumbar puncture)
- Muscle biopsy.

Management

Medical

- **Anti-glutamates:** It prevents the damage that can result from the nerve cell being overexcited by glutamate, an amino acid that affects nerves that sends messages from the brain to muscles. For example, riluzole, etc.
- **Anticonvulsants:** It helps in easing cramps. For example, phenytoin sodium, diazepam, etc.
- **Anti-spastic agent:** It helps in relieving stiffness in limbs and the throat. For example, lioresal, gablofen, etc.

Nursing

- Promote adequate nutritional intake
- Establish effective means of communication

- Initiate use of word boards or letter board if unable to use arms
- Keep them as active as possible
- Encourage verbalization of feelings.

BELL'S PALSY

Definition

The temporary paralysis of one or both the facial nerves which results due to damage or trauma may finally lead to inability to control facial muscles on the affected side is known as Bell's palsy.

Etiology

- Acute mononeuropathy (disease involving only one nerve)
- Idiopathic
- Viral infections (Herpes simplex 1 type)
- Bacterial infections
- Auto immune disorders.

Risk Factors

- Stress
- Lack of sleep
- Minor illness
- Physical trauma
- Upper respiratory tract infections
- Diabetes
- Pregnancy during third trimester
- Upper respiratory tract infections.

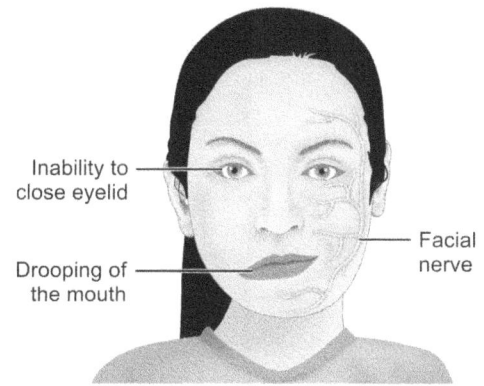

Fig. 1.3: Depicts the cardinal features of Bell's palsy.

Pathophysiology

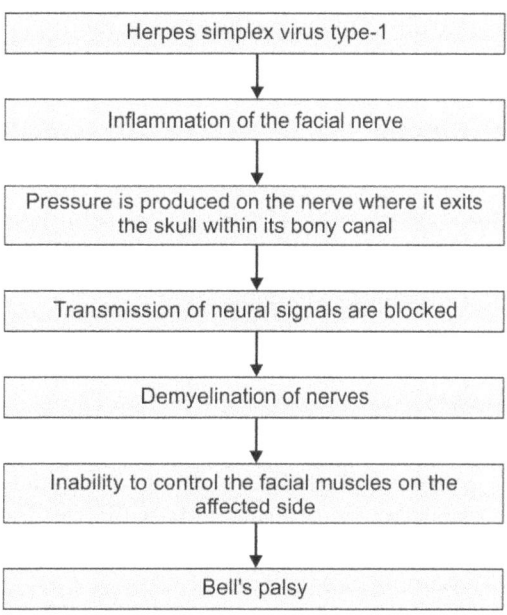

Clinical Features

- Facial drooping on the affected side
- Facial tingling
- Pain persists behind the ears
- Vertigo
- Dizziness
- Hearing loss
- Severe headache
- Neck pain
- Memory problems
- Balance problems
- Ipsilateral limb paresthesia
- Ipsilateral limb weakness
- Sense of clumsiness
- Swollen and tender lymph nodes.

Complications

- Corneal damage
- Poor nutrition
- Depression
- Ageusia (loss of taste)
- Chronic facial spasm
- Crocodile tear syndrome (the client shed their tears while they are eating)

Disorders of Nervous System

- Irreversible damage to facial nerves
- Synkinesis
- Misdirected regrowth of nerve fibers.

Diagnostic Tests

- History
- Physical examination
- Electromyography
- X-ray
- Magnetic resonance imaging
- Computerized tomography.

Management

Medical

- **Corticosteroids:** It helps to reduce inflammation and edema and this inturn reduces vascular compression and permits restoration of blood circulation to the nerve. For example, prednisone.
- **Analgesics:** It helps to relieve facial pain. For example, ibuprofen, acetaminophen, aspirin, etc.
- **Antiviral agents:** It helps to prevent any secondary infection due to a viral agent. For example, valacyclovir, famciclovir, acyclovir, etc.

Nursing

- Encourage to maintain adequate nutritional status.
- Encourage to maintain appropriate oral hygiene.
- Protect the eye using lubricating eye drops during the day and an eye ointment at night.
- Apply moist heat by putting a wash cloth soaked in warm water on your face several times a day.
- Massage and exercise the face to relax the facial muscles.

BRAIN ABSCESS

Definition

Brain abscess is an accumulation of pus within the brain tissue that can result from a local or a systemic infection.

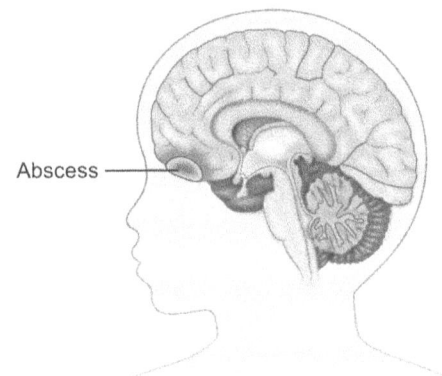

Fig. 1.4: Shows the abscess formation in the ventricles due to brain abscess.

Etiology

- Pulmonary infection
- Bacterial endocarditis
- Skull fracture
- Brain trauma
- Surgery
- Sinus infection
- Spread of infection from nearby sites such as ears, teeth, etc. (Otitis media, dental sepsis, etc.).

Risk Factors

- White race
- Advanced age
- Exposure to radiations
- Exposure to chemicals
- Family history of brain tumor.

Pathophysiology

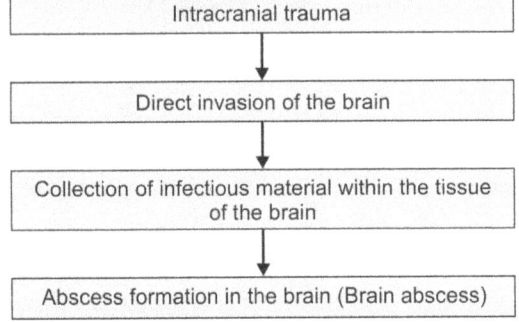

Clinical Features

- Headache usually worse in the morning
- Decreased vision

- Drowsiness
- Confusion
- Seizures
- Weakness of the extremity
- Fever
- Nausea
- Vomiting
- Irritability
- Disoriented behavior.

Complications
- Weakness
- Vision changes
- Headache
- Personality changes
- Hearing loss
- Seizure.

Diagnostic Tests
- History
- Physical examination
- Computed tomography
- Magnetic resonance imaging scan.

Management

Medical

- **Antimicrobial therapy:** It helps to reduce its virulence. For example, penicillin-G, Chloramphenicol, etc.
- **Corticosteroids:** It helps to reduce the inflammatory cerebral edema. For example, dexamethasone.
- **Antiepileptics:** It helps to prevent the attack of seizures. For example, phenytoin, phenobarbital, etc.

Surgical

Surgical incision and aspiration.

Nursing

- Provide symptomatic treatment
- Prepare client for surgery, if indicated
- Maintain the blood pressure at 150/100 mm Hg or less than that to facilitate perfusion.
- Provide complete bed rest.

CEREBRAL INFARCTION

Definition

A cerebral infarction is an ischemic stroke resulting from a disturbance in the blood vessels supplying blood to the brain.

Etiology

- Atherosclerotic occlusion of large vessels
- Embolic occlusion of distal vessels
- Vasculitis

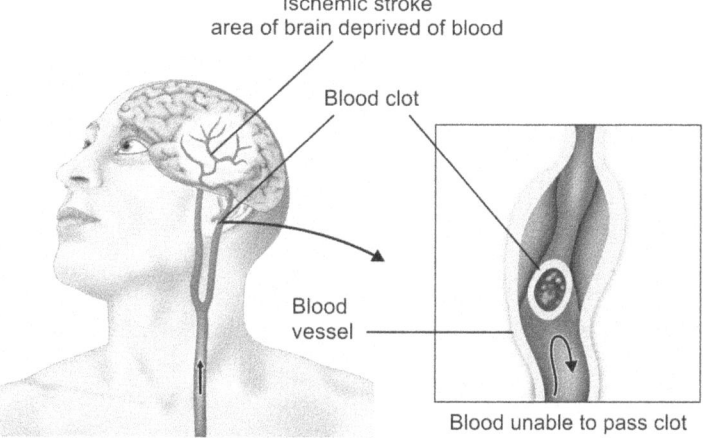

Fig. 1.5: Shows the cerebral infarction in the brain.

- Arterial spasm
- Sickle cell disease
- Inherited metabolic disorders
- Systemic lupus erythematosus
- Meningitis
- Hypercoagulability
- Fibromuscular dysplasia.

Risk Factors

- High blood pressure
- Diabetes mellitus
- Hyperlipoproteinemia
- Hypercholesterolemia
- Tobacco smoking
- Obesity.

Types

There are three types of cerebral infarction as follows:

1. ***Atherosclerotic cerebral infarction:*** It is caused by the cerebrovascular cavity blockage or narrowing. It is the result of ischemic necrosis due to an insufficient blood supply to the brain. Patient may suffer aphasia, hemiplegia or other cerebral damages. It may take several days for symptoms to peak, but also can occur within minutes or seconds.
2. ***Hemorrhagic cerebral infarction:*** It is due to thrombosis or embolism that occurs to a major cerebral artery or branch. Blood leaks out of the artery and enters cerebral tissues. Cerebral tissues suffer anoxia, diffuse ischemia and weakened vessel and blood capillary walls. It was reported that up to 75% of hemorrhagic cerebral infarction patients incur another incident within 7 days of the initial occurrence. The sooner the opening occurs, the quicker the another hemorrhage will occur.
3. ***Lacunar cerebral infarction:*** It refers to old or new infarctions deep within the brain. When this occurs, lacunas or holes are formed. Depending on the infracted blood vessels, symptoms like limb numbness, dizziness, headache,

aphasia and clumsiness may occur. This is due to the small arteries being blocked. Middle-aged and old people are at risk due to decreased blood flow as a result to body changes including increased blood lipids, enhanced platelet aggregation and increased blood viscosity.

Pathophysiology

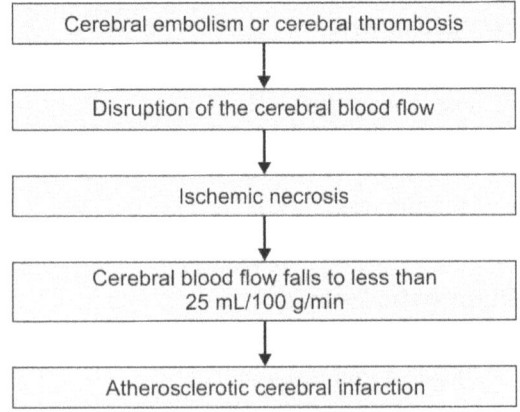

Clinical Features

- Abrupt onset of weakness or paralysis of an arm, leg, side of the face or any part of the body
- Numbness
- Swallowing difficulties or drooling
- Loss of memory
- Aphasia
- Dysarthria
- Ataxia
- Diplopia
- Vertigo
- Loss of balance or coordination
- Personality changes
- Drowsiness
- Mood changes.

Complications

- Myocardial infarction
- Pneumonia
- Renal insufficiency
- Dementia
- Contractures
- Depression.

Diagnostic Tests

- History
- Physical examination
- Neurologic examination
- Blood test
- CT scan—to determine whether the event is ischemic or hemorrhagic
- Arteriography
- Echocardiography
- Carotid ultrasound
- Cerebral angiography
- Transcranial Doppler flow studies
- Magnetic resonance imaging of the brain.

Management

Medical

- **Blood thinning agents:** It reduces the likelihood of having cerebral infarction through restoring blood flow to the brain. For example, aspirin, warfarin, heparin, clopidogrel, etc.
- **Platelet inhibiting agents:** It helps in preventing platelets, blood cells and the vessels from using adenosine that helps in forming a clot and also has the potential to vasodilate the vessels that carry the blood to allow more blood and particles to flow through. For example, dipyridamole, ticlopidine, etc.
- **Dehydrating hyperosmolar agents:** It helps to reduce brain swelling and pressure. For example, mannitol, urea, etc.
- **Analgesics:** It helps to block the flow of pain signals from the central nervous system. For example, voveran, gabapentin, pregabaline, topiramate.
- **Calcium channel blockers:** It helps in blocking the entry of calcium into muscle cells in artery walls. For example, verapamil, diltiazem, etc.
- **Antihypertensive agents:** It helps in reducing the rate of recurrent cerebral ischemia. For example, atenolol, propranolol, etc.

Surgical

- **Carotid angioplasty or stenting:** It is a procedure in which a small metal coil, called a stent is placed in the clogged artery and to prop the artery open to prevent the occurrence of cerebral infarction through increasing the blood flow in areas blocked by plaque and also decreases the chance of it narrowing again.
- **Carotid endarterectomy:** It is the surgical removal of an atherosclerotic plaque or thrombus from the carotid artery.
- **Decompressive hemicraniectomy:** It is the surgical removal of the bone flap including the frontal, parietal and temporal squamous bone was removed. The temporal squama was removed to the middle cranial fossa floor to reduce the chance of subsequent cerebral infarction.
- **Extracranial-intracranial arterial bypass:** To establish collateral blood supply to allow surgery on the aneurysm (a localized dilation of the wall of a blood vessel).

Nursing

- Elevate the head of the bed (15° to 20°) to promote venous drainage and to lower increased ICP.
- Maintain the blood pressure at 150/100 mm Hg or less than that to facilitate perfusion.
- Provide complete bed rest
- Promote the use of intermittent compression stockings to prevent deep vein thrombosis.
- Instruct the patient to maintain normoglycemia (blood glucose level between 80 to 120 mg/dL).

COMA

Definition

Coma is a state of unarousable unconsciousness due to dysfunction of the brain's ascending reticular activating system (ARAS), which is responsible for arousal and the maintenance of wakefulness.

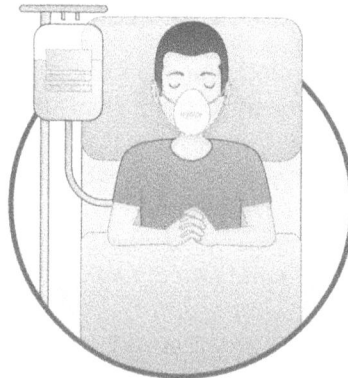

Fig. 1.6: Depicts the patient with coma.

Etiology

- Drug or alcohol intoxication
- Stroke
- Hemorrhage
- Infections involving brain
- Seizures
- Brain damage caused by a lack of oxygen for too long
- Brain tumor
- Traumatic head injury
- Diabetes.

Risk Factors

- Severe illness
- Liver, kidney or cardiovascular disease
- Chemotherapy
- Tendency to have blood clots.

Types

- ***Toxic-metabolic encephalopathy:*** This is an acute condition of brain dysfunction with symptoms of confusion or delirium. The condition is usually reversible and causes are varied. They include systemic illness, infection, organ failure, and other conditions.
- ***Anoxic brain injury:*** This is a brain condition caused by total lack of oxygen to the brain. Lack of oxygen for a few minutes causes cell death to brain tissues. Anoxic brain injury may result from heart attack (cardiac arrest), head injury or trauma, drowning, drug overdose, or poisoning.
- ***Persistent vegetative state:*** This is a state of severe unconsciousness. The person is unaware of his or her surroundings and incapable of voluntary movement. With a persistent vegetative state, someone may progress to wakefulness but with no higher brain function. With persistent vegetative state, there is breathing, circulation, and sleep-wake cycles.
- ***Locked-in syndrome:*** It is a rare condition where the person is totally paralyzed except for the eye muscles, but remains awake and alert and with a normal mind.
- ***Brain death:*** This is an irreversible cessation of all brain function and brain death may result from any lasting or widespread injury to the brain.

Stages of Coma and Recovery

- ***Stage 1:*** No response stage—The person is in a coma and appears to be asleep and restless. He or she does not respond to sound, sights, touch or movement
- ***Stage 2:*** Generalized response stage—The person is semicomatose. He or she begins to respond to sounds, sights, touch or movement. Response is slow, inconsistent or occurs after a delay. The person responds or mimics what is heard, seen or felt. Response may include—chewing, sweating, breathe faster, moaning, moving or increased blood pressure.
- ***Stage 3:*** Localized response stage—The person appears more alert. He or she reacts to what is seen, heard or felt. For example, the person may follow you with his or her eyes or turn the head towards sound. When the person feels pain, an arm or leg may move, and he or she may cry out. The person may follow simple commands, like "close your eyes". The person may show signs of knowing family or friends.
- ***Stage 4:*** Confused and agitated stage—This stage can be difficult for families and friends. The person may not understand what is happening (gets confused) and be scared. He or she may try to remove

all restraints, kick, and hit or bite others, pull out tubes and crawl out of bed. The person may overreact due to confusion by screaming or say things that are not appropriate. He or she may make up stories to overcome internal confusion and fear. Often, the person's attention span is very short and he or she may lack short-term recall. Memory may be limited only to past events. The person may be focused on basic needs like eating, going to the bathroom, or dressing and need help with these activities.

- **Stage 5:** Confused and inappropriate stage—During this stage, the person is not as explosive or combative. The person is more alert and can follow simple commands most of the time. Complex or multiple step commands may lead to frustration and upset. Attention to any task may be limited. Long-term memory of past events may be better than short-term recall of daily events. To fill in the gaps of memory, the person may make up stories. He or she may have confusion due to problems learning or organizing information. He or she is better able to understand physical injury than problems with thinking or memory.
- **Stage 6:** Confused and appropriate stage— At this stage, a person's behavior is more functional. He or she can remember time, events of the day and major life events. There is improvement in the care of basic needs. The person can follow simple commands more consistently and can keep attention for 30 minutes on a task. It is easier to learn information at this stage, but details may be forgotten. Response time to finish activities may still be slow. May have trouble connecting thoughts with specific words or say things without thinking.
- **Stage 7:** Automatic and appropriate stage— At this stage, most daily activities are done automatically when tasks have structure. Concentration, judgment and problem solving may be difficult. Safety is a concern. The person may feel "better", but lacks judgment for some activities. Learning new information is possible, but it takes time and practice to retain.
- **Stage 8:** Purposeful and appropriate stage—At this stage, the person has purpose in daily living. He or she can recall and integrate past and present. Carryover for new learning is evident. The person needs no supervision once activities are learned and can be independent at home and in the community. The person may continue to show decreased abilities, reasoning, judgment, stress tolerance, and emotional and intellectual capacity compared to preinjury, yet be functional in society.

Pathophysiology

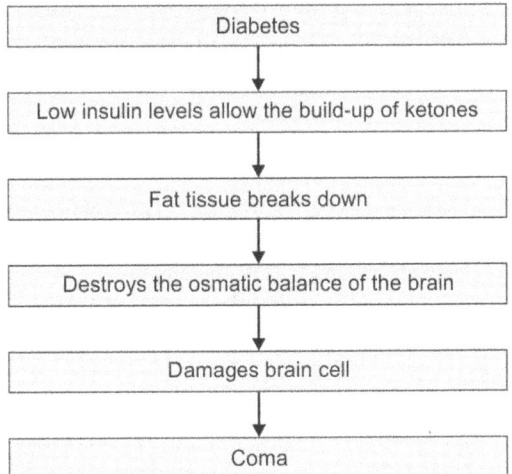

Clinical Features

- Inability to be aroused to consciousness
- Lack of self-awareness
- Lack of sleep-wake cycle
- Lack of purposeful movements
- Lack of suffering
- Impaired breathing.

Complications

- Permanent brain damage
- Persistent vegetative state
- Seizures
- Cognitive problems
- Sensory disturbances

- Lung damage
- Bladder infections.

Diagnostic Tests

- History
- Physical examination
- Blood tests
- Lumbar puncture
- Computerized tomography (CT) scan
- Magnetic resonance imaging (MRI) scan
- Electroencephalography (EEG).

Management

Medical

- Intravenous administration of glucose in the case of hypoglycemia
- Intravenous administration of Nalaxone in the case of a heroin overdose
- Antibiotics in the case of any infection
- An intravenous line to provide fluids and drugs
- An oxygen mask is required to administer oxygen
- Pumping of the stomach, if the person ate or drank something poisonous
- Urinary bladder catheterization
- A respirator if the person is unable to breathe by themselves.

Surgical

Craniotomy: It is a surgical procedure in which the observed masses are removed to decrease pressure on the brain.

Nursing

- Reposition the patient once in every two hours
- Turn the patient gently because they cannot verbalize pain
- Provide safety of the patient by always keeping the side-rails up
- Do not restrain the patient
- Facilitate enteral feeding
- Provide oral care atleast twice daily
- Do suctioning whenever needed
- Encourage passive range of motion exercises.

DECOMPRESSION SICKNESS

Definition

Decompression sickness (Also known as generalized barotrauma or the Bends and Caisson disease) refers to injuries caused by a rapid decrease in the pressure that surrounds us, either in air or water.

Etiology

- Reduction in ambient pressure
- Formation of gas bubbles in the blood and tissues
- Severe changes in altitude.

Risk Factors

- Congenital birth defects
- Being older than 30 years
- Being female
- Low cardiovascular fitness
- High percentage of body fat
- Use of alcohol or tobacco
- Fatigue, seasickness or lack of sleep
- Injuries
- Diving in cold water
- Lung disease.

Types

Type I Decompression Sickness

It is the least serious form of decompression sickness. It normally involves only pain in the body and is not immediately life-threatening. It is important to note that this may be warning signs of more serious problems.

- **Cutaneous decompression sickness:** This is when the nitrogen bubbles come out of solution in skin capillaries. This normally results in a red rash, often on the shoulders and chest.
- **Joint and limb pain decompression sickness:** This type is characterized by aching in the joints. It is not known exactly what causes the pain as bubbles in the joint would not have this effect. The common theory is that it is caused by the bubbles aggravating bone marrow, tendons, and

Disorders of Nervous System

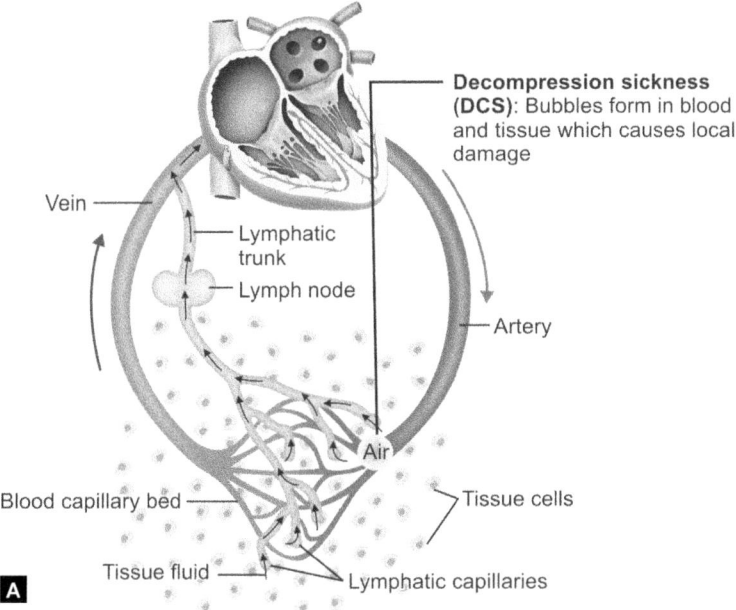

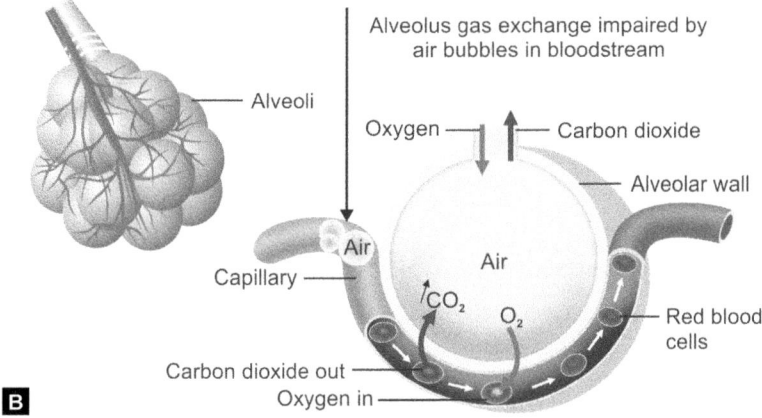

Figs. 1.7A and B: (A) Decompression sickness; (B) Arterial gas embolism.

joints. The pain can be in one place or it can move around the joint. It is unusual for bisymmetrical symptoms to occur.

Type II Decompression Sickness

Type II decompression sickness is the most serious and can be immediately life-threatening. The main effect is on the nervous system.

- ***Neurological decompression sickness:*** When nitrogen bubbles affect the nervous system, they can cause problems throughout the body. This type of decompression sickness normally shows as tingling, numbness, respiratory problems, and unconsciousness. Symptoms can spread quickly and if left untreated can lead to paralysis or even death.

- **Pulmonary sickness:** This is a rare form of decompression sickness that occurs when bubbles form in lung capillaries. Fortunately, the majority of the time bubbles dissolve naturally through the lungs. However, it is possible for them to interrupt blood flow to the lungs which can lead to serious and life-threatening respiratory and heart problems.
- **Cerebral decompression sickness:** It is possible for bubbles that make their way into the arterial blood stream to move to the brain and to cause an arterial gas embolism. This is extremely dangerous and can be identified by symptoms such as blurred vision, headaches, confusion, and unconsciousness.

Pathophysiology

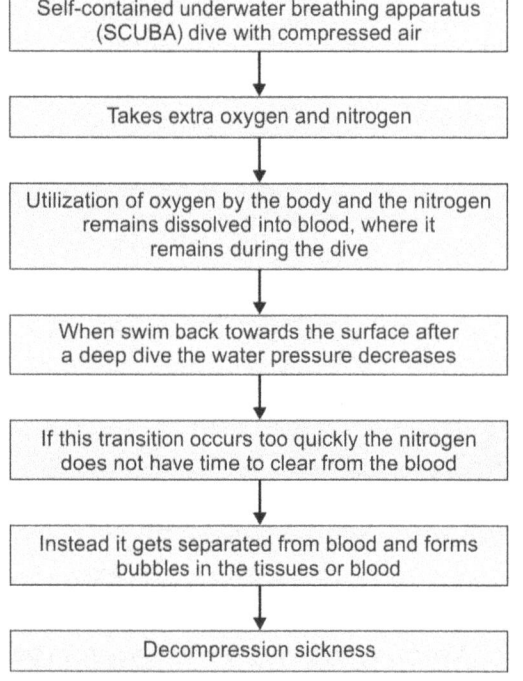

Clinical Features

- Extreme fatigue
- Joint and limb pain
- Tingling
- Numbness
- Red rash on skin
- Respiratory problems
- Heart problems
- Dizziness
- Blurred vision
- Confusion
- Unconsciousness
- Stomach sickness.

Complications

- Headache
- Oxygen toxicity
- Pain
- Vertigo
- Hearing loss
- Thoracic myelopathy.

Diagnostic Tests

- History
- Physical examination
- Blood examination.

Management

Medical

Hyperbaric oxygen chamber: It is the use of high-pressure chamber in which the patient receives 100% oxygen. It reverses the pressure changes that allowed gas bubbles to form and it drives nitrogen back into its liquid form so that it can be cleared more gradually over a period of hours.

Nursing

- Instruct to avoid alcohol especially before diving
- Encourage to dive and rise slowly in the water
- Instruct them not to stay the deepest depth longer than recommended
- Instruct them to avoid flying within 24 hours after diving
- Make sure that they are well hydrated, well rested and prepared before the dive.
- Instruct them to avoid hot baths after diving.

DELIRIUM

Definition
Delirium or acute confusional state is an acute and relatively sudden (developing over hours to days) decline in attention-focus, perception and cognition.

Etiology
- Infections (Pneumonia and urinary tract infections) and immune disorders
- Metabolic problems and endocrine abnormalities
- Nutritional deficiencies
- Heart and lung problems
- Anoxia
- Brain tumor
- Subdural hematoma
- Poisoning
- Any reaction to medications
- Trauma
- Cerebral hemorrhage
- Acute vascular disease (stroke, MI, pulmonary embolism and heart failure).

Risk Factors
- Old age
- Family history
- Dementia
- Severe chronic or terminal illness
- Alcohol use
- Cholesterol
- High estrogen levels
- Homocysteine blood levels
- Smoking.

Types
Delirium is classified as follows:
- **Hyperactive delirium:** It is observed in patients with alcohol withdrawal or intoxication
- **Hypoactive delirium:** It is observed in patients with hepatic encephalopathy and hypercapnia
- **Mixed delirium:** It is observed in clients with daytime sedation with nocturnal agitation and behavioral problems.

Pathophysiology

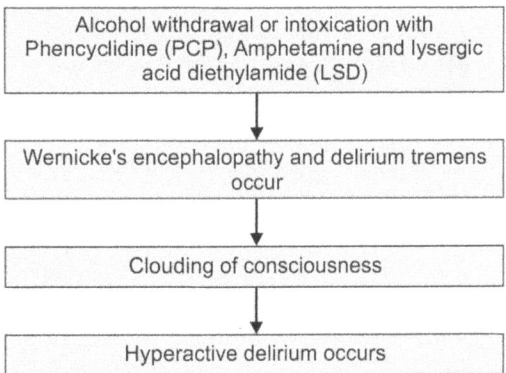

Clinical Features
- Memory loss
- Decreased attention span
- Waxing and waning type of confusion
- Personality changes
- Inappropriate behavior
- Agitation
- Illusions
- Tremor
- Hallucinations
- Dysphasia
- Dysarthria
- Asterixis
- Motor abnormalities.

Complications
- General decline in health
- Loss of ability to function or care for self

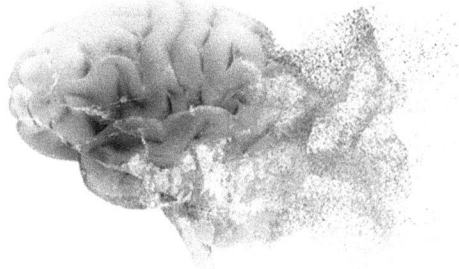

Fig. 1.8: Shows the delirium in elderly patients.

- Loss of ability to interact
- Progression to stupor or coma
- Increased risk of death.

Diagnostic Tests
- History
- Physical examination
- Mental status examination
- Neurological examination
- Brain imaging.

Management

Medical
- **Dopamine blockers:** It causes less sedation and reduce the risks of exacerbating delirium. For example, haloperidol, olanzapine, risperidone, clozapine, etc.
- **Mood stabilizers:** It is used to treat mood disorders characterized by intense and sustained mood shifts, typically bipolar disorder. For example, imipramine, fluoxetine, citalopram, etc.
- **Sedatives:** It is used prophylactically to prevent delirium tremens. For example, clonazepam, diazepam, lorazepam, etc.
- **Serotonin affecting agent:** It is used for the management of anxiety disorders or for the short-term relief of the symptoms of anxiety. For example, trazadone, buspirone, etc.
- **Thiamine hydrochloride:** It is used for alcohol withdrawal and Wernicke's encephalopathy. For example, Thiamilate, etc.

Nursing
- Encourage a balanced intake
- Provide a environment which is stable, quiet and well-lighted
- Correct the sensory deficits with eye glasses and hearing aids
- Avoid physical restraints
- Never leave the patient alone or unattended.

DEMENTIA

Definition

Dementia is the progressive decline in cognitive function due to any damage or disease in the body beyond what might be expected from normal aging.

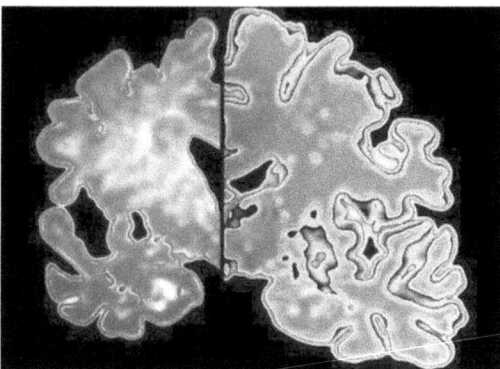

Fig. 1.9: Depicts the progressive decline in cognitive function due to dementia.

Etiology
- Advanced Parkinson's disease
- Alzheimer's disease
- Multiple sclerosis
- Huntington's disease
- Lyme disease
- Pick's disease
- Progressive supranuclear palsy.

Risk Factors
- Old age
- Chronic alcohol abuse
- Normal pressure hydrocephalus
- Use of cimetidine and cholesterol lowering medications
- Low vitamin B12 levels.

Types
- *Cortical dementia:* This type of dementia occurs where the brain damage primarily affects the brain's cortex or outer layer. It tends to cause problems with memory, language, thinking and social behavior.
- *Subcortical dementia:* This type of dementia affects parts of the brain below the cortex. It tends to cause changes in emotions and movement in addition to problems with memory.
- *Progressive dementia:* This type of dementia gets worse over time, gradually interfering with more and more cognitive abilities.

Disorders of Nervous System

- *Primary dementia:* This type of dementia results due to Alzheimer's disease and not due to any other disease.
- *Secondary dementia:* This type of dementia occurs as a result of a physical disease or injury.

Pathophysiology

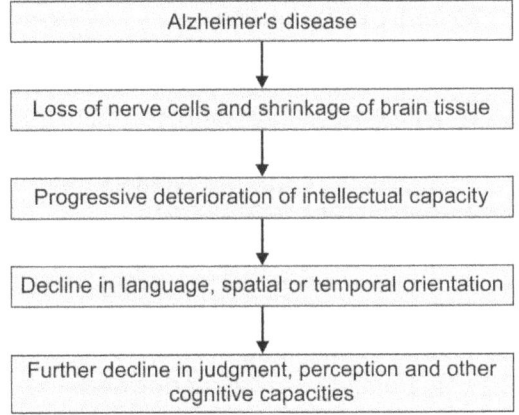

Clinical Features

- Difficulty performing more than one task at a time
- Difficulty solving problems or making decisions
- Forgetting recent events or conversations
- Taking longer time to perform more difficult mental activities
- Getting lost on familiar routes
- Language problems, such as trouble finding the name of familiar objects
- Losing interest in things you previously enjoyed, flat mood
- Misplacing items
- Personality changes and loss of social skills, which can lead to inappropriate behaviors
- Change in sleep patterns, often waking up at night
- Having delusions, depression, agitation
- More difficulty reading or writing
- Poor judgment and loss of ability to recognize danger
- Using the wrong word, not pronouncing words correctly, speaking in confusing sentences
- Withdrawing from social contact.

Complications

- Abuse by an overstressed caregiver
- Loss of ability to function or care for self
- Loss of ability to interact
- Severe injury
- Reduced life span.

Diagnostic Tests

- History
- Physical examination
- Neurological examination
- Cognitive and neuropsychological test
- CT scan
- MRI scan
- Positron emission tomography
- Single photon emission computed tomography
- Blood examination
- Urine analysis
- Analysis of thyroid and thyroid stimulating hormones
- CSF analysis.

Management

Medical

- **Acetyl cholinesterase inhibitors:** It is used for the treatment of dementia induced by Alzheimer's disease. For example, tacrine, donepezil, galantamine, rivastigmine etc.
- **Amyloid deposit inhibitors:** It helps to reduce amyloid deposits in the brain of person with Alzheimer's disease. For example, minocycline, clioquinoline, etc.
- **Antipsychotic drugs:** It helps to decrease psychotic symptoms and agitation. For example, haloperidol, risperidone, olanzapine, quetiapine, etc.
- **Antidepressant drugs:** It helps in alleviating cognitive and behavioral symptoms by reuptaking neurotransmitter regulation through reuptake of serotonin, noradrenaline and dopamine. For example, trazodone, agomelatine, etc.
- **Anxiolytic agents:** It helps in treating anxiety which is of mild to moderate

anxiety. For example, diazepam, buspirone, etc.
- **N-methyl-D-aspartate blockers:** It is used in combination with acetylcholinesterase inhibitors. For example, Memantine.
- **Antioxidant:** It slows down the development of dementia by preventing free radical damage. For example, Selegiline.

Nursing

- Maintain patient's usual routines as much as possible
- Communicate clearly to the patient
- Reduce stressors such as fatigue, overstimulation or pain
- Involve family members in care
- Keep them active-physically, mentally and socially.

ENCEPHALITIS

Definition

Encephalitis is an acute inflammation of the brain which often coexists with inflammation of the covering of the brain and spinal cord and commonly results due to a viral infection.

Etiology

- Herpes simplex virus
- Arbovirus
- Allergies to vaccinations
- Autoimmune diseases
- Cancer involving the brain tissue
- Rabies virus.

Risk Factors

- People who live in warm and moist climates
- Children's and young adults.

Types

- *Primary encephalitis:*
  - It results due to viral infection of the brain and spinal cord
  - It may occur in isolated cases (sporadic) or occur in many people at the same time in the same area (epidemic).
- *Herpes simplex encephalitis:*
  - It results due to herpes simplex virus
  - It carries a high risk for serious neurological damage and death and can occur in newborns if the virus is passed from mother to the infant during birth.
- *Arboviral encephalitis:*
  - It results due to arthropod-borne viruses
  - Mosquitoes are the most common agents of transmission and most cases occur during warmer weather, when the insects are more active.
- *Secondary encephalitis:* It results due to a complication of a viral infection or reactivation of a latent virus.
- *Acute disseminated encephalitis:* It results due to a variola virus infection following smallpox vaccination or reactivation of another viral infection.

Pathophysiology

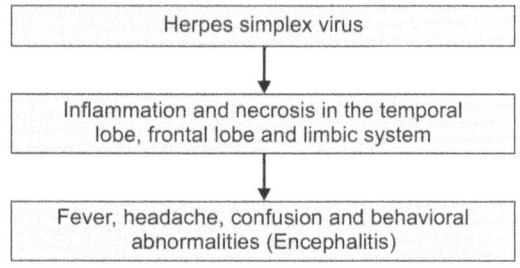

Clinical Features

- Sudden fever
- Fatigue

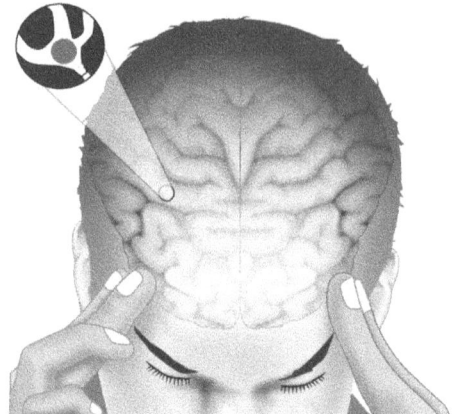

Fig. 1.10: Depicts the inflammation and necrosis in the temporal lobe of the brain.

- Sore throat
- Stiff neck and back
- Behavioral changes (lethargy, confusion, etc.)
- Headache
- Irritability
- Vomiting
- Unsteady gait
- Drowsiness
- Visual sensitivity to light.

Complications

- Seizures
- Paralysis
- Memory loss
- Sudden impaired judgment
- Poor responsiveness.

Diagnostic Tests

- History
- Physical examination
- Neurological examination
- Blood examination
- CSF examination
- Electroencephalography
- Urine examination
- ELISA test
- CT scan
- Magnetic resonance imaging (MRI) scan
- Spinal tap or lumbar puncture
- Polymerase chain reaction technique.

Management

Medical

- **Antiviral agents:** It inhabitants the replication of viral DNA and used specifically for treating viral infections. For example, acyclovir, foscartnet sodium, etc.
- **Antifungal agents:** It is a drug that selectively eliminates fungal pathogens from a host with minimal toxicity to the host. For example, amphotericin-A, fluconazole, flucytosine, etc.
- **Osmodiuretics:** It helps to reduce cerebral oedema. For example, mannitol, etc.
- **Corticosteroids:** It suppresses the immune system which mistakenly attacks its own tissues. For example, dexamethasone, prednisone, etc.
- **Anticonvulsants:** It helps to prevent the occurrence of seizures. For example, phenobarbital, sodium valproate, etc.

Nursing

- Elevate the head of the bed 30° to 45°
- Turn the patient frequently
- Provide support to the patient and family members to cope with the illness
- Prevent the patient from any injury
- Restrict environmental stimuli in the patients room.

EPILEPSY OR SEIZURE

Definition

Seizures are episodes of abnormal motor, sensory, autonomic or psychic activity resulting from sudden excessive discharge from cerebral neurons.

Etiology

Prenatal Factors

- Genetic predisposition
- Development defects
- Fetal infections
- Maternal diseases.

Perinatal Factors

- Hypoxemia
- Trauma
- Jaundice
- Infection
- Prematurity
- Drug withdrawal.

Postnatal Factors

- Primary infections of the CNS
- Head injury
- Infectious disease of the childhood with encephalopathy
- Brain tumors
- Renal disease
- Degenerative disease
- Allergies

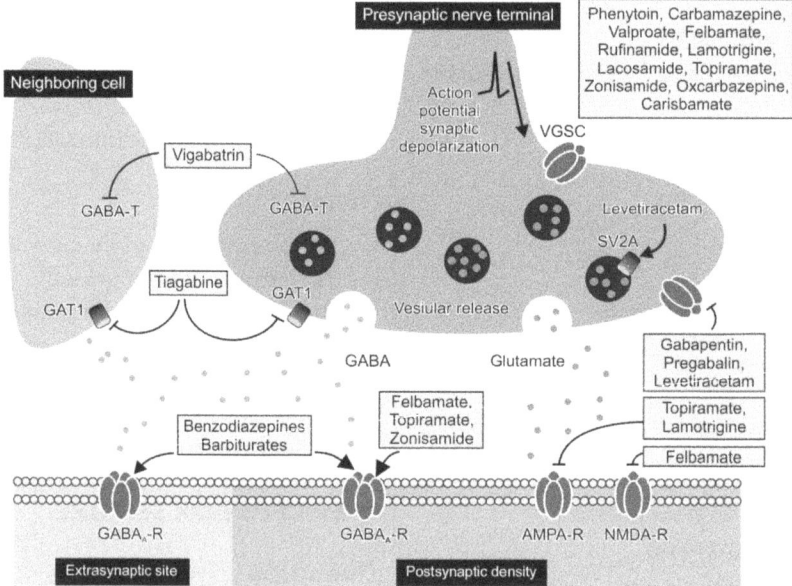

Fig. 1.11: Depicts the abnormal motor, sensory, autonomic or psychic activity resulting from sudden excessive discharge from cerebral neurons.

- Metabolic and toxic condition
- Hypertension
- Cerebrovascular diseases
- Anoxia.

Types

- Generalized seizures
- Partial seizures.

Generalized Seizures

- This type involves electrical discharges in the whole brain
- It may be of tonic-clonic, absence, myoclonic or atonic type
  - **Tonic clonic seizures**
    - It begins with an aura (a sensation that warns the client of the impending seizure).
    - The tonic phase involves the stiffening or rigidity of the muscles of the arms and legs and usually lasts 10 to 20 sec, followed by loss of consciousness.
    - The clonic phase consists of hyperventilation and jerking of the extremities and usually lasts about 30 sec.
    - In this type, full recovery from the seizure may take several hours.
  - **Absence seizures**
    - This type of seizure is more common in children
    - It is a brief seizure lasting for few seconds and the individual may or may not lose consciousness.
    - In this type, no loss or change in the muscle tone
    - It may occur several times during a day
    - The victim appears to be day-dreaming.
  - **Myoclonic seizures**
    - It is a seizure that presents as a brief generalized jerking or stiffening of extremities
    - The victim may fall to ground due to seizure.
  - **Atonic seizures**
    - It is a sudden momentary loss of muscle tone
    - The victim may fall to ground as a result of the seizure.

Partial Seizures

- This type of seizure begins in one part of the brain
- It may be of simple partial (or) complex partial:
  - **Simple partial seizures**
    - It produces sensory symptoms accompanied by motor symptoms that are localized or confined to a specific area
    - The client remains conscious and may report an aura.
  - **Complex partial seizures**
    - It is a psychomotor seizure
    - The area of the brain most involved is the temporal lobe
    - It is characterized by periods of altered behavior
    - The client loses consciousness for a few second.

Phases of Epilepsy

- **Aura phase:** A sensation that warns the client of the impending seizure.
- **Preictal phase:** It refers to the time immediately before a seizure occurs.
- **Ictal phase:** It refers to the time during the seizure.
- **Interictal phase:** It refers to the time between seizure activities.
- **Postictal phase:** It refers to the time immediately after a seizure as the patient recovers.

Pathophysiology

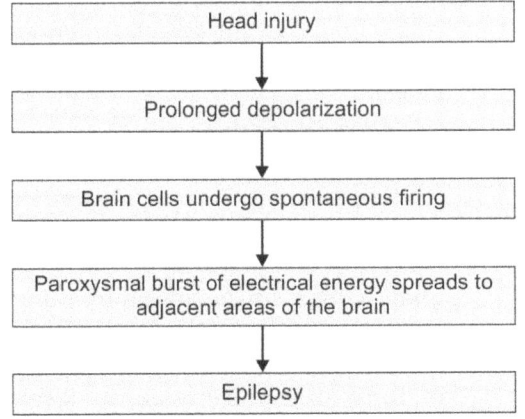

Clinical Features

- Aura—a peculiar sensation that precedes seizures
- Loss of consciousness
- Tachycardia
- Diaphoresis
- Warm skin
- Pallor, flushing (or) cyanosis
- Continuous muscle contractions
- Extreme muscle rigidity lasting for about 5 to 15 seconds
- Lethargy
- Confusion and headache
- Bowel and bladder incontinence
- Mood changes
- Irritability
- Insomnia.

Complications

- Pulmonary aspiration
- Injury
- Hypoxia
- Status epilepticus.

Diagnostic Tests

- History
- Physical examination
- Magnetic resonance imaging (MRI): It is used to detect lesions in the brain, focal abnormalities, cerebrovascular abnormalities and cerebral degenerative changes.
- Electroencephalogram: To probe the action of single brain cells.
- EEG telemetry: To determine the type of seizure.
- Single photon emission computed tomography (SPECT): It is useful for identifying the epileptogenic zone so that the area in the brain gives rise to seizures can be removed.

Management

Medical

- **Anticonvulsants:** It is used to depress abnormal neuronal discharges and prevent the spread of seizures. For example,

diazepam, carbamazepine, gabapentin, phenobarbital, phenytoin, sodium valproate etc.
- **Hydantoin:** It blocks synaptic potentiation and propagation of electrical discharges in the motor cortex and blocks sodium transport and stabilize membrane sensitivity. For example, phenytoin, mephenytoin, etc.
- **Barbiturates:** It depress postsynaptic excitatory discharge. For example, phenobarbital, primidone, etc.
- **Succinimides:** It depresses motor cortex and raises threshold to stimuli and is used to manage absence seizures. For example, ethosuximide.
- **Benzodiazepines:** It is used to treat absence seizures. For example, diazepam, clonazepam, etc.
- **Oxazolidinediones:** It is used to treat absence seizures. For example, tiagabine.
- **Valproates:** It is used to treat tonic-clonic, partial, myoclonic and psychomotor seizures. For example, sodium valproate, topiramate, etc.
- **Iminostilbenes:** It is used to treat seizure disorders that have not responded to other anticonvulsants. For example, lamotrigine.

Surgical

- **Hemispherectomy:** It is the surgical removal of the lateral half of the cerebrum.
- **Tumor resection:** It is the surgical removal of the intracranial tumors.
- **Corpus callosotomy:** It is the surgical opening which is made in the transverse band of nerve fibers joining the cerebral hemisphere.

Nursing

- Maintain a patent airway (do not force the jaws open)
- Turn the client's head to the side
- Do not restrain the client
- Push aside any furniture that may injure the patient during the seizure
- Provide privacy and safeguard the patient from curious onlookers
- Place the client on the floor and protect the head and body
- Loosen the clothing of the patient
- Administer oxygen as prescribed
- Prepare for suctioning of the patient
- Place the bed in the lowest position
- Side-rails should be raised
- Place a pillow under the head
- Instruct the client to avoid alcohol, excessive stress and fatigue.

FLOPPY INFANT SYNDROME (HYPOTONIA)

Definition

It is a state of low muscle tone (the amount of tension or resistance to stretch in a muscle) often involving reduced muscle strength.

Etiology

- Down syndrome
- Muscular dystrophy
- Cerebral palsy
- Achondroplasia
- Tay-Sachs disease
- Isopropyl alcohol poisoning
- After shave poisoning.

Risk Factors

- Being infants
- Previous family history.

Types

- *Congenital hypotonia:*
  - It is present at birth
  - It is usually an inherited or genetic condition that affects nerves, brain or muscles.
  - Some conditions that cause this type of hypotonia are Down's syndrome, Marfan syndrome, dyspraxia, cerebral palsy, etc.
- *Acquired hypotonia:*
  - It develops after birth as a result of an underlying medical condition, injury or trauma.
  - Conditions that may lead to hypotonia include muscular dystrophy, brain

Disorders of Nervous System

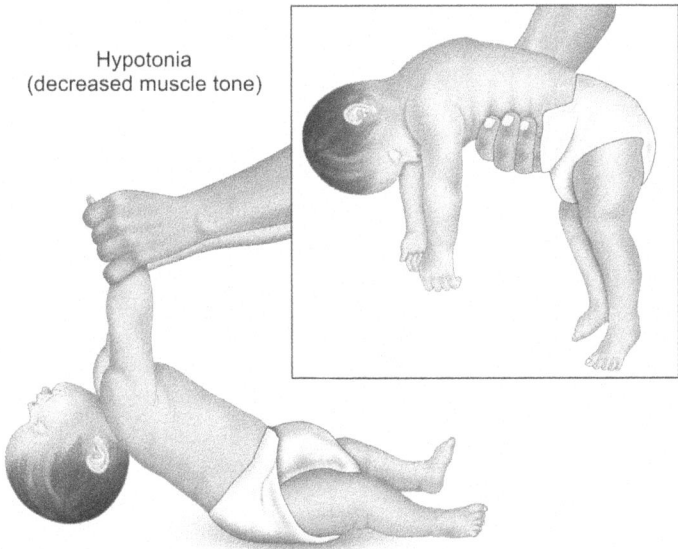

Fig. 1.12: Depicts the decreased muscle tone (hypotonia) resulting from floppy infant syndrome.

infections like meningitis or encephalitis, head injury and myasthenia gravis.

Pathophysiology

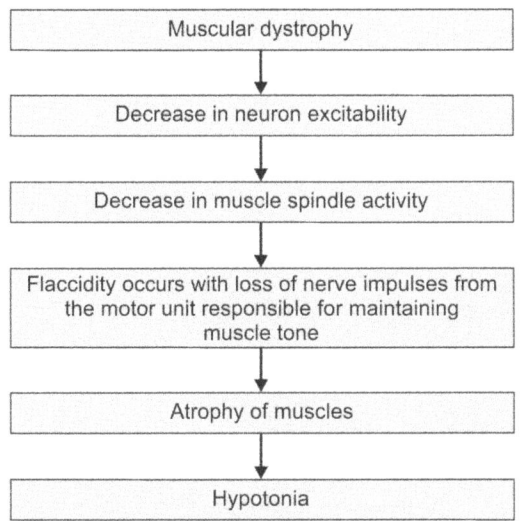

Clinical Features

- Becoming clumsy
- Falling frequently
- Difficulty with getting up from a lying or sitting position
- An unusual high degree of flexibility in the hips, elbows and knees
- Difficulty reaching for or lifting an object.

Complications

- Respiratory insufficiency
- Recurrent pneumonia
- Orthopedic deformities
- Poor nutritional status.

Diagnostic Tests

- History
- Physical examination
- Blood examination
- CT scan
- MRI scan
- CSF examination
- Muscle biopsy
- Nerve conduction velocity
- Electroencephalogram
- Electromyography.

Management

Medical

- **Anticholinesterase agents:** It prevents acetyl choline destruction and increase the accumulation of acetylcholine at neuromuscular junctions which improves the ability of the muscles to contract. For example, neostigmine, pyridostigmine, etc.

Surgical

- **Plasmapheresis:** It is a surgical procedure in which blood is withdrawn and passed through a series of filters that separate the different type of blood cells. The blood cells are then suspended in donor or synthetic plasma and returned to the patient's body. The patient's plasma is discarded
- **Immunoglobulin:** It is a procedure in which large doses of immunoglobulin given intravenously helps to shorten the duration of symptoms. It is preferred over Plasmapheresis because it does not require insertion of a large venous catheter.

Nursing

- Maintain maximum muscle function and reduce secondary deformities
- Place the patient in a comfortable and clean environment
- Proper turning from time to time must be done in order to prevent accumulation of moisture on the back of the patient.
- Encourage to comply with medications
- Encourage balanced diet to prevent tissue and muscle breakdown.

GILLES DE LA TOURETTE SYNDROME

Definition

Gilles de la Tourette syndrome (GTS) is a childhood onset neuropsychiatric movement disorder characterized by multiple motor tics and one or more vocal/phonic tics, lasting longer than a year.

Etiology

- Autoimmune disease
- Idiopathic
- Heredity
- Brain abnormalities
- Exposure to stimulants (methylphenidate, amphetamines and lamotrigine)
- Maternal stress.

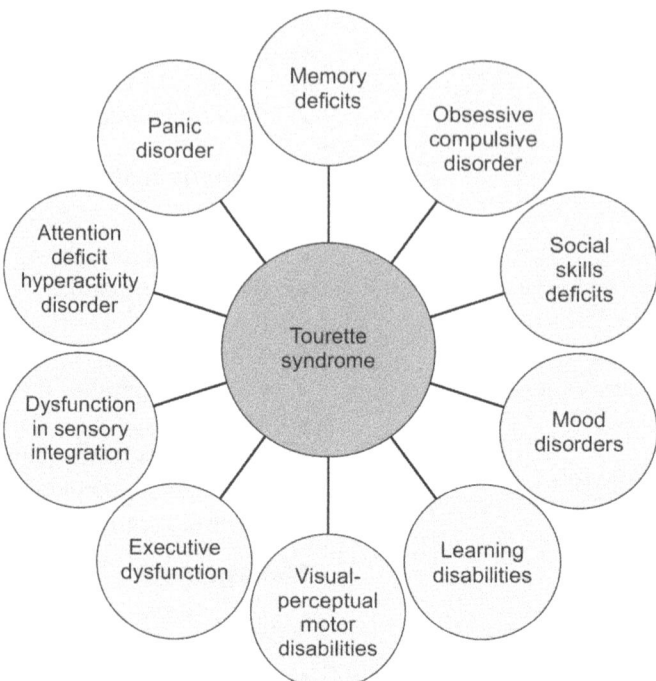

Fig. 1.13: Shows the complex clinical spectrum of Tourette syndrome.

Risk Factors

- More common in boys than in girls by a ratio of five to one
- Smoking
- Obstetric complications.

Pathophysiology

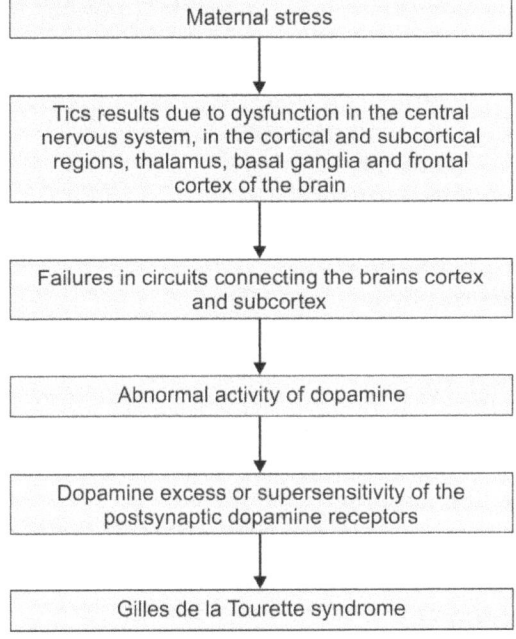

Clinical Features

The main symptoms are tics. Some are so mild they are not even noticeable. Others happen often and obvious. The more severe ones can be embarrassing and can affect our social life and work. Traditionally, tics have been divided in two main groups:
1. Motor tics
2. Vocal tics

The following are examples of tics commonly seen in persons with Tourette's:

- ***Simple motor tics:***
  - Eye blinking
  - Shoulder rotation or elevation
  - Head jerking
  - Lip contractions
  - Closing of the eyes
  - Eyes rolling in the orbits
  - Torticollis (turning the neck to one side)
  - Opening and closing of the mouth
  - Abdominal contractions
  - Stretching of arms and legs
- ***Complex motor tics:***
  - Jumping
  - Kicking
  - Touching objects
  - Retching
  - Trunk bending or rotation
  - Burping
  - Socially inappropriate movements
  - Obscene gestures
  - Imitation of other peoples' gestures
- ***Simple phonic tics:***
  - Grunting
  - Clearing throat
  - Coughing
  - Meaningless sounds or utterances
- ***Complex phonic tics:***
  - Complex and loud sounds
  - Phrase out of context
  - Phrases with obscenities
  - Cursing
  - Repetition of other person's phrases.

Complications

- Attention deficit hyperactivity disorder (ADHD)
- Anger control issues
- Impulsive behavior
- Obsessive-compulsive disorder
- Poor social skills.

Diagnostic Tests

- History
- Physical examination
- Blood tests
- Neuroimaging studies
- Magnetic resonance imaging (MRI) scan.

Management

Medical

- **Neuroleptics:** It blocks dopamine receptors in the brain and the periphery and thereby relaxing the muscle tissues.

For example, haloperidol, risperidone, pimozide, sulpiride, tiapride, aripiprazole, etc.
- **Benzodiazepines:** It enhances the effect of the neurotransmitter gamma-aminobutyric acid (GABA) at the GABA receptor resulting in sedative, hypnotic, anxiolytic, anticonvulsant and muscle relaxant properties. For example, clonazepam, diazepam, etc.
- **Neurotoxin:** It inhibits acetylcholine release at the neuromuscular junction, which results in paralysis of muscle tissue. For example, botulinum toxin, etc.
- **Central adrenergic inhibitors:** It prevents brain from sending signals to the nervous system to speed up the heart rate and narrowing of blood vessels. For example, clonidine, guanfacine, methyldopa, etc.

Surgical

Deep brain stimulation: It is a procedure in which battery-operated medical device (neurostimulator) is implanted in the brain to deliver electric stimulation to targeted areas that control movement.

Nursing

- Provide counseling to reduce stress and anxiety, as well as to maintain optimal mental health.
- Educate them tics usually gets better as age advances
- Instruct the family members to nurture their patients to build self-esteem
- Encourage them to go out in public and engage in social activities.

GUILLAIN-BARRE SYNDROME

Definition

Guillain-Barre syndrome (GBS) is an inflammatory disorder of the peripheral nerves usually in response to an infection or other illness and these are nerves which convey sensory information (pain, temperature) from the body to the brain and motor (movement) signals from the brain to the body.

Etiology

- Autoimmune disease
- Idiopathic
- Infection with *Campylobacter jejuni*
- Systemic lupus erythematosus
- Severe illness
- Porphyria
- Viral hepatitis.

Risk Factors

- Viral infections (AIDS, herpes simplex, mononucleosis, etc.)
- Minor surgery
- Influenza immunization
- Hodgkin's disease.

Stages

- *Acute stage:* In this stage, the symptoms show between one to three weeks.
- *Plateau stage:* In this stage, the symptoms show between several days to two weeks.
- *Recovery stage:* This is the stage wherein there is remyelination which may last up to two years.

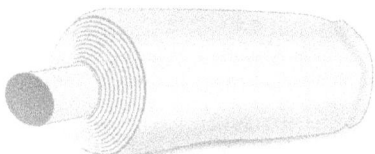 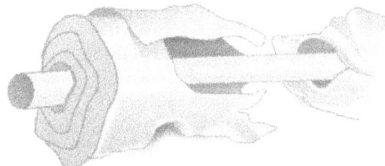

Fig. 1.14: Shows the comparison of normal motor neuron axons with axons of Guillain-Barre syndrome.

Pathophysiology

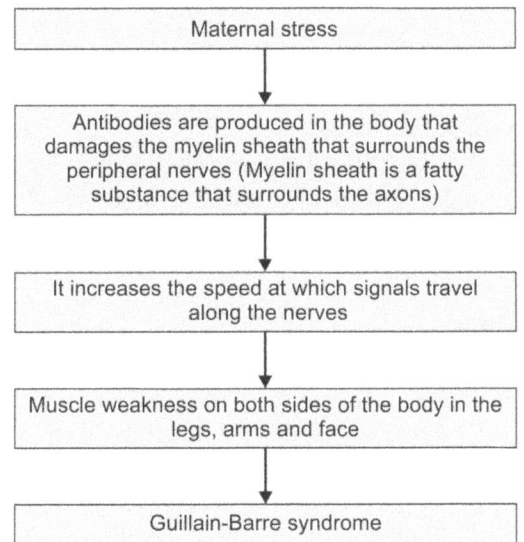

Clinical Features

- Varying degrees of weakness or tingling sensations in the toes and fingers and occasionally around the mouth and lips.
- Muscle weakness on both sides of the body in the legs, arms and face
- Difficulty in speaking, chewing and swallowing
- Numbness
- Paralysis of arms and legs
- Inability to move the eyes
- Back pain
- Mild difficulty in walking, requiring crutches or a walking stick.

Complications

- Paralysis of respiratory muscles
- Pneumonia
- Blood clot in the legs
- Urinary tract infection
- Residual weakness
- Severe disability
- Relapse.

Diagnostic Tests

- History
- Physical examination
- Lumbar puncture
- Electromyogram (EMG)
- Nerve conduction velocity (NCV) test—to figure out how well nerves are sending signals down to the arms and legs.

Management

Medical

- **Analgesics:** It helps to treat severe pain. For example, acetaminophen with hydrocodone, etc.
- **Muscle relaxants:** It helps to relax the muscles thereby reducing pain in the muscles. For example, diazepam, etc.
- **Corticosteroids:** It helps to reduce the severity of the autoimmune disorder. For example, prednisolone, etc.
- **Anticonvulsants:** It helps to relieve against seizures. For example, gabapentin, sodium valproate, etc.

Surgical

- **Plasmapheresis:** It is a surgical procedure in which blood is withdrawn and passed through a series of filters that separate the different type of blood cells. The blood cells are then suspended in donor or synthetic plasma and returned to the patient's body. The patient's plasma is discarded.
- **Immunoglobulin:** It is a procedure in which large doses of immunoglobulin given intravenously helps to shorten the duration of symptoms. It is preferred over Plasmapheresis because it does not require insertion of a large venous catheter.

Nursing

- Place the patient in a comfortable and clean environment
- Provide ventilator support when needed
- Proper turning from time to time must be done in order to prevent accumulation of moisture on the back of the patient
- Encourage to comply with steroid medications
- Encourage balanced diet to prevent tissue and muscle breakdown.

HEADACHE

Definition

A headache is a condition of pain in the head, scalp or neck.

Etiology

- Tension
- Eye strain
- Dehydration
- Migraine
- Hypermastication
- Sinusitis
- Meningitis
- Encephalitis
- Cerebral aneurysm
- Brain tumor
- Fluctuating estrogen during menstrual years
- Chocolate, cheese and monosodium glutamate
- Stroke or transient ischemic attack
- Head injury.

Risk Factors

- Anxiety
- Stress
- Consumption of caffeine

- Extremely high blood pressure
- Low blood sugar
- Overexerting oneself
- Missing meals
- Poor sleep position
- Over working
- Holding your head in one position for a long time, like at a computer, microscope or typewriter
- Using alcohol or drugs.

Types

1. **Migraine headache (vascular)**
   - It is a severe form of headache which occurs with other symptoms such as visual disturbances or nausea.
   - The pain will be throbbing, pounding or pulsating.
   - It tends to begin on one side of the head and may spread to both sides.
   - The pain usually gets worse when you try to move around
   - It is more common in women.
2. **Myogenic or muscular headache**
   - It is caused by tight, contracted muscles in your shoulders, neck, scalp and jaw.
   - It tend to occur on both sides of the head
   - They often start at the back of your head and spread forward
   - The pain may be of squeezing or dull type like a tight band
   - The shoulders, neck or jaw may feel tight and sore
   - The pain is usually persistent, but does not get worse with activity.
3. **Cervicogenic headache**
   - It originates from disorders of the neck, including the anatomical structures innervated by the cervical roots C1 to C3.
   - It is often precipitated by neck movement or sustained awkward head positioning.
   - It is often accompanied by restricted cervical range of motion, ipsilateral neck, and shoulder or arm pain.

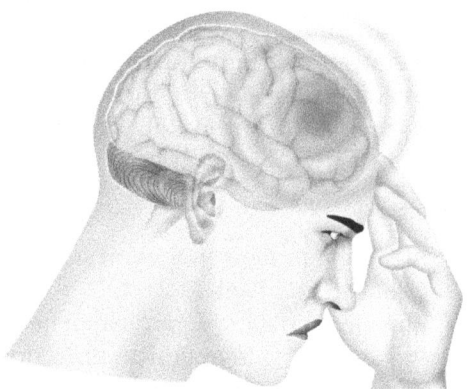

Fig. 1.15: Depicts the different kinds of headache and its understanding.

4. **Traction headache**
   - The headache is the symptom of other disorders ranging from stroke to sinus infection.
5. **Inflammatory headache**
   - In can serve as a warning signal for most serious disorders
   - It may result due to any inflammatory conditions such as meningitis, diseases of the sinuses, spine, neck, ears and teeth.
6. **Cluster headache**
   - These are sharp and extremely painful headaches that tend to occur several times per day for months then go away for the similar period.
   - It is a less common type.
7. **Sinus headache**
   - This type of headache cause pain in front of your head and face.
   - They are due to inflammation in the sinus passage that lie behind the cheeks, nose and eyes.
   - The pain tends to be worse when you bend forward and when you first wake up in the morning.

Other Types

1. Idiopathic intracranial hypertension
2. Ictal headache
3. Brain freeze type (also known as ice cream headache)
4. Thunderclap headache
5. Toxic headache
6. Coital cephalgia (also known as sex headache)
7. Rebound headache (also known as medication overuse headache)
8. Red wine headache
9. Hemicrania continua type
10. Spinal headache (post-dural puncture headache)
11. Hangover type (caused by heavy alcohol consumption)
12. Temporal arteritis type (these are headache which is experienced after 50 years of age for the first time

Pathophysiology

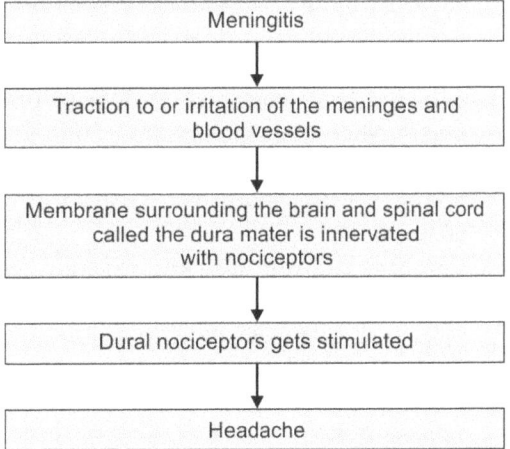

Clinical Features

- Stiff neck
- Fever
- Convulsions
- Confusion
- Pain in the eye or ear.

Complications

- Status migrainosus
- Migrainosus infarction
- Migraine seizure
- Persistent aura without infarction.

Diagnostic Tests

- History
- Physical examination
- Blood examination
- Magnetic resonance imaging
- Computed tomography scan of the brain or sinuses
- X-ray examination
- Temporal artery biopsy
- Lumbar puncture

Management

Medical

- **Nonsteroidal anti-inflammatory drug (NSAID):** It helps to relieve headache. For example, paracetamol, acetaminophen, ibuprofen, etc.
- **Antidepressants:** It helps to relieve tension or migraine headache. For example, nortriptyline, amitriptyline, fluoxetine, etc.
- **Beta blockers:** It helps to relieve migraine headache. For example, propranolol, atenolol, etc.
- **Calcium channel blockers:** It helps to relieve migraine headache. For example, verapamil, diltiazem, etc.
- **Antiepileptic drugs:** It helps to control seizures. For example, topiramate, sodium valproate, etc.

Nursing

- Strictly prohibit long-term use of painkillers
- Encourage to keep a headache diary to identify the source or trigger of your symptoms.
- Instruct to take adequate rest
- Encourage to perform relaxation technique using meditation, deep breathing, yoga or other techniques.
- Encourage to take healthy diet
- Stress to do regular exercise
- Instruct to stretch the neck and upper body, if the work involves typing or using a computer.
- Instruct to stop smoking
- Educate regarding proper usage of posture
- Instruct to wear proper eye glasses.

■ HERNIATED DISC

Definition

A herniated disc is a medical condition affecting the spine in which a tear in the outer fibrous ring of an intervertebral disc allows the soft central portion to bulge out and it may result in the release of inflammatory chemical reactors which may directly cause severe pain even in the absence of nerve root compression.

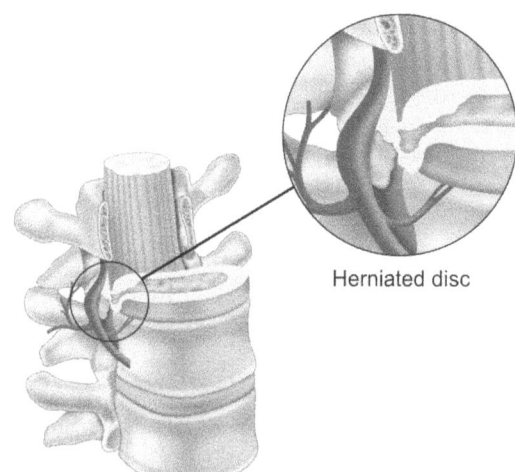

Fig. 1.16: Shows the disc protrusion and herniated disc.

Etiology

- Falls
- Accidents
- Spinal stenosis
- Wear and tear of the disc due to aging.

Risk Factors

- Repeated strenuous activities
- Sudden pressure
- Improper lifting
- Excessive body weight that places added stress on the disc
- Smoking.

Stages of Disc Herniation

- ***Disc degeneration stage:*** The chemical changes associated with aging causes discs to weaken, but without a herniation.
- ***Prolapse stage:*** It is a form or position of the disc changes with some slight impingement into the spinal canal.
- ***Extrusion stage:*** The gel-like nucleus pulposus breaks through the tire-like wall (annulus fibrosus) but remains within the disc.

- *Sequestration stage:* The nucleus pulposus breaks through the annulus fibrosus and lies outside the disc in the spinal canal.

Pathophysiology

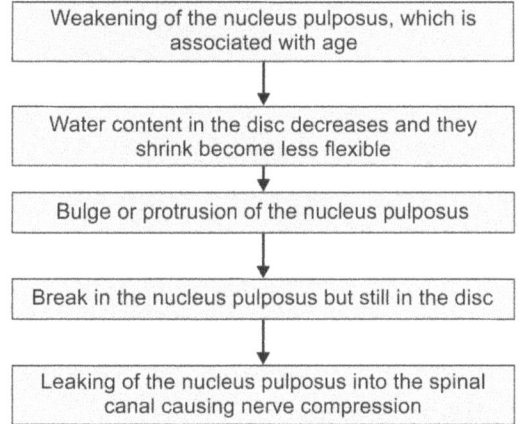

Clinical Features

- Sciatica (a herniated disc in the lower back leading to pain and numbness in the buttock and down the leg)
- Electric shock pain
- Tingling and numbness
- Low back pain
- Paresthesia
- Muscle weakness on both legs.

Complications

- Cauda equina syndrome
- Saddle anesthesia
- Chronic back pain
- Permanent nerve damage.

Diagnostic Tests

- History
- Physical examination
- Nerve conduction studies
- Magnetic resonance imaging (MRI) scan
- X-rays
- Computed tomography (CT) scan
- Myelogram
- Electromyogram.

Management

Medical

- **High dose corticosteroids:** It helps to reduce the acute effects of spinal cord herniation. For example, methylprednisolone, dexamethasone, etc.
- **Nonsteroidal anti-inflammatory drugs:** It is used to reduce swelling and inflammation that occur as a result of disc herniation. For example, ibuprofen, aspirin, diclofenac sodium, etc.
- **Muscle relaxants:** It eases muscle tension and pain within few hours. For example, diazepam, cyclobenzaprine, carisoprodol, etc.
- **Injected corticosteroids:** It can reduce inflammation, relieving pain and improving function and mobility. For example, betamethasone, methylprednisolone, etc.

Surgical

The goal of surgery is to make the herniated disc stop pressing on and irritating the nerves, causing symptoms of pain and weakness

- **Laminotomy/Microdiscectomy:** It is a surgical procedure in which an opening is made in the spinal canal (laminotomy) in order to visualize the pinched nerve root followed by careful protection of nerve root with a special retractor and protruding disc fragments along with remaining loose or degenerated disc material which are then removed with a small grasping device (microdiscectomy). The small hole left in the annulus will generate in 4 to 6 weeks and fill in with new disc material.
- **Discectomy:** It involves removing all or part of the damaged disc in order to relieve pressure on the spinal nerves. A discectomy can be performed as "open surgery" (open Discectomy) or "minimally invasive surgery"(microdiscectomy).
- **Laminectomy:** It is a surgical procedure which involves removing a parts of the

vertebrae called the lamina in order to make more room for the spinal nerves, relieving pressure on them and reducing pain.
- **Spinal fusion:** It is a procedure in which bone is grafted onto the spine, creating a solid unit between two or more vertebrae. It stabilizes the spine and relieves pressure on them and reducing pain.
- **Artificial disc surgery:** It is the surgical replacement of a diseased or herniated lumbar disc with a manufactured disc.
- **Hemilaminectomy:** It is a surgical procedure that decompresses impinged nerve roots being pinched by the lamina bone and other tissues of the spinal processes.
- **Disc arthroplasty:** It is a surgical procedure in which the painful degenerated disc is removed and replaced by an artificial mobile disc that mimics the movement of a normal disc.

Nursing
- Provide bed rest
- Instruct to maintain a healthy body weight
- Instruct not to remain seated for longer periods
- Encourage to use safe lifting techniques
- Encourage use of a lumbosacral back support.

HUNTINGTON'S DISEASE

Definition
It is an inherited, progressive, degenerative disease that causes certain nerve cells in the brain to waste away and it may lead to uncontrolled movements, emotional disturbances and mental deterioration.

Etiology
Genetic defect on chromosome 4.

Risk Factors
- Family history
- Those aged between 30 to 40 years
- Children of people with the disorder.

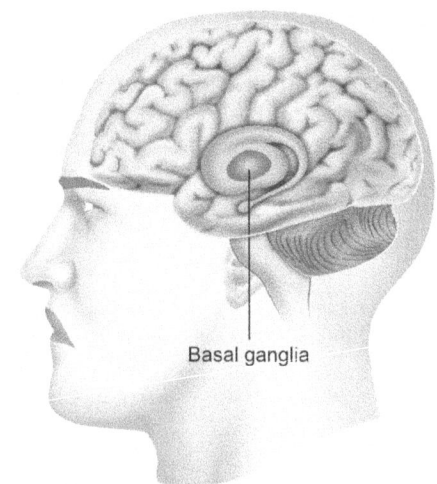

Fig. 1.17: Shows the degeneration of neurons in Huntington's disease affecting the basal ganglia of brain.

Pathophysiology

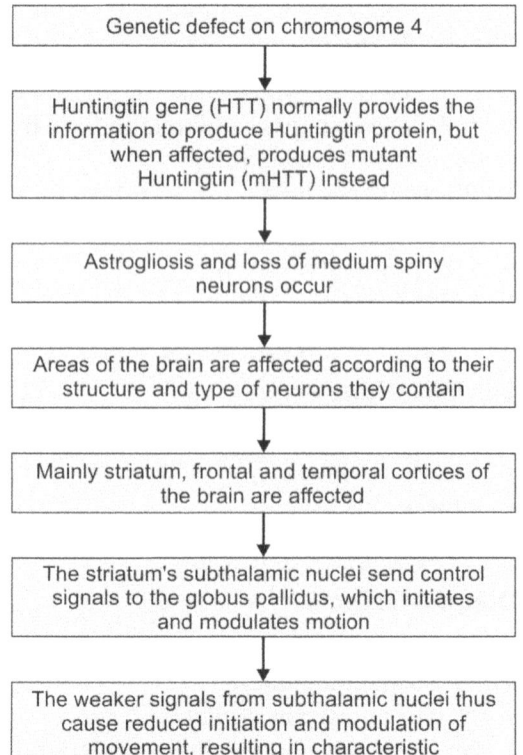

Clinical Features

Physical
- Uncontrolled movement of the arms, legs, head, face and upper body

- Impaired gait, posture and balance
- Slow or abnormal eye movements
- Difficulty in speech
- Difficulty in swallowing.

Cognitive
- Decline in thinking and reasoning skills including memory, concentration, judgment and ability to plan and organize
- Inability to start a task or conversation
- Difficulty focusing on a task for long periods
- Difficulty in learning new information
- Lack of awareness of one's own behaviors and abilities.

Psychiatric
- Alterations in mood especially depression and anxiety
- Uncharacteristic anger and irritability
- Obsessive-compulsive behavior, leading a person to repeat the same question or activity over and over
- Loss of interest in normal activities
- Social withdrawal
- Insomnia or excessive sleeping
- Reduced sexual drive.

Complications
- Loss of ability to care for self
- Loss of ability to interact
- Injury to self or others
- Increased risk of infection
- Depression
- Death.

Diagnostic Tests
- History
- Physical examination
- Psychological examination
- Blood examination
- Embryonic screening
- CT scan of head
- MRI scan of head.

Management

No treatments can alter the course of Huntington's disease. But medications can lessen some symptoms of movement and psychiatric disorders and multiple interventions can help a person adapt to changes in his or her abilities for a certain amount of time.

Medical
- **Antiepileptics:** It helps to prevent the attack of seizures. For example, phenytoin, phenobarbital, etc.
- **Monoamine depletors:** It helps in reducing the amount of certain chemicals in the body that are overly active people with Huntington's disease. For example, nitoman, xenazine, etc.
- **Antipsychotics:** It is used to treat psychosis. For example, haloperidol, chlorpromazine, etc.
- **Anti-depressants:** It is used for the treatment of major depressive disorder. For example, fluoxetine, sertraline hydrochloride, etc.
- **Tranquilizers:** It is used in the treatment of anxiety, tension, panic attacks and insomnia. For example, benzodiazepines, paroxetine, etc.
- **Mood stabilizers:** It is used to treat mood disorders characterized by intense and sustained mood shifts. For example, lithium, carbamazepine, etc.

Nursing
- Provide talk therapy to help a person manage behavioral problems, develop coping strategies, manage expectations during progression of the disease and facilitate effective communication among family members
- Provide speech therapy to improve the ability to speak
- Provide physical therapy to enhance strength, flexibility, balance and coordination.
- Recommend for genetic counseling
- Provide multidisciplinary treatment plan to maintain a person's quality of life.
- Instruct to maintain a healthy body weight as it is essential to it

- Medication should be reviewed regularly to ensure it remains effective in treating symptoms over the course of the illness.
- Maintain a person's mental wellbeing through exercise, social and psychological support.

HYDROCEPHALUS

Definition

Hydrocephalus is a condition where an abnormal build-up of cerebrospinal fluid (CSF) causes an increase in pressure in the ventricles or subarachnoid space of the brain.

Etiology

- Aqueductal obstruction (stenosis)
- Myelomeningocele
- Intraventricular hemorrhage
- Head trauma
- Tumors
- Arachnoid cysts
- Dandy-Walker syndrome (enlargement of the 4th ventricle).

Risk Factors

- Being children
- Pre-eclampsia
- Alcohol use during pregnancy
- Poor antenatal care
- Low birth weight infants
- Family history of hydrocephalus
- Cranial bleeding
- Infections of the central nervous system
- Uterus infection during pregnancy.

Types

- ***Obstructive (non-communicating) hydrocephalus:*** It occurs when cerebrospinal

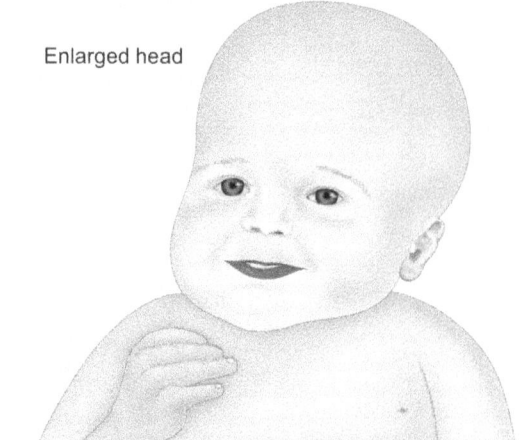
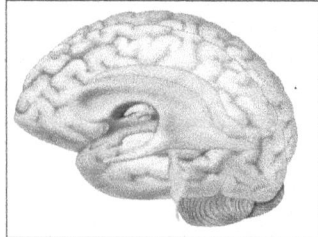
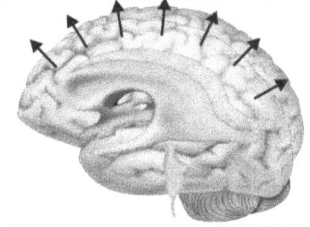

Fig. 1.18: Shows the comparison of brain with normal ventricles and brain with enlarged ventricles due to hydrocephalus.

fluid flow is blocked within the ventricular system.
- *Non-obstructive (communicating) hydrocephalus:* It occurs where there is inadequate cerebrospinal fluid absorption.
- *Normal pressure hydrocephalus:* It results due to an increase in the amount of cerebrospinal fluid in the brain's ventricles with little or no increase in the pressure inside the head and is most often seen in adults over 60 years of age.

Pathophysiology

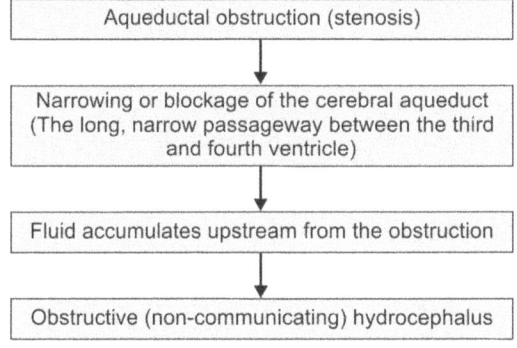

Clinical Features

In Infants

- Abnormally large head
- Bulge fontanelle (soft spot) on the top of the head
- Rapid increase in the head size
- Eyes fixed downward (sunsetting of the eyes)
- Irritability
- Seizures
- Separated sutures
- Sleepiness
- Vomiting
- Delays in development.

In Older Children

- Gait disturbances
- Chronic headache followed with vomiting
- Mild dementia
- Impairment in bladder control
- Brief, shrill, high-pitched cry
- Eyes fixed downward (sunsetting of the eyes)
- Excessive sleepiness
- Irritability
- Muscle spasm
- Retarded growth
- Nausea
- Lack of energy
- Impaired performance at school.

Complications

- Obstruction
- Infection (meningitis or encephalitis)
- Physical disabilities
- Intellectual impairment
- Nerve damage.

Diagnostic Tests

- History
- Physical examination
- Neuropsychological testing
- Blood examination
- Cranial ultrasound
- Lumbar puncture
- Isotopic cisternography
- Skull X-ray examination.
- Computed Tomography (CT) scan
- Magnetic resonance imaging (MRI) scan.

Management

Medical

- **Dehydrating hyperosmolar agents:** It helps to reduce brain swelling and pressure. For example, mannitol, glycerol, urea, etc.
- **Antibiotics:** It helps to prevent secondary infections. For example, benzyl penicillin, ampicillin, piperacillin, vancomycin, cephalosporin, etc.
- **Corticosteroids:** It helps to reduce the mortality rate by reducing brain swelling and pressure. For example, dexamethasone, prednisolone, etc.

- **Anticonvulsants:** It helps to prevent seizure occurrence. For example, phenytoin, sodium valproate, etc.
- **Diuretics:** It helps to reduce intracranial pressure and cerebrospinal fluid production. For example, furosemide, etc.

Surgical

- **Shunt placement:** It is a surgical procedure that involves implanting a tube, called a shunt, in the brain to remove the excess cerebrospinal fluid (CSF) in the brain through the shunt to another part of the body, usually the abdomen.
- **Ventriculostomy:** It is a surgical procedure in which a hole is created in the bottom or base of one of the ventricles, in order to allow the fluid to flow toward the base or bottom of the brain, where absorption that normally occurs.

Nursing

- Women of child-bearing age should have folate regularly in the diet before becoming pregnant to help prevent the development of neural tube defects.
- Encourage the pregnant women to go for a regular hospital visit to reduce the risk of premature birth.
- Instruct the patient to wear appropriate protective gear when traveling in a bike to avoid severe head injury.
- Provide physical therapy to enhance strength, flexibility, balance and coordination.
- Medication should be reviewed regularly to ensure it remains effective in treating symptoms over the course of the illness.

INCREASED INTRACRANIAL PRESSURE

Definition

The pressure exerted by the cranium on the brain tissue, cerebrospinal fluid and the brain's circulating volume and this phenomena is known as increased intracranial pressure.

Etiology

- Severe head injury
- Brain tumor
- Stroke
- Encephalitis
- Aneurysm rupture
- Intraventricular hemorrhage
- Subdural or epidural hematoma
- Sinus thrombosis
- Heart failure
- Hydrocephalus
- Meningitis
- Subarachnoid hemorrhage
- Choroid plexus tumor
- Cerebral venous thrombosis
- Acute liver failure.

Risk Factors

- Tobacco smoking
- Obesity
- High blood pressure
- Diabetes mellitus
- Hypercholesterolemia.

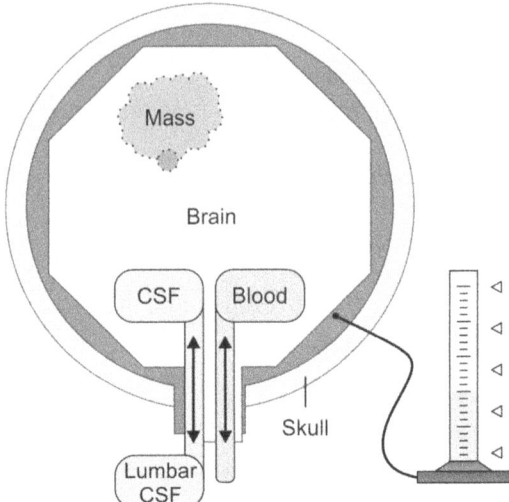

Fig. 1.19: Shows the raised intracranial pressure.

Pathophysiology

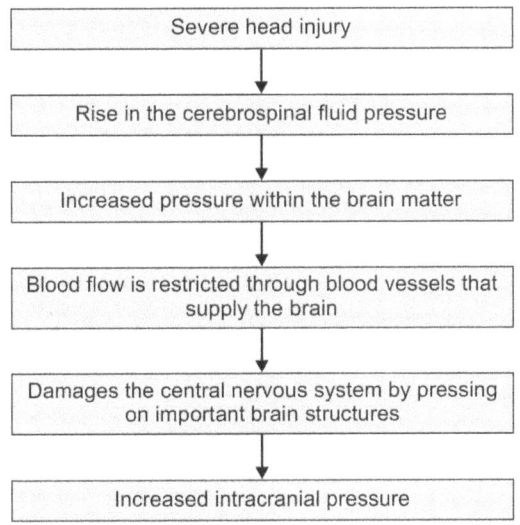

Clinical Features

- Headache
- Nausea
- Vomiting
- Dizziness
- Increased blood pressure
- Shallow breathing
- Behavioral changes
- Progressive decreased consciousness
- Lethargy
- Ocular palsy
- Poor memory
- Restlessness
- Decreased mental abilities
- Papilledema
- Bradycardia
- Hyperventilation.

Complications

- Seizures
- Stroke
- Permanent neurologic problems
- Coma
- Death.

Diagnostic Tests

- History
- Physical examination
- Magnetic resonance imaging (MRI) scan
- Computed tomography (CT) scan
- Spinal tap or lumbar puncture
- X-ray of head
- Electroencephalogram
- Radio isotope scan
- Cerebral angiography.

Management

Medical

- **Dehydrating hyperosmolar agents:** It helps to reduce brain swelling and pressure. For example, mannitol, urea, etc.
- **Calcium channel blockers:** It helps in blocking the entry of calcium into muscle cells in artery walls. For example, verapamil, diltiazem, etc.
- **Anti-hypertensive agents:** It helps in reducing the increased blood pressure. For example, atenolol, propranolol, etc.

Surgical

- **Extraventricular drain:** It is a procedure in which a catheter is inserted into the brain's lateral ventricles to drain the cerebrospinal fluid in order to decrease the intracranial pressure.
- **Craniotomy:** It is a surgical procedure in which holes are drilled in the skull to relieve pressure from parts of the brain.
- **Decompressive craniectomy:** It is a surgical procedure in which a part of the skull is removed and the dura mater is expanded to allow the brain to swell without crushing it or causing herniation.

Nursing

- Ensure adequate airway, breathing and oxygenation
- Elevate the head of the bed (15° to 20°) to promote venous drainage and to lower increased ICP.
- Maintain the blood pressure at 150/100 mm Hg or less than that to facilitate perfusion.

- Provide complete bed rest
- Instruct the patient to maintain normoglycemia (blood glucose level between 80 to 120 mg/dL).

KENNEDY'S DISEASE (ALSO KNOWN AS SBMA)

Definition

Kennedy's disease also known as spinal bulbar muscular atrophy (SBMA) is a rare inherited neuromuscular disorder that causes progressive weakening and wasting of the muscles, particularly the arms and the legs.

Etiology

Mutations in the androgen receptor gene on the X chromosome.

Risk Factors

- Males
- Those between 20 to 50 years.

Pathophysiology

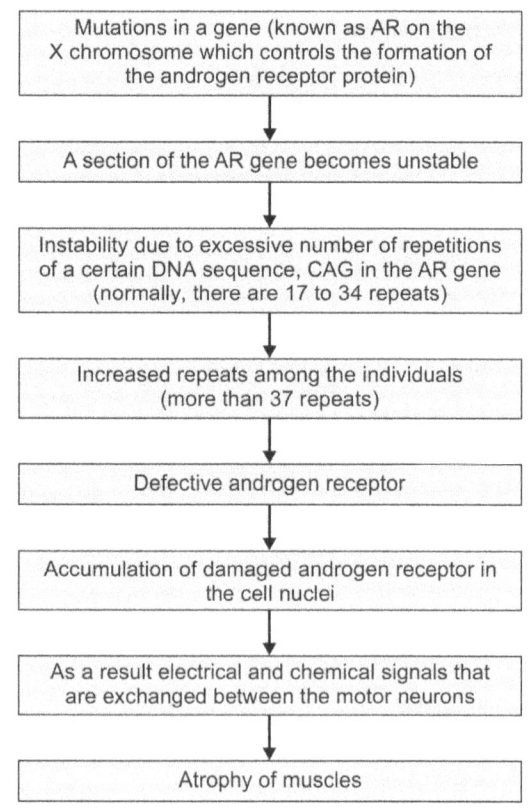

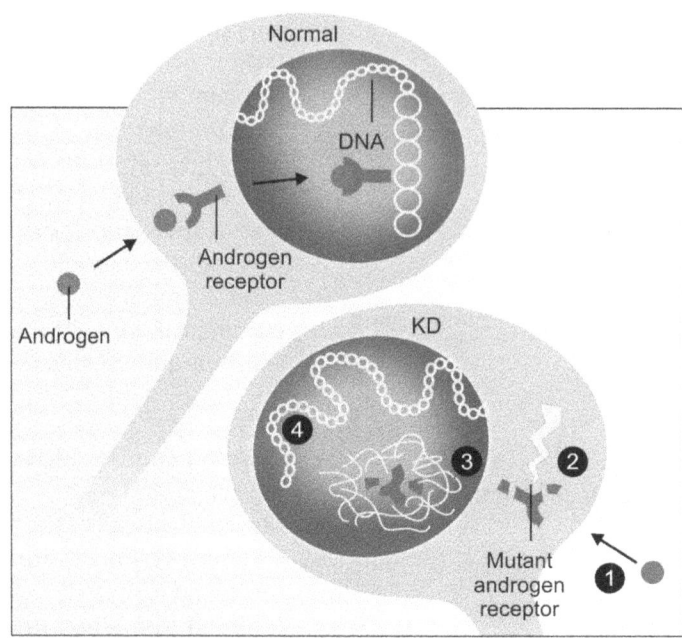

Fig. 1.20: Shows the defective androgen receptor seen in Kennedy's disease.

Clinical Features

- Weakness of tongue and mouth muscles
- Difficulty swallowing
- Poor articulation
- Changes in voice and speech (harsh or strained voice)
- Numbness
- Hand tremors
- Decreased of absent deep tendon reflexes
- Twitching of muscles when at rest (fasciculations)
- Cramps
- Increased calf size due to cramps
- Loss of muscle bulk
- Erectile dysfunction
- Impotence
- Shrunken testicles
- Low sperm count.

Complications

- Gynecomastia (swelling of the breasts)
- Gonadal atrophy
- Diabetes.

Diagnostic Tests

- History
- Physical examination
- Blood tests—to check for elevated serum creatine kinase (CPK)
- DNA blood tests—to check whether the Kennedy's disease gene is present or not.
- Neurophysiological examination—to identify normal peripheral nerve conduction.
- EMG test—to detect chronic denervation
- Muscle biopsy—to detect chronic denervation.

Management

Medical

There is no cure for Kennedy's disease, because medical science does not know how to regenerate muscle neurons and the treatment aims at easing the symptoms.

Nursing

- Encourage to do regular stretching to help in reducing muscle cramps
- Encourage to do gentle and regular aerobic exercises
- Instruct to take healthy balanced diet
- Instruct to take plenty of rest to avoid exhaustion.

MENINGITIS

Definition

Meningitis is a medical condition in which there is an infection and inflammation of the protective membranes which covers around the brain and spinal cord, known collectively as the meninges.

Etiology

- Viral infection (Enterovirus, herpes simplex virus, etc.)
- Bacterial infection (Group B *Streptococcus, Escherichia coli, Neisseria,* etc.).
- Fungal infection (*Cryptococcus neoformans*)
- Parasitic infection (*Naegleria fowleri*)
- Spread of cancer to meninges
- Certain drugs (NSAIDs, antibiotics and intravenous immunoglobulins)
- Sarcoidosis
- Systemic lupus erythematosus
- Vasculitis
- Migraine headache.

Risk Factors

- It usually affects children, teens and young adults
- Old age group of people
- People with long-term illness
- People with weakened immune system
- Tobacco use
- Viral upper respiratory tract infections
- Otitis media
- Mastoiditis
- Skull fractures

Disorders of Nervous System

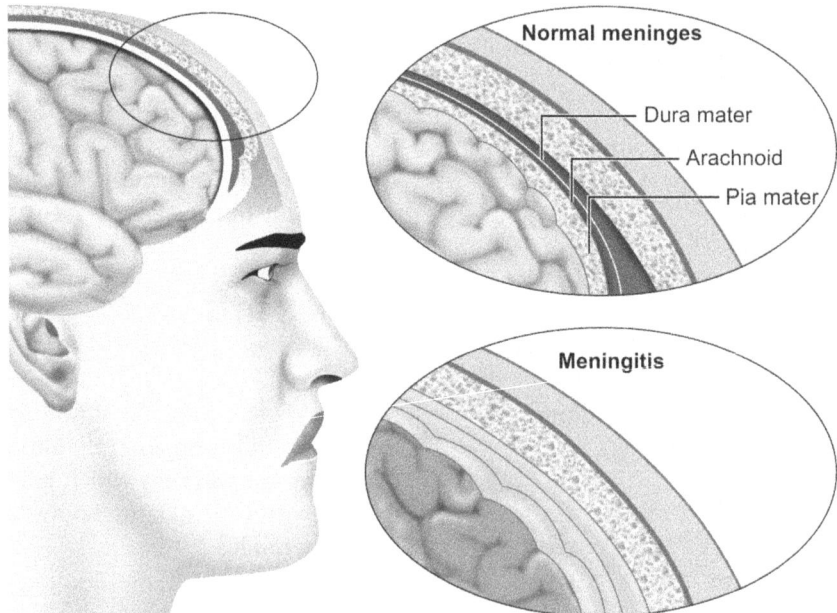

Fig. 1.21: Shows the comparison of normal meninges with that of inflammatory meninges in the brain.

- Brain or spinal surgery
- Use of nasal sprays.

Types

There are two types of meningitis as follows:
1. **Viral meningitis (aseptic meningitis):** This type is fairly common and does not cause any serious illness.
2. **Bacterial meningitis:** This type is rare, but is usually serious and can be life-threatening if it is not treated right away.

Pathophysiology

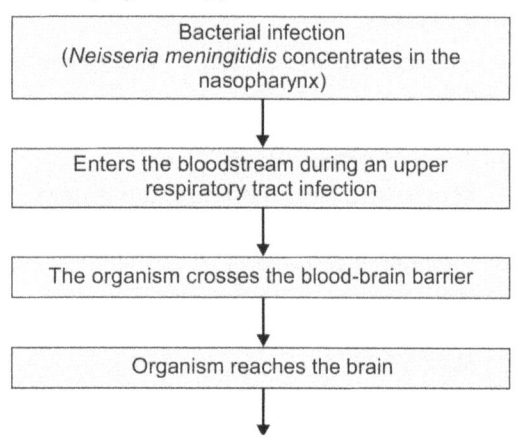

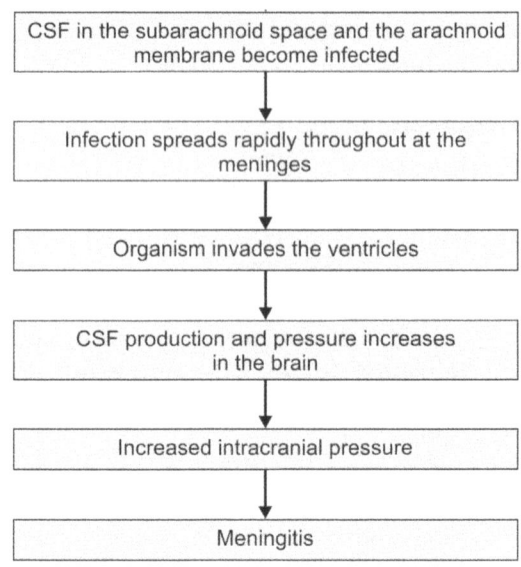

Clinical Features

- Severe headache
- Nuchal rigidity (stiffness of neck) especially when they try to touch their chin to the chest
- Sudden high fever
- Altered mental status

- Photophobia (inability to tolerate bright light)
- Phonophobia (inability to tolerate loud noises)
- A positive Kernig's sign occurs when the patient lies supine with both hips and knee flexed to 90° pain limits passive extension of the knee.
- A positive Brudzinski's sign occurs when flexion of the neck causes involuntary knee and hip flexion.
- Trouble staying awake
- Irritability
- Delirium
- Bulging of the fontanelle (soft spot)
- Pain over the legs
- Cold extremities
- Abnormal skin color
- Nausea and vomiting
- Red, macular rash
- Tachycardia
- Short attention span
- Generalized muscle aches and pains
- Seizures
- Increased intracranial pressure
- Disorientation and memory impairment
- Lethargy
- Unresponsiveness
- Coma
- High fever.

Complications

- Gangrene formation
- Sepsis
- Systematic inflammatory response syndrome (fall in blood pressure, fast heart rate, high or abnormally low temperature and rapid breathing).
- Disseminated intravascular coagulation (excessive activation of blood clotting).
- Hearing loss
- Encephalitis
- Cerebral vasculitis
- Cerebral venous thrombosis
- Hydrocephalus
- Hemiparesis and hemianopia
- Subdural effusion.

Diagnostic Tests

- History
- Physical examination
- Jolt accentuation maneuver—A test in which the headache is not worsened by rapidly (2 to 3 times per second) rotating the head horizontally, meningitis is unlikely
- Lumbar puncture or spinal tap
- Blood examination
- Blood culture
- Computed tomography (CT) scan
- Magnetic resonance imaging (MRI) scan
- CSF culture
- Latex agglutination test
- Limulus lysate test
- Polymerase chain reaction test
- Electroencephalogram
- X-ray examination of the skull
- Urine routine.

Management

Medical

- **Antibiotics:** It helps to prevent secondary infections. For example, benzyl penicillin, ampicillin, piperacillin, vancomycin, cephalosporin, etc.
- **Corticosteroids:** It helps to reduce the mortality rate by reducing edema.
- **Antiviral agents:** For example, acyclovir. It helps to prevent any viral infection. For example, dexamethasone, prednisolone, etc.
- **Antifungal agents:** It helps to prevent any fungal infection. For example, amphotericin B, flucytosine, etc.
- **Anticonvulsants:** It helps to prevent seizure occurrence. For example, phenytoin, etc.
- **Osmodiuretics:** It helps to reduce cerebral edema. For example, mannitol, etc.

Nursing

- Assess neurologic status and vital signs constantly
- Elevate the head of the bed 30° and avoid neck flexion and extreme hip flexion.
- Ensure that the airway is patent and adequate ventilation is established.

- Prevent stimulation and restrict visitors
- Institute infection control precautions until 24 hours after initiation of antibiotic therapy.
- Protect the patient from injury secondary to seizure activity
- Reduce high fever to decrease load on heart and brain from oxygen demands.
- Provide foods as per the likes of the patient.

MOEBIUS SYNDROME

Definition
Moebius syndrome is an extremely rare congenital neurological disorder that typically affects the sixth and seventh cranial nerves. These nerves affect the face and eye muscles and cause facial paralysis.

Etiology
- Underdevelopment of the VI and VII cranial nerves
- Temporary vascular abnormalities during early intrauterine life
- Cocaine abuse during pregnancy
- Use of ergotamine
- Use of Misoprostol during early pregnancy life
- Use of teratogen thalidomide
- Exposure to infections
- Alcohol consumption during pregnancy
- Idiopathic.

Risk Factors
- Heredity
- Both male and female are affected equal in number
- Toxins.

Stages
There are four types of stages as follows:
1. *Group-I:* It was characterized by small or absent brain stem nuclei that control the cranial nerves.
2. *Group-II:* It was characterized by loss and degeneration of neurons in the facial peripheral nerve.
3. *Group-III:* It was characterized by loss and degeneration of neurons and other brain cells, microscopic areas of damage and hardened tissue in the brain stem nuclei and
4. *Group-IV:* It was characterized by muscular symptoms in spite of a lack of lesions in the cranial nerve.

Pathophysiology

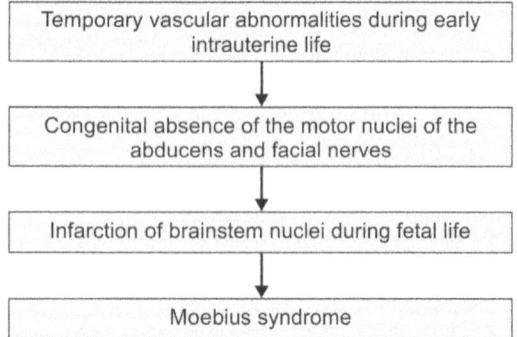

Clinical Features
- Mask like expression when crying is the hallmark feature
- Motor delays due to upper body weakness
- Strabismus (crossed eyes)
- Dry eyes and irritability
- Dental problems
- High palate
- Cleft palate
- Hand and feet problems including club foot and missing or fused fingers (syndactyly)

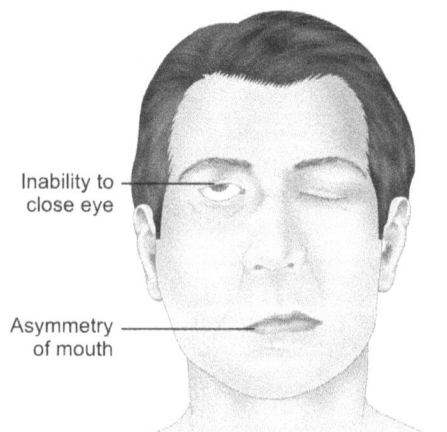

Fig. 1.22: Depicts the cardinal features of Moebius syndrome.

- Hearing problems
- Poland's syndrome (chest wall and upper limb anomalies)
- Inability to smile.

Complications

- Micrognathia (small chin)
- Microstomia (small mouth).

Diagnostic Tests

- History
- Physical examination
- Magnetic resonance imaging of the brain and brain stem
- Computerized axial tomography (CAT) scan.

Management

Surgical

There is no cure for this and the treatment plan aimed at managing and minimizing their symptoms to the greatest extent possible.

- **Static slings:** It is a procedure in which a piece of the child's own tissue that is transplanted in order to prop up the drooping skin around the lips (the "smile area") or eyelids.
- **Smile surgery (functional muscle transfer):** It is a surgical procedure in which the muscle is taken from elsewhere in the child's body (usually the thigh) and grafts it onto the corners of their mouth, giving them the ability to smile.
- **Tarsorrhaphy:** It is a surgical procedure in which the eyelids are partially closed in facilitating the eyes to blink properly.

Nursing

- Encourage the patient to use alternative ways to communicate emotion such as body language, posture and their tone of voice.
- Encourage patient to maintain proper eye care
- Teach friends and family how to easily pick up on the emotional cues of a person with this syndrome.
- Keep them active-physically, mentally and socially.

MULTIPLE SCLEROSIS

Definition

Multiple sclerosis is an immune-mediated, chronic, progressive, non-contagious, degenerative disease of the CNS characterized by demyelinization of the neurons.

Etiology

- Viral infection (Epstein-Barr virus)
- Autoimmune response

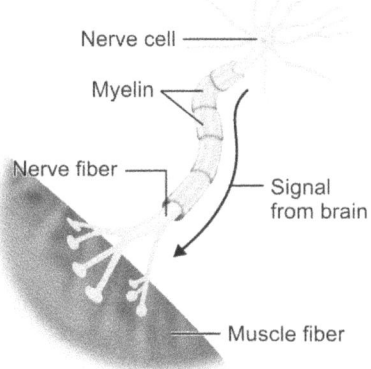
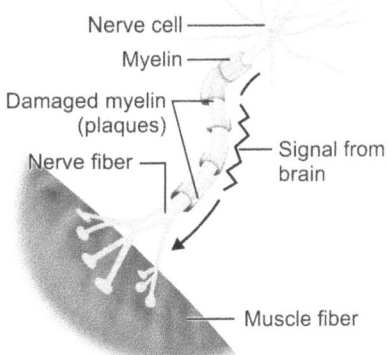

Fig. 1.23: Shows the comparison of normal myelin with that of damaged myelin seen in multiple sclerosis.

- Trauma
- Genetic predisposition.

Risk Factors

- Being women
- Those who live in cold environment
- Vitamin D deficiency
- Those who born in spring or late spring season
- More common in whites, particularly those with Northern European ancestry
- Second generation (grand children) in a family with multiple sclerosis
- Smoking
- Those who are between 20 to 40 years of age
- Stress
- Pregnancy
- Fatigue
- Lack of sleep.

Pathophysiology

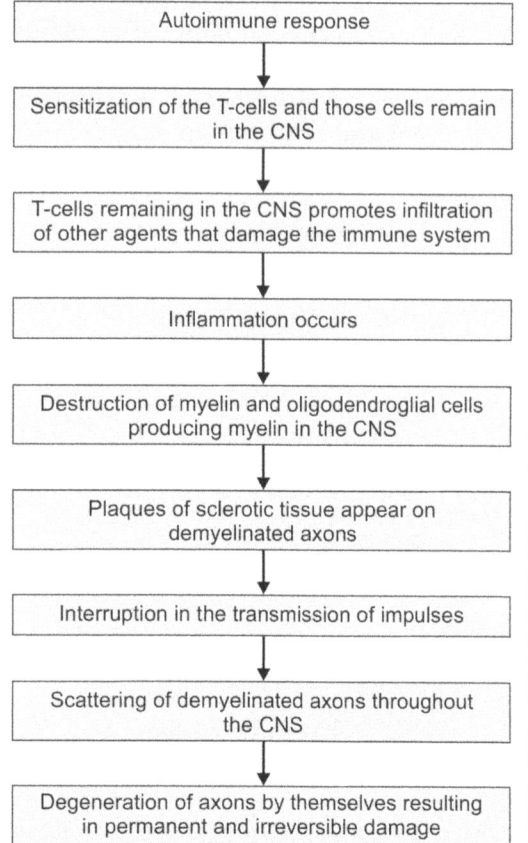

Clinical Features

- Paresthesia
- Blurred vision
- Diplopia
- Nystagmus
- Fatigue
- Weakness
- Ataxia
- Vertigo
- Dysphasia
- Positive Babinski reflex
- Tremors and spasticity (muscle hypertonicity) of the lower extremities
- Decreased perception to pain, touch and temperature
- Bladder and bowel disturbances
- Memory changes and confusion
- Irritability
- Numbness and tingling on the face or extremities
- Slurred speech
- Loss of short-term memory
- Poor judgment and inability to solve problems effectively.

Complications

- Quadriparesis
- Cognitive dysfunction
- Urinary tract infections
- Constipation
- Pressure ulcers
- Contractive deformities
- Dependent pedal edema
- Pneumonia
- Reactive depression
- Decreased bone mass.

Diagnostic Tests

- History
- Physical examination
- Magnetic resonance imaging
- Electrophoresis of CSF
- Urodynamic studies
- Neuropsychological testing
- CSF analysis
- Evoked response test
- Computed tomography (CT) scan.

Management

Medical

- **Corticosteroids:** It helps to reduce the severity of the disease by relieving nerve inflammation. For example, prednisone, methylprednisolone.
- **Muscle relaxants:** It relaxes muscle stiffness or spasms particularly in the legs. For example, baclofen, cyclobenzaprine, tizanidine, etc.
- **Beta interferons:** It controls the growth of lesions and reduce symptoms. For example, avonex, betaseron, copaxone, etc.
- **Immunosuppressant agents:** It blocks the movement of potentially damaging immune cells from the bloodstream to the brain and spinal cord. For example, natalizumab, alemtuzumab, mitoxantrone, etc.
- **Benzodiazepines:** It helps to treat the spasm. For example, diazepam, etc.
- **Beta-adrenergic blockers:** It is used to treat high blood pressure. For example, inderal, etc.
- **Antineoplastic agents:** It reduces the number of relapses a person is experiencing. For example, mitoxantrone, etc.
- **Nonsteroidal anti-inflammatory drugs (NSAID):** It blocks the enzyme prostaglandins which are chemicals produced by the body that promote pain and inflammation. For example, ibuprofen, naproxen, etc.
- **Anti-seizure agents:** It helps to prevent and control seizures. For example, neurontin, etc.

Surgical

Plasmapheresis or plasma exchange: It is a procedure in which blood is removed from the body and blood cells are separated from the liquid portion of the blood (plasma). Then acetylcholine receptor antibodies are removed and blood cells are diluted with artificial plasma (usually a solution of saline and sterilized human albumin protein) and infused back into the body.

Nursing

- Provide bed rest during exacerbation
- Encourage regular exercise and rest
- Protect the patient from injury by providing safety measures
- Promote regular elimination by bladder and bowel training
- Encourage independence activities
- Instruct the patient to balance activity with rest periods
- Instruct the patient to have more fluids and roughages in the diet
- Instruct the patient to avoid fatigue, stress and infection
- Instruct safety measures to the patient.

MYASTHENIA GRAVIS (MG) (GOLDFLAM DISEASE)

Definition

Myasthenia gravis (MG) is a chronic autoimmune neuromuscular disease which is characterized by varying degrees of skeletal

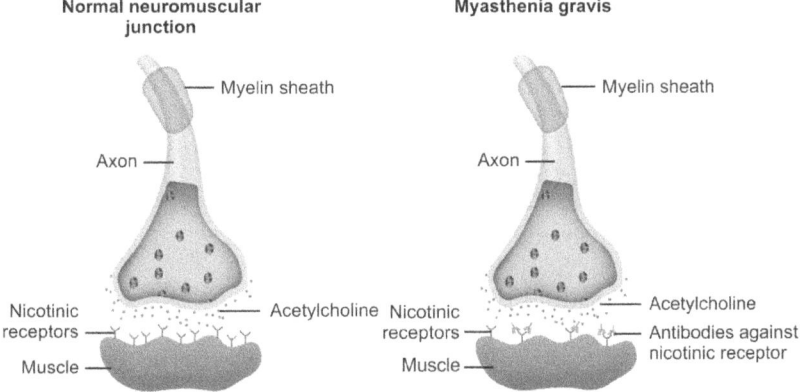

Fig. 1.24: Shows the comparison of normal neuromuscular junction with that of damaged neuromuscular junction seen in myasthenia gravis.

muscle weakness at the neuromuscular junction. Skeletal muscles are primarily muscle fibers that contain bands or striations that are connected to bone.

Etiology
- Autoimmune response
- Thymus gland tumors
- Genetic predisposition.

Risk Factors
- Being women
- Being children
- Emotional stress
- Exposure to extreme temperatures
- Low levels of potassium in blood
- Illness
- Being overtired
- Medications like muscle relaxants, anti-convulsants and certain antibiotics
- Overexertion
- Scleroderma.

Types
It is classified based on which skeletal muscles are affected:
- *Generalized myasthenia gravis:*
  - It contributes to 85–90% of the cases
  - It is characterized by weakness in the trunk, arms, and legs.
- *Ocular myasthenia gravis:*
  - It contributes to 10–15% of the cases
  - It is characterized by weakness only in the muscles that control eye movement.
- *Congenital myasthenia gravis:*
  - It develops at or shortly after birth and causes generalized symptoms
  - It is an inherited condition caused by genetic defect and transient neonatal that occurs in infants born to mothers who have myasthenia gravis
- *Transient neonatal myasthenia gravis:*
  - It develops in 10–20% of infants born to mothers who have myasthenia gravis.
  - It is caused by circulation of the mother's antibodies through the placenta and it lasts as long as the mother's antibodies remain in the infant (usually a few weeks after birth).

Pathophysiology

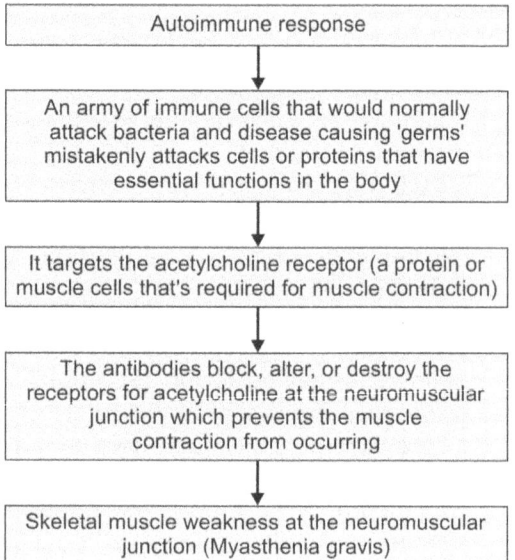

Clinical Features
- Weakness of the eye muscles
- Difficulty in swallowing
- Slurred speech or impaired speech (dysarthria)
- Drooping of one or both eyelids (ptosis)
- Blurred or double vision (diplopia)
- Unstable or waddling gait
- Weakness in the arms, hands, fingers, legs and neck
- Changes in facial expression
- Shortness of breath.

Complications
- Respiratory failure
- Systemic lupus erythematosus
- Rheumatoid arthritis
- Hyperthyroidism
- Grave's disease.

Diagnostic Tests
- History
- Physical examination
- Blood examination
- Electrodiagnostic testing
- Tensilon test
- Electromyography

- Magnetic resonance imaging
- X-ray examination of chest
- Computed tomography (CT) scan.

Medical

- **Anticholinesterase:** It prevents acetyl choline destruction and increase the accumulation of acetyl-choline at neuromuscular junctions which improves the ability of the muscles to contract. For example, neostigmine, pyridostigmine, etc.
- **Corticosteroids:** It suppresses the antibodies that block antichoiine receptors at the neuromuscular junction. For example, Prednisolone.
- **Immunosuppressants:** It is used to treat generalized myasthenia gravis. For example, azothioprine, cyclophosphamide, etc.

Surgical

- **Plasmapheresis or plasma exchange:** It is a procedure in which blood is removed from the body and blood cells are separated from the liquid portion of the blood (plasma). Then acetylcholine receptor antibodies are removed and blood cells are diluted with artificial plasma (usually a solution of saline and sterilized human albumin protein) and infused back into the body.
- **Thymectomy:** It is a procedure in which thymus gland is surgically removed.

Nursing

- Encourage the patient to eat more frequent and smaller meals throughout the day.
- Instruct the patient to break up tasks into small pieces and to take adequate rest.
- Instruct the patient to prevent eyes become overstrained by giving them rest.
- Instruct the patient to avoid fatigue, stress and infection
- Instruct safety measures to the patient
- Instruct the patient to take a soft or bland diet
- Protect the patient from injury by providing safety measures.

MYOGLOBINURIA

Definition

Myoglobinuria is the presence of myoglobin in the urine, usually associated with rhabdomyolysis or muscle destruction. Myoglobin is present in muscle cells as a reserve of oxygen.

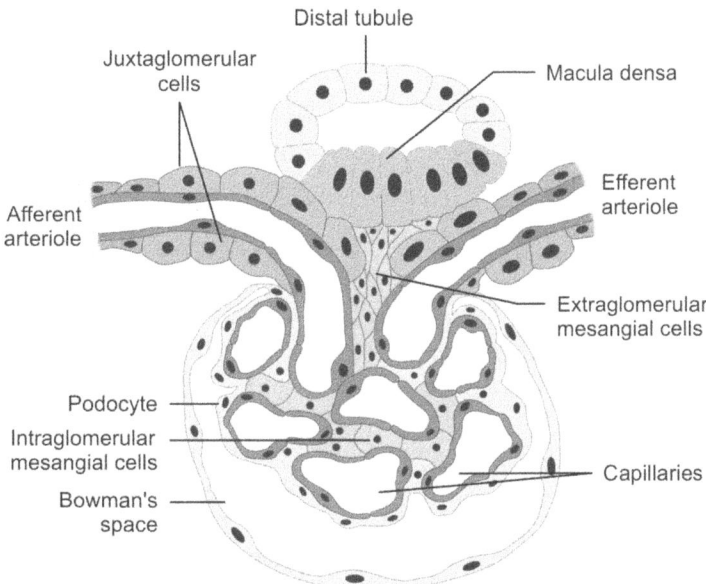

Fig. 1.25: Depicts the breakdown of striated muscle followed by the leakage of the muscle protein myoglobin into the blood.

Etiology

- Trauma, burns and compartment syndromes
- Vascular problems
- Malignant hyperthermia
- Status epilepticus
- Neuroleptic malignant syndrome
- McArdle's disease
- Polymyositis.

Risk Factors

- Alcohol abuse
- Certain drugs (Erythromycin, corticosteroids, heroin, cocaine, atropine, statins, etc.)
- Lactate dehydrogenase deficiency
- Phosphofructokinase deficiency
- Carnitine palmitoyltransferase II deficiency.

Pathophysiology

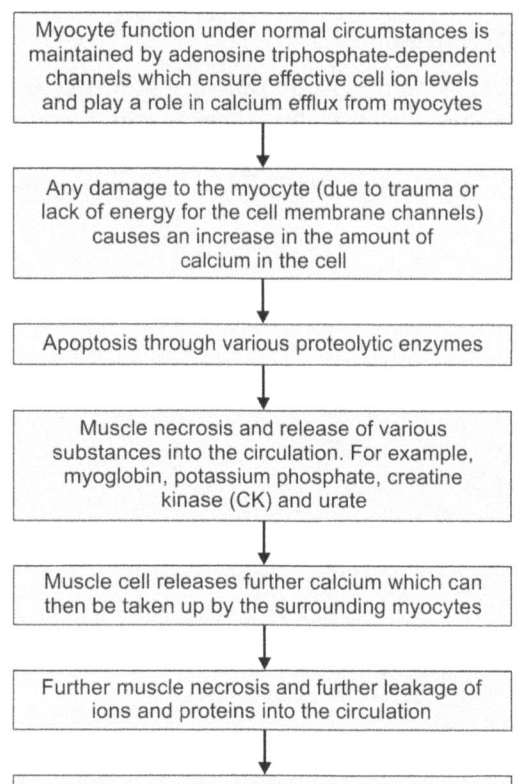

Clinical Features

- Delirium among elderly individuals
- Swollen and painful muscles
- Fever
- Nausea
- Vomiting
- Myalgia
- Dark (tea or cola-colored) urine
- Decrease in calcium ions.

Complications

- Acute kidney injury
- Hyperkalemia
- Metabolic acidosis
- Rhabdomyolysis
- Hypocalcaemia
- Hepatic failure
- Ventricular fibrillation
- Disseminated intravascular coagulation
- Compartment syndrome.

Diagnostic Tests

- History
- Physical examination
- Blood examination
- Urine examination
- Muscle biopsy
- Genetic testing.

Management

Medical

- **Intravenous hydration:** For example, isotonic saline boluses of 20 mL/kg were initially administered, with repeat boluses depending on the hydration status of the patient and it was followed by continued hydration with IV fluids given at a rate of 2–3 times maintenance and thereby achieving a urine output of 2–3 mL/kg/hour.
- **Osmotic diuretics:** It promotes urinary flow and prevent obstructive myoglobin casts. For example, mannitol, etc.
- **Alkalinizing agents:** It minimizes the breakdown of myoglobin into its

nephrotoxic metabolites and to reduce crystallization of uric acid and thereby decreasing damage to the tubule cells. For example, sodium bicarbonate, etc.

Nursing

- Instruct the patient that they require extensive rehabilitation for muscle damage.
- Enforce the importance of prompt fluid resuscitation among patients with crystalloids.
- Instruct the patient to avoid exercising in the heat
- Educate the patient to lower pre-exercise core temperature thereby increasing heat storage capacity among patients.

NEUROSARCOIDOSIS

Definition

Neurosarcoidosis is a chronic inflammatory granulomatous disease that affects various tissues, involving the central nervous system (brain and spinal cord).

Etiology

- Abnormal immune response
- Infective agent or an allergy combined with susceptible genes
- Idiopathic.

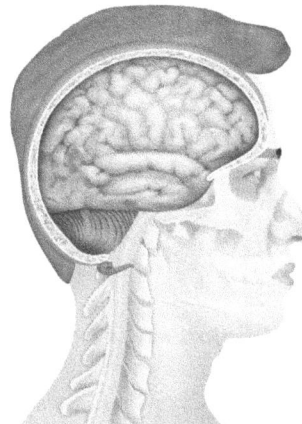

Fig. 1.26: Shows the organization of responding cells into granulomas seen in neurosarcoidosis.

Risk Factors

- People of African and Scandinavian descent
- Being Black Americans
- Irish immigrants in London
- Natives of Martinique living in France
- Family history of neurosarcoidosis
- Being women
- Exposure to dusty or moldy environments
- People between 20 to 40 years of age.

Pathophysiology

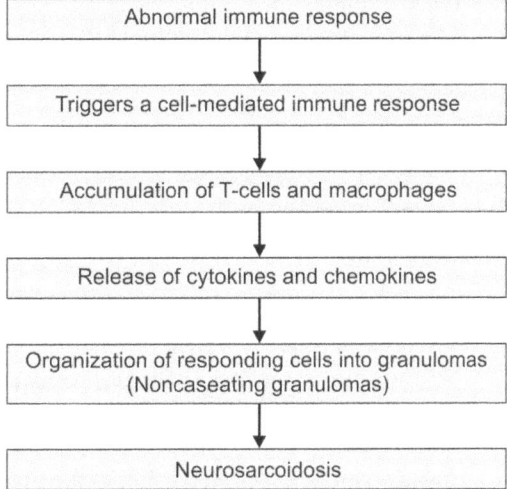

Clinical Features

- Cranial neuropathy
- Myopathy
- Facial palsy, which is characterized by weakness or drooping of the facial muscles
- Myelopathy
- Depression
- Insomnia
- Confusion
- Disorientation
- Dementia
- Delirium
- Hearing loss
- Dizziness
- Vertigo
- Double vision
- Headache
- Seizures.

Complications
- Permanent loss of neurological function
- Blindness
- Peripheral neuropathy
- Meningitis.

Diagnostic Tests
- History
- Physical examination
- Blood examination
- Spinal tap (lumbar puncture)
- Chest X-ray examination
- Nerve biopsy
- Magnetic resonance imaging (MRI) scan of the brain
- Eye tests
- Neurological tests
- Electrocardiogram (ECG)
- Echocardiogram.

Management

Medical
- **Corticosteroids:** It helps to turn down the immune system's activity and reduces the severity of the disease. For example, prednisone, etc.
- **Immunosuppressants:** It inhibits the production of disease-fighting white blood cells. For example, azothioprine, cyclosporin, cyclophosphamide, etc.
- **Immunomodulators:** It may ease symptoms and prevent further organ damage. For example, methotrexate, thalidomide, etc.
- **Antimalarial agents:** It may help with neurosarcoidosis that involves the skin or joints and prevent further organ damage. For example, hydroxychloroquine, chloroquine, etc.
- **Nonsteroidal anti-inflammatory drugs:** They used to treat musculoskeletal discomfort with neurosarcoidosis that involves the joints. For example, ibuprofen, aspirin, etc.

Nursing
- Encourage the patient to eat a well-balanced diet with a variety of fresh fruits and vegetables.
- Encourage the patient to take plenty of fluids
- Encourage the patient to do regular exercise when have trouble breathing as they can improve the overall strength and endurance.
- Ensure 6 to 8 hours of sleep for the patient at each night
- Instruct the patients to avoid the intake of excessive amounts of calcium and vitamin-D rich foods.

PARANEOPLASTIC SYNDROMES

Definition
Paraneoplastic syndromes are a group of rare disorders that are triggered by an abnormal immune system response to a cancerous tumor known as a "neoplasm".

Etiology
- Small cell lung cancer
- Gynecological malignancies
- Hematological malignancies.

Risk Factors
- It occur most often in people with cancers of the lung, ovary, breast, testis or lymphatic system.
- More common in older patients
- Family history of autoimmune disorders
- Occupational carcinogens
- Genetics
- Chronic obstructive pulmonary disease (COPD)
- Obesity
- Air pollution.

Types
There are many types of paraneoplastic neurological syndrome and examples include:
- **Lambert-Eaton myasthenic syndrome:** In which muscles around the hip and shoulder become weak. Swallowing and vision may also be affected. This form of paraneoplastic syndrome is often associated with lung cancer.

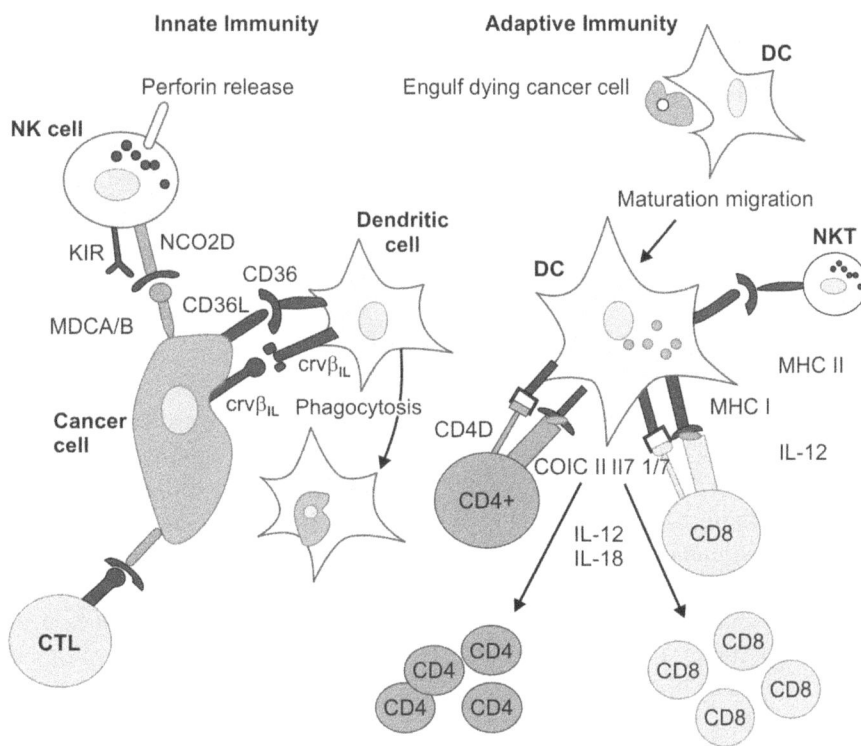

Fig. 1.27: Shows the abnormal immune system response to a cancerous tumor.

- *Myasthenia gravis:* It produces severe muscle weakness, sometimes causing breathing difficulties.
- *Cerebellar degeneration:* It causes loss of balance, unsteady limb movements and problems with speech and swallowing.
- *Limbic encephalitis:* It is a paraneoplastic syndrome that involves swelling of the brain, often causing depression, seizures and irritability.
- *Sensory neuropathy:* It involves progressive loss of skin sensation in the limbs.
- *Stiff person syndrome:* In which muscles, particularly in the legs and spine, become stiff or rigid.
- *Opsoclonus-myoclonus syndrome:* It is a type of paraneoplastic syndrome that is sometimes associated with neuroblastoma in children. It involves rapid irregular eye movements with muscle jerks and poor coordination.

Pathophysiology

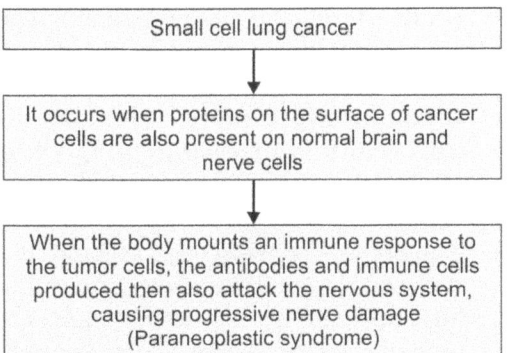

Clinical Features

- Difficulty in walking
- Dysphagia
- Loss of muscle tone
- Loss of fine motor coordination
- Slurred speech
- Memory loss
- Vision problems
- Sleep disturbances

- Dementia
- Seizures
- Sensory loss in the limbs
- Vertigo or dizziness.

Complications

- Thrombocytosis
- Thrombocytopenia
- Peripheral neuropathy
- Cachexia
- Hypercalcemia
- Myositis.

Diagnostic Tests

- History
- Physical examination
- Neurologic examination
- Blood examination
- Spinal tap (lumbar puncture)
- Computerized tomography (CT) scan
- Magnetic resonance imaging (MRI) scan
- Positron emission tomography (PET) scan.

Management

Medical

- **Physical therapy:** It helps to regain some muscle function that have been damaged.
- **Corticosteroids:** It inhibits inflammation and reduces the severity of the disease. For example, prednisone, etc.
- **Immunosuppressants:** It inhibits the production of disease-fighting white blood cells. For example, azothioprine, cyclophosphamide, etc.
- **Anti-seizure agents:** It helps in controlling the seizures associated with syndromes affecting nerve cells in the brain. For example, carbamazepine, valproic acid, etc.
- **Anticholinesterase agents:** It enhance the release of a chemical messenger that transmits a signal from nerve cells to muscles. For example, pyridostigmine, 3,4-diaminopyridine, etc.

Surgical

- **Plasmapheresis or plasma exchange:** It is a procedure in which blood is removed from the body and blood cells are separated from the liquid portion of the blood (plasma). Then acetylcholine receptor antibodies are removed and blood cells are diluted with artificial plasma (usually a solution of saline and sterilized human albumin protein) and infused back into the body.
- **Intravenous immunoglobulin (IVIG):** It is a blood product prepared from the serum of between 1000 and 15000 donors per batch. It is the treatment of choice for patients with antibody deficiencies. For this indication, IVIG is used at a 'replacement dose' of 200–400 mg/kg body weight, given approximately 3-weekly. In contrast, 'high dose' IVIG (hdIVIG), given most frequently at 2 g/kg/month, is used as an 'immunomodulatory' agent in an increasing number of immune and inflammatory disorders.

Nursing

- Assist patients to manage medications and achieve concordance
- Encourage to comply with steroid medications
- Encourage healthy diet rich in fruits, vegetables and fruits
- Instruct the patient to break up tasks into small pieces and to take adequate rest.
- Instruct the patient to prevent eyes become overstrained by giving them rest.
- Instruct the patient to avoid fatigue, stress and infection
- Instruct safety measures to the patient
- Encourage the patient to communicate using strategies such as by shouting or using short sentences.

PARKINSON'S DISEASE

Definition

Parkinson's disease is a slowly progressing neurologic movement disorder which results due to the depletion of dopamine, which interferes with the inhibition of excitatory impulses.

Etiology

- Genetic mutations
- Idiopathic
- Viral infections
- Chronic antipsychotic medication use
- Injury to mid brain
- Ischemia of the basal ganglia.

Risk Factors

- Advanced age
- Family history
- Being a men
- Exposure to toxins (Agricultural herbicide and pesticide)
- Low levels of B-vitamin folate
- Declining estrogen levels.

Pathophysiology

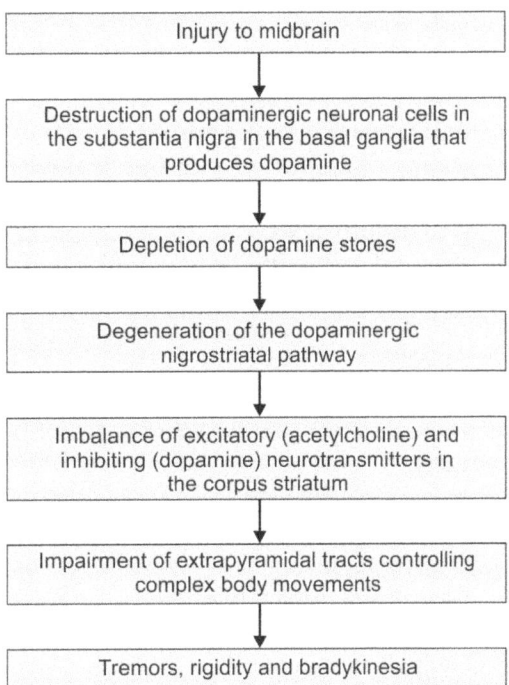

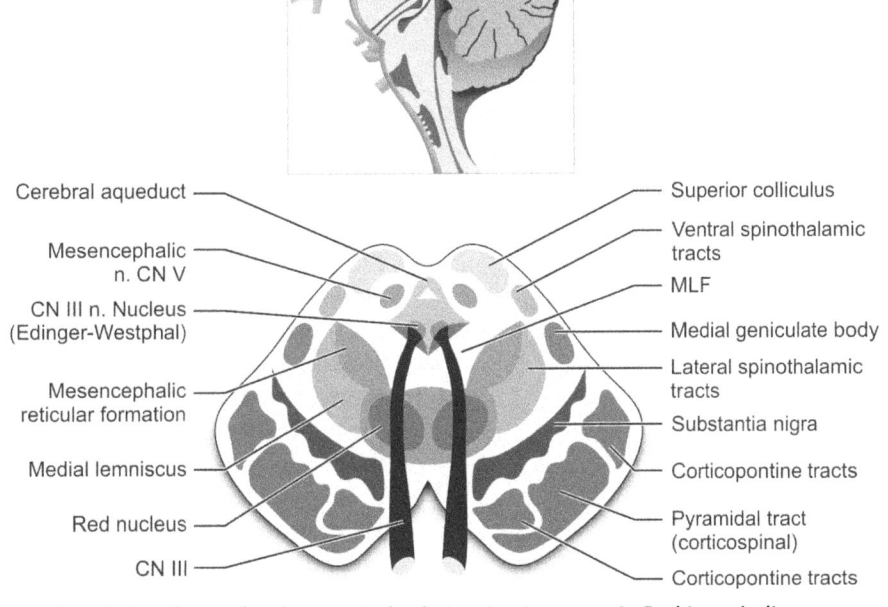

Fig. 1.28: Shows the depreciated substantia nigra seen in Parkinson's disease.

Clinical Features

- Tremor of the hands, arms, legs, jaw and face
- Rigidity or stiffness of the limbs and trunk
- Bradykinesia or slowness of movement
- Aching shoulders and arms
- Handwriting that becomes progressively smaller (micrographia)
- Gait disturbances
- Postural instability or impaired balance and coordination
- Dysphonia (soft, slurred and less audible speech)
- Excessive and uncontrolled sweating
- Dementia (progressive mental deterioration)
- Paroxysmal flushing
- Orthostatic hypotension
- Constipation
- Gastric and urinary retention
- Sexual disturbances
- Sleep disturbances.

Complications

- Oculogyric crisis
- Blepharospasm
- Depression and anxiety
- Dementia
- Injury from falls.

Diagnostic Tests

- History
- Physical examination
- PET scan
- Neurologic examination
- Genetic testing
- Single-photon emission computed tomography (SPECT)
- Autonomic system testing
- Olfactory system testing.

Management

Medical

- **Anti-parkinsonian agents:** It precipitate oxidation, which further damages the substantia nigra and eventually speeds disease progression. For example, levodopa, carbidopa, etc.
- **Anti-cholinergic agents:** It blocks nerve impulses that control muscle movement and is effective in controlling tremor and rigidity. For example, cycrimine, procyclidine, biperiden, etc.
- **Antiviral agents:** It acts by releasing dopamine from neuronal storage sites. For example, amantadine hydrochloride, etc.
- **Dopamine agonists:** It acts as a dopamine receptor agonist and slows down the progression of the disease. For example, ropinirole, pramipexole, etc.
- **Monoamine oxidase inhibitors (MAO inhibitors):** It inhibits dopamine breakdown and slows down the progression of the disease. For example, selegiline, rasagiline, etc.
- **Catechol-O-methyl transferase (COMT) inhibitors:** It reduces motor fluctuations in patients with advanced Parkinson's disease. For example, entacapone, tolcapone, etc.
- **Anti-depressants:** It has both anti-cholinergic and anti-depressant action and reduces tremors. For example, amitriptyline, etc.
- **Anti-histamines:** It reduces tremors in patients with advanced Parkinson's disease. For example, diphenhydramine hydrochloride, orphenadrine citrate, etc.

Surgical

- **Thalamotomy:** A stereotactic electrical stimulator destroys part of the vendor lateral portion of the thalamus in an attempt to reduce tremor.
- **Pallidotomy:** It involves destroying part of the ventral aspect of the medical globus pallidus through electrical stimulation in patients with advanced disease.
- **Neural transplantation:** It is a surgical implantation of adrenal medullary tissue into the corpus striatum is performed in an effort to re-establish normal dopamine release.
- **Deep brain stimulation:** An electrode is placed in the thalamus and connected to a pulse generator implanted in a

subcutaneous subclavicular or abdominal pouch. The battery powered pulse generator sends high frequency electrical impulses through a wire placed under the skin to a lead anchored to the skull. The electrode blocks nerve pathways in the brain that cause tremors.

Nursing

- Assist patients to manage medications and achieve concordance.
- Minimize stress and discomfort that the person regularly experiences.
- Monitor the weight of the patient
- Ensure that medication are given 30 to 45 minutes before food as it may have an impact upon by protein in the diet.
- Encourage the patient to communicate using strategies such as by shouting or using short sentences.

PRION DISEASE

Definition

Prion diseases [transmissible spongiform encephalopathies(TSEs)] are a group of progressive neurodegenerative conditions which exist both in animals and humans.

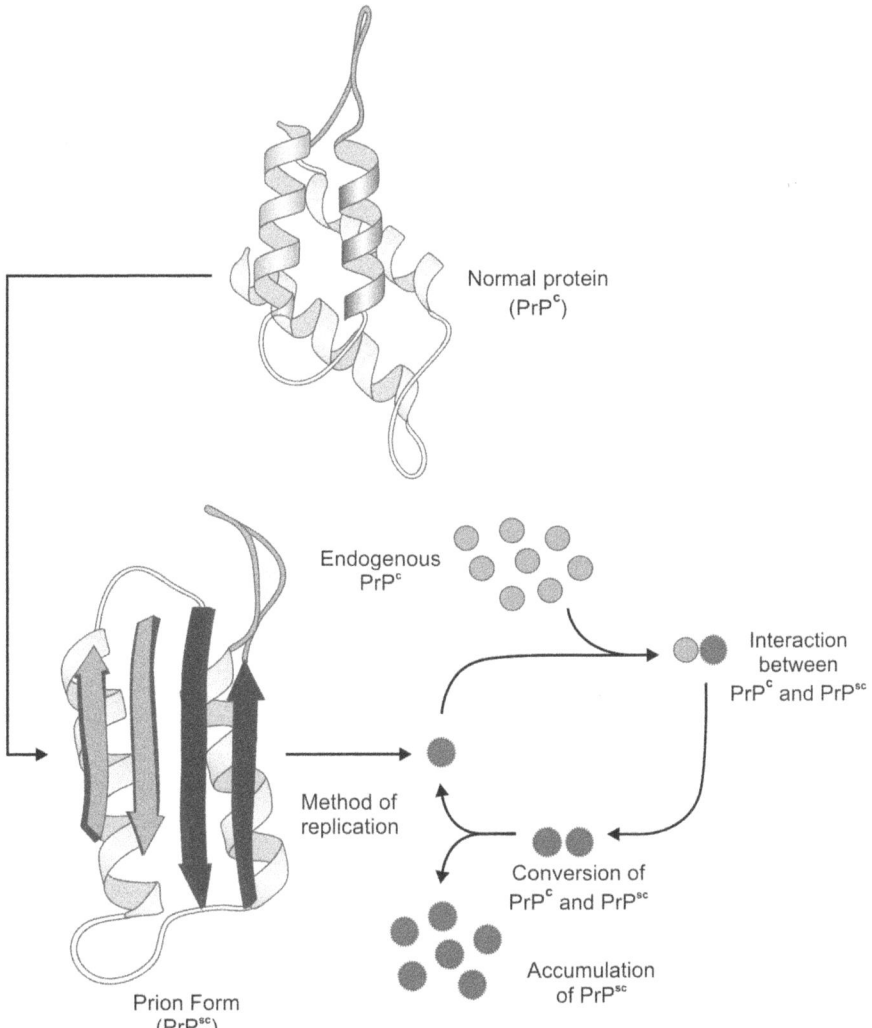

Fig. 1.29: Shows the abnormal accumulation of protein in the brain seen in Prion disease.

Etiology

- Consumption of diseased meat
- Contaminated surgical tools
- Idiopathic
- Heavy metal poisoning.

Risk Factors

- Immunocompromised people
- Genetic mutation.

Types

- ***Iatrogenic Creutzfeldt-Jakob disease (CJD):*** This condition is inherited or develops suddenly without any known risk factors. Most cases of CJD are sporadic and tend to strike people around age 60. Symptoms of CJD quickly lead to severe disability and death. In most cases, death occurs within a year.
- ***Variant Creutzfeldt-Jakob disease (CJD):*** This is an infectious type of the disease that is related to "mad cow disease." Eating diseased meat may cause the disease in humans. The meat may cause normal human prion protein to develop abnormally. It spreads to people receiving cornea transplants from infected donors and from contaminated medical equipment. This type of the disease usually affects younger people.
- ***Kuru Creutzfeldt-JaKob disease (CJD):*** This disease has largely been seen in New Guinea. It's caused by eating human brain tissue contaminated with infectious prions. It is a rare type of prion disease.

Pathophysiology

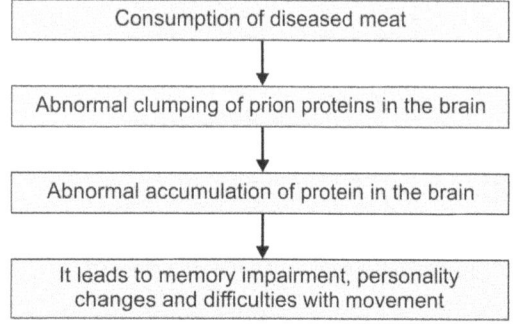

Clinical Features

- Rapidly developing dementia
- Difficulty walking and changes in gait
- Hallucinations
- Muscle stiffness
- Confusion
- Fatigue
- Difficulty speaking.

Complications

- Severe mental impairment
- Inability to move
- Inability to speak
- Death.

Diagnostic Tests

- History
- Physical examination
- Computed tomography (CT) scan
- Magnetic resonance imaging
- Electroencephalography
- Cerebrospinal fluid (CSF) examination
- Tonsil biopsy
- Brain biopsy.

Management

Medical

- **Selective serotonin reuptake inhibitors (SSRI):** It is used for the treatment of depression. For example, citalopram, escitalopram, etc.
- **Anti-convulsants:** It is used to treat epilepsy. For example, levetiracetam, sodium valproate, etc.
- **Anti-psychotics:** It inhibits communication among nerves of the brain. It does this by blocking receptors on the nerves for several neurotransmitters, the chemicals that nerves use to communicate with each other. It is thought that its beneficial effect is due to blocking of the dopamine type 2 (D2) and serotonin type 2 (5-HT2) receptors. For example, quetiapine, etc.

Nursing

- Restrict the activity to maximum extent
- Provide calm and quiet environment as much as possible

- Provide adequate support to the individual and also keep them safe
- Position the individual using correct body alignment.

SPINAL CORD INJURY

Definition

A spinal cord injury (SCI) is damage to the spinal cord or the spinal nerve roots within the spinal canal and resulting in temporary or permanent loss of movement or feeling.

Etiology

- Trauma due to automobile crashes
- Domestic and work-related accidents
- Self-harm
- Sports injuries
- Gunshot wound
- Falls
- War injuries
- Tumor such as meningiomas, ependymomas, astrocytomas and metastatic cancer.
- Spina bifida
- Friedreich's ataxia
- Meningomyelocele
- Spinocerebellar ataxia
- Multiple sclerosis.

Risk Factors

- Being males
- Being older than 65 years
- Being athletes
- Alcohol consumption
- Engaging in risky behavior
- Being between the ages of 15 to 30 years
- Having a bone or joint disorder
- Lifting heavy articles.

Types

Spinal cord injury is classified into 5 types by the American Spinal Injury Association and the International Spinal Cord Injury Classification System and Frankel has given the grading for functional recovery based on the motor and sensory deficits as follows:

1. "A" indicates, a complete paralysis in which motor or sensory function is not preserved.
2. "B" indicates, an incomplete paralysis in which sensory function only is preserved below the injury level.
3. "C" indicates, an incomplete paralysis in which partial motor function only is preserved below the injury level.
4. "D" indicates, an incomplete paralysis in which fair to good motor function only is preserved below the injury level.
5. "E" indicates, a normal function in which both motor and sensory scores are normal.

Pathophysiology

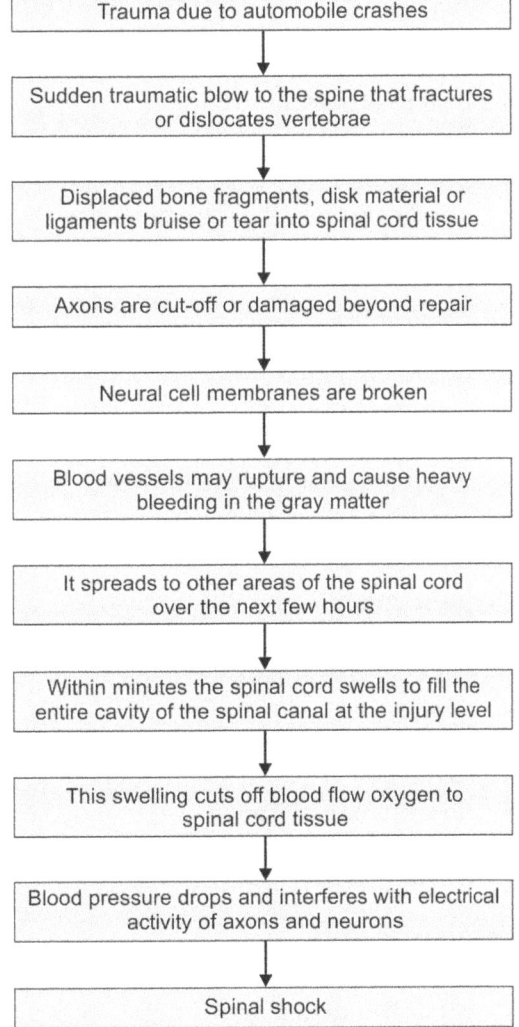

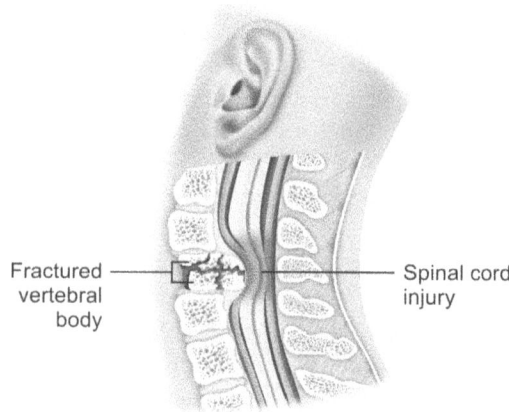

Fig. 1.30: Shows the fractured vertebral body seen in spinal cord injury (SCI).

Clinical Features

- Pain and numbness or burning sensation
- Headache
- Inability to move the extremities or walk
- Sensitivity to stimuli
- Loss of reflexes
- Weakness
- Changes in sexual function
- Muscle spasms
- Loss of bladder or bowel control
- Difficulty breathing
- Unnatural positioning of the head
- Inability to maintain balance
- Chronic pain.

Complications

- Autonomic dysreflexia
- Deep vein thrombosis
- Hypotension
- Sublesional osteoporosis
- Spasticity
- Heterotopic ossification
- Respiratory failure
- Pressure sores.

Diagnostic Tests

- History
- Physical examination
- Blood examination
- Urinalysis
- X-ray spine
- Myelogram
- Somatosensory evoked potential (SSEP)
- Computerized tomography (CT) scan
- Magnetic resonance imaging (MRI) scan
- Lumbar puncture.

Management

Medical

- **High dose corticosteroids:** It helps to reduce the acute effects of spinal cord injury. For example, methylprednisolone, dexamethasone, etc.
- **Non-steroidal anti-inflammatory drugs:** It is used to reduce swelling and inflammation that occur as a result of spinal cord injury. For example, ibuprofen, aspirin, diclofenac sodium, etc.
- **Muscle relaxants:** It eases muscle tension and pain within few hours. For example, diazepam, cyclobenzaprine, carisoprodol, etc.
- **Injected corticosteroids:** It can reduce inflammation, relieving pain and improving function and mobility. For example, betamethasone, methylprednisolone, etc.

Surgical

- **Laminotomy/Microdiscectomy:** It is a surgical procedure in which an opening is made in the spinal canal (laminotomy) in order to visualize the pinched nerve root followed by careful protection of nerve root with a special retractor and protruding disk fragments along with remaining loose or degenerated disk material which are then removed with a small grasping device (microdiscectomy).
- **Laminectomy:** It is a surgical procedure which involves removing a parts of the vertebrae called the lamina in order to make more room for the spinal nerves, relieving pressure on them and reducing pain.
- **Spinal fusion:** It is a procedure in which bone is grafted onto the spine, creating a

solid unit between two or more vertebrae. It stabilizes the spine and relieves pressure on them and reducing pain.
- **Hemilaminectomy:** It is a surgical procedure that decompresses impinged nerve roots being pinched by the lamina bone and other tissues of the spinal processes.
- **Nerve transfer:** It is a procedure in which the nerves with the best control are transferred to the most important muscle groups to improve function in that limb.
- **Tendon transfer:** It is a procedure in which a tendon is moved from one point to another to improve joint function.
- **Selective peripheral neurotomy:** It is a procedure in which the nerves are trimmed to reduce spasticity.
- **Spinal cord stimulation:** It is a procedure in the electrodes are placed in the space outside of the thick membrane that surrounds the spinal cord (the dura) to reduce pain and spasticity through nerve stimulation and also it helps in controlling the movement.

Nursing

- Encourage a comprehensive program of physical and occupational therapy.
- Instruct the patient to wear seat belt and to follow the rules of the road.
- Ask the patient to avoid cell phone usage during driving.
- Ask the patient not to drive the vehicle under the influence of alcohol or drugs.
- Encourage the patient to eat a well-balanced diet.
- Instruct the patient to perform exercise regularly to maintain the muscle tone and balance.
- Instruct the patient to wear appropriate gear when participating in sports activities.

STROKE (CEREBROVASCULAR ACCIDENT)

Definition

A stroke is an abnormal condition of the brain characterized by occlusion by an embolus, thrombus, or cerebrovascular hemorrhage or vasospasm, resulting in ischemia of the brain tissues normally perfused by the damaged vessels.

Etiology

- Large artery thrombosis
- Spasm in the arteries of the brain
- Embolism
- Hemorrhage from rupture of a vessel
- Transient ischemic attack (TIA)
- Arteriovenous malformation
- Aneurysm.

Risk Factors

- Personal or family history of stroke
- Advanced age
- High cholesterol
- Hypertension
- Anticoagulation therapy
- Diabetes mellitus

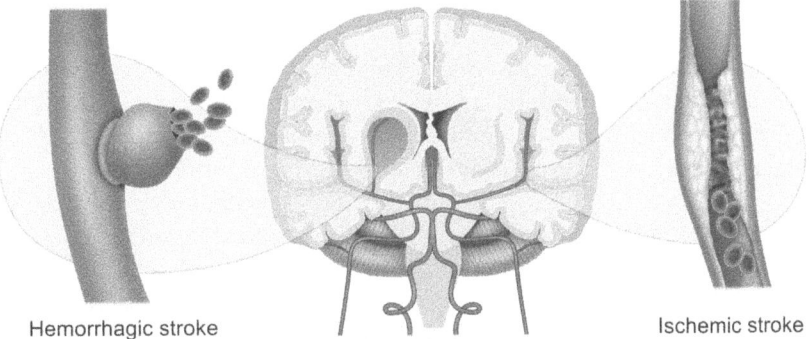

Hemorrhagic stroke   Ischemic stroke

Fig. 1.31: Shows the two types of stroke.

- Stress
- Obesity
- Physical inactivity
- Oral contraceptives
- Cigarette smoking or exposure to second hand smoke
- Use of illicit drugs such as cocaine and methamphetamines
- Excessive alcohol consumption.

Types

There are two types of CVA as follows:
1. *Ischemic stroke:*
   - Due to vascular occlusion
   - It constitutes 85% of the cases.
2. *Hemorrhagic stroke:*
   - Due to extravasation of blood into the brain
   - It constitutes about 15% of the cases.

Pathophysiology

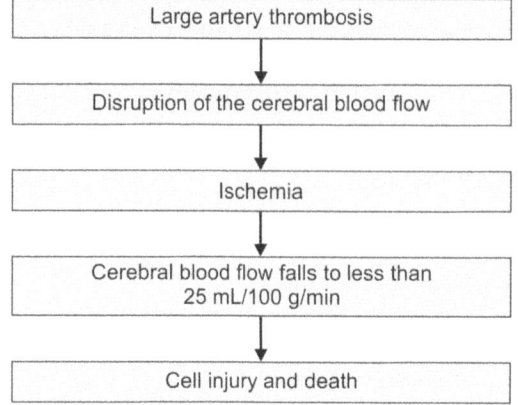

Clinical Features

- Numbness or weakness of the face, arm or leg especially on one side of the body.
- Confusion or change in the mental status
- Sudden severe headache
- Hemiplegia (paralysis of one side of the body)
- Hemiparesis (weakness of one side of the body)
- Dysarthria (difficulty in speaking)
- Aphasia (loss of speech)
- Apraxia (inability to perform a previously learned action)
- Hemianopsia (loss of half of the visual field)
- Dysphagia (difficulty in swallowing)
- Ataxia (staggering, unsteady gait)
- Loss of peripheral vision
- Diplopia
- Memory loss
- Decreased attention span
- Inability to concentrate
- Depression
- Slow and bounding pulse
- Cheyne-Stokes respiration
- Hypertension
- Nausea
- Vomiting
- Nuchal rigidity

Complications

- Paralysis or loss of muscle movement
- Decreased cerebral blood flow due to increased ICP
- Inadequate oxygen delivery to the brain
- Difficult talking or swallowing
- Pneumonia
- Vasospasm
- Seizures
- Hydrocephalus
- Hemorrhage
- Memory loss or trouble with understanding
- Pain
- Changes in behavior and selfcare.

Diagnostic Tests

- History
- Physical examination
- Neurological examination
- Blood examination
- Carotid Doppler examination
- Carotid artery angiography
- Holter monitoring
- Echocardiogram
- Electrocardiogram
- Computerized tomography (CT) scan
- Computerized tomography (CT) angiography

- Magnetic resonance imaging (MRI) scan
- Magnetic resonance angiography (MRA)
- Cerebral angiography
- Electroencephalography
- Transcranial Doppler ultrasound
- Single photon emission computed tomography
- Positron emission tomography.

management

- ***Blood thinning agents:*** It prevents or destroy blood clots and reduces the risk of stroke in survivors who have had transient ischemic attack. For example, aspirin, warfarin, heparin, clopidogrel, etc.
- ***Platelet inhibiting agents:*** It helps in preventing platelets, blood cells and the vessels from using adenosine that helps in forming a clot and also has the potential to vasodilate the vessels that carry the blood to allow more blood and particles to flow through. For example, dipyridamole, ticlopidine, etc.
- ***Osmotic diuretics:*** It helps to reduce brain swelling and pressure. For example, mannitol, urea, etc.
- ***Analgesics:*** It helps to block the flow of pain signals from the central nervous system. For example, voveran, gabapentin, pregabaline, topiramate.
- ***Calcium channel blockers:*** It helps in blocking the entry of calcium into muscle cells in artery walls. For example, verapamil, diltiazem, etc.
- ***Angiotensin II receptor blockers (ARBs):*** These are drugs that relax blood vessels by blocking a chemical (angiotensin II) that causes blood vessels to narrow, constrict or tighten and this action allows blood to flow more easily through the blood vessels and thus, helps to lower blood pressure. For example, losartan, candesartan, etc.
- ***Angiotensin converting enzyme (ACE) inhibitors:*** These are drugs that relax blood vessels by reducing the production of an enzyme required to produce a chemical (angiotensin II) that causes blood vessels to narrow, constrict or tighten and this action allows blood to flow more easily through the blood vessels and thus, helps to lower blood pressure. For example, enalapril, captopril, ramipril, etc.
- ***Beta blockers:*** These are drugs that slow down the rate of the heart, the pumping force of the heart and the amount of blood pumped by the heart per minute and thus, helps to lower blood pressure. For example, propranolol, metoprolol, atenolol, etc.
- ***Statins or HMG-CoA reductase inhibitors:*** These are drugs used to lower blood cholesterol by inhibiting the enzyme HMG-CoA reductase. It also helps the body to reabsorb cholesterol that has accumulated in plaques in the artery walls, helps in preventing further blockage in the blood vessels. For example, atorvastatin, lovastatin, simvastatin, etc.

Surgical

- *Carotid endarterectomy:* It is the surgical removal of an atherosclerotic plaque or thrombus from the carotid artery
- *Surgical evacuation:* It is the surgical removal of the cerebellar hemorrhage if the diameter exceeds 3 cm
- *Extracranial-intracranial arterial bypass:* To establish collateral blood supply to allow surgery on the aneurysm (a localized dilation of the wall of a blood vessel).

Nursing

- Elevate the head of the bed (15 to 20°) to promote venous drainage and to lower increased ICP.
- Maintain the blood pressure at 150/100 mm Hg or less than that to facilitate perfusion.
- Provide complete bed rest
- Administer oxygen 4–8 L/min as prescribed
- Provide suctioning as prescribed, but never suction nasally and for no longer than 10 sec, to prevent increasing ICP

- Change the position every 2 hours
- Encourage passive exercise to have a full range of motion and to maintain joint mobility
- Encourage fluids and high-fiber diet
- Encourage independence in activities of daily living
- Provide gait training
- Make sure that external stimuli are kept to a minimum
- Thigh-high elastic compression stockings should be prescribed to decrease the incidence of deep vein thrombosis resulting from immobility.

SUSAC'S SYNDROME

Definition
Susac's syndrome is an autoimmune disease in which the smallest blood vessels in the brain, retina, and inner ear become blocked, causing these organs to suffer due to decreased blood flow.

Etiology
- Autoimmune endotheliopathy
- Idiopathic.

Risk Factors
- Females
- Those between the ages 20 to 40 years.

Pathophysiology

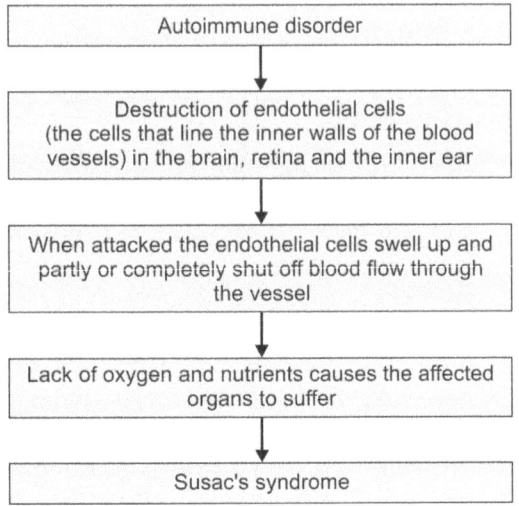

Clinical Features
It is not necessary for all three components of the disease to appear at the same time. Any one of the above symptoms may be the first sign of

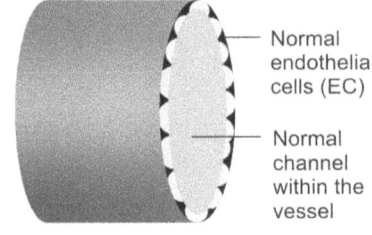

Normal small blood vessel

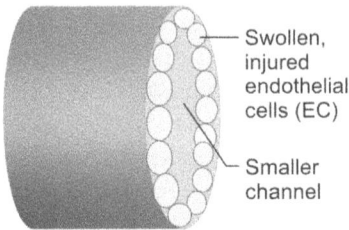

Microvascular endotheliopathy (injured endothelial cell)

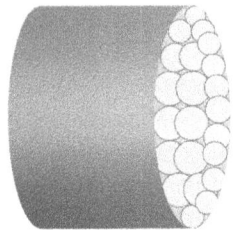

No blood flow and no oxygen or nutrients can get through this vessel

Fig. 1.32: Depicts the destruction of endothelial cells in the brain, retina and the inner ear seen in Susac's syndrome.

Susac's syndrome. It may take weeks, months, or even years for all three parts to show up. Some patients never have more than two of the components.

Brain Symptoms

- Severe headache accompanied with vomiting
- Problems with thinking (short-term memory loss, confusion, slow thought processing and reduced ability to solve problems)
- Inability to remain alert or focused
- Slurred speech
- Changes in personality
- Psychiatric problems (depression, psychosis, aggression, anxiety or withdrawal).

Eye Symptoms

- Dark area in one part of the visual field
- Visual disturbances
- Loss of peripheral (side) vision.

Inner Ear Symptoms

- Hearing loss
- Dizziness (vertigo)
- Ringing in the ears (tinnitus).

Complications

- Dementia
- Blindness
- Deafness.

Diagnostic Tests

- History
- Physical examination
- Magnetic resonance imaging
- Fluorescein angiography
- Hearing examination.

Management

Medical

- **Immunosuppressive agents:** It suppresses the activity of the immune system. For example, prednisone, azathioprine, cyclophosphamide, etc.
- **Intravenous immunoglobulin (IVIG):** It is a blood product prepared from the serum of between 1000 and 15000 donors per batch. It is the treatment of choice for patients with antibody deficiencies. For this indication, IVIG is used at a 'replacement dose' of 200–400 mg/kg body weight, given approximately 3-weekly. In contrast, 'high dose' IVIG (hdIVIG), given most frequently at 2 g/kg/month, is used as an 'immunomodulatory' agent in an increasing number of immune and inflammatory disorders.

Nursing

- Place the patient in a comfortable and clean environment
- Encourage to comply with steroid medications
- Encourage healthy diet rich in fruits, vegetables and fruits
- Instruct to take adequate rest.

SYNCOPE (SUDDEN FAINTING)

Definition

Syncope is the temporary loss of consciousness due to a sudden decline in blood flow to the brain.

Etiology

- Heart problem
- Changes in the blood volume
- Changes in blood distribution
- Violent coughing spells
- Neurological disorders
- Psychiatric disorders
- Metabolic disorders
- Lung disorders
- Cardiomyopathy
- Coronary artery disease.

Risk Factors

- Advanced age
- Prior heart attack
- An abnormal electrocardiogram
- Ventricular dysfunction
- Emotional stress
- Being in hot an stuffy places

Disorders of Nervous System

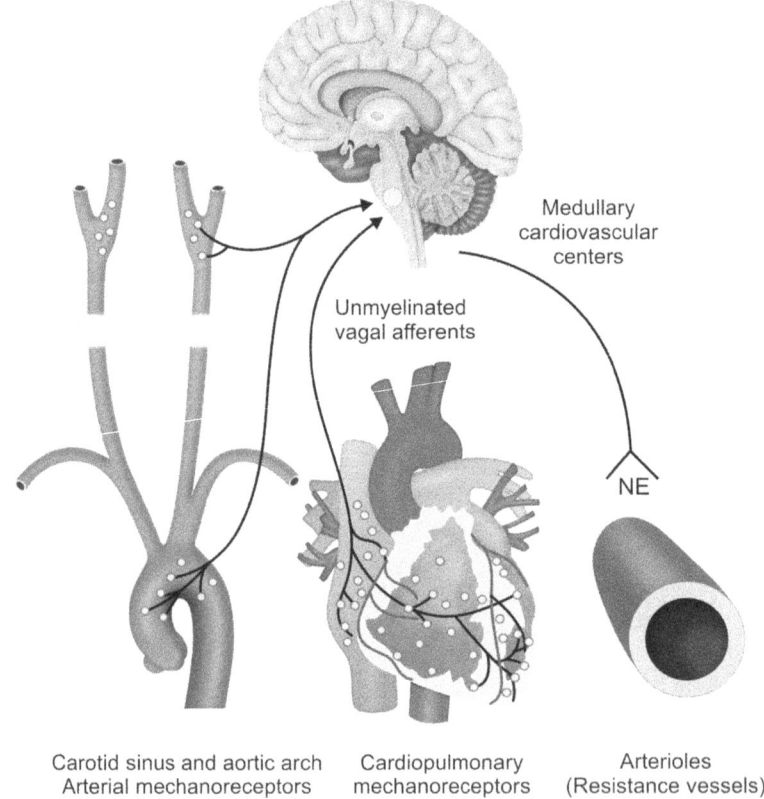

Fig. 1.33: Depicts the decline in blood flow to the brain seen in syncope.

- Dehydration
- Heavy sweating
- Long period standing still.

Pathophysiology

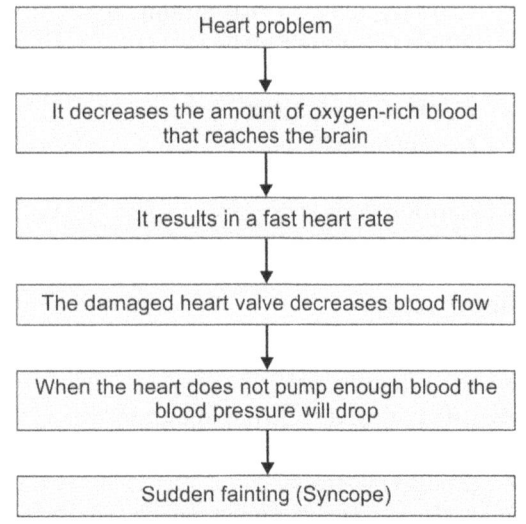

Clinical Features

- Weakness
- Nausea
- Dimmed vision
- Sweating
- Light headedness
- Fast heart beat
- Diaphoresis
- Epigastric discomfort
- Chest pain
- Dyspnea
- Low back pain
- Palpitations
- Pallor
- Paresthesia.

Complications

- Falls
- Stroke
- Cardiovascular disease.

Diagnostic Tests

- History
- Physical examination
- Electrocardiogram
- Holter monitoring
- Echocardiogram
- Electrophysiologic studies (EPS)
- Tilt table test
- Chest radiography
- Magnetic resonance imaging
- Computed tomography (CT) scan.

Management

Medical

- **Nonsteroidal anti-inflammatory drugs (NSAIDs):** It helps to block the flow of pain signals from the central nervous system and reduces pain. For example, ibuprofen, naproxen, etc.
- **Antihypertensive agents:** It helps in treating hypertension. For example, atenolol, propranolol, etc.

Nursing

- Instruct the patient not to stand for a long time
- Ask the patient to lie down until they feel better in about 20 to 30 minutes.
- Instruct the patient to avoid driving
- Ask the patient to get up slowly after they have been lying down
- Encourage the patient to drink plenty of fluids, especially when exercising and during hot weather.

SYRINGOMYELIA

Definition

Syringomyelia is a condition characterized by a fluid-filled cavity or cyst known as a syrinx that forms within the spinal cord and is a chronic condition that can expand over time compressing or destroying the surrounding nerve tissue.

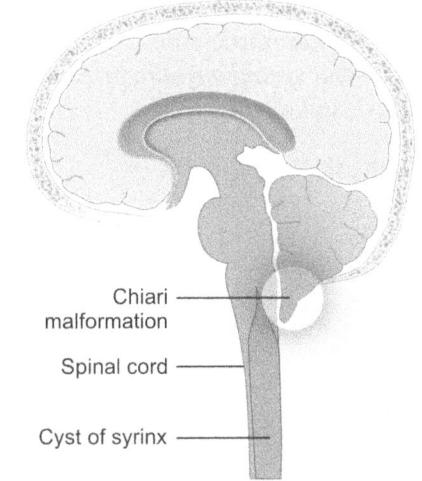

Fig. 1.34: Shows the cystic enlargement of spinal cord.

Etiology

- Chiari malformation
- Spinal cord injury (SCI)
- Obstruction or disruption of the flow of cerebrospinal fluid (CSF)
- Spinal cord tumor
- Meningitis
- Spinal arachnoiditis
- Spinal dysraphism (spinal bifida occulta)
- Spinal vertebrae misalignment
- Spina bifida
- Idiopathic.

Risk Factors

- Young adults between 20 to 40 years of age
- More common in males than females.

Types

There are three types of syringomyelia as follows:
1. **Congenital syringomyelia:** It is mostly seen in Arnold-Chiari malformation. In this type, the bottom part of the brain (cerebellum) lies in the upper part of the neck, instead of within the skull.
2. **Traumatic syringomyelia:** It includes any trauma, tumors and infections (such as

meningitis, HIV, etc.) and where there is severe cord compression.
3. ***Idiopathic syringomyelia:*** In this type, the cause is unknown.

Pathophysiology

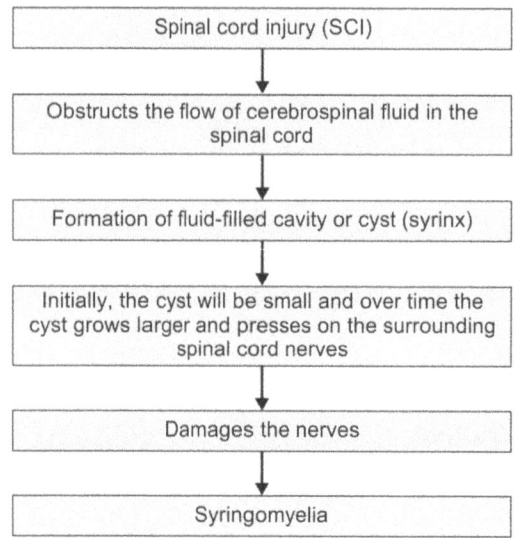

Clinical Features

- Severe chronic pain
- Loss of sensitivity to hot and cold
- Numbness and tingling
- Muscle weakness
- Spasticity
- Paralysis
- Sweating
- Sexual dysfunction
- Bowel and bladder function may be affected.

Complications

- Syringobulbia
- Scoliosis
- Horner syndrome
- Respiratory failure
- Tongue wasting
- Painless ulcer on the hands
- Charcot joints.

Diagnostic Tests

- History
- Physical examination
- Magnetic resonance imaging
- CT scanning
- Myelography
- Plain X-rays
- Lumbar puncture.

Management

Surgical

Surgery is the only viable treatment for syringomyelia, but not all patients will advance to the stage where surgery is needed. Evaluation of the condition is often difficult because SM can remain stationary for long periods of time, and in some cases progress rapidly.

- **Posterior fossa decompression:** This is a procedure that allows the cerebellar tonsils to move into a normal position, restoring the normal flow among persons with Chiari malformation. After this procedure, the syrinx will often reduce or resolve on its own. This can take months and may never completely collapse the syrinx.
- **Thecoperitoneal shunting:** It is a procedure in which a thin tube is inserted into the cyst to drain the fluid into the abdominal cavity. The shunt contains a one-way valve to prevent backflow.
- **Laminectomy and duraplasty:** It is a procedure in which a tumor or a bony growth that hinders the normal flow of cerebrospinal fluid is surgically removed for restoring the normal flow and allow fluid to drain from the syrinx.

Nursing

- Instruct the patients not to delay the treatment as it may lead irreversible spinal cord injury.
- Instruct the patient that physical therapy is an important part of a nonsurgical approach to restore, maintain, and promote overall health.
- Instruct the patient that exercise is a vital part of improving and maintaining a normal healthy back.
- Encourage the patient to maintain good posture as it supports muscles and

Disorders of Nervous System

ligaments during movement or weight-bearing activities.

THORACIC OUTLET SYNDROME

Definition

Thoracic outlet syndrome (TOS) is a syndrome involving compression at the superior thoracic outlet resulting from excess pressure placed on a neurovascular bundle passing between the anterior scalene and middle scalene muscles.

Etiology

- Abnormal compression from the clavicle and shoulder girdle
- Pancoast tumor
- Physical trauma from a car accident
- Repetitive occupational movements (playing a keyboard)
- Anatomic defects such as having an extra rib
- Pressure on the joints
- Anomalous tissue overgrowth.

Risk Factors

- Breast implants
- Scalene muscle hypertrophy from athletic activities
- Rapid weight loss associated with vigorous physical activity
- Poor posture
- Pregnancy
- Sleep disorders
- Sports-related activities
- Weight lifting.

Pathophysiology

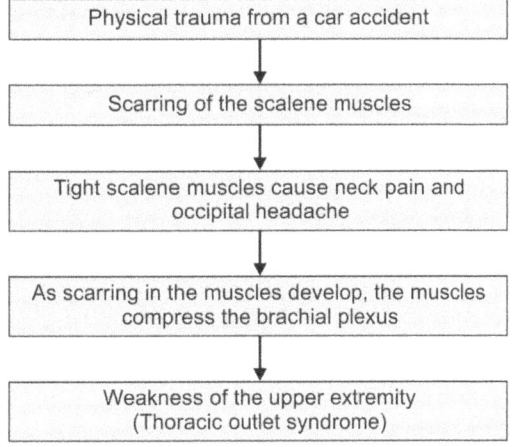

Types

- ***Neurogenic thoracic outlet syndrome:*** It is a form of thoracic outlet syndrome

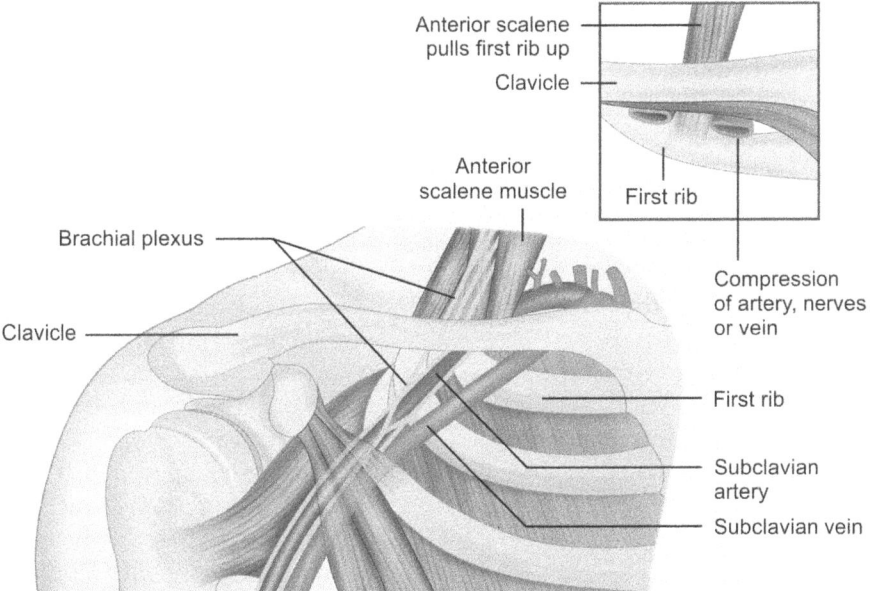

Fig. 1.35: Shows the compression of the nerves, arteries or veins in the passageway from the neck to the armpit.

which is characterized by compression of the brachial plexus. The brachial plexus is a network of nerves that arise from the spinal cord and control muscle movements and sensation in the shoulder, arm and hand. In majority cases, the symptoms are neurogenic.
- ***Vascular thoracic outlet syndrome:*** It occurs when one or more of the veins (venous thoracic outlet syndrome) or arteries (arterial thoracic outlet syndrome) under the collarbone (clavicle) are compressed.
- ***Nonspecific-type thoracic outlet syndrome:*** It is also called disputed thoracic outlet syndrome. People with nonspecific-type thoracic outlet syndrome have chronic pain in the area of the thoracic outlet that worsens with activity, but the specific cause of the pain cannot be determined.

Clinical Features
- Wasting in the fleshy base of the thumb
- Numbness or tingling in the arms or fingers
- Pain or aches in the neck, shoulder or hand
- Weakening grip
- Discoloration of the hand (bluish color)
- Arm pain and swelling, possibly due to blood clots
- Blood clot in veins or arteries in the upper area of the body
- Lack of color (pallor) in one or more fingers or entire hand
- Weak or no pulse in the affected arm
- Cold fingers, hands or arms
- Arm fatigue after activity
- Numbness or tingling in the fingers
- Weakness of arm or neck
- Throbbing lump near the collarbone.

Complications
- Injury to the brachial plexus
- Recurrence
- Bleeding
- Lymphatic fluid leakage
- Pneumothorax.

Diagnostic Tests
- History
- Physical examination
- Electromyogram
- Angiogram X-ray
- Nerve conduction study
- Arteriography and venography
- Magnetic resonance imaging (MRI) scan
- Computed tomography (CT) scan
- Ultrasound scan.

Management

Medical
- **Thrombolytics:** It helps in dissolving blood clots into the veins or arteries. For example, reteplase, urokinase, etc.
- **Anticoagulants:** It helps in decreasing the blood's ability to clot and keep more clots from forming. For example, warfarin, heparin, etc.
- **Nonsteroidal anti-inflammatory drugs:** It helps in decreasing inflammation, reduce pain and encourage muscle relaxation. For example, Ibuprofen, etc.

Surgical
- **Physical therapy:** It is the first line of treatment to learn how to do exercises that strengthen and stretch shoulder muscles.
- **Transaxillary approach:** It is a procedure in which an incision is made in the chest to access the first rib and to remove a portion of it to relieve compression.
- **Supraclavicular approach:** It is a procedure in which repair is done on the compressed blood vessels by removing the muscles causing compression.
- **Infraclavicular approach:** It is a procedure in which an incision is made under the collar bone and across the chest to treat compressed veins that require extensive repair.

Disorders of Nervous System

Nursing

- Instruct the patient to avoid prolonged positions with their arms held out or overhead.
- Restrict them from lifting heavy objects
- Instruct to avoid sleeping on their stomach with their arms above the head
- Encourage weight reduction
- Encourage them to do exercises.

TRANSIENT ISCHEMIC ATTACK (MINI-STROKE)

Definition

A transient ischemic attack is the same as a stroke, except that the symptoms last for a short amount of time and no longer than 24 hours.

Etiology

- Large artery thrombosis
- Spasm in the arteries of the brain
- Embolism
- Hemorrhage from rupture of a vessel
- Arteriovenous malformation
- Aneurysm.

Risk Factors

- Advanced age
- High cholesterol
- Hypertension
- Diabetes mellitus
- Family history of transient ischemic attack
- Stress
- Obesity
- Physical inactivity
- Oral contraceptives
- Cigarette smoking or exposure to second hand smoke
- Use of illicit drugs such as cocaine and methamphetamines
- Excessive alcohol consumption.

Pathophysiology

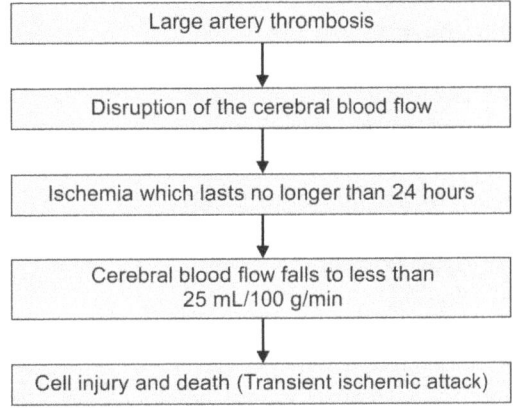

Clinical Features

- Numbness or weakness of the face, arm or leg especially on one side of the body

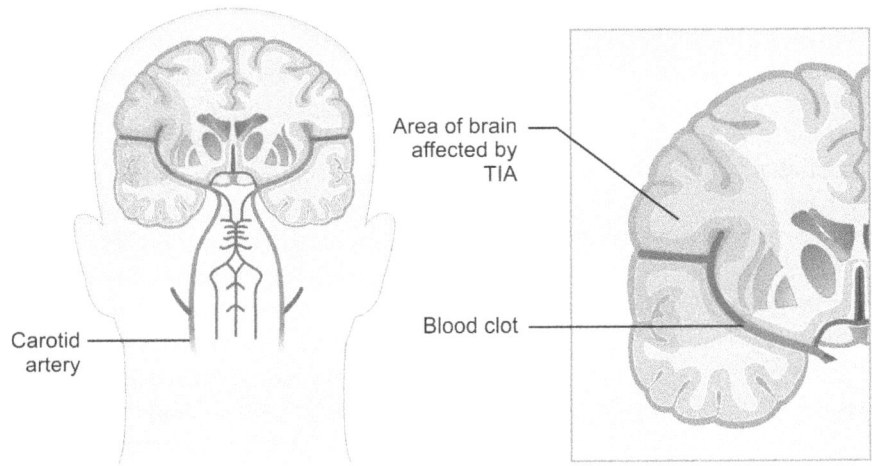

Fig. 1.36: Shows the area of brain affected by transient ischemic attack (TIA).

- Confusion or change in the mental status
- Sudden severe headache
- Hemiplegia (paralysis of one side of the body)
- Hemiparesis (weakness of one side of the body)
- Dysarthria (difficulty in speaking)
- Aphasia (loss of speech)
- Apraxia (inability to perform a previously learned action)
- Hemianopsia (loss of half of the visual field)
- Dysphagia (difficulty in swallowing)
- Ataxia (staggering, unsteady gait)
- Loss of peripheral vision
- Diplopia
- Memory loss
- Decreased attention span
- Inability to concentrate
- Depression
- Slow and bounding pulse
- Cheyne-Stokes respiration
- Hypertension
- Nausea
- Vomiting
- Nuchal rigidity.

Complications

- Paralysis or loss of muscle movement
- Decreased cerebral blood flow due to increased ICP
- Inadequate oxygen delivery to the brain
- Difficult talking or swallowing
- Pneumonia
- Vasospasm
- Seizures
- Hydrocephalus
- Hemorrhage
- Memory loss or trouble with understanding
- Pain
- Changes in behavior and self care.

Diagnostic Tests

- History
- Physical examination
- Neurological examination
- Blood examination
- Carotid Doppler examination
- Carotid artery angiography
- Holter monitoring
- Echocardiogram
- Electrocardiogram
- Computerized tomography (CT) scan
- Computerized tomography (CT) angiography
- Magnetic resonance imaging (MRI) scan
- Magnetic resonance angiography (MRA)
- Cerebral angiography
- Electroencephalography
- Transcranial Doppler ultrasound
- Single photon emission computed tomography
- Positron Emission Tomography.

MANAGEMENT

Medical

- **Blood thinning agents:** It prevents or destroy blood clots and reduces the risk of stroke in survivors who have had transient ischemic attack. For example, aspirin, warfarin, heparin, clopidogrel, etc.
- **Platelet inhibiting agents:** It helps in preventing platelets, blood cells and the vessels from using adenosine that helps in forming a clot and also has the potential to vasodilate the vessels that carry the blood to allow more blood and particles to flow through. For example, dipyridamole, ticlopidine, etc.
- **Osmotic diuretics:** It helps to reduce brain swelling and pressure. For example, mannitol, urea, etc.
- **Analgesics:** It helps to block the flow of pain signals from the central nervous system. For example, voveran, gabapentin, pregabaline, topiramate.
- **Calcium channel blockers:** It helps in blocking the entry of calcium into muscle cells in artery walls. For example, verapamil, diltiazem, etc.
- **Angiotensin II receptor blockers (ARBs):** These are drugs that relax blood vessels by blocking a chemical (angiotensin II) that causes blood vessels to narrow, constrict or tighten and this action allows blood to

flow more easily through the blood vessels and thus, helps to lower blood pressure. For example, losartan, candesartan, etc.
- **Angiotensin converting enzyme (ACE) inhibitors:** These are drugs that relax blood vessels by reducing the production of an enzyme required to produce a chemical (angiotensin II) that causes blood vessels to narrow, constrict or tighten and this action allows blood to flow more easily through the blood vessels and thus, helps to lower blood pressure. For example, enalapril, captopril, ramipril, etc.
- **Beta blockers:** These are drugs that slow down the rate of the heart, the pumping force of the heart and the amount of blood pumped by the heart per minute and thus, helps to lower blood pressure. For example, propranolol, metoprolol, atenolol, etc.
- **Statins or HMG-CoA reductase inhibitors:** These are drugs used to lower blood cholesterol by inhibiting the enzyme HMG-CoA reductase. It also helps the body to reabsorb cholesterol that has accumulated in plaques in the artery walls, helps in preventing further blockage in the blood vessels. For example, atorvastatin, lovastatin, simvastatin, etc.

Surgical
- **Carotid endarterectomy:** It is the surgical removal of an atherosclerotic plaque or thrombus from the carotid artery.
- **Surgical evacuation:** It is the surgical removal of the cerebellar hemorrhage if the diameter exceeds 3 cm.
- **Extracranial-intracranial arterial bypass:** To establish collateral blood supply to allow surgery on the aneurysm (a localized dilation of the wall of a blood vessel).

Nursing
- Elevate the head of the bed (15° to 20°) to promote venous drainage and to lower increased ICP.
- Maintain the blood pressure at 150/100 mm Hg or less than that to facilitate perfusion.
- Provide complete bed rest
- Administer oxygen 4–8 L/min as prescribed
- Provide suctioning as prescribed, but never suction nasally and for no longer than 10 sec, to prevent increasing ICP.
- Change the position every 2 hours
- Encourage passive exercise to have a full range of motion and to maintain joint mobility.
- Encourage fluids and high-fiber diet
- Encourage independence in activities of daily living
- Provide gait training
- Make sure that external stimuli are kept to a minimum
- Thigh-high elastic compression stockings should be prescribed to decrease the incidence of deep vein thrombosis resulting from immobility.

TRAUMATIC BRAIN INJURY

Definition
Traumatic brain injury (TBI) is any damage to the brain caused by a blow to the head and its severity may range from minor, with few or no lasting consequences, to major, resulting in profound disability or death [Cerebral concussion is a brief (seconds to minutes) loss of consciousness caused by a blow to the head]

Etiology
- Falls
- Vehicle accidents
- Assaults

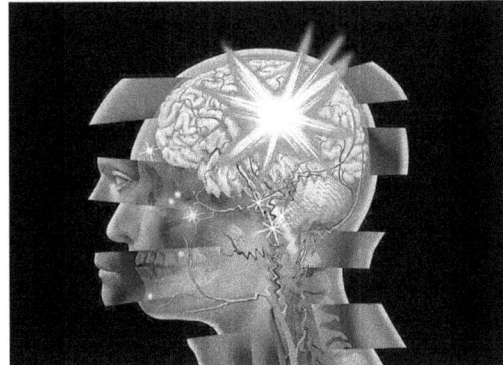

Fig. 1.37: Shows the sudden damage to the brain caused by a blow to the head.

- Bicycle accidents
- Construction work related and industrial accidents
- Child abuse
- Suicidal attempt
- Firearms
- Blast injuries from explosions
- War injury
- Sports injuries.

Risk Factors

- Professional athletes
- Participants in recreational activities
- Young children (aged 0 to 4 years)
- Older adults
- Being males
- Striking or being struck by something
- Construction workers.

Types

The severity of traumatic brain injury is classified into three levels as follows:

1. **Mild type**
   - The traumatic brain injury with a Glasgow coma scales of 13 or above are mild type.
   - In this type, the duration of post-traumatic amnesia is less than an hour.
   - In this type, the duration of loss of consciousness is less than 30 minutes.
   - The common features found in mild TBI were headache, vomiting, nausea, lack of motor coordination, dizziness, difficulty balancing, lightheadedness, blurred vision, vertigo, bad taste in the mouth, fatigue, behavioral or mood changes and changes in sleep patterns.
2. **Moderate type**
   - The traumatic brain injury with a Glasgow coma scales ranging within 9 to 12 are moderate type.
   - In this type, the duration of post-traumatic amnesia ranges between 60 minutes to 24 hours.
   - In this type, the duration of loss of consciousness ranges between 1 to 24 hours.
   - The common features found in moderate TBI were headache that gets worsened, repeated vomiting, nausea, convulsions or seizures, an inability to awaken from sleep, dilation of one or both pupils of the eyes, slurred speech, weakness or numbness in the limbs, loss of coordination, increased confusion, restlessness or agitation.
3. **Severe type**
   - The traumatic brain injury with a Glasgow coma scales of less than 8 are severe type.
   - In this type, the duration of post-traumatic amnesia is more than a day
   - In this type, the duration of loss of consciousness is more than 24 hours
   - The common features found in severe TBI were increased intracranial pressure, unequal size of pupil (Anisocoria), abnormal posturing.

The traumatic brain injury is classified into two based on area of confinement as follows:

Focal Type of TBI

- A focal brain injury is confined to a specific area of the brain and causes localized damage that can be detected with a CT scan or X-ray.
- It is of following types:

1. **Contusions**
   - Focal contusions are bruises that cause swelling, bleeding, and destruction of brain tissue.
   - It occurs in the frontal and temporal lobes, where memory and behavior centers are located.
   - The clinical features of contusions are abnormal sensations, behavior impairment, loss of vision, loss of coordination and memory impairment.
2. **Hemorrhage**

A cerebral or intracranial (inside the skull) hemorrhage occurs when blood leaks from a damaged vessel into brain tissue.

Diffuse Type of TBI

A diffuse axonal injury causes shearing of large nerve fibers and stretching of blood vessels in many areas of the brain and in addition it can trigger a biochemical cascade of toxic substances in the brain during the days following the initial injury.

Pathophysiology

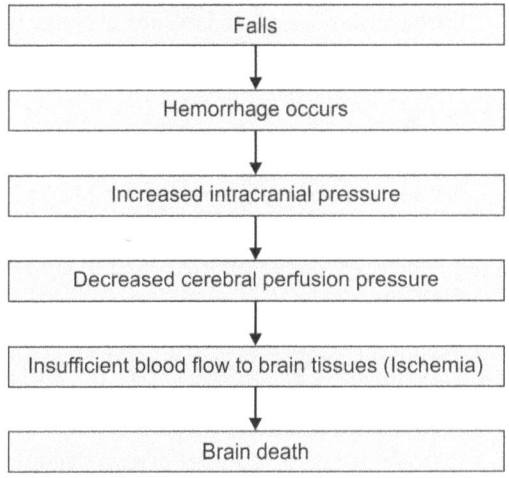

Clinical Features

- Anxiety
- Nervousness
- Difficulty in controlling urges (Disinhibition)
- Impulsiveness
- Inappropriate laughter
- Irritability
- Diplopia
- Depression
- Difficulty in concentrating or thinking
- Aphasia
- Dysphagia
- Dizziness
- Headache
- Incoordination of movements
- Light headedness
- Loss of balance
- Loss of memory
- Muscle stiffness or spasm
- Seizure
- Difficulty in sleep
- Tingling, numbness, or pain sensation
- Slurred speech
- Sense of spinning (Vertigo)
- Weakness in one or more limbs, facial muscles or on an entire side of the body
- Unequal size of pupil (Anisocoria).

Complications

- Hydrocephalus
- Seizures
- Spasticity
- Heterotopic ossification
- Neuroendocrine dysfunction
- Urinary incontinence.

Diagnostic Tests

- History
- Physical examination
- Neuroimaging
- Neurological examination
- CT scan
- CT angiography
- X-rays
- Magnetic resonance imaging
- Cerebral angiography
- Electroencephalography
- Transcranial Doppler ultrasound
- Single photon emission computed tomography
- Positron emission tomography.

Management

Medical

- **Acetylcholinesterase inhibitors:** It reduces the rate at which acetylcholine is broken down, thereby increasing the concentration of acetylcholine in the brain and combating the loss of acetylcholine caused by the death of cholinergic neurons. For example, donepezil, galantamine, rivastigmine, etc.
- **N-Methyl D-Aspartate receptor antagonist:** It acts on the glutamatergic system by blocking NMDA receptors and inhibiting their overstimulation by glutamate. For example, memantine, etc.

- **Selective serotonin reuptake inhibitors:** It helps in improving cognitive ability. For example, sertraline, fluvoxamine, citalopram, fluoxetine, etc.
- **Neuroleptics:** It helps to reduce aggression and improves cognitive behavior. For example, haloperidol, loxapine, risperidone, olanzapine, etc.
- **Antioxidants:** It slows down progression of the disease by preventing nerve cell damage by destroying toxic free radicals. For example, vitamin-C, vitamin-A, selegiline, etc.

Surgical

- **Craniotomy:** It is the prompt surgical procedure performed to remove subdural hematomas in the cranium in less than 4 hours for an optimal outcome by making a hole in the skull to remove a bone flap. In this procedure, the surgeon repairs the damage (skull fracture, bleeding vessel, remove large blood clots, etc.) and the bone flap is replaced in its normal position and secured to the skull with plates and screws.
- **Decompressive craniectomy:** It is a surgical procedure that involves removing a large section of bone so that the brain can swell and expand. This is typically performed when extremely high intracranial pressure becomes life threatening. At that time, the patient is taken to the operating room where a large portion of the skull is removed to give the brain more room to swell. A special biologic tissue is placed on top of the exposed brain and the skin is closed. The bone flap is stored in a freezer. One to 3 months after the swelling has resolved and the patient has stabilized from the injury, the bone flap is replaced in another surgery, called cranioplasty.

Nursing

- Raise the head of bed to 30 to 45° as it would reduce intracranial pressure.
- Turn the patient regularly and frequently with careful observation of the intra cranial pressure.
- Keep the head and neck of the patient in a neutral position as it would improve cerebral venous drainage and in turn reduces intracranial pressure.
- Provide eye care, mouth and skin hygiene.
- Avoiding compression of internal or external jugular veins with tight cervical collar or tight tape fixation of the endotracheal tube that would impede cerebral venous drainage and result in an increase in the intracranial pressure.

2
CHAPTER

Disorders of Endocrine

CHAPTER OUTLINE

- Addison's disease
- Cushing's syndrome
- Diabetes insipidus
- Diabetes mellitus
- Diabetic ketoacidosis
- Hyperaldosteronism
- Hyperosmolar hyperglycemic nonketotic syndrome
- Hyperparathyroidism
- Hyperpituitarism
- Hyperthyroidism
- Hypoglycemia
- Hypoparathyroidism
- Hypopituitarism
- Hypothyroidism
- Syndrome of Inappropriate anti-diuretic hormone (SIADH) secretion

ADDISON'S DISEASE

Definition

Addison's disease is a severe or total deficiency of the hormones made in the adrenal cortex, caused by its destruction.

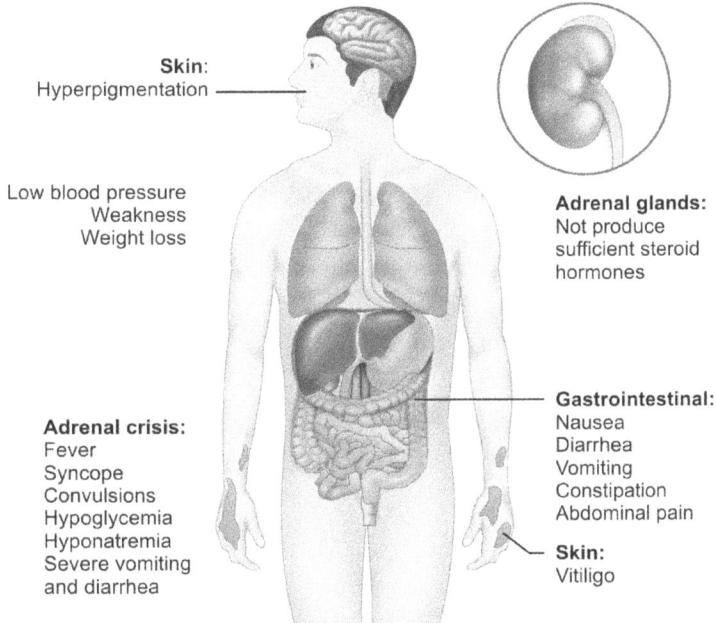

Fig. 2.1: Shows the cardinal signs and symptoms of Addison's disease.

Etiology

- Destruction of the cortex
- Autoimmune diseases
- Idiopathic atrophy of adrenal glands
- Surgical removal of both adrenal glands
- Infection of the adrenal glands
- Tuberculosis
- Histoplasmosis
- Congenital defects
- Inadequate secretion of ACTH from the pituitary gland
- Therapeutic use of corticosteroids.

Risk Factors

- Chronic thyroiditis
- Dermatitis herpatiformis
- Grave's disease
- Hypoparathyroidism
- Hypopituitarism
- Myasthenia gravis
- Pernicious anemia
- Type I diabetes
- Testicular dysfunction
- Vitiligo
- Tumors.

Pathophysiology

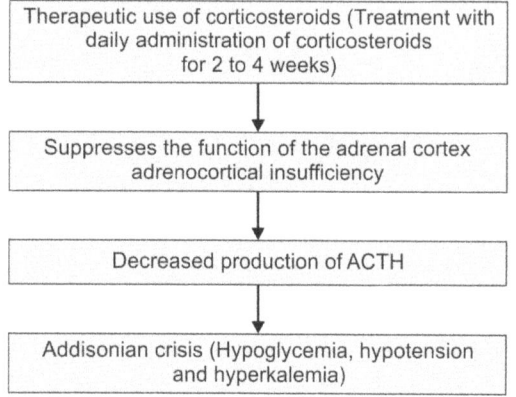

Clinical Features

- Chronic diarrhea
- Nausea
- Vomiting
- Dark pigmentation of the skin
- Emaciation
- Low serum sodium levels
- High serum potassium level
- Increased plasma ACTH
- Dizziness when standing up
- Paleness
- Muscle weakness
- Mouth lesions on the inside of the cheek
- Salt craving
- Weight loss with reduced appetite.

Complications

- Adrenal crisis (addisonian crisis)
- Osteoporosis
- Hypoglycemia
- Hypotension
- Low levels of cortisol.

Diagnostic Tests

- History
- Physical examination
- Blood examination
- ACTH stimulation test
- Antibody blood tests
- Tuberculin skin test
- Insulin-induced hypoglycemia test
- Computerized tomography (CT) scan.

Management

Medical

- **Hormone replacement therapy:** These are medications that are supplementing or replacing the hormones that the adrenal glands are not making. Hydrocortisone is used to replace cortisol, and fludrocortisone is used to replace aldosterone. The dose of each medication is adjusted to meet the individual's need.
- **Antibiotics:** It helps to reduce the risk of secondary infections. For example, Ciprofloxacin, etc.
- **Glucocorticoids:** It helps to correct any metabolic imbalance.
- **Mineralocorticoids:** It helps to correct any electrolyte imbalance.

Nursing

- Ask them to wear a medical alert bracelet that informs people of their condition

- Encourage them to take high protein and carbohydrate diet
- Encourage them to drink plenty of oral fluids
- Instruct them to take their medication every day at the right time of the day
- Instruct them to carry spare medications while at work or in travel.

CUSHING'S SYNDROME

Definition

Cushing's syndrome is a debilitating endocrine disorder characterized by excessive cortisol levels in the blood which may be the result of a tumor of the pituitary gland, adrenal glands (located above the kidneys) or from tumors or cancer arising elsewhere in the body.

Etiology

- Excessive production of corticosteroids by the adrenal cortex
- Frequent use of corticosteroid medications
- Hyperplasia of the adrenal cortex
- Tumor of the adrenal cortex
- Ectopic ACTH (a tumor in the body not associated with pituitary)
- Ectopic CRH (a tumor in the body not associated with hypothalamus)
- Multiple Endocrine Neoplasia Type 1 (MEN 1).

Risk Factors

- Being women
- Those who were between 20 to 50 years of age
- Obesity
- Type 2 diabetes
- Poorly controlled blood sugar levels and high blood pressure.

Pathophysiology

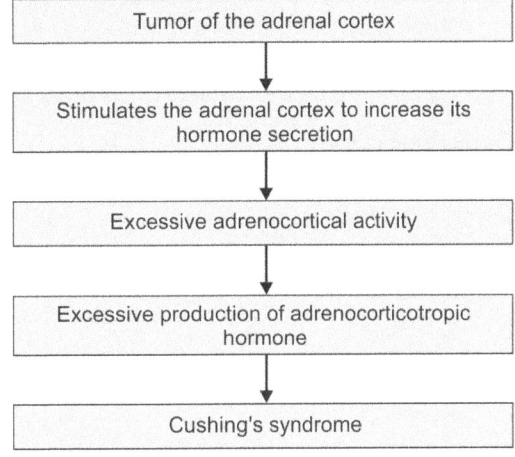

Clinical Features

- A 'buffalo' hump of fat high on the back
- Round, red and puffy-looking face ('moon face')
- Obese trunk with relatively thin arms and legs

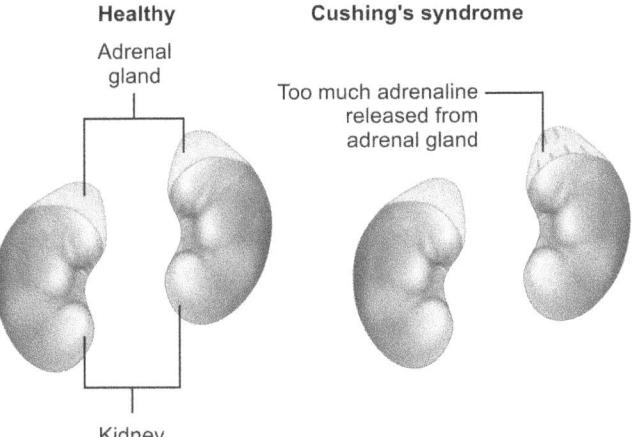

Fig. 2.2: Resembles the kidneys which are healthy and with Cushing's syndrome.

- Hypokalemia
- Elevated plasma cortisol level
- Decreased libido
- Mood swings to psychosis
- Muscular weakness
- Hirsutism
- Amenorrhea in women
- Osteoporosis
- Ecchymoses (bruises)
- Acne
- Increased susceptibility to infections
- Weight gain around the abdomen
- Elevated white blood cell count
- Purple striae on the breast and abdomen.

Complications

- High blood pressure
- Diabetes
- Obesity
- High cholesterol and triglycerides
- Infertility.

Diagnostic Tests

- History
- Physical examination
- Blood examination
- 24 hour urinary free cortisol level
- Midnight plasma cortisol and late-night salivary cortisol measurements
- Low dose dexamethasone suppression test (LDDST)
- Dexamethasone-corticotropin releasing hormone (CRH) stimulation test
- High dose dexamethasone suppression test (HDDST)
- Petrosal sinus (veins that drain the pituitary) blood sampling
- Computerized tomography (CT) scan
- Magnetic resonance imaging (MRI) scan.

Management

Medical

- **Adrenal enzyme inhibitors:** These are medications that are used to reduce hyperadrenalism. For example, ketoconazole, mitotane, amioglutethimide, metyrapone, etc.
- **Antibiotics:** It helps to reduce the risk of secondary infections. For example, ciprofloxacin, cephalosporins, etc.
- **Hormone replacement therapy:** These are medications that are supplementing or replacing the hormones that the adrenal glands are not making. Hydrocortisone is used to replace cortisol and the dose of it is adjusted to meet the individual's need.

Surgical

- **Adrenalectomy:** It is a surgical procedure in which the entire adrenal gland is surgically removed as it helps stopping over production of its secretions.
- **Transsphenoidal hypophysectomy:** It is a surgical procedure in which the pituitary tumors are removed.
- **Bilateral adrenalectomy:** It is the surgical removal of both the adrenal glands.

Nursing

- Emphasize the importance of regular medical follow up
- Stress the importance of wearing a medical alert bracelet for the sake of notifying others
- Emphasize the need to keep and adequate supply of the corticosteroid to prevent skipping a dose of it
- Ensure safe environment for them with minimal stress and risk for falls
- Instruct them not to stop the medications abruptly without the medical advice.

DIABETES INSIPIDUS

Definition

Diabetes insipidus is a condition that results from insufficient production of the anti-diuretic hormone (ADH), a hormone that helps the kidneys and body conserve the correct amount of water. Normally, the anti-diuretic hormone controls the kidneys' output of urine. It is secreted by the hypothalamus (a small gland located at the base of the brain) and stored in the pituitary gland and then released into the bloodstream.

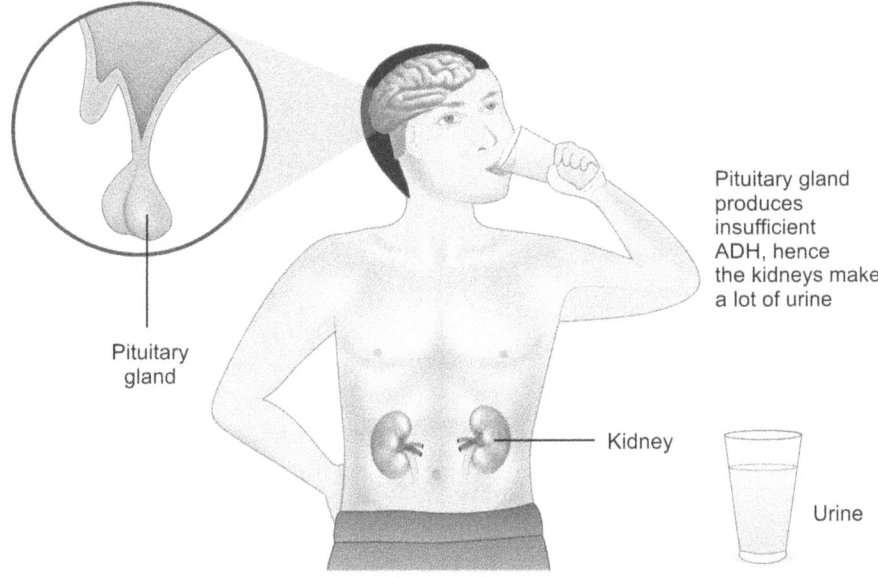

Fig. 2.3: Shows the pathophysiological aspects of diabetes insipidus.

Etiology

- Head injury
- Malfunctioning hypothalamus
- Damage to hypothalamus or pituitary gland during surgery
- Tumor
- Tuberculosis
- Blockage in the arteries leading to the brain
- Irradiation of the head
- Sarcoidosis.

Risk Factors

- Kidney disease
- Brain surgery
- Encephalitis
- Meningitis
- Family history of diabetes insipidus.

Types

- ***Central diabetes insipidus:*** It happens when damage to a person's hypothalamus or pituitary gland causes disruptions in the normal production, storage, and release of vasopressin. The disruption of vasopressin causes the kidneys to remove too much fluid from the body, leading to an increase in urination.
- ***Nephrogenic diabetes insipidus:*** It occurs when the kidneys do not respond normally to vasopressin and continue to remove too much fluid from a person's bloodstream. It can result from inherited gene changes, or mutations, that prevent the kidneys from responding to vasopressin.
- ***Dipsogenic diabetes insipidus:*** It is a defect in the thirst mechanism, located in a person's hypothalamus, causes dipsogenic diabetes insipidus. This defect results in an abnormal increase in thirst and liquid intake that suppresses vasopressin secretion and increases urine output.
- ***Gestational diabetes insipidus:*** In the gestational form of this disorder, the placenta makes a certain enzyme that competes against ADH. The job of the placenta is to nourish the baby and remove waste to filter out through the mother's kidneys. In gestational diabetes insipidus, this process is somewhat interrupted, but the reason remains unknown.

Pathophysiology

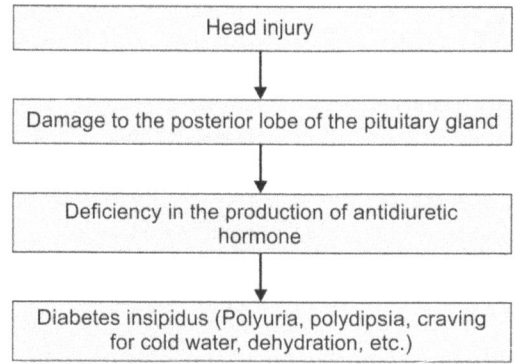

Clinical Features

- Polydipsia (increased thirst 2 to 20 liters of fluid daily)
- Polyuria (5 to 25 liters per day)
- Craving for cold water
- Colorless urine instead of pale yellow
- Waking frequently through the night to urinate
- Dry skin
- Constipation
- Weak muscles
- Hypernatremia
- Wetting the bed at night.

Complications

- Chronic dehydration
- Accelerated heart rate
- Weight loss
- Fatigue
- Sluggishness
- Frequent headaches
- Kidney damage
- Brain damage.

Diagnostic Tests

- History
- Physical examination
- Blood examination
- Urinalysis
- Fluid deprivation test
- Vasopressin test
- Hypertonic saline infusion test
- Magnetic resonance imaging (MRI) scan
- Computerized tomography (CT) scan.

Management

Medical

- **Anti-diuretic hormone replacement:** It helps to prevent loss of water from the body by reducing urine output and helping kidneys reabsorb water into the body. For example, desmopressin, vasopressin tannate, etc.
- **Hypolipidemic agent:** It helps in lowering cholesterol and triglyceride levels in the blood. For example, clofibrate, etc.
- **Thiazide diuretics:** It inhibits sodium and chloride reabsorption in the distal tubule of the kidney, resulting in increased urinary excretion of sodium and water. For example, chlorothiazide, hydrochlorothiazide, chlorthalidone, indapamide, metolazone, etc.
- **Antibiotics:** It helps to reduce the risk of secondary infections. For example, ciprofloxacin, cephalosporins, etc.
- **Prostaglandin inhibitors:** They act on lipid compounds known as prostaglandins, found throughout the body to regulate muscle contractions. For example, aspirin, ibuprofen, etc.

Nursing

- Instruct them not to drive or operate heavy machinery
- Instruct the patient to wear a medical alert wristband
- Instruct them not to stop the medications abruptly without the medical advice
- Instruct them to monitor their weight on daily basis
- Encourage them to take a diet high in fiber and low in sodium.

DIABETES MELLITUS

Definition

Diabetes mellitus is a chronic metabolic disease characterized by hyperglycemia resulting from inherited or acquired deficiency in production of insulin by the pancreas or by the ineffectiveness of the insulin produced or both.

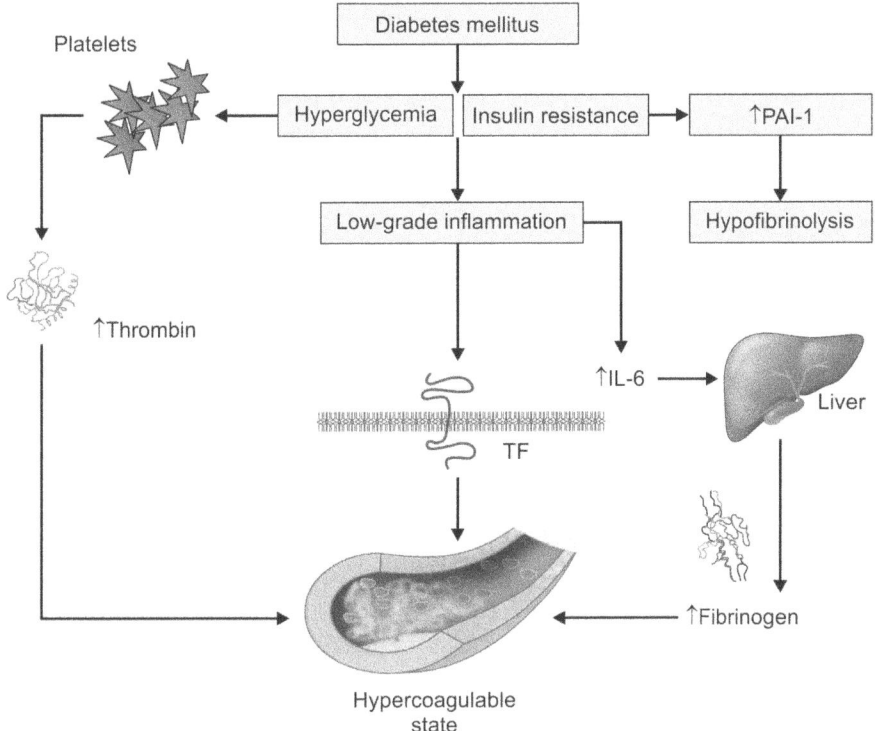

Fig. 2.4: Shows the pathophysiological aspects of diabetes mellitus.

Etiology

- Genetic predisposition
- Pancreatitis
- Polycystic ovary syndrome (PCOS)
- Cushing's syndrome
- Glucagonoma
- Steroid-induced diabetes
- Overweight
- Unidentified component causing autoimmune reaction
- Chemical toxins within food
- Viral or bacterial infection.

Risk Factors

- Family history of diabetes
- Overweight
- Unhealthy diet
- Physical inactivity
- Increasing age
- High blood pressure
- Ethnicity
- Impaired glucose tolerance
- History of gestational diabetes
- Poor nutrition during pregnancy.

Types

- ***Type 1 diabetes (formerly known as insulin-dependent):*** It is a form in which the pancreas fails to produce the insulin which is essential for survival. It develops most frequently in children and adolescents, but is being increasingly noted later in life.
- ***Type 2 diabetes (formerly named non-insulin-dependent):*** It results from the body's inability to respond properly to the action of insulin produced by the pancreas. Type 2 diabetes is much more common and accounts for around 90% of all diabetes cases worldwide. It occurs most frequently in adults, but is being noted increasingly in adolescents as well.

Pathophysiology

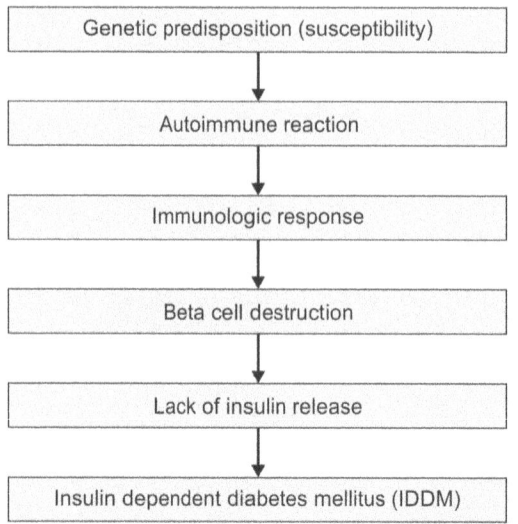

Clinical Features

- Frequent urination
- Excessive thirst
- Increased hunger
- Weight loss
- Tiredness
- Lack of interest and concentration
- A tingling sensation or numbness in the hands or feet
- Blurred vision
- Frequent infections
- Slow-healing wounds.

Complications

- Diabetic neuropathy
- Diabetic nephropathy
- Diabetic retinopathy
- Diabetic ketoacidosis
- Hypertension
- Stroke
- Hyperosmolar hyperglycemic nonketotic syndrome (HHNS)
- Gastroparesis.

Diagnostic Tests

- History
- Physical examination
- Blood examination
- Oral glucose tolerance test
- Glycated Hemoglobin (HbA1c).

Management

Medical

- **Sulfonylureas:** They bind to specific sulfonylurea receptors on pancreatic beta cells and increases insulin secretion. For example, chlopropamide, tolbutamide, gliclazide, glipizide, etc.
- **Meglitinide analogs:** It act on separate non-sulfonylurea receptor binding sites on beta cell and enhance insulin secretion. For example, repaglinide, nateglinide, etc.
- **Biguanides:** It decreases hepatic glucose production and improves peripheral glucose disposal while suppressing appetite and promoting weight reduction. For example, metformin, phenformin, etc.
- **Thiazolidinediones:** It acts by improving insulin sensitivity in adipose tissue and skeletal muscles. For example, pioglitazone, rosiglitazone, etc.
- **Alpha glucosidase inhibitors:** It acts by competitively inhibiting alpha-glucosidase, the enzyme in the small intestine brush border, which breaks down oligosaccharides and disaccharides into monosaccharides. For example, acarbose, etc.
- **Insulin:** It is used to treat people with type 2 diabetes who require long-acting insulin to control diabetes. For example, Human actrapid, etc.

Nursing

- Instruct them to keep the diabetes under control with the help of medications, diet and exercise
- Instruct them not to smoke
- Encourage them to take a balanced and healthy diet
- Ask to engage with 30 minutes of regular exercise
- Encourage them to participate in the weight reduction program in case of overweight
- Instruct them not to stop the medications abruptly without the medical advice
- Ask them to limit the take away and processed foods
- Encourage them to have a regular check-up
- Encourage them to keep their weight under control

- Strictly instruct them to avoid the intake of alcohol
- Encourage them to take high-fiber, low fat and low calorie diet.

DIABETIC KETOACIDOSIS

Definition

Diabetic ketoacidosis (DKA) is a life-threatening metabolic disorder resulting from decreased effective circulating insulin, insulin resistance and increased production of counter-regulatory hormones.

Etiology

- Poor insulin compliance
- Long-term complication of diabetes
- Psychiatric disorders (Eating disorders)
- Pancreatitis

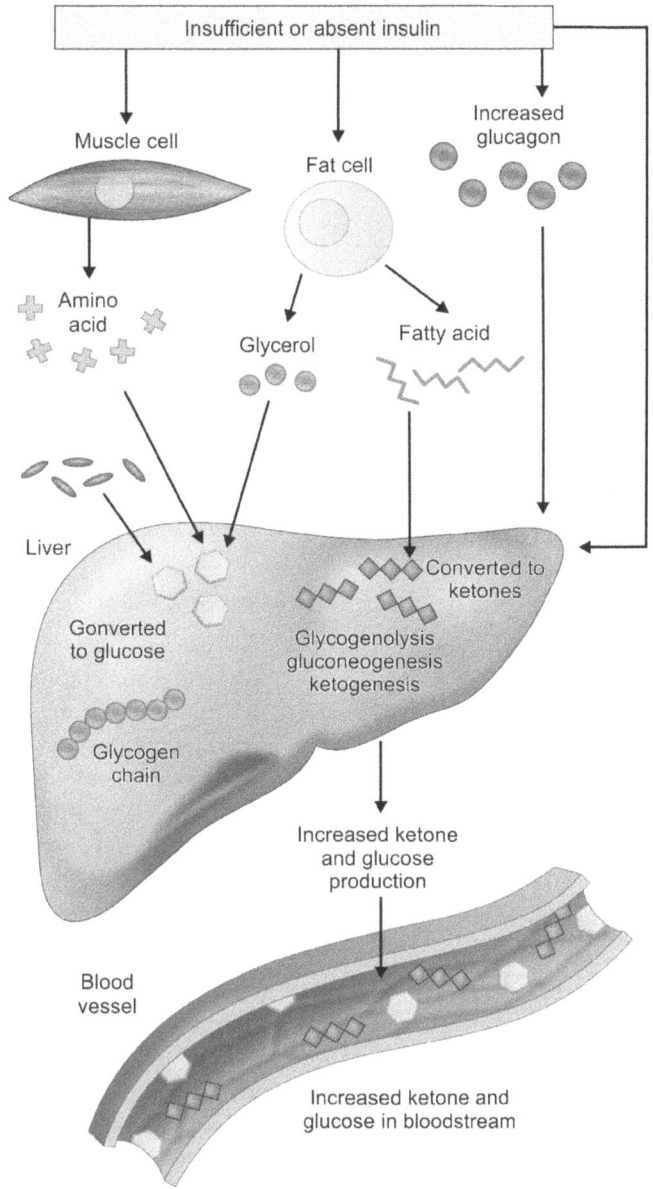

Fig. 2.5: Shows the pathophysiological aspects of diabetic ketoacidosis.

- Medications (high dose glucocorticoids, antipsychotics, diazoxide, and immunosuppressives)
- Sepsis
- Burns
- Trauma.

Risk Factors

- Young age (<5 years)
- First degree relative with type 1 diabetes
- Lower socioeconomic status
- Poor metabolic control
- Pregnancy
- Gastroenteritis
- Stroke
- Silent myocardial infection
- Previous episode of diabetic ketoacidosis
- Female adolescents.

Pathophysiology

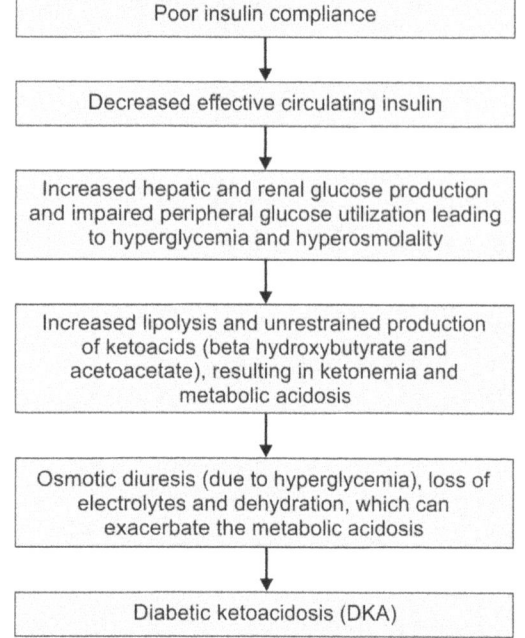

Clinical Features

- Hyperglycemia
- Ketosis and acidosis
- Dehydration
- Electrolyte imbalance
- Feeling unwell for a short period, often less than 24 hours
- Polydipsia and increased thirst
- Polyuria/Nocturia
- Polyphagia
- Weight loss
- Nausea and vomiting
- Abdominal pain due to dehydration and acidosis
- Weakness
- Neurologic signs (restlessness, agitation, lethargy, drowsiness and coma)
- Visual disturbances due to hyperglycemia
- Deep and rapid breathing (Kussmaul breathing)
- Signs of hypovolemia (tachycardia, hypotension, postural hypotension, etc.)
- Signs of dehydration (reduced skin turgor, dry mucus membranes, etc.)
- Mild hypothermia due to acidosis-induced peripheral vasodilation.

Complications

- Hypoglycemia or hyperglycemia due to inadequate insulin therapy
- Hypokalemia
- Fluid overload, non-cardiogenic pulmonary edema
- Acute respiratory distress syndrome (ARDS)
- Pancreatitis
- Rhabdomyolysis.

Diagnostic Tests

- History
- Physical examination
- Blood examination
- Arterial blood gas (ABG) analysis
- Urinalysis
- Glycated hemoglobin (HbA1c)
- Liver function tests.

Management

Medical

- **Oxygenation/Ventilation:** Airway and breathing remain the first priority. If the patient presents with reduced consciousness/coma (GCS <8) consider intubation and ventilation. Airway, breathing and level of consciousness have to be monitored throughout the treatment of diabetic ketoacidosis.

- **Fluid replacement:** Circulation is the second priority. These patients are severely dehydrated and can be in hypovolemic shock. Fluid replacement should be initiated immediately. Fluid resuscitation reduces hyperglycemia, hyperosmolality and counter regulatory hormones, particularly in the first few hours, thus reducing the resistance to insulin. Insulin therapy is therefore most effective when it is preceded by initial fluid and electrolyte replacement.
- **Electrolyte replacement:** Dehydration and osmotic diuresis cause enormous electrolyte shifts in cells and serum. Potassium is the major intracellular positive ion, responsible for maintenance of the electro- potential gradient of the cell membrane. Hyperkalemia may result from reduced renal function, but the patient is more likely to have total body potassium depletion. Early hyponatremia in diabetic ketoacidosis does not usually require specific treatment, it is an artefact arising from dilution by the hyperglycemia-induced water shifts. As excess water moves out of the extracellular space with the correction of hyperglycemia, the sodium level will return to normal. Total body phosphate can be low due to loss from osmotic diuresis. Phosphate will move into cells with glucose and potassium once insulin therapy has started.
- **Insulin therapy:** Insulin therapy is very crucial to diabetes ketoacidosis management. It facilitates glucose uptake into the cell, correction of cell metabolism and acidosis. Insulin is initially given as an intravenous bolus of 0.1 units/kg or a bolus of 5 or 10 units. Then a continuous insulin infusion of 50 units of Actrapid in 50 mL N/Saline is commenced.
- **Sulfonylureas:** They bind to specific sulfonylurea receptors on pancreatic beta cells and increases insulin secretion. For example, chlopropamide, tolbutamide, gliclazide, glipizide, etc.
- **Meglitinide analogs:** It act on separate non-sulfonylurea receptor binding sites on beta cell and enhance insulin secretion. For example, repaglinide, nateglinide, etc.
- **Biguanides:** It decreases hepatic glucose production and improves peripheral glucose disposal while suppressing appetite and promoting weight reduction. For example, metformin, phenformin, etc.
- **Thiazolidinediones:** It acts by improving insulin sensitivity in adipose tissue and skeletal muscles. For example, pioglitazone, rosiglitazone, etc.
- **Alpha glucosidase inhibitors:** It acts by competitively inhibiting alpha-glucosidase, the enzyme in the small intestine brush border, which breaks down oligosaccharides and disaccharides into monosaccharides. For example, acarbose, etc.

Nursing

- Strictly maintain fluid balance
- Give reassurance to relieve anxiety
- Provide comfort measures and manage pain
- Provide oral hydration with ice chips and frequent oral hygiene
- Advise insertion of an arterial line due to frequent blood sampling
- Monitor vital signs (temperature, pulse, respiration, blood pressure) at regular intervals
- Keep patient nil by mouth until acidosis is reversed
- Check urine for ketones every 2nd hourly.

HYPERALDOSTERONISM

Definition

Hyperaldosteronism is a disease caused by an excess production of the normal adrenal hormone, aldosterone. This hormone is responsible for sodium and potassium balance, which then directly controls water balance to maintain appropriate blood pressure and blood volume.

Etiology

- Benign tumor of adrenal gland
- Over activity of both adrenal glands
- Adrenal cortical cancer

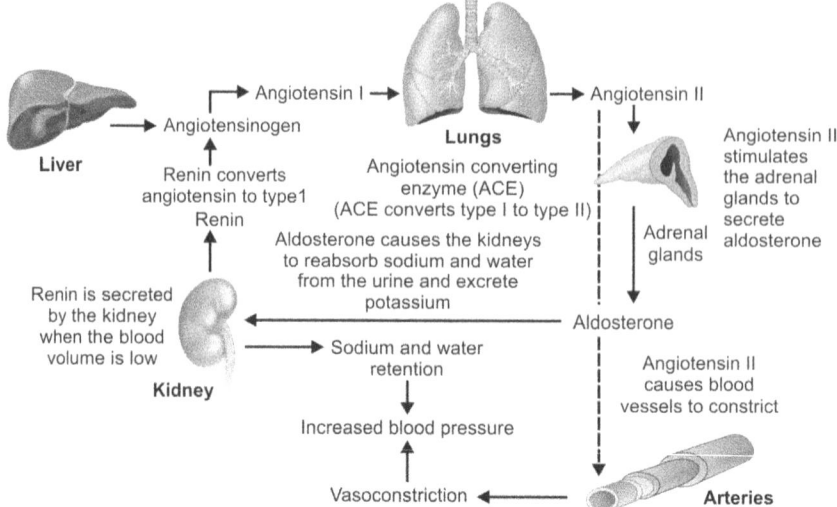

Fig. 2.6: Shows the pathophysiological aspects of hyperaldosteronism.

- Obstruction of the renal artery or renal artery stenosis
- Liver cirrhosis
- Nephrotic syndrome.

Risk Factors

- Being women
- Alcohol abuse
- Enlarged heart
- People between the ages of 30 and 50 years old.

Pathophysiology

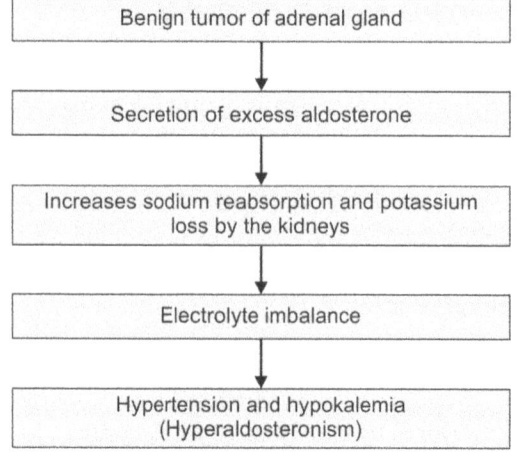

Clinical Features

- Hypertension
- Headaches
- Blurred vision
- Dizziness
- Hypokalemia
- Fatigue
- Numbness
- Intermittent paralysis
- Increased urination
- Increased thirst
- Muscle cramps
- Muscle weakness.

Complications

- Impotence
- Gynecomastia (in men)
- Gastrointestinal distress
- Menstrual irregularities (in women).

Diagnostic Tests

- History
- Physical examination
- Blood examination
- 24 hours urinary excretion of aldosterone test
- Oral salt loading test
- Saline suppression test

- Captopril suppression test (CST)
- Abdominal computerized tomography (CT) scan
- Adrenal vein sampling test
- PAC: PRA ratio.

Management

Medical

- **Mineralocorticoid receptor antagonists:** It blocks the action of aldosterone in the body and helps in correcting high blood pressure and low potassium level. For example, aldactone, eplerenone, etc.

Surgical

- **Adrenalectomy:** It is a surgical procedure in which the entire adrenal gland is surgically removed as it helps stopping over production of its secretions.
- **Bilateral adrenalectomy:** It is the surgical removal of both the adrenal glands.

Nursing

- Encourage them to maintain a healthy body weight
- Instruct them to keep the blood pressure under control with the help of medications, diet and exercise
- Instruct them not to smoke
- Strictly avoid the intake of alcohol
- Ask to engage with 30 minutes of regular exercise
- Instruct them not to stop the medications abruptly without the medical advice
- Encourage them to take a diet high in fiber and low in sodium.

HYPEROSMOLAR HYPERGLYCEMIC NONKETOTIC SYNDROME (HHNS)

Definition

Hyperosmolar hyperglycemic nonketotic syndrome (HHNS) is a metabolic complication of diabetes mellitus characterized by hyperglycemia, extreme dehydration, hyperosmolar plasma and altered consciousness.

Etiology

- First presentation of diabetes mellitus (unsuspected and undiagnosed)
- Pancreatitis
- Cushing's syndrome
- Stroke
- Recent surgery
- Heart attack
- Impaired kidney function.

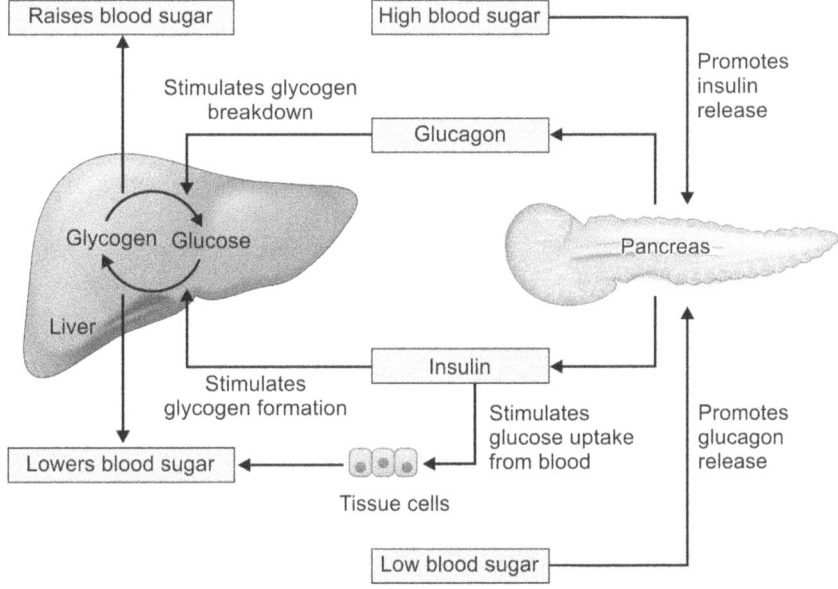

Fig. 2.7: Shows the pathophysiological aspects of hyperosmolar hyperglycemic nonketotic syndrome.

Risk Factors

- Old-aged people with type 2 diabetes mellitus
- Acute infections and other medical conditions
- Drugs that impair glucose tolerance (glucocorticoids) or increase fluid loss (diuretics)
- Nonadherence to diabetes treatment
- Children with long-term steroid use
- Dementia
- Sedative drugs
- Heat waves
- Propensity to infection
- Inappropriate diuretic use
- Certain medications (Beta-blockers, Phenytoin, etc.).

Pathophysiology

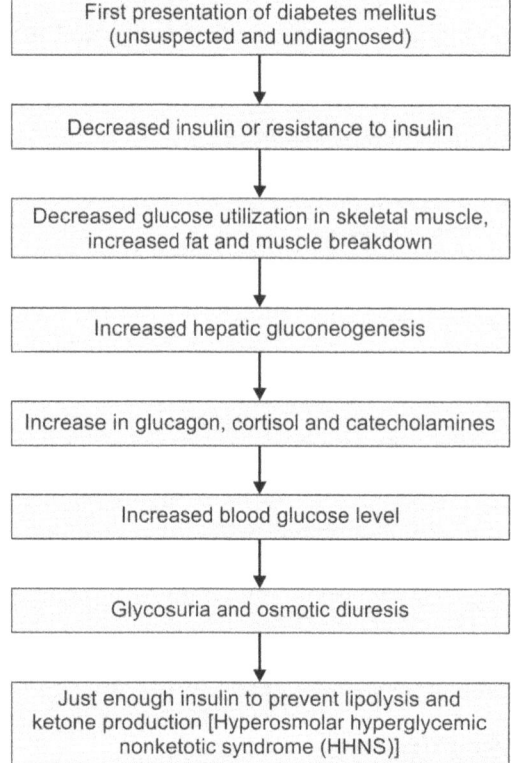

Clinical Features

- Blood glucose level over 600 mg/dL
- Dry, parched mouth
- Extreme thirst
- Polyuria
- Warm, dry skin that does not sweat
- High urine output
- High fever (>101°F)
- Sleepiness
- Confusion
- Loss of vision
- Hallucinations (seeing or hearing things that are not there)
- Speech impairment
- Weight loss
- Weakness on one side of the body
- Progressive dehydration.

Complications

- Coma
- Seizures
- Death
- Blood clots
- Heart attack
- Stroke.

Diagnostic Tests

- History
- Physical examination
- Blood examination
- Arterial blood gas (ABG) analysis
- Urinalysis
- Glycated hemoglobin (HbA1c)
- Liver function tests.

Management

Medical

- **Sulfonylureas:** They bind to specific sulfonylurea receptors on pancreatic beta cells and increases insulin secretion. For example, chlorpropamide, tolbutamide, gliclazide, Glipizide, etc.
- **Meglitinide analogs:** It act on separate non-sulfonylurea receptor binding sites on beta cell and enhance insulin secretion. For example, repaglinide, nateglinide, etc.
- **Biguanides:** It decreases hepatic glucose production and improves peripheral glucose disposal while suppressing appetite and promoting weight reduction. For example, metformin, phenformin, etc.

- **Thiazolidinediones:** It acts by improving insulin sensitivity in adipose tissue and skeletal muscles. For example, pioglitazone, rosiglitazone, etc.
- **Alpha glucosidase inhibitors:** It acts by competitively inhibiting alpha-glucosidase, the enzyme in the small intestine brush border, which breaks down oligosaccharides and disaccharides into monosaccharides. For example, acarbose, etc.
- **Insulin:** It is used to treat people with type 2 diabetes who require long-acting insulin to control diabetes. For example, human actrapid, etc.

Nursing

- Ask them to wear a medical alert bracelet that informs people of their condition
- Instruct them to take their medication every day at the right time of the day
- Encourage them to maintain a healthy body weight
- Instruct them to keep the diabetes mellitus under control with the help of medications, diet and exercise
- Instruct them not to smoke
- Strictly avoid the intake of alcohol
- Encourage them to do exercise regularly
- Instruct them not to stop the medications abruptly without the medical advice
- Encourage them to take a healthy diet
- Instruct them to monitor their blood glucose levels at regular intervals.

HYPERPARATHYROIDISM

Definition

Hyperparathyroidism is a condition in which the parathyroid glands, located in the neck, secrete too much parathyroid hormone (PTH). Parathyroid hormone regulates the amount of calcium and phosphorus in the body, by controlling how much calcium is taken from bones, absorbed in the intestines and lost in urine.

Etiology

- Benign tumors in the parathyroid glands
- Parathyroid hyperplasia (excessive growth of normal parathyroid cells)
- Chronic kidney disease
- Anticonvulsant drugs
- Parathyroid cancer
- Multiple endocrine neoplasia (MEN) syndrome.

Risk Factors

- Being elders
- Being women
- Previous neck irradiation
- Depression
- Obesity
- Long-term lithium therapy.

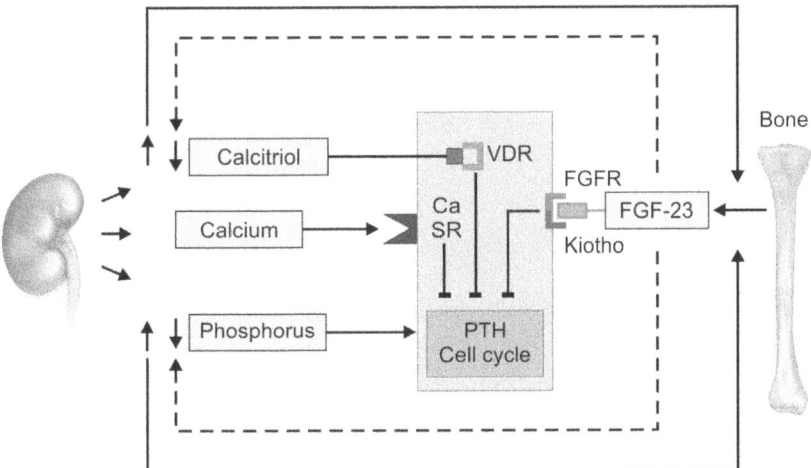

Fig. 2.8: Shows the pathophysiological aspects of hyperparathyroidism.

Pathophysiology

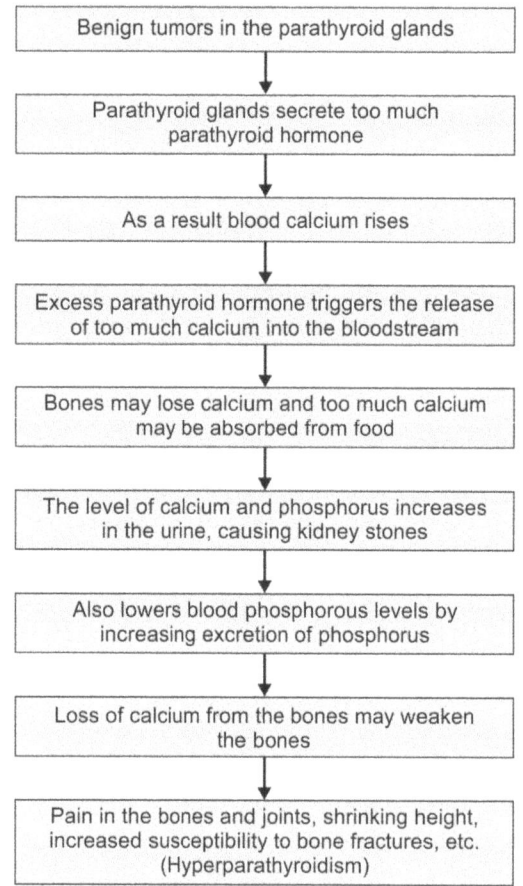

Clinical Features

- Pain in the bones and joints
- Increased susceptibility to bone fractures
- Shrinking height
- Backache
- Muscle aches
- Thirst
- Frequent urination
- Abdominal pain
- Fatigue
- Nausea
- Loss of appetite
- Constipation
- Memory loss
- Depression and other personality changes.

Complications

- Bone fractures
- Kidney stones
- Nervous system complaints
- Osteoporosis and osteopenia
- Peptic ulcers
- Pancreatitis.

Diagnostic Tests

- History
- Physical examination
- Blood examination
- 25-hydroxy-vitamin D blood test
- Bone mineral density test
- Ultrasound scan
- Computerized tomography (CT) scan
- Urine examination.

Management

Medical

- **Calcimimetics:** They suppress the secretion of parathyroid hormone by sensitizing the parathyroid calcium receptor to serum calcium. For example, Cinacalcet, etc.
- **Bisphosphonates:** These are drugs used to slow down or prevent bone damage. For example, bonefos, clasteon, loron, etc.
- **Estrogen receptor modulators:** These are agents that bind to estrogen receptors but act either as agonists or antagonists in different tissues. For example, clomid, osphena, raloxifene, etc.

Surgical

- **Total parathyroidectomy:** It is a surgical procedure in which the entire parathyroid glands are removed.
- **Partial parathyroidectomy:** It is a surgical procedure in which at least one parathyroid gland is left intact to help the body regulate calcium.

Nursing

- Encourage them to eat calcium rich foods
- Instruct them to avoid refined foods
- Ask them to limit their intake of carbonated beverages
- Ask them to strictly avoid coffee and other stimulants (alcohol and tobacco)
- Encourage them to drink 6 to 8 glasses of filter water daily

- Encourage them to do exercise regularly
- Instruct them to reduce the intake of foods rich in trans-fatty acids.

HYPERPITUITARISM

Definition

Hyperpituitarism is characterized by an excessive secretion of pituitary hormones (growth hormone, adrenocorticotropic hormone and prolactin) in the blood due to over activity of the gland or as a result of an adenoma.

Etiology

- Benign pituitary adenomas
- Over activity of the pituitary gland
- Hypothalamic disorders
- Pituitary carcinomas
- Peptic ulcer disease
- Multiple endocrine neoplasia type 1.

Risk Factors

- Between 35 to 60 years
- Being women
- Previous history of hyperpituitarism
- Family history of hyperpituitarism
- Genetic predisposition.

Types

- ***Acromegaly (adults):*** It is an excess growth of hormone in adults, results in bone and soft tissue deformities and enlargement of the viscera without an increase in height.
- ***Gigantism (children):*** In children, over secretion of growth hormone results in gigantism, with a person reaching 7 or even 8 feet tall. Conversely insufficient secretion of growth hormone during childhood results in generalized limited growth and dwarfism.

Pathophysiology

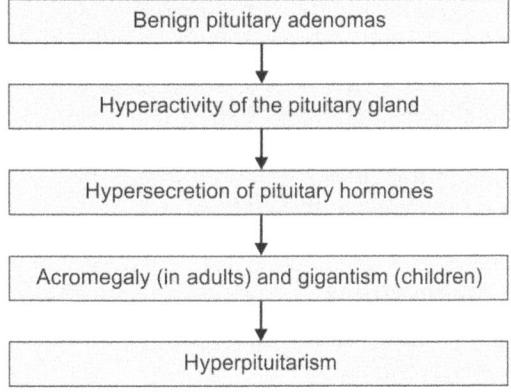

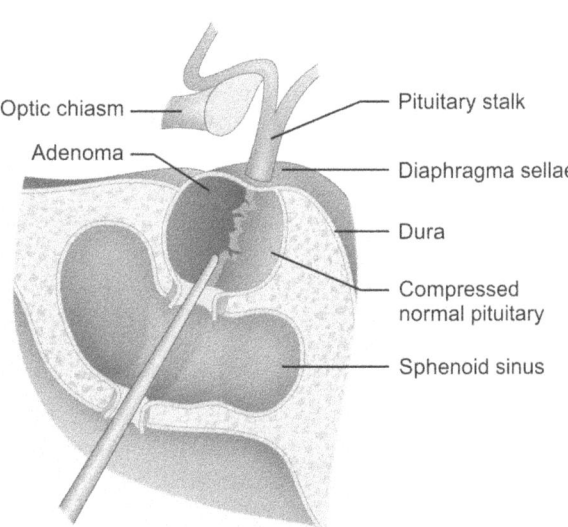

Fig. 2.9: Shows the physiologic changes seen in hyperpituitarism.

Clinical Features

- Coarse body hair
- Deep, husky voice
- Erectile dysfunction
- Exaggerated facial features
- Excessive sweating and often an offensive body odor
- Headache
- Irregular menstrual cycles (in women)
- Irritability
- Joint pain
- Protrusion of the jaw
- Swelling of the hands and feet
- Thickening of the ribs, creating a barrel chest
- Weakness in the arms and legs
- Widening of spaces between teeth
- Depression
- Increased soft tissue and bone thickness
- Increased growth hormone, corticotropic or prolactin
- Enlarged hands and feet
- Glycosuria.

Complications

- Carpal tunnel syndrome
- Osteoporosis
- Kyphosis
- Osteoporosis and osteopenia
- Diabetes mellitus
- Severe psychological stress
- Hypertension
- Glucose intolerance.

Diagnostic Tests

- History
- Physical examination
- Blood examination
- Urine examination
- Human growth hormone tests
- Bone X-rays
- Ultrasound scan
- Computed tomography (CT) scan
- Magnetic resonance imaging (MRI) scan.

Management

Medical

- **Somatostatin analogues:** They inhibit the secretion of growth hormone. For example, octreotide acetate, lanreotide acetate, etc.
- **Dopamine agonists:** These drugs are used to slow down or prevent bone damage. For example, cabergoline, etc.
- **Growth hormone receptor antagonist:** They bind to the growth hormone receptor and make it non-functional and are used in the treatment of acromegaly. For example, pegvisomant, somavert, etc.

Surgical

- **Transsphenoidal hypophysectomy:** It is the surgical removal of the hypophysis (pituitary gland).
- **Stereotactic radiosurgery:** It is a form of radiation therapy that focuses high-power energy on a small area of the body (pituitary gland).

Nursing

- Allow the patient to verbalize their concerns and feelings
- Prepare the patient and family for possible surgery
- Encourage the patient to participate in care as much as possible to maximize function
- Provide reassurance that mood changes result from hormonal imbalances and can be reduced with treatment
- Monitor blood glucose levels as indicated to evaluate for possible altered glucose levels
- Assist the patient with range of motion exercises
- Institute safety precautions to reduce the risk of injury.

HYPERTHYROIDISM

Definition

Hyperthyroidism is a condition which results from an excessive output of thyroid hormones caused by abnormal stimulation of the thyroid gland by circulating immunoglobulins.

Etiology

- Grave's disease
- Hyperfunctioning thyroid nodules

Disorders of Endocrine

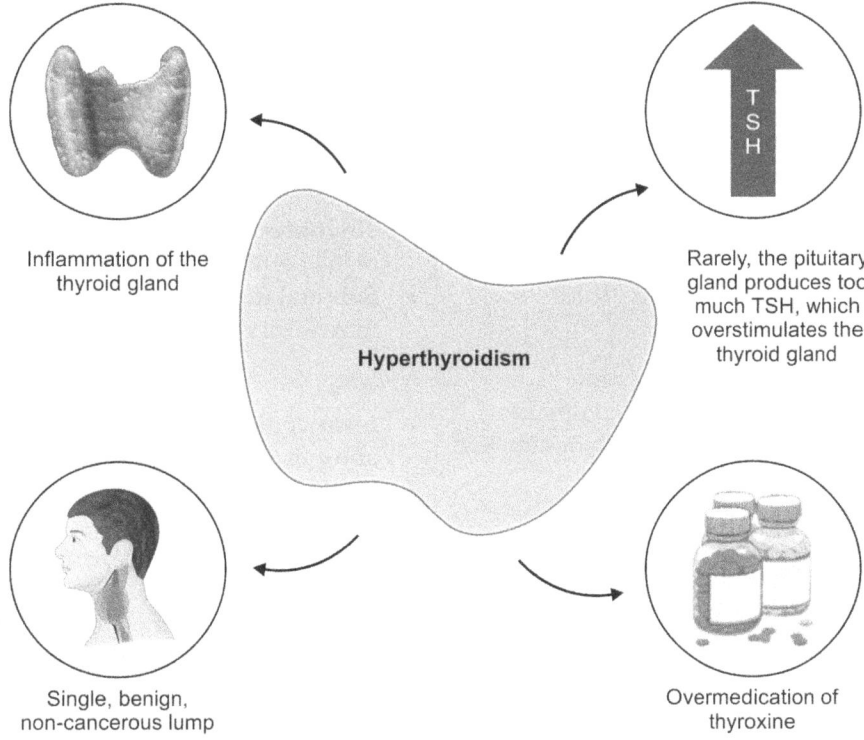

Fig. 2.10: Shows the etiological aspects of hyperthyroidism.

- Excessive ingestion of thyroid hormone
- Benign tumors of the thyroid
- Excessive iodine
- Thyroiditis
- Emotional shock
- Stress
- Infection
- Tumors of the ovaries or testes.

Risk Factors

- Old age population
- Being women
- Japanese ancestry
- Family history of Grave's disease
- Recent pregnancy
- Previous history of thyroid problems
- Consuming significant amounts of iodine through food or medication.

Pathophysiology

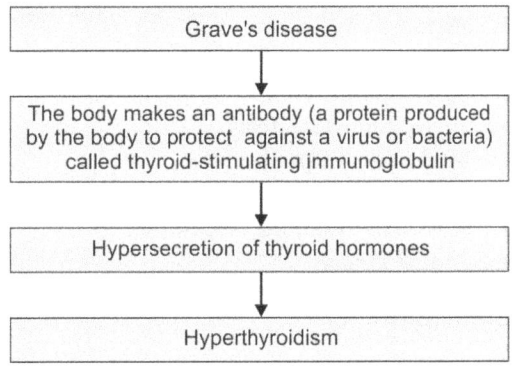

Clinical Features

- Fatigue or muscle weakness
- Polyphagia
- Mood swings
- Nervousness or anxiety

- Heat intolerance
- Exopthalmus (bulging eyes)
- Increased systolic blood pressure
- Increased temperature
- Rapid heart beat
- Heart palpitations
- Dryness of skin
- Tachypnea
- Hand tremors
- Diaphoresis
- Trouble sleeping
- Increased basal metabolic rate
- Increased radioactive thyroid uptake
- Increased T_3 and T_4 (triiodothyronine and thyroxine) level
- Increased frequency of bowel movements
- Progressive weight loss
- Light periods or skipped periods (in women).

Complications

- Thyroid storm (thyrotoxic crisis)
- Arrhythmia
- Cardiac dilation
- Sudden cardiac arrest
- Hypertension
- Osteoporosis.

Diagnostic Tests

- History
- Physical examination
- Blood examination
- Thyroid function tests
- Radioiodine uptake test
- Thyroid scan
- Thyroid stimulating hormone test
- T_3 and T_4 tests.

Management

Medical

- **Anti-thyroid drugs:** These drugs work by interfering with the gland's ability to use iodine. For example, carbimazole (CMZ), propylthiouracil (PTU), etc.
- **Radioactive iodine therapy:** It helps to damage the cells that make thyroid hormones. For example, iodine 131, Iodine 123, etc.
- **Beta-blockers:** It helps in relieving some of the symptoms of an overactive thyroid including tremor, rapid heart beat and hyperactivity. For example, propranolol, atenolol, etc.

Surgical

- **Thyroidectomy:** It is the surgical removal of the partial or total thyroid gland.
- **Subtotal thyroidectomy:** It is the surgical removal of about 5/6th of the thyroid tissue.

Nursing

- Instruct them not to stop the medications abruptly without the medical advice
- Allow the patient to verbalize their concerns and feeling
- Instruct the patient to avoid alcohol and tobacco
- Encourage the patient to do exercise regularly for 30 minutes
- Instruct them to reduce the intake of foods rich in trans fatty acids
- Encourage them to eat foods rich in antioxidants
- Ask them to avoid refined foods
- Encourage them to eat foods rich vitamin B and iron.

HYPOGLYCEMIA

Definition

Hypoglycemia is a condition in which there is an abnormally low level of glucose (sugar) in the blood (below 4 mmol/L or 72 mg/dL).

Etiology

- Hormone deficiencies
- Critical organ failure (heart, kidney or liver)
- Fasting
- Recovery from gastrointestinal surgery
- Certain medication (Beta-blockers, angiotensin converting enzymes inhibitors)
- Prolonged illness.

Risk Factors

- Advanced age
- Postponing or skipping a meal

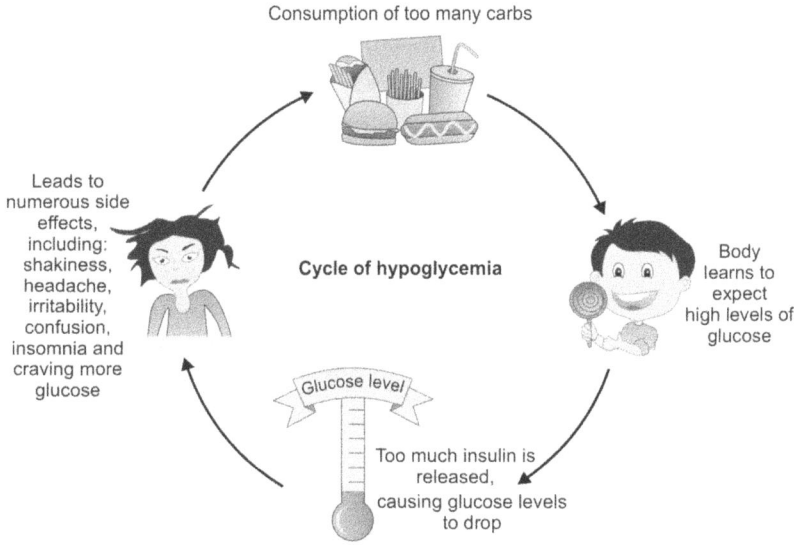

Fig. 2.11: Shows the cycle of hypoglycemia.

- Strenuous exercise
- Eating smaller meals
- Drinking too much alcohol
- Longer duration diabetes
- Peripheral neuropathy
- Obesity
- Cognitive dysfunction.

Types

The Canadian diabetes association classifies hypoglycemia as follows:
- ***Mild hypoglycemia (below 70 mg/dL):*** It consists of the following symptoms—an urgent need to eat, perspiration, nervousness and shakiness. The individual is able to self treat and the cause is due to the release of extra adrenaline.
- ***Moderate hypoglycemia (below 55 mg/dL):*** It consists of the following symptoms—dizziness, sleepiness, confusion, difficulty speaking and feeling anxious or weak. The symptoms caused by the release of extra adrenaline and by lack of glucose getting to the brain both occur but the individual is able to self-treat.
- ***Severe hypoglycemia (below 40 mg/dL):*** It consists of the following symptoms—seizures/convulsions, loss of consciousness and coma. The individual requires the assistance of another person.

Pathophysiology

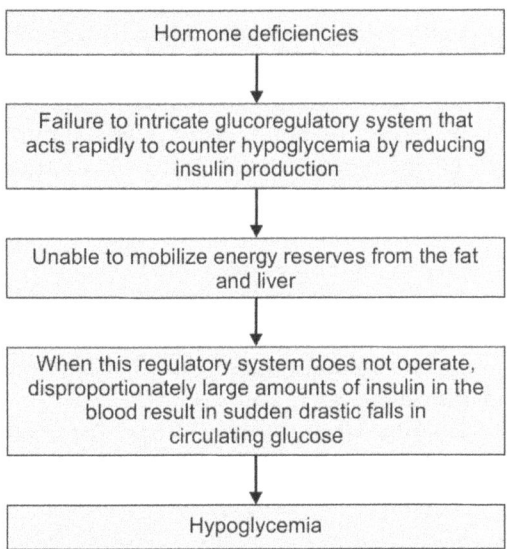

Clinical Features

- Shakiness
- Nervousness or anxiety
- Irritability or impatience
- Blurred/impaired vision
- Tingling or numbness in the lips or tongue

- Confusion
- Sleepiness
- Light headedness or dizziness
- Rapid/fast heart beat
- Hunger and nausea
- Weakness or fatigue
- Nightmares or crying out during sleep
- Lack of coordination
- Sweating
- Tremors.

Complications

- Seizures
- Loss of consciousness
- Death.

Diagnostic Tests

- History
- Physical examination
- Blood examination
- Oral glucose tolerance test.

Management

Medical

- **Follow the 15–15 rule:** Eat or drink something from the list followed equal to 15 g of carbohydrate (3 glucose tablets, 4 ounces of fruit juice, 5 to 6 ounces of regular soda, and 1 tbsp of sugar or jelly). Rest for 15 minutes then re-check the blood glucose and if it is still low (less than 70 mg/dL) repeat the first step as mentioned above.
- **Glucose elevating agents:** It can act in the pancreas or the peripheral tissues to increase blood glucose levels. For example, glucagon, etc.
- **Insulin secretion inhibitors:** These are drugs that inhibits insulin secretion in the blood. For example, diazoxide, octreotide, etc.
- **Glucose supplement:** It helps to raise the patient's serum glucose. For example, dextrose (Glucose D), etc.

Nursing

- Ensure them eat enough food for the medication they are taking
- Encourage them to monitor their blood glucose at regular intervals
- Teach them to be aware of the time of day (when they take insulin, the blood sugar will be the lowest before a meal)
- Ensure that they eat and take the medications on time
- Instruct them not to stop the medications abruptly without the medical advice
- Encourage them to eat more to cover unplanned exercise which may lower the blood sugar too much
- Ask them to report all unexplained hypoglycemia episodes to the physician
- Encourage them to be prepared and carry some form of carbohydrates with them in case there is a meal delay
- Instruct the patient to avoid alcohol.

HYPOPARATHYROIDISM

Definition

Hypoparathyroidism is a rare condition in which the parathyroid glands fail to produce sufficient amounts of parathyroid hormone or the parathyroid hormone produced lacks biologic activity.

Etiology

- Removal or damage to the parathyroid glands
- Congenital hypoparathyroidism
- Radiation therapy to thyroid gland
- Metabolic alkalosis
- Addison's disease
- Wilson's disease
- Too much iron in tissues
- Low levels of magnesium in blood
- Adrenal insufficiency.

Risk Factors

- Family history of parathyroid disorder
- Taking medications that suppress the parathyroid gland
- Autoimmune condition
- Recent thyroid or neck surgery
- DiGeorge syndrome.

Disorders of Endocrine

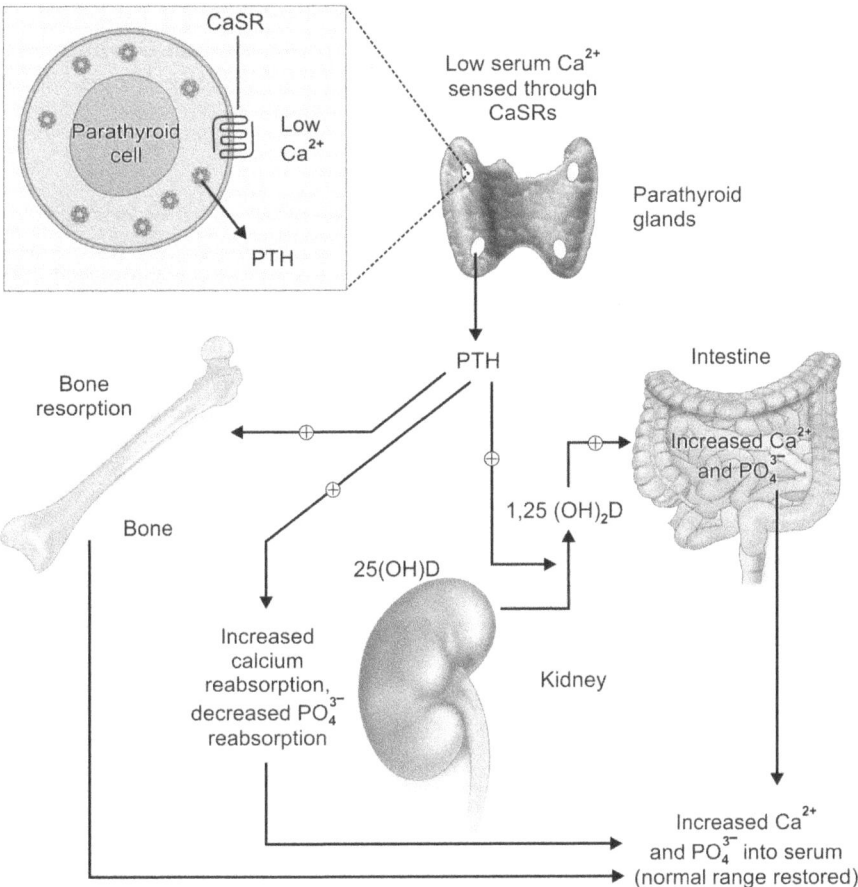

Fig. 2.12: Shows the pathophysiological aspects of hypoparathyroidism.

Types

- **Post-operative hypothyroidism:** It is the most common form of hypoparathyroidism. This is where a surgery in the neck has either removed the parathyroids or damaged them, or damaged their blood supply.
- **Idiopathic hypoparathyroidism:** It is a type in which the cause for the hypoparathyroidism is unknown.
- **Congenital hypoparathyroidism:** It is a disorder that exists at or before birth usually through heredity or acquired at birth or during uterine development usually as a result of environmental influences.
- **Pseudohypoparathyroidism:** It is a type of hypoparathyroidism which is characterized by hypocalcemia and hyperphosphatemia.

Pathophysiology

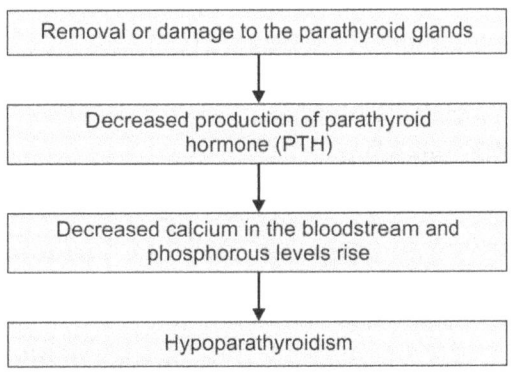

Clinical Features

- Tingling lips, hands and feet
- Muscle cramps
- Pain in the face, legs and feet

- Abdominal pain
- Dry hair
- Convulsions (seizures)
- Painful menstruations
- Hand or foot spasms
- Decreased consciousness
- Low serum calcium level
- High serum phosphorus level
- Low serum parathyroid hormone level
- Dry hair and brittle nails
- Psoriasis (dry, red, flaky patches of skin)
- Cataracts (cloudy vision)
- Soft tissue calcification
- Headaches
- Memory problems
- Depression.

Complications
- Tetany
- Kidney diseases
- Stunted growth
- Malformed teeth
- Pernicious anemia
- Parkinson's disease
- Addison's disease.

Diagnostic Tests
- History
- Physical examination
- Blood examination
- 24 hours urine examination
- X-ray examination
- Computed tomography (CT) scan
- Echocardiogram
- Genetic studies.

Management

Medical
- **Recombinant parathyroid hormone (rPTH):** The use of a recombinant parathyroid hormone is to control hypoglycemia in people with hypothyroidism.
- **Vitamin D:** It increases the intestines ability to absorb calcium. For example, cholecalciferol, vitamin D_2, vitamin D_3, etc.
- **Calcium:** It helps to increase the calcium level in blood. For example, calcium carbonate, calcium citrate, etc.
- **Calcitriol:** It is a prescription form of activated vitamin D which increases the calcium level in blood. For example, rocaltrol, etc.

Nursing
- Encourage them to take good sources of calcium and vitamin D
- Ask them to wear a medical alert bracelet that informs people of their condition
- Instruct them to take their medication every day at the right time of the day
- Instruct them not to stop the medications abruptly without the medical advice
- Encourage them to have a regular check-up.

HYPOPITUITARISM (SIMMOND'S DISEASE)

Definition
The total absence of pituitary hormones due to the deficiency of one or more anterior pituitary hormones is known as pan hypopituitarism (or) Simmond's disease.

Etiology
- Tumors in or near the pituitary gland
- Radiation treatment for a tumor
- Chemotherapy
- Brain surgery
- Traumatic brain injury
- Tuberculosis or meningitis
- Sheehan's syndrome (necrosis of the pituitary)
- Lymphocytic hypophysitis
- Sarcoidosis
- Hemochromatosis
- Histiocytosis X.

Risk Factors
- History of childhood cancer
- Type 1 diabetes
- Infection
- Sickle cell anemia
- Hypovolemia
- Genetic predisposition
- Severe bleeding in the brain or severe blood loss during childbirth

Disorders of Endocrine

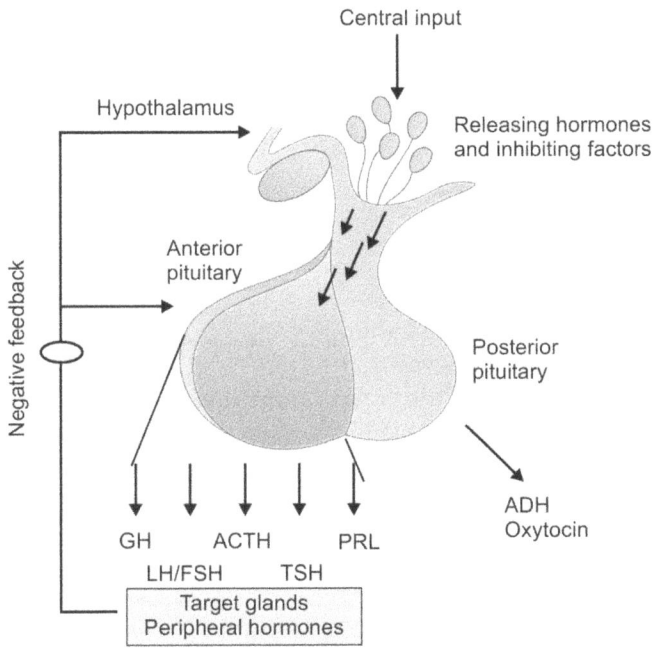

Fig. 2.13: Shows the mechanism of secretion of parathyroid hormone.

- Adrenal insufficiency
- Diabetes insipidus.

Pathophysiology

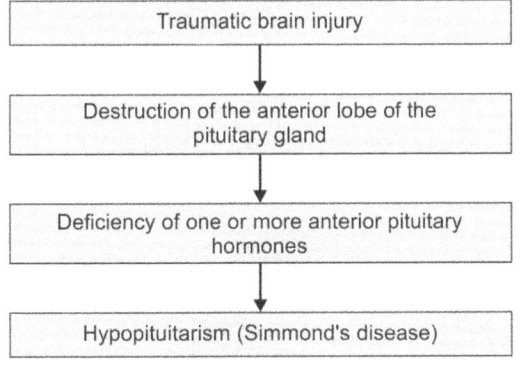

Clinical Features

- Headache and dizziness
- Excessive thirst and urination
- Extreme weight loss
- Emaciation
- Lethargy
- Loss of strength and libido
- Decreased tolerance for cold
- Hair loss
- Hypometabolism
- Hypoglycemia
- Decreased temperature
- Decreased blood pressure
- Visual disturbances
- Stiffness in the joints.

Complications

- Amenorrhea
- Failure to develop puberty
- Hypothyroidism
- Hypotension
- Impotence
- Osteoporosis
- Short stature.

Diagnostic Tests

- History
- Physical examination
- Blood examination
- Visual acuity test
- Growth hormone-releasing hormone (GHRH) test
- Arginine stimulation test

- Clonidine stimulation test
- Insulin tolerance test
- Adrenocorticotropic hormone (ACTH) stimulation test
- Computerized tomography (CT) scan
- Magnetic resonance imaging (MRI) scan.

Management

Medical

- **Replacement of hormones:** It enables the patient to live a normal life, feel well and not have the consequences of hormone deficiency and restores fertility in men and women. For example, testosterone, estrogen, etc.
- **Anti-diuretic hormone:** It is a synthetic analog of vasopressin with low vasopressor activity. For example, desmopressin, etc.
- **Corticosteroids:** It closely resemble and replace cortisol, a hormone that the adrenal glands produce naturally in the body. For example, hydrocortisone, etc.

Nursing

- Instruct them to take their medication every day at the right time of the day
- Instruct them not to stop medication just because they feel better
- Instruct them to carry spare medications while at work or in travel
- Ask them to wear a medical alert bracelet that informs people of their condition
- Encourage them to take high protein and low calorie and fiber food
- Instruct the patient when sleeping with head elevation position to reduce trauma to the eye
- Wet the eye with sterile water to provide comfort to the eye
- Give skin care and encourage patient to perform regular skin care.

HYPOTHYROIDISM (MYXEDEMA)

Definition

Hypothyroidism is a condition which is characterized by decreased production of thyroid hormone in response to decreased thyroid stimulating hormone due to the occurrence of any primary thyroid disease.

Etiology

- Hashimoto's thyroiditis
- Decreased production of thyroid stimulating hormone
- Congenital thyroid agenesis
- Sarcoidosis
- Tumor of the pituitary gland
- Genetic defects
- Certain medications (Amiodarone, Interferon-alpha, Interleukin-2, Lithium, etc.).

Risk Factors

- Being an older women
- Family history of thyroid disease

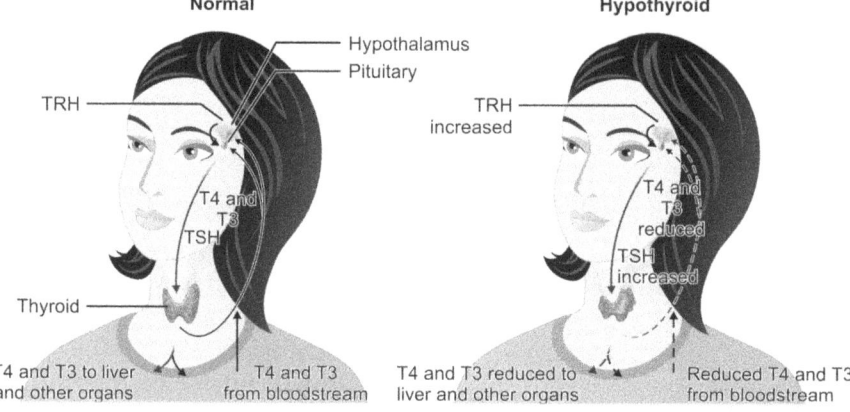

Fig. 2.14: Shows the pathophysiological aspects of normal and hypothyroidism individual.

- Type 1 diabetes
- Rheumatoid arthritis
- Treatment with radioactive iodine
- Thyroid surgery
- Exposure to radiations in the chest or upper neck area.

Types

- **Cretinism:** It is a type of hypothyroidism most commonly seen in infants and young children.
- **Hypothyroidism without myxedema:** It is a type of hypothyroidism seen with mild degree of thyroid failure in older children and adults.
- **Hypothyroidism with myxedema:** In this type, there will be severe degree of thyroid failure in older individuals.

Pathophysiology

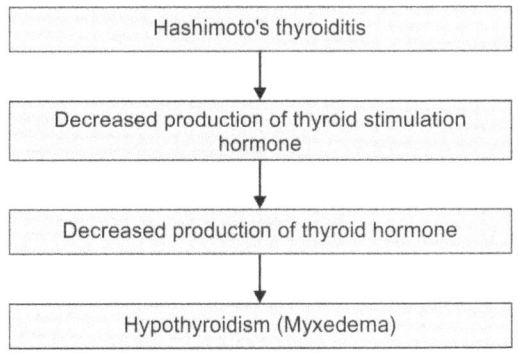

Clinical Features

- Fatigue
- Weakness
- Hoarseness of voice
- Weight gain or difficulty losing weight
- Coarse, dry hair and dry skin
- Hair loss
- Sensitivity to cold
- Muscle cramps and aches
- Constipation
- Depression
- Irritability
- Memory loss
- Decreased libido
- Apathy
- Loss of appetite
- Bradycardia
- Enlarged tongue
- Thinning of lateral eyebrows
- Decreased basal metabolic rate
- Decreased levels of T3 and T4
- Lack of facial expression
- Abnormal menstrual cycles (in women).

Complications

- Birth defects
- Goiter
- Infertility
- Heart problems
- Myxedema
- Depression.

Diagnostic Tests

- History
- Physical examination
- Blood examination
- Thyroid function test
- Lipid profile test.

Management

Medical

- **Corticosteroids:** Hydrocortisone, etc. It helps to treat the insufficiency of adrenocorticotropic hormone.
- **Hormone replacement therapy:** These are medications that are supplementing or replacing the hormones that the thyroid glands are not making (thyroxine).
- **Synthetic levothyroxine:** It helps in treating hypothyroidism and to suppress nontoxic goiters. For example, synthroid, levothroid, etc.

Nursing

- Ask them to wear a medical alert bracelet that informs people of their condition
- Encourage them to avoid fatty rich diet
- Encourage them to drink plenty of oral fluids
- Instruct them to take their medication every day at the right time of the day

- Instruct them to carry spare medications while at work or in travel
- Encourage them to include more roughages in their diet.

SYNDROME OF INAPPROPRIATE ANTI-DIURETIC HORMONE (SIADH) SECRETION

Definition

The syndrome of inappropriate antidiuretic hormone secretion (SIADH) is a clinical syndrome in which enhanced secretion or action of antidiuretic hormone (ADH) due to various disease processes and medications causes persistent hyponatremia and inappropriately elevated urine osmolality.

Etiology

- People with a diseased hypothalamus
- Meningitis
- Encephalitis
- Malignancy
- Psychosis
- Damage to the hypothalamus or pituitary gland during surgery
- Thyroid or parathyroid hormone deficiencies
- Head trauma
- Guillain-Barre Syndrome (GBS)
- HIV
- Hereditary diseases.

Risk Factors

- Advancement in age
- Being female
- Premenopausal women
- People with a heart failure
- History of endurance exercise
- Certain medications (Thiazide diuretics, anti-depressants, etc.)

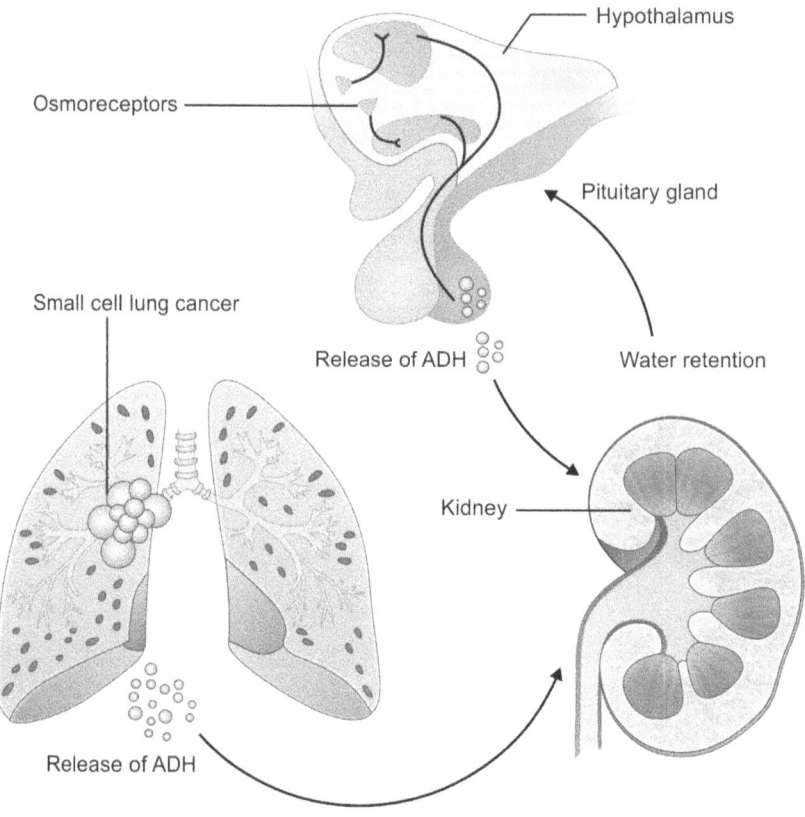

Fig. 2.15: Shows the pathophysiological aspects of syndrome of inappropriate anti-diuretic hormone (ADH) secretion.

- Nursing home residence
- Presence of a postoperative state
- Presence of pulmonary conditions
- Alcohol withdrawal.

Pathophysiology

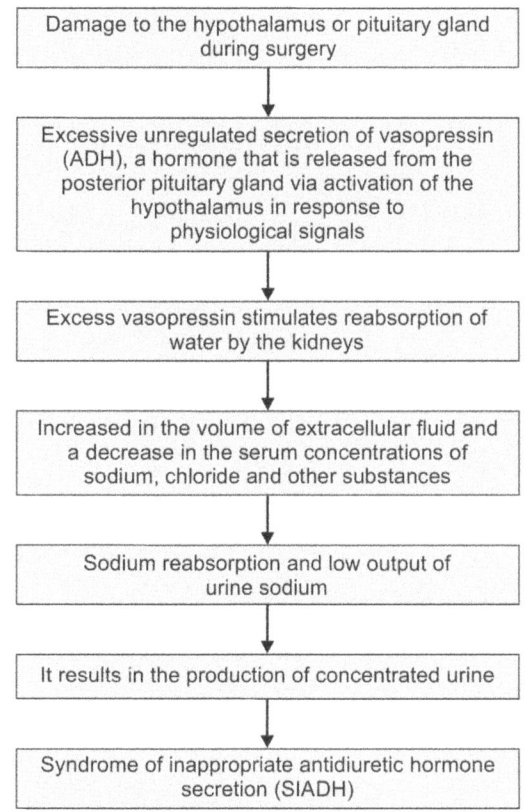

Clinical Features

- Nausea
- Vomiting
- Headache
- Increased thirst
- Cramps or tremors
- Tiredness
- Weakness
- Dark colored urine
- Loss of appetite
- Depressed mood
- Memory impairment
- Irritability
- Personality changes (combativeness, confusion and hallucinations)
- Ataxia
- Persistent hyponatremia
- Elevated urine osmolality.

Complications

- Seizures
- Stupor or coma
- Brainstem herniation
- Central pontine myelinolysis
- Death.

Diagnostic Tests

- History
- Physical examination
- Blood examination
- Urine examination
- Chest X-ray
- Computed tomography (CT) scan
- Liquid challenge test.

Management

Medical

- History
- **Fluid restriction:** This is a common management strategy for increasing serum sodium concentrations, at least time being, whilst the underlying cause is sought and treated. Usually, the fluid restriction is between 500 to 1000 mL per day.
- **Replacing sodium:** Another general management strategy for treating hyponatremia is to replace sodium by giving normal saline 0.9% as a slow infusion. This has to be done with great care, as if the sodium concentration is corrected too rapidly it can result in the devastating complication
- **Vasopressin receptor antagonists:** It is a V2 selective vasopressin receptor antagonists that is used to treat hyponatremia in SIADH. For example, tolvaptan, vaptans, etc.
- **Tetracycline antibiotics:** Demeclocycline, etc. It reduces the sensitivity of the ADH receptors on the distal tubules of the kidneys, as a result of this partially blocks the effects of ADH on the kidneys, essentially creating a partial nephrogenic diabetes insipidus.

Nursing

- Maintain proper intake output chart
- Encourage them to drink water in moderate amount
- Instruct them to take precautions during high-intensity activities
- Instruct them to take their medication every day at the right time of the day
- Instruct them to avoid salty foods
- Monitor weight at regular intervals
- Provide frequent mouth care to the patient.

CHAPTER 3

Disorders of Eye

CHAPTER OUTLINE

- Age-related macular degeneration
- Blepharitis
- Cataract
- Chalazion
- Conjunctivitis
- Correctable refractive errors
- Diabetic retinopathy
- Eye trauma
- Glaucoma
- Hordeolum (Stye)
- Keratitis
- Retinal detachment
- Strabismus
- Visual impairment (Blindness)

AGE-RELATED MACULAR DEGENERATION (AMD)

Definition

Age-related macular degeneration (AMD) is a chronic painless eye disease that causes damage to macula, the central part of the retina at the back of the eye that allows us to see fine details clearly.

Etiology

- Idiopathic
- Certain genes
- Repeated eye exposure to sunlight.

Risk Factors

- Increased age
- Family history of macular degeneration
- White race

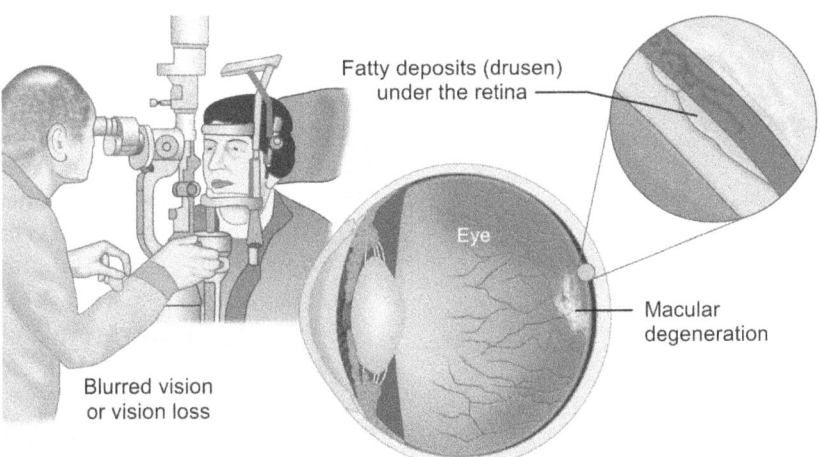

Fig. 3.1: Shows the fatty deposits under the retina due to damaged macula (the central part of the retina at the back of the eye that allows us to see fine details clearly).

- Females
- Being obese
- Smoking cigarette
- High blood pressure
- High cholesterol
- Unhealthy diet
- Cardiovascular disease.

Types

- *Wet age-related macular degeneration:* It occurs when abnormal blood vessels behind the retina start to grow under the macula. These new blood vessels tend to be very fragile and often leak blood and fluid. The blood and fluid raise the macula from its normal place at the back of the eye. The most common symptom of wet age-related macular degeneration is straight lines will appear wavy.
- *Dry age-related macular degeneration:* It occurs when the light-sensitive cells in the macula slowly breakdown, gradually blurring central vision in the affected eye. As it gets worse blurred spot is seen in the center of the vision. Over time, macula functions, central vision in the affected eye will be lost gradually. The most common symptom of dry age-related macular degeneration is blurred vision, difficulty recognizing faces, need light for reading and other tasks.

Pathophysiology

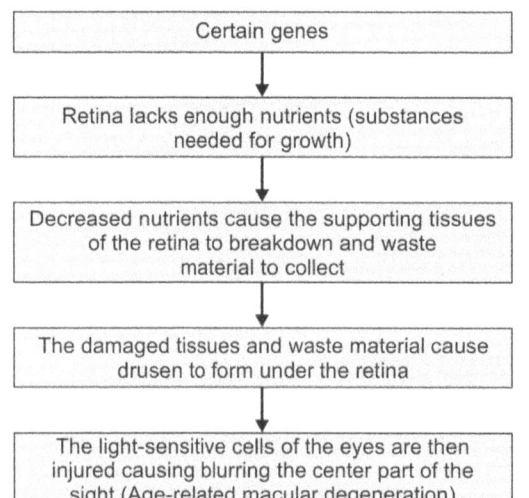

Clinical Features

- Blurry vision
- Distorted vision
- Painless worsening of vision
- Straight lines appear wavy
- Objects may appear as the wrong shape or size
- The loss of clear, correct colors
- Difficulty reading
- A dark, empty area in the center of vision.

Complications

- Blindness
- Choroidal neovascularization
- Retinal drusen
- Maculopathy
- Vitreous hemorrhage.

Diagnostic Tests

- History
- Physical examination
- Ophthalmic examination
- Amsler grid test
- Visual acuity test
- Slit-lamp test
- Dilated eye examination
- Fluorescein angiography
- Optical coherence tomography (OCT) scan.

Management

Medical

- **Antioxidant vitamins and minerals:** It helps to protect the body cells from damage and keeps the disease from getting worse and improves the vision. For example, vitamin C and E, beta carotene, zinc, etc.
- **Anti-vascular endothelial growth factor:** It stops blood vessels from growing and leaking and keeps the disease from getting worse and improves the vision. For example, anti-VEGF injections, etc.

Surgical

- **Laser photocoagulation:** It is a procedure in which a thermal (heat) laser is directed

at leaking blood vessels in the retina and seals the leaking blood vessels to prevent more damage to the retina.
- **Photodynamic therapy:** It is a procedure in which a shot of medicine is injected into the vein (blood vessel) and the medicine gets collected in the leaking blood vessel in the eye.

Nursing
- Instruct the patient to have enough lighting into the room to see the objects better
- Instruct the patient not to smoke
- Motivate the patient to have their blood pressure and cholesterol checked regularly
- Instruct the patient to maintain a healthy weight
- Encourage the patient to wear sunglasses with ultraviolet protection lenses to protect the eyes when outdoors.

BLEPHARITIS

Definition
Blepharitis is an ocular disease characterized by inflammation of the eyelid margins which results due to low-grade bacterial infection or a generalized skin condition.

Etiology
- A bacterial infection
- Recurrent conjunctivitis

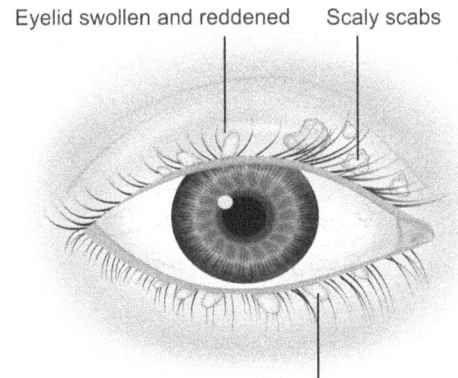

Fig. 3.2: Shows the inflamed and reddened eyelid margins resulting from bacterial infections.

- Malfunctioning oil glands present in the posterior eyelids (Meibomian glands)
- Acne rosacea (a skin condition characterized by facial redness)
- Seborrheic dermatitis (dandruff of the scalp and eyebrows)
- Eyelash mites (tiny organisms in the eyelash follicles)
- Trichiasis.

Risk Factors
- Advanced age
- Cosmetic makeup
- Diabetes
- Poor hygiene
- Chemical irritants
- Contact allergies.

Types
There are two types of blepharitis as follows:
1. ***Anterior blepharitis:*** It affects the anterior margin (front) of the eyelids near the roots of the eyelashes. It is caused by Seborrheic dermatitis and *Staphylococcus* infection.
2. ***Posterior blepharitis:*** It affects the posterior margin (back) of the eyelids, the part that makes contact with the eyes. It is caused by the irregular oil production by the glands of the eyelids (Meibomian glands) which create a favorable environment for bacterial growth present in the eyelid region. It develops as a result of other skin conditions such as acne rosacea and scalp dandruff.

Pathophysiology

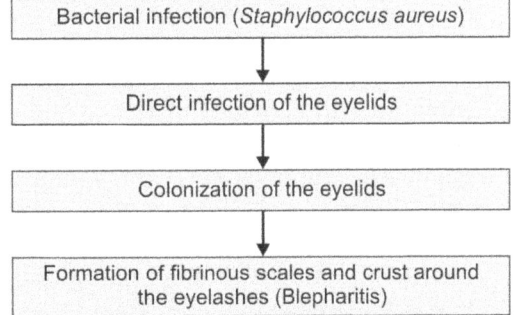

Clinical Features

- Watery eyes
- Red eyes
- A gritty, burning sensation in the eye
- Greasy eyelids
- Itchy eyelids
- Red swollen eyelids
- Flaking of the skin around the eyes
- Crusted eyelashes upon awakening
- Sensitivity to light
- Loss of eyelashes.

Complications

- Stye or hordeolum
- Chalazion
- Chronic pink eye (conjunctivitis)
- Ulceration of the cornea
- Misdirected eyelashes
- Scarring of eyelids.

Diagnostic Tests

- History
- Physical examination
- Ophthalmic examination
- Visual acuity test
- Slit-lamp test

Management

Medical

- **Antibiotics:** It helps to control ulcerative lid margin disease and helps in blocking staphylococcal lipase production. For example, azithromycin, chloramphenicol, Tetracycline, etc.
- **Weak topical steroids:** It helps in controlling eye and eyelid inflammation for short-term treatment. For example, fluorometholone, loteprednol, etc.
- **Anti-fungal agents:** It is used to treat infections in any part of the eye that is caused by the fungus. For example, natamycin, amphotericin B, voriconazole, etc.
- **Omega 3 fatty acids:** It helps in aiding healthy function of meibomian glands that provide essential lubrication for eye and eyelid comfort. For example, flaxseed oil, etc.

Nursing

- Instruct the patient to rinse the lids with warm water and pat gently with a clean, dry towel
- Enforce the patient to wash the hands thoroughly before touching the eyelids
- Educate the patient to avoid using cosmetic makeup
- Instruct the patients to wash the hair and face at regular intervals.

CATARACT

Definition

Cataract is a clouding that develops in the crystalline lens of the eye or in its envelope, varying in degree from slight to complete opacity and obstructing the passage of light.

Etiology

- Long-term exposure to ultraviolet light radiations
- Secondary to diseases such as diabetes, hypertension, etc.
- Eye injury or physical trauma
- Denaturation of lens proteins
- Genetic factors
- Nutritional deficiencies
- Persons exposed to infrared radiation, such as glassblowers
- Exposure to microwave radiations
- Certain drugs such as Corticosteroids and Ezetimibe.

Risk Factors

- Advanced age
- Positive family history
- Smoking
- People with flying jobs
- Tobacco use
- Obesity
- Heavy drinking
- Exposure to radiation from X-rays and cancer treatment
- Exposure to lead.

Disorders of Eye

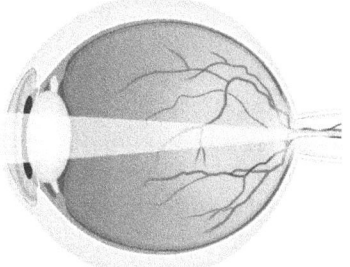
Normal eye

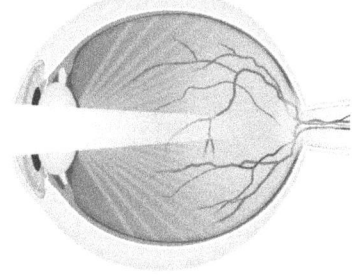
Cataract eye

A healthy lens allows for all parts of the retina to receive the image

A cloudy lens scatters light, causing an image that's out of focus and hazy

Fig. 3.3: Shows the comparison of normal eye with that of cataract eye.

Types

1. ***Age-related cataract***
   - These are cataracts which occur due to aging (old age)
   - Its types are as follows: hypermature senile cataract (HMSC), mature senile cataract (MSC) and immature senile cataract (IMSC).
2. ***Congenital cataract***
   - These are cataracts which occur on babies' right from the birth most often in both eyes
   - Its types are as follows: sutural cataract, lamellar cataract, zonular cataract and total cataract.
3. ***Secondary cataract***
   - These are cataracts which occur in people secondary to any diseases such as diabetes, hypertension, uveitis, etc.
   - Its types are as follows: drug-induced cataract (e.g. Corticosteroids).
4. ***Traumatic cataract***
   - These are cataracts which develop soon after an eye injury or years later
   - Its types are as follows: blunt trauma cataract and penetrating trauma cataract.

Pathophysiology

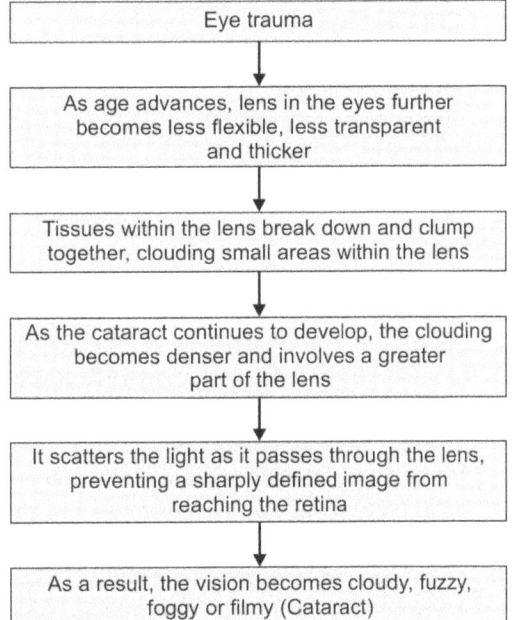

Clinical Features

- Cloudy, fuzzy, foggy or filmy vision
- Decreased vision in bright or low light
- Altered color appreciation
- Problems driving at night because headlights seem too bright

- Problems with glare from lamps or the sun
- Rapid changes in the power of glasses
- Sometimes pain, redness and watering will occur
- Double or multiple visions
- Seeing many images of one object
- Pearly white appearance of pupils
- Change in the eye's refractive error.

Complications

- Infection
- Endophthalmitis
- Bleeding
- High pressure inside the eye (Glaucoma)
- Inflammation (Pain, redness and swelling)
- Haziness of the cornea
- Detachment of the retina
- Posterior capsular opacification.

Diagnostic Tests

- History
- Physical examination
- Visual acuity test
- Tonometric examination
- Slit lamp examination
- Ultrasound of the eye.

Management

Surgical

1. **Extra-capsular cataract extraction:** It is a procedure in which the lens is removed leaving the majority of lens capsule intact. High frequency sound waves (Phacoemulsification) may be used to break up the lens before extraction.
2. **Intra-capsular cataract extraction:** It is a procedure in which the entire lens of the eye is removed.
3. **Phacoemulsification with foldable IOL:** It is a procedure in which very small incision (3.2 mm) is made into the clear part of the eye (cornea) and the hard core (nucleus) of the lens is converted into a soft pulp using high frequency sound waves (not LASER) and sucked out. Then a foldable lens (IOL) is injected through the small incision and positioned into capsular bag.
4. **Small incision cataract surgery (SICS) with intraocular lens (IOL) implantation:** It is a procedure in which slightly larger incision (5-6 mm) is made and the nucleus is removed using fluid pressure, so no stitches are required and the recovery is much faster.

Nursing

- Instruct the patient to limit their night driving
- Instruct the patient not to smoke
- Motivate the patient to have their blood pressure and cholesterol checked regularly
- Instruct the patient to maintain a healthy weight
- Encourage the patient to wear sunglasses with ultraviolet protection lenses to protect the eyes when outdoors
- Educate the patient to improve lighting in their home with more brighter lamps
- Educate the patient to choose a healthy diet that includes plenty of fruits and vegetables.

CHALAZION

Definition

It is a benign, painless bump or nodule present inside the upper or lower eyelid caused by chronic inflammation of one of the small oil producing glands (Meibomian glands).

Etiology

- Chronic blepharitis
- Acne rosacea
- Seborrhea
- Tuberculosis
- Viral infection
- Any obstruction in the opening of the meibomian gland
- Uncorrected refractive errors.

Risk Factors

- Uncontrolled diabetes
- Long hours of work on computers
- Previous history of chalazion
- Family history of chalazion
- Oily skin.

Disorders of Eye

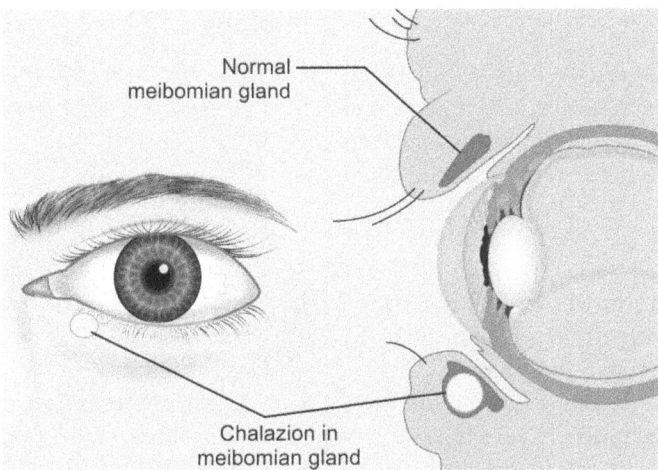

Fig. 3.4: Shows the formation of lump in the eyelid causing inflammation and scar tissue (Chalazion).

Pathophysiology

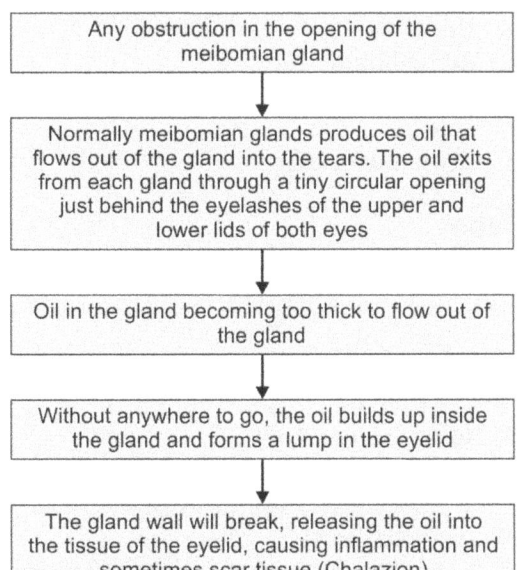

Clinical Features

- Small lump on the eyelid
- Burning feeling in the eyelid
- Drooping of the eyelid
- Swelling on the eyelid
- Eyelid tenderness
- Increased tearing
- Heaviness of the eyelid
- Itching of the eye or eyelid
- Trouble seeing
- Sensitivity to light.

Complications

- Astigmatism due to pressure on the cornea
- Hypopigmentation
- Sebaceous cell carcinoma
- Orbital cellulitis
- Recurrence.

Diagnostic Tests

- History
- Physical examination
- Biopsy test
- Swab examination
- Ophthalmic examination.

Management

Medical

- **Watchful waiting:** It may be advised if the chalazion is not causing any problems, since 25–50% of people get better without any treatment. However, the condition can take between 2 and 6 months or more to resolve.
- **Antibiotics:** It helps to control the infection, which will inturn reduces the swelling and facilitates the meibomian gland to open and allow the oily fluid that had collected there to drain. For example, doxycycline, minocycline, tetracycline, etc.
- **Weak topical steroids:** It helps in controlling eye and eyelid swelling of a chalazion. For example, fluorometholone, loteprednol, triamcinolone, etc.

Surgical

- **Surgical drainage:** It is a surgical procedure in which the eyelid is numbed and a small cut is made on the inside of the eyelid to release the contents of the cyst (a fluid-filled swelling).

Nursing

- Encourage the patient to place warm compresses over the eyelid for 10 to 15 minutes at least four times a day
- Educate the patient to do gentle massage to express the glandular secretions
- Instruct the patient not to rub their eyes as this can irritate the eyes and let it bacteria into it
- Instruct the patient to protect their eyes from dust and air pollution with the help of safety glasses
- Instruct the patient to avoid eye makeup especially mascara as it can grow bacteria in it.

CONJUNCTIVITIS

Definition

Conjunctivitis (also known as pink eye or red eye) is the redness and inflammation of the membranes (conjunctiva) covering the whites of the eyes and the membranes on the inner part of the eyelids.

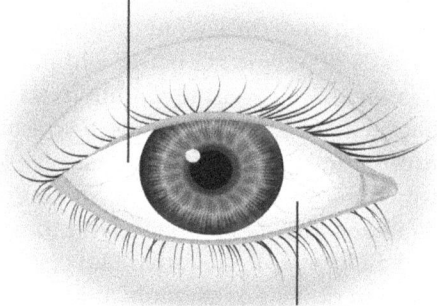

Fig. 3.5: Depicts the uninflamed and inflamed conjunctiva (conjunctivitis).

Etiology

- Virus infection (Adenovirus infection)
- Bacterial infection (Staphylococcal infection)
- Allergy provoking agents
- Irritants
- Toxic agents
- Use of marijuana
- Use of contact lenses (especially extended-wear lenses)
- Household dust
- Pollen from trees and grass
- Mold spores
- Animal dander.

Risk Factors

- People who work in health care settings
- Children's
- Upper respiratory tract infection
- Air pollution
- Skin medicines
- Smoke
- Use of perfumes.

Types

1. **Allergic conjunctivitis:**
   - It is an itchy type leading to eyelid swelling
   - Chronic allergy often causes itching and irritation.
2. **Viral conjunctivitis:**
   - It is often associated with infection of the upper respiratory tract, common cold or a sore throat
   - Its features include watery discharge and variable itching
   - It usually begins with one eye and later spreads to the other very easily.
3. **Bacterial conjunctivitis:**
   - It is often associated with pyogenic infections
   - Its features include eye pain, swelling, redness and a moderate to large amount of discharge usually yellow or red in color.

4. ***Irritant or toxic conjunctivitis:***
   - It is caused due to any toxic agents or eye irritants
   - Its features include irritable and painful eyes when an eye is pointed far down and far up.

Pathophysiology

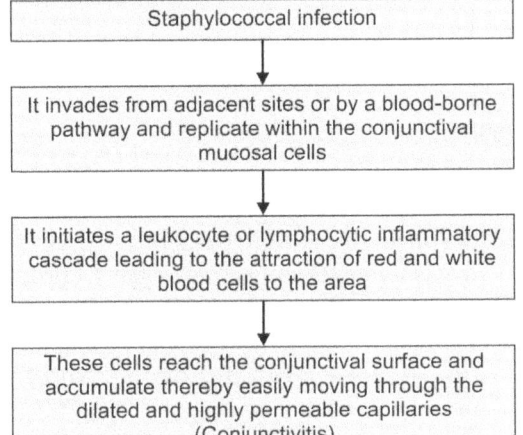

Clinical Features

- Pink or red color in the white of the eye (Hyperemia)
- Eye pain
- Blurred vision
- Crusts that form on the eyelid overnight
- Gritty feeling in the eyes
- Watery eyes (Epiphora)
- Itchy or scratchy eyes
- Sensitivity to light
- Irritation (Chemosis).

Complications

- Spreading the condition to others
- Scarring of the cornea
- Recurrence
- Abscess around the eye.

Diagnostic Tests

- History
- Physical examination
- Smear examination
- Visual acuity test
- Ophthalmic examination
- Immunoassay test
- Biomicroscopic examination.

Management

Medical

- **Antibiotics:** It helps to control the infections, which will inturn reduces the swelling and redness in conjunctivitis. For example, fusidic acid, chloramphenicol, etc.
- **Corticosteroids:** It helps in controlling the inflammation and swelling of conjunctival infection as a short-term measure. For example, dexamethasone, fluorometholone acetate, medrysone, etc.
- **Mast cell stabilizer:** It blocks the calcium channel essential for mast cell degranulation, stabilizing the cell and thereby preventing the release of histamine and related mediators in conjunctivitis. For example, cromolyn sodium, nedocromil sodium, lodoxamide tromethamine, etc.
- **Anti-histamine agonist:** It serves to reduce or eliminate effects mediated by histamine, an endogenous chemical mediator released during allergic reactions in conjunctivitis. For example, Emedastine Difumarate drops, etc.
- **Antihistamine/mast cell stabilizer:** It helps in preventing the release of histamine and other chemicals made by the body during an allergic reaction in conjunctivitis. For example, ketotifen fumarate, olopatadine hydrochloride, etc.

Nursing

- Instruct the patient not to rub the infected eye
- Encourage the patients to wear glasses instead of contact lenses
- Instruct the patient to avoid sharing common articles such as unwashed towels, cups and glasses
- Make the patient to wash their hands often with soap and warm water
- Enforce the patient not to use eye drops that were used for an infected eye to a non-infected eye.

CORRECTABLE REFRACTIVE ERRORS

Definition
Refraction error is a condition in which the shape of the eye does not bend light correctly, resulting in a blurred image.

Etiology
- *Eye length:* If the eye is too long, light is focused before it reaches the retina, causing nearsightedness. If the eye is too short, light is not focused by the time it reaches the retina. This causes farsightedness or hyperopia.
- *Curvature of the cornea:* If the cornea is not perfectly spherical, then the image is refracted or focused irregularly to create a condition called astigmatism. A person can be nearsighted or farsighted with or without astigmatism.
- *Curvature of the lens:* If the lens is too steeply curved in relation to the length of the eye and the curvature of the cornea, this causes nearsightedness. If the lens is too flat, the result is farsightedness.

Risk Factors
- Frequent performance of work requiring extensive use of close vision
- Advanced age
- Presence of uncorrected hyperopia
- Accidents affecting the crystalline lens
- Diabetes
- Multiple sclerosis.

Types
The following are the common refractive errors:
- *Myopia (Nearsightedness):* A myopic eye is longer than normal or has a cornea that is too steep, as a result of which the light rays focus in front of the retina. Close objects look clear, but distant objects appear blurred.
- *Astigmatism (Cylindrical error):* It is a condition in which the eye does not focus

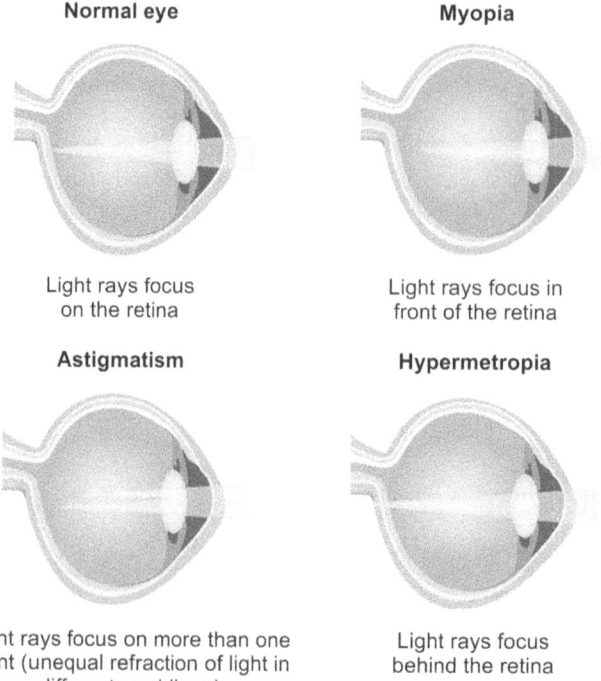

Fig. 3.6: Portrays the different types of correctable refractive errors.

light evenly onto the retina, the light-sensitive tissue at the back of the eye. This can cause images to appear blurry and stretched out.
- *Hypermetropia (Farsightedness):* Hypermetropia is a condition of farsightedness. The causes of an eye that is too short or a cornea that is too flat, as a result of which images focus at a point behind the retina. People with hypermetropia can usually see distant objects well, but have trouble focusing on nearby objects.
- *Presbyopia:* It is an age-related condition in which the ability to focus up close becomes more difficult. As the eye ages, the lens can no longer change shape enough to allow the eye to focus close objects clearly.

Pathophysiology

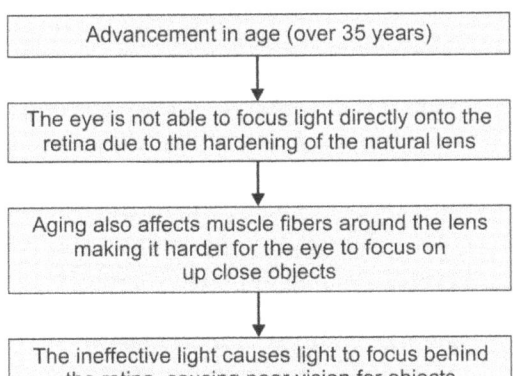

Clinical Features

- Blurred vision
- Double vision
- Haziness
- Glare or halos around bright lights
- Squinting
- Headache
- Eye strain.

Complications

- Macular degeneration
- Retinal detachment
- Glaucoma
- Strabismus or amblyopia
- Vision difficulty.

Diagnostic Tests

- History
- Physical examination
- Examination of the retina
- Muscle integrity test
- Refraction test
- Visual acuity test
- Slit lamp test.

Management

Surgical

- **Eye glasses:** Myopia may be corrected using a concave lens, and hyperopia may be corrected using a convex lens. Both lenses focus light rays on the retina, correcting poor distance vision or near vision, respectively. Astigmatism may be corrected using lenses which correspond especially to the patient's corneal deformations. Eyeglasses are the simplest and safest means of correcting presbyopia. Eyeglasses for presbyopia have higher focusing power in the lower portion of the lens. This allows us to read through the lower portion of the lens and see properly at distant through the upper portion of the lens.
- **Contact lenses:** In the cases of myopia, hyperopia, and astigmatism, contact lenses often provide a better correction of both visual acuity and peripheral vision than glasses. If suffering from myopia or hyperopia, we can use either soft or hard contact lenses. Astigmatism may be corrected either by hard contact lenses or soft tonic contact lenses, which operate on the same principles as glasses.
- **Photorefractive keratectomy (PRK):** It is the surgical removal of the superficial corneal cell layer, called the epithelium, and the reshaping of the cornea just below with a computer-controlled laser. This procedure flattens the cornea in myopic patients and rounds it in hyperopic

patients, permitting light rays to converge on the retina rather than in front of or behind it.

- **Laser in-situ keratomileusis (LASIK):** It is a surgical technique designed to decrease the cornea's thickness in order to modify its refraction capacity. The procedure involves the creation of a corneal flap which is raised to expose the cornea. The laser then sculpts the cornea to the desired thickness. Following the surgery, visual recovery is quick, and most patients experience a major improvement in their vision within a day. It is used to treat myopia, astigmatism, and hyperopia.
- **Laser epithelial keratomileusis (LASEK):** It is a surgical procedure in which the cornea of the eye is reshaped using a laser with a flap of tissue being cut as part of the procedure.
- **Epi-LASIK:** It is a refractive surgery technique designed to reduce a person's dependency on eyeglasses and contact lenses.
- **Intraocular implants:** These are optic lenses of varying power, made of synthetic material, which are either placed in front of the crystalline lens or used to replace it. They permit the restoration of near or distance vision, depending on the eye condition they are used to correct. After the surgery, an instrument called an optic biometer will be used to measure the length of the eye and calculate how powerful the implant is. This will ensure that the capsule surrounding the crystalline lens remains intact. This procedure is generally performed on patients with severe myopia or hyperopia, for whom laser procedures do not yield satisfactory results. Moreover, in patients whose cornea is too thin for laser treatment, an intraocular implant may be the best solution.
- **Radial keratotomy:** It is a surgical procedure which is used to correct myopia (nearsightedness). The procedure involves making microscopic, radial incisions (keratotomies) in the cornea to alter the curvature of the cornea, thus, correcting light refraction.
- **Astigmatic keratotomy:** It is a surgical procedure, which is used to correct astigmatism (an irregularly-shaped cornea which causes blurring). Instead of using a radial pattern of incisions, the incisions were made in a curved pattern when performing this procedure.
- **Automated lamellar keratoplasty (ALK):** It is a surgical procedure that is used for hyperopia (farsightedness) and severe cases of myopia (nearsightedness). A person with hyperopia has shorter-than-normal eyes or has a corneal that is too flat, causing objects up close to look blurry. Although each procedure varies slightly, in general, surgery for myopia involves cutting a flap across the front of the cornea with a microkeratome (surgical instrument). The flap is folded to the side and a thin slice of tissue is removed from the surface of the cornea. The removal of tissue flattens the central cornea, or optical zone, reducing refraction. The flap is then put back in place, where it adheres without sutures. During surgery for hyperopia, deeper incision is made into the cornea with the microkeratome (a surgical instrument) to create a flap. The internal pressure in the eye causes the corneal surface to stretch and bulge. The bulging cornea improves the optical power, correcting the hyperopia. The flap is then put back in place, where it adheres without sutures.
- **Laser thermal keratoplasty (LTK):** It is a surgical procedure in which heat is applied from a laser to the periphery of the cornea to shrink the collagen fibers, and reshaping the cornea. When the tissue is treated thermally, it contracts the tissue and causes the central cornea to steepen.
- **Conductive keratoplasty (CK):** It is a surgical procedure which uses heat from low-level, radio frequency waves, rather than laser or scalpel, to shrink the collagen

and change the shape of the cornea. A probe that is smaller than a strand of hair is used to apply the radio waves around the outer cornea. This creates a constrictive band that increases the curve of the cornea and improves vision.
- **Intracorneal rings or Intacs:** It is a micro-thin intracorneal ring that is implanted into the cornea. Intacs produces a reshaping of the curvature of the cornea, thus improving vision. Intacs are rarely available in few developed countries for low degrees of myopia.

Nursing

- Encourage the patients to wear glasses instead of contact lenses
- Encourage the patient to wear sunglasses with ultraviolet protection lenses to protect the eyes when outdoors
- Educate the patient to improve lighting in their home with more brighter lamps
- Educate the patient to choose a healthy diet that includes plenty of fruits and vegetables.

DIABETIC RETINOPATHY

Definition

Diabetic retinopathy is a condition occurring in persons with diabetes, which causes progressive damage to the retina, the light sensitive lining at the back of the eye.

Etiology

High blood glucose level.

Risk Factors

- Poorly controlled diabetes
- High blood pressure
- American race with diabetes
- Pregnant mothers with diabetes
- Long-term duration of diabetes
- Elevated blood cholesterol levels
- Sleep apnea
- Smoking.

Stages

It has four stages as follows:
1. *Mild nonproliferative retinopathy:*
   - In this stage, microaneurysm occurs
   - They are small areas of balloon like swelling in the retina's tiny blood vessels.
2. *Moderate nonproliferative retinopathy:*
   - In this stage, blood vessels that nourish the retina are blocked.
3. *Severe nonproliferative retinopathy:*
   - Much more blood vessels are blocked depriving several areas of the retina with their blood supply
   - These areas of the retina send signals to the body to grow new blood vessels for nourishment.
4. *Proliferative retinopathy:*
   - In this advanced stage, the signals sent by the retina for nourishment will trigger the growth of new blood vessels

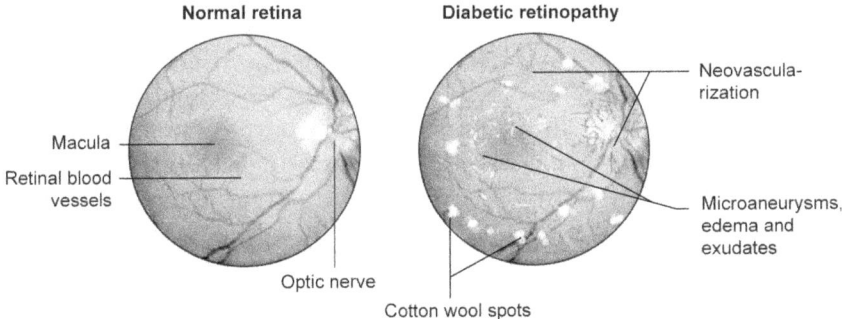

Fig. 3.7: Shows the comparison of normal retina with that of diabetic retinopathy.

- These new blood vessels are abnormal and fragile and they grow along the surface of the clear, vitreous gel that fills the inside of the retina
- If these blood vessels leak severe vision loss may occur leading to blindness.

Pathophysiology

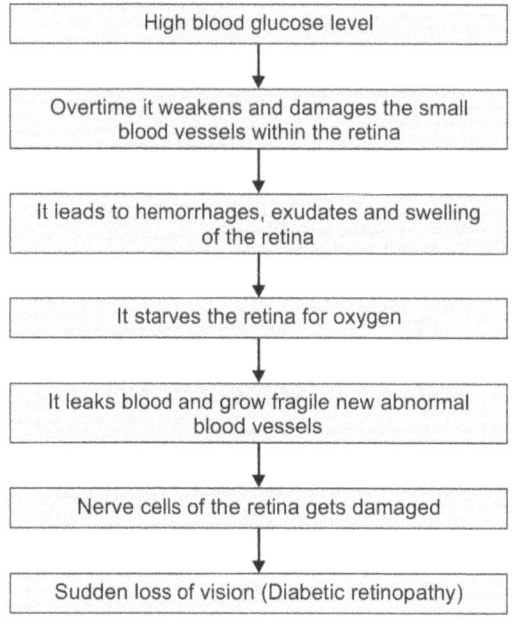

Clinical Features

- Blurred vision
- Flashes of light in the field of vision
- Loss of vision
- Blotches or spots in vision
- Eye strain
- Headache
- Impairment of color vision
- Poor night vision.

Complications

- Retinal detachment
- Glaucoma
- Sudden loss of vision.

Diagnostic Tests

- History
- Physical examination
- Dilated eye examination
- Fluorescein angiography
- Color fundus photography
- Fundoscopic examination
- Ocular coherence tomography (OCT) scan
- Tonometric examination
- Slit lamp test.

Management

Medical

- **Anti-VEGF therapy:** It involves the injection of the medication into the back of the eye. The medication is an antibody designed to bind to and remove the excess VEGF (vascular endothelial growth factor) present in the eye that is causing the diabetic retinopathy. For example, ranibizumab, bevacizumab, etc.
- **Intraocular steroid agents:** It helps reduce the amount of fluid leaking into the retina, resulting in visual improvement. For example, dexamethasone, triamcinolone, prednisone, etc.

Surgical

- **Laser photocoagulation:** It is a surgical procedure in which a laser is focused on the damaged retina to seal leaking retinal vessels. For abnormal blood vessel growth (neovascularization), the laser treatments are delivered over the peripheral retina. The small laser scars that result will reduce abnormal blood vessel growth and help bond the retina to the back of the eye, thus preventing retinal detachment. Laser surgery can greatly reduce the chance of severe visual impairment.
- **Pan retinal photocoagulation (PRP):** It creates burns in the retina with the hope of reducing the retina's oxygen demand and hence the possibility of ischemia and also destroys the abnormal blood vessels that form in the retina.
- **Vitrectomy:** It is a microsurgical procedure that is performed to remove the blood-filled vitreous and replace it with a clear solution.

Nursing

- Instruct the patient not to smoke
- Motivate the patient to have their blood pressure and cholesterol checked regularly
- Instruct the patient to maintain a healthy weight
- Educate the patient to choose a healthy diet that includes plenty of fruits and vegetables.

EYE TRAUMA

Definition

Eye trauma refers to any damage caused by a direct blow to the eye and can be a serious threat to vision if not treated appropriately and in a timely fashion.

Etiology

- Foreign bodies in the eye (such as dirt, pebbles, insects, etc)
- Unsafe storage of chemicals
- Aerosol exposure
- Fingernails
- Toys
- Fighting with each other
- Falling
- Accidentally struck by a person or object
- Car crash
- Fireworks.

Risk Factors

- Being distracted
- Using tools
- Tool malfunction
- Performing an unfamiliar task
- Being rushed
- Working overtime
- Feeling fatigued
- Excessive bright lights or ultraviolet rays
- Dusty environment
- Compressed air
- Use of contact lenses.

Types

- ***Corneal abrasion:*** It is a scratch or injury to the cornea, the clear, dome-shaped surface that covers the front of the eye. It most commonly occurs in children.
- ***Chemical burns:*** It occurs when any type of chemicals exposed into the eye accidentally. Chemical burns are a medical emergency, and your child should receive immediate medical care. It can result in a loss of vision and even a loss of the eye itself, if not treated promptly and accurately.
- ***Hyphema:*** It refers to blood in the anterior chamber of the eye. The anterior chamber is the front section of the eye's interior where fluid flows in and out, providing nourishment to the eye and surrounding tissues.
- ***Ecchymosis (black eye or bruising):*** It usually occurs from some type of injury to the eye, causing the tissue around the eye to become bruised.
- ***Fractures of the orbit:*** The orbit is the bony structure around the eye. When

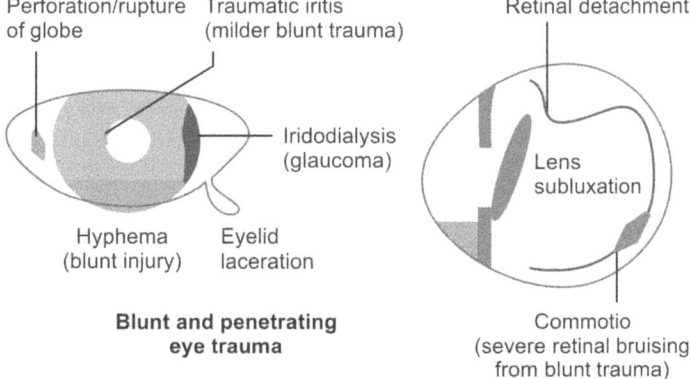

Fig. 3.8: Depicts blunt and penetrating eye trauma.

one or more bones surrounding the eye are broken, the condition is called orbital fracture. An orbital fracture usually occurs after some type of injury or a strike to the face. Depending on where the fracture is located, it can be associated with severe eye injury and damage.
- **Eyelid lacerations:** These are cuts to the eyelid caused by injury.

Pathophysiology

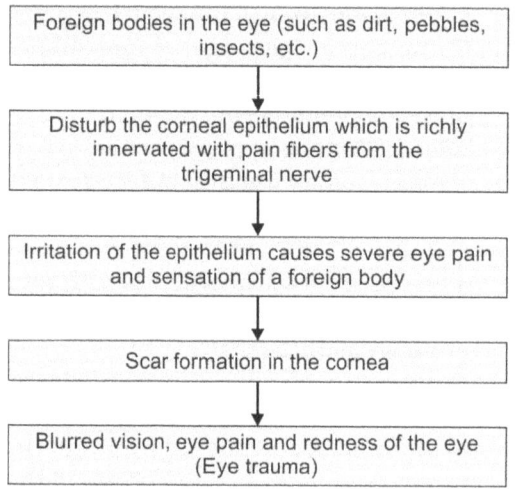

Clinical Features

- Blurred vision
- Eye pain or stinging and burning in the eye
- Feeling like something is in the eye.
- Sensitivity to light
- Redness of the eye
- Swollen eyelids
- Watery eyes or increased tearing.

Complications

- Corneal scarring
- Hyphema
- Iridodialysis
- Post-traumatic glaucoma
- Uveitis cataract
- Vitreous hemorrhage
- Retinal detachment.

Diagnostic Tests

- History
- Physical examination
- Seidel's test
- Dilated eye examination
- Ophthalmic examination
- Slit lamp test.

Management

Medical

- **Irrigation:** It is the first line of management for chemical injuries and performs copious irrigation of eye with isotonic saline or sterile water.
- **Patching:** Depending on the type of ocular injury, either a pressure patch or shield patch is applied.
- **Suturing:** It may be a part of appropriate management in cases of eyelid laceration.

Nursing

- Instruct the patient to maintain equipments and make sure all safety devices including guards or shields are in good working order.
- Encourage to use water to dampen dusty environment.
- Instruct the patient to keep adequate first aid equipment in the first aid kit.
- Instruct the patient to wear safety goggles at all times when using hand or power tools or chemicals, during high impact sports or during other activities where they may get an eye injury.
- Instruct the patient to be careful while using household cleansers.

GLAUCOMA

Definition

Glaucoma refers to a group of disorders that lead to damage to the optic nerve, the nerve that carries visual information from the eye to the brain.

Etiology

- Infection
- Inflammation
- Tumors
- Cataracts
- Migraine
- Retinal detachment

Disorders of Eye

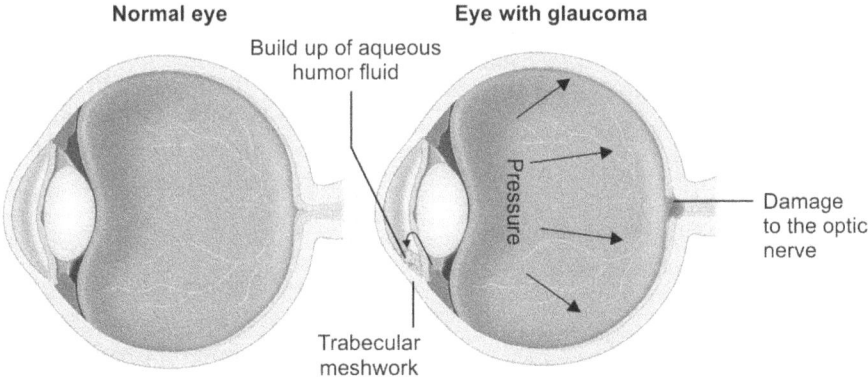

Fig. 3.9: Shows the comparison of normal eye with that of an eye with glaucoma.

- Bad diet
- Wearing contact lenses
- Too much reading or reading in low light.

Risk Factors

- Over 60 years of age
- Elevated eye pressure
- Hypothyroidism or diabetes
- African American descent
- Food sensitivities
- Stress
- Sedentary lifestyle
- Thin cornea
- Family history of glaucoma
- Nearsightedness or farsightedness
- Past injuries to the eyes
- Steroid use
- History of severe anemia or shock.

Types

- ***Open-angle glaucoma:*** It is the most common type of glaucoma in Caucasians (people of white skin). It occurs when the aqueous humor (the clear liquid that nourishes the inside of the front of the eye) does not drain properly, causing the pressure in the eye to rise and eventually damage the optic nerve.
- ***Angle-closure glaucoma:*** It is the most common form of glaucoma in some Asian populations. It occurs when the peripheral part of the iris (the colored part of the eye) blocks the outflow pathways. It can be sudden in onset or develop slowly over time.
- ***Normal-tension glaucoma:*** It is a type of glaucoma without high eye pressure; it occurs when there is progressive optic nerve damage and loss of peripheral vision, despite the eye pressures being within normal range for the population.
- ***Secondary glaucoma:*** It can develop as a result of other conditions such as eye injuries, cataracts, diabetes and inflammation of the eye or the use of certain medications (particularly those containing steroids).
- ***Congenital glaucoma:*** It is a rare form of glaucoma present at birth or that develops in infants. It is caused by the improper development of the baby's drainage channels and can lead to the eyes expanding in size, with excessive eye watering and light intolerance.

Pathophysiology

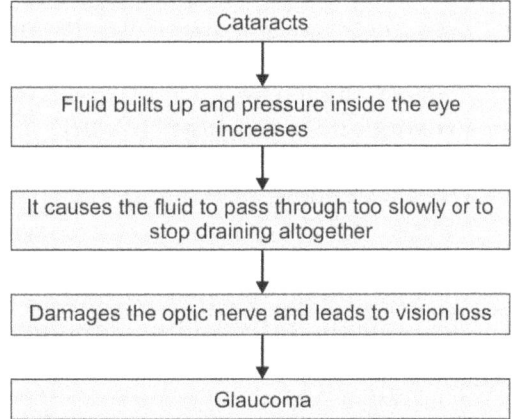

Clinical Features

- Unusual trouble adjusting to dark rooms
- Difficulty focusing on near/distant objects
- Squinting or blinking due to unusual sensitivity to light or glare
- Change in color of iris
- Red-rimmed, encrusted or swollen lids
- Recurrent pain in or around eyes
- Double vision
- Dark spot at the center of viewing
- Lines and edges appear distorted or wavy
- Excess tearing or watery eyes
- Dry eyes with itching or burning
- Seeing spots, ghost-like images.

Complications

- Sudden loss of vision in one eye
- Sudden hazy or blurred vision
- Flashes of light or black spots
- Halos or rainbows around light.

Diagnostic Tests

- History
- Physical examination
- Visual acuity test
- Visual field test
- Dilated eye exam
- Tonometric examination
- Pachymetric examination
- Ophthalmic examination.

Management

Medical

- **Beta blockers:** It reduces the amount of fluid being secreted into the eye. For example, timolol, etc.
- **Prostaglandin analogs:** It works by increasing the drainage of fluid out of the eye. For example, latanoprost, travatan, lumigan, etc.
- **Sympathomimetics:** It reduces the amount of fluid secreted into the eye. For example, brimonidine, lopidine, etc.
- **Carbonic anhydrase inhibitors:** It reduces the secretion of fluid into the eye. For example, dorzolamide, etc.
- **Miotics or cholinergic agents:** It increases the drainage of fluid out of the eye. For example, pilocarpine, etc.

Surgical

- **Trabeculectomy:** It is a surgical procedure that involves an incision to remove a piece of tissue to allow fluid to drain from the eye.
- **Tube-shunt surgery:** It is a surgical procedure that involves an incision to place a tube in the eye to allow fluid to drain.
- **Laser trabeculoplasty:** It is a surgical procedure in which the tissue is burnt to create an opening that allows fluid to drain from the eye.
- **Sclerostomy:** It is a surgical procedure which removes a piece of the white part of the eye to allow fluid to drain.
- **Iridotomy:** It is a surgical procedure that involves making puncture-like openings through the iris without the removal of iris tissue.
- **Iridectomy:** It is a surgical procedure that involves the removal of a portion of iris tissue.
- **Viscocanalostomy:** It is a surgical procedure in which Schlemm's canal is exposed by making a large and very deep scleral flap.
- **Goniotomy:** It is a surgical procedure that involves cutting the fibers of the trabecular meshwork to allow aqueous fluid to flow more freely from the eye.

Nursing

- Encourage the patient to eat a healthy diet to maintain the health.
- Instruct the patient to sleep with heads elevated to reduce intra ocular pressure.
- Instruct the patient to avoid intake of caffeine drinks as it increase the intraocular pressure.
- Encourage the patient to do regular exercise as it reduces intraocular pressure.

HORDEOLUM (STYE)

Definition

A hordeolum or stye is a bacterial infection of the mucus secreting sebaceous glands at the base of the eyelashes either on the inner surface or on the margin of the eyelid.

Etiology

- Bacterial infection (*Staphylococcus aureus*)
- Blepharitis
- Ocular rosacea
- Meibomian gland dysfunction
- Wearing contact lenses
- Make-up or cosmetic application.

Risk Factors

- Stress
- Poor nutrition
- Using the same razor to shave
- It is most common in infants.
- Poor eyelid hygiene.

Types

- *External hordeolum:* It emerges along the edge of the eyelid. It can become yellow, filled with pus and painful when touched. It is also called an external stye.
- *Internal hordeolum:* It develops inside the eyelid. It is much more painful. It is also called an internal stye.

Pathophysiology

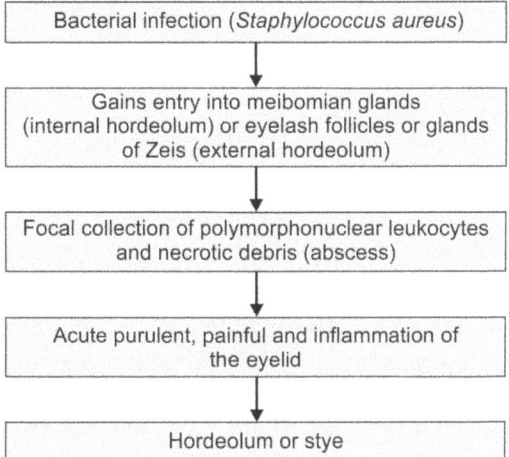

Clinical Features

- Tenderness, pain and redness in the affected area
- Itching
- Swelling
- Watering of the eye
- Sensitivity to light
- Discomfort when blinking
- Sometimes a yellowish bump develops in the affected area.

Complications

- Decreased vision
- Hyperopia
- Meibomian cyst
- Pre-orbital cellulitis (Pre-septal cellulitis)
- Chalazion
- Cosmetic deformity.

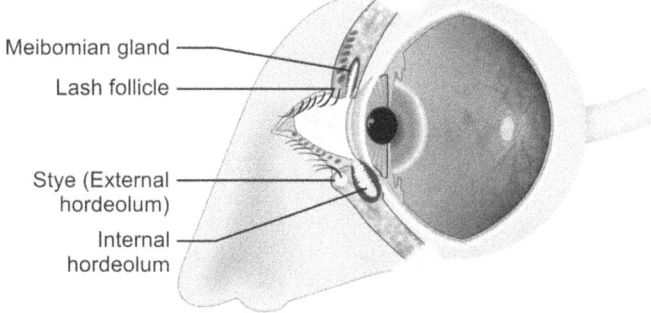

Fig. 3.10: Depicts an eye with hordeolum or stye.

Diagnostic Tests

- History
- Physical examination
- Visual acuity test
- Slit lamp test
- Dilated fundoscopic examination.

Management

Medical

- **Topical antibiotics:** It interferes with bacterial cell wall synthesis by inhibition of the regeneration of phospholipid receptors involved in peptidoglycan synthesis. For example, Bacitracin zinc, polymyxin B sulfate, erythromycin, etc.

Surgical

- **Draining of hordeola or stye:** It is a surgical procedure which is performed on hordeola or sties that do not respond to any type of therapies. The procedure consists of making a small incision on the inner or outer surface of the eyelid, depending if the stye is pointing externally or not. After the incision is made, the pus is drained out of the gland, and very small and unnoticeable sutures are used to close the lesion.

Nursing

- Instruct the patient not to squeeze or open the hordeola.
- Provide information to the patient that most hordeola will heal spontaneously within 1-2 weeks, after swelling, breaking open and draining on their own.
- Encourage the patient to maintain good eyelid hygiene.
- Assist the patient with 4-5 warm compresses per day to promote drainage and resolution of these lesions.
- Instruct the patient not to rub the eyes.
- Instruct the patient to wash the hands before touching the eyes.

KERATITIS

Definition

Keratitis is a condition in which the cornea of the eye becomes inflamed and is often accompanied by a moderate to intense pain which leads to impaired eyesight.

Etiology

- Injury to the cornea
- Contaminated contact lenses
- Herpes viruses
- Contaminated water.

Risk Factors

- Wearing contact lenses
- Reduced immunity
- Warm climate
- Use of corticosteroids
- Eye injury.

Types

- **Amoebic keratitis:** It is due to amoebic infection in the cornea.

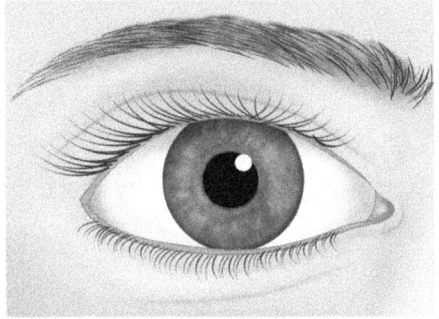
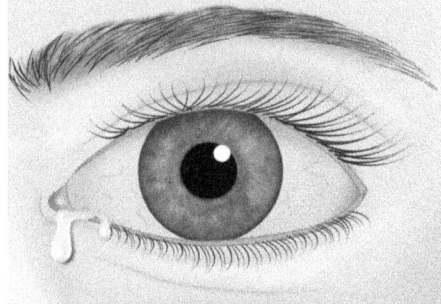

Healthy eye   Keratitis

Fig. 3.11: Shows the comparison of healthy eye with that of an eye with keratitis.

- **Bacterial keratitis:** It is due to bacterial infection in the cornea.
- **Fungal keratitis:** It is due to fungal infection in the cornea.
- **Viral keratitis:** It is due to viral infection in the cornea.
- **Onchocercal keratitis:** It is due to onchocerciasis.
- **Exposure keratitis:** It is due to exposure to certain chemicals.
- **Photo keratitis:** It is due to intense ultraviolet radiation exposure.
- **Vernal keratitis:** It is due to severe allergic response.
- **Ulcerative keratitis:** It is due to ulceration of the cornea.
- **Nonulcerative sterile keratitis:** It is due to colonization of gram negative bacteria on contact lenses.

Pathophysiology

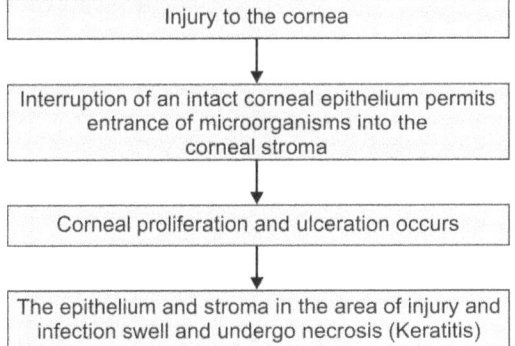

Clinical Features

- Inflamed conjunctiva
- Sensitivity to light (Photophobia)
- Reddened eyes
- Excess tears or other discharge from the eye
- Difficulty opening the eyelid because of pain or irritation
- Intense eye pain
- Blurred vision
- Decreased vision
- A feeling that something is in the eye
- Pus formation may occur in later stages.

Complications

- Chronic corneal inflammation
- Chronic or recurrent viral infections of the cornea
- Corneal ulcers
- Corneal swelling and scarring
- Temporary or permanent reduction in the vision
- Blindness
- Astigmatism
- Endophthalmitis.

Diagnostic Tests

- History
- Physical examination
- Blood examination
- Biopsy examination
- Penlight examination
- Slit lamp examination
- Smear examination
- Culture examination.

Management

Medical

- **Antibiotics:** It works by blocking bacteria from reproducing in the eye. For example, levofloxacin, ofloxacin, etc.
- **Anti-viral agents:** It is used to treat eye infections caused by the herpes simplex virus. For example, acyclovir, valacyclovir, etc.
- **Corticosteroids:** It helps in suppressing the inflammatory response and inhibits the body's defense mechanism against infection. For example, maxitrol, neomycin sulfate, etc.
- **Muscarinic receptor antagonists:** It blocks muscarinic receptors in the eye causing pupil dilation and difficulty for near vision accommodation. For example, atropine, scopolamine, etc.

Nursing

- Instruct the patient to follow strict aseptic technique of handwashing to prevent

spreading organisms from one eye to the other.
- Modify the patient environment or activities for safety.
- Encourage the patient to comply with the prescribed therapy.
- Promote appropriate health-seeking behaviors among patients.

RETINAL DETACHMENT

Definition

A retinal detachment is a disorder of the eye in which the retina of the eye peels away from its underlying layer of support tissue within the eye as a result of retinal break, hole or tear.

Etiology

- Lattice degeneration of the retina
- Trauma to the eye
- Cataract surgery
- Proliferic diabetic retinopathy
- Shrinkage or contraction of the vitreous
- Advanced diabetes
- An inflammatory eye disorder.

Risk Factors

- Being over 40 years old
- Highly nearsighted people (myopic)
- Use of pilocarpine eye drops
- Prior retinal detachment in the other eye
- Family history of retinal detachment.

Types

- ***Rhegmatogenous retinal detachment:*** It is a type of retinal detachment which occurs due to a hole, tear or break in the retina that allows fluid to pass from the vitreous space into the subretinal space between the sensory retina and the retinal pigment epithelium.
- ***Exudative, serous, or secondary retinal detachment:*** It is a type of retinal detachment which occurs due to inflammation, injury or vascular abnormalities that result in fluid accumulating underneath the retina without the presence of a hole, tear or break.
- ***Tractional retinal detachment:*** It is a type of retinal detachment which occurs when fibrovascular tissue, caused by an injury, inflammation or neovascularization pulls the sensory retina and retinal pigment epithelium.

Pathophysiology

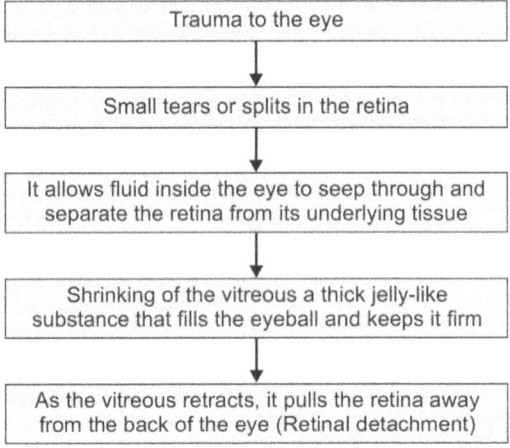

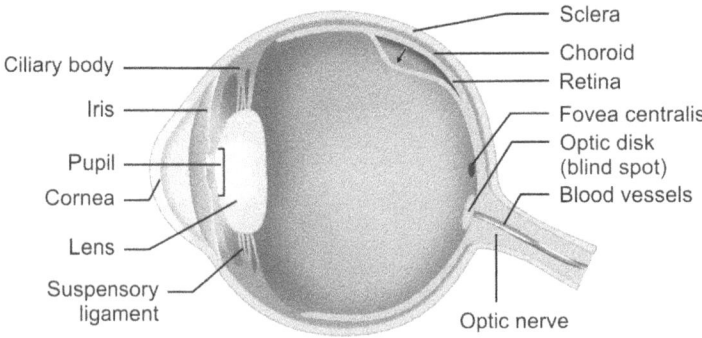

Fig. 3.12: Shows the traumatic eye with retinal detachment.

Clinical Features

- Flashing lights (Photopsia)
- Sudden increase in the number of floater
- Dense shadow appearance that starts in the peripheral vision and slowly progressing towards the central vision
- Feeling of heaviness in the eye
- A ring of floaters or hairs on the temporal side of the central vision
- Impression of a veil or curtain was drawn over the field of vision
- Straight lines will suddenly appear curved
- Central visual loss.

Complications

- Bleeding into the eyeball
- Built-up of pressure inside the eyeball
- Cataract formation.

Diagnostic Tests

- History
- Physical examination
- Retinal examination
- Peripheral fundus examination
- Visual acuity test
- Ultrasound scan
- Indirect ophthalmoscopy
- Direct fundoscopy
- Slit lamp examination.

Management

Surgical

- **Photocoagulation laser surgery:** It is a surgical procedure in which a laser is used to seal the tears by burning the retina. This makes scar tissue form. A scar helps to anchor the retina to the back of the eye.
- **Cryopexy:** It is a surgical procedure in which a small, extremely cold instrument called a cryoprobe prompts the retina to produce scar tissue. This tissue seals the tear, and helps to anchor the retina to the back of the eye.
- **Pneumatic retinopexy:** It is a surgical procedure in which a gas bubble is injected into the vitreous cavity and treats the tear (s) with either laser or cryotherapy (freezing). The bubble presses the retina flat against the wall of the eye and the laser or freezing sticks the retina down. The gas gradually disappears over the days or weeks following the surgery.
- **Scleral buckling:** It is a surgical procedure in which the fluid under the retina is drained and sutured (sews) a specially shaped piece of silicone rubber to the outer wall of the eye (the sclera). The silicone creates an indent, which closes the tear and holds it in place while the cryotherapy seal has time to form.
- **Vitrectomy:** It is a surgical procedure in which under an operating microscope, the vitreous is removed using very fine instruments. It treats any tears with laser or cryotherapy and fill the eye with gas or silicone oil. Poor vision will be experienced while the eye is filled with gas. However, if the surgery is successful, the vision will improve as the gas reabsorbs and is replaced with the eye's own clear fluid.

Nursing

- Educate the patient to improve lighting in their home with more brighter lamps.
- Encourage the patient to use glasses that are specifically prescribed for the effects of retinal detachment to optimize the vision.
- Discuss with the patient the allowed and restricted activities at home.
- Instruct the patient to avoid heavy lifting, deep bending or otherwise injuring the head.

STRABISMUS (SQUINT EYES) (CROSSED EYES)

Definition

It is the misalignment or wandering of one or both eyes either inward (esotropia), outward (exotropia), up (hypertropia) or down (hypotropia).

Etiology

- Thyroid eye disease
- Cataract

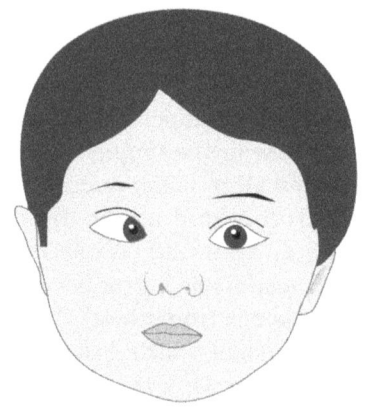

Fig. 3.13: Shows an eye with strabismus or squint eyes.

- Eye injuries
- Cranial nerve palsies
- Myasthenia gravis
- Traumatic brain injury
- Botulism
- Diabetes
- Guillain-Barre syndrome
- Shellfish poisoning.

Risk Factors

- Family history of strabismus
- Refractive error
- Down's syndrome
- Cerebral palsy
- Stroke
- Head injury.

Pathophysiology

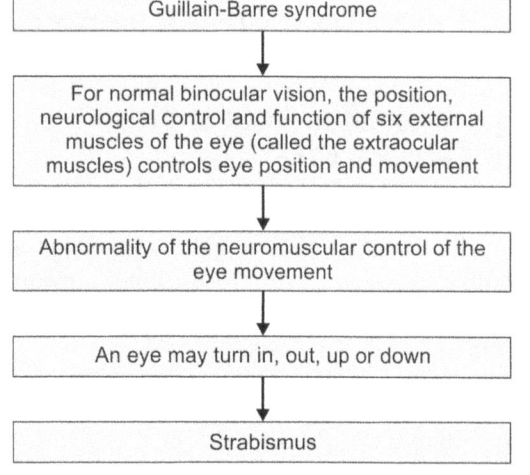

Clinical Features

- Crossed eyes
- Double vision
- Eyes that do not align in the same direction
- Uncoordinated eye movements (eyes do not move together)
- Loss of vision or depth perception.

Complications

- Infection
- Slipped muscles
- Scleral perforation
- Endophthalmitis.

Diagnostic Tests

- History
- Physical examination
- Retinal examination
- Cover/uncover test
- Visual acuity test
- Corneal light reflex examination
- Simultaneous red reflex test
- Alternate-cover test
- Ophthalmic examination.

Management

Medical

- **Antibiotics:** It works by blocking the release of acetylcholine, so muscle contractions are reduced and thus temporarily decreases muscle activity in strabismus. For example, botox, ofloxacin, etc.
- **Eye glasses or contact lenses:** This is the first step in treating strabismus. The glasses should be worn all the time to treat the vision and the strabismus. It may help people who have crossed eyes due to an uncorrected farsightedness.
- **Patching:** It works by strengthening the weakened eye. It is advised to patch the good eye to encourage the squinting eye to work. Patching must be done in the first seven years of life while the eyes are still developing. The earlier the patching is started the better the result.

- **Prism lenses:** These are special lenses that have a prescription for prism power in them. The prisms alter the light entering the eye and assist in reducing the amount of turning, the eye has to do to look at objects. Sometimes, the prisms are able to fully compensate for and eliminate the eye turning.
- **Vision therapy:** It is a structured program of visual activities prescribed to improve eye coordination and eye focusing abilities. Vision therapy trains the eyes and brain to work together more effectively. These eye exercises help remediate deficiencies in eye movement, eye focusing and eye teaming and reinforce the eye–brain connection.

Surgical

- **Eye muscle surgery:** It can change the length or position of the muscles around the eye in an attempt to better align the eyes. Eye muscle surgery may be able to physically align the eyes so they appear straight. Often a program of vision therapy may also be needed to develop a functional improvement in eye coordination and to keep the eyes from reverting back to their previous condition of misalignment.

Nursing

- Instruct the patient to wear eye glasses or contact lenses for refraction error and to improve strabismus.
- Teach the patient the reason for using patching or corrective lenses and the expected results of it.
- Encourage the patient to use prism lenses that are specifically prescribed for the effects of strabismus to optimize the vision.
- Encourage the patient to comply with the prescribed therapy.

VISUAL IMPAIRMENT (BLINDNESS)

Definition

It refers to a loss of vision that cannot be corrected with glasses or contact lenses.

Fig. 3.14: Depicts an eye with visual impairment (Blindness).

Etiology

- Cataract
- Glaucoma
- Age-related macular degeneration
- Corneal opacities
- Onchocerciasis
- Childhood blindness
- Diabetic retinopathy
- Trachoma
- Injuries
- Infections
- Genetic diseases
- Poisoning
- Blocked blood vessels
- Retrolental fibroplasias (complications of premature birth)
- Complications of eye surgery
- Lazy eye (Amblyopia)
- Stroke
- Optic neuritis
- Retinoblastoma and optic glioma
- Retinitis pigmentosa.

Risk Factors

- Increased age
- Being female
- Living in developing countries
- Tobacco use
- Exposure to ultraviolet radiation
- High body mass index
- Vitamin A deficiency
- Metabolic disorders.

Types

- **Strabismus:** It is a condition in which the eyes look in different directions and

do not focus simultaneously on a single point.
- **Congenital cataract:** It is a condition in which the lens of the eye is cloudy.
- **Retinopathy of prematurity:** It is a condition that occurs in premature babies when the light-sensitive retina hasn't developed sufficiently before birth.
- **Retinitis pigmentosa:** It is a rare inherited disease that slowly destroys the retina.
- **Coloboma:** It is a condition where a portion of the structure of the eye is missing.
- **Optic nerve hypoplasia:** It is a condition that is caused by underdeveloped fibers in the optic nerve and which affects depth perception, sensitivity to light and acuity of vision.
- **Cortical visual impairment (CVI):** It is a condition which is caused by damage to the part of the brain related to vision, not to the eyes themselves.

Pathophysiology

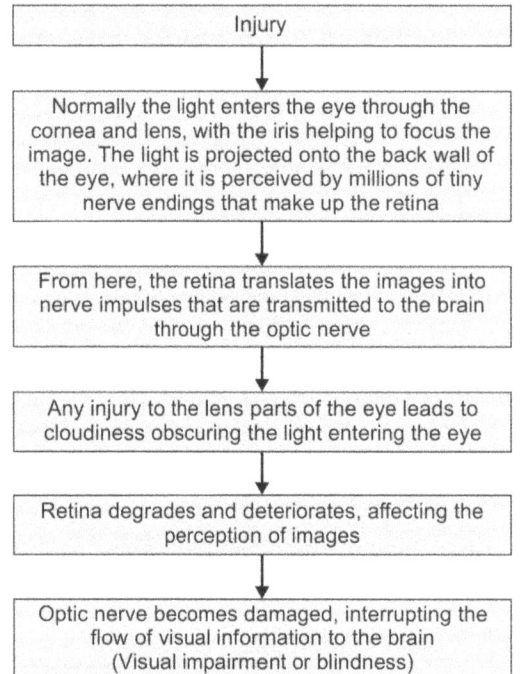

Clinical Features

- Leaning against the wall when walking
- Running into objects
- Difficulty in walking on uneven surfaces
- Difficulty in getting food onto a utensil
- Frequently spilling food
- Frequently knocking over items while reaching for something else
- Inability to read without holding an object very near the face or at an odd angle
- Difficulty in writing on the lines of a piece of paper
- Handwriting that is becoming less clear
- Frequently complaining that the lighting is inadequate for reading or writing
- Wearing mismatched clothing.

Complications

- Partial loss of vision
- Legal blindness
- Locked-in-syndrome.

Diagnostic Tests

- History
- Physical examination
- Ophthalmic examination
- Snellen test
- Visual field test
- Tonometric test
- Ocular motility assessment
- Electroretinogram (ERG)
- Visually evoked potential (VEP)
- Electrooculogram (EOG).

Management

Medical

- **White canes with a red tip:** It is used to extend the user's range of touch sensation. It is usually swung in a low sweeping motion, across the intended path of travel, to detect obstacles. However, techniques for cane travel can vary depending on the user and/or the situation. Some visually impaired persons do not carry these kinds of canes, opting instead for the shorter, lighter identification (ID) cane. Still others require a support cane. The choice depends on the individual's vision, motivation, and other factors.
- **Guide dogs:** A small number of people employ guide dogs to assist in mobility.

These dogs are trained to navigate around various obstacles, and to indicate when it becomes necessary to go up or down a step. However, the helpfulness of guide dogs is limited by the inability of dogs to understand complex directions.
- **GPS devices:** It can assist blind people with orientation and navigation, but it is not a replacement for traditional mobility tools such as white canes and guide dogs.
- **Computer adaptations:** There are numerous ways to modify a computer to make it usable by a person with visual impairment. For example, software programs can change the text size, screen background color, or text color. Screen readers speak everything on the screen, including text, graphics, control buttons, and menus in a computerized voice.

Surgical

- **Corneal transplantation made in the laboratory:** The corneas are made in the laboratory from recombinantly produced human collagen that is chemically treated and moulded into the shape of a normal cornea. Once the patient's damaged tissue is removed and the biosynthetic corneas are placed, the patient's own nerves and cells grow into the implant and begin to work properly.
- **Microchip implants:** The implant receives images from a camera mounted on a pair of glasses the person wears and then sends information directly to the brain through the optic nerves.
- **Modified osteo-odonto-keratoprosthesis (MOOKP):** It can give sight to people blinded by severe corneal damage by inserting one of their own teeth into their eye.

Nursing

- Instruct the patient to have enough lighting into the room to see the objects better.
- Instruct the patient to avoid falls by making some relatively small changes.
- Encourage the patient to wear sunglasses with ultraviolet protection lenses to protect the eyes when outdoors.
- Provide orientation and mobility training to the patient which will help him to move safely in or out of his home.

4
CHAPTER

Disorders of Ear, Nose and Throat

CHAPTER OUTLINE

- Acute pharyngitis
- Cerumen impaction
- Deviated nasal septum
- Epistaxis
- Hearing loss
- Labyrinthitis
- Mastoiditis
- Meniere's disease
- Nasal polyps
- Otitis media
- Otosclerosis
- Peritonsillar abscess
- Rhinitis
- Sinusitis
- Tonsillitis

ACUTE PHARYNGITIS (SORE THROAT)

Definition

Acute pharyngitis is a sudden onset of infection or inflammation of the mucous membranes of the oropharynx or nasopharynx.

Etiology

- Viral infection (e.g., Adenovirus, influenza, coronavirus, rhinovirus, enterovirus, Epstein-Barr virus, Herpes simplex virus, etc.)

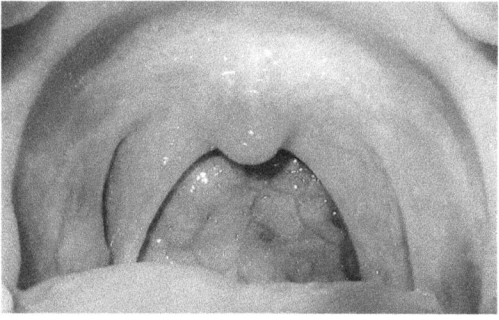

Fig. 4.1: Depicts acute pharyngitis.

- Bacterial infection (e.g., Group A beta-hemolytic streptococci, *Chlamydia pneumoniae*, *Neisseria gonorrhoeae*, etc.)
- Fungal infection (*Candida albicans*)
- Allergic rhinitis
- Sinusitis with postnasal drip
- Mouth breathing
- Trauma
- Gastroesophageal reflux disease (GERD).

Risk Factors

- Previous episodes of pharyngitis or tonsillitis
- Smoking
- Overcrowding
- Weakened immune system
- Use of corticosteroids
- Oral sex
- Diabetes mellitus
- Cold and flu seasons
- Having close contact with someone who has a sore throat or cold.

Pathophysiology

```
Viral infection (e.g., Adenovirus, influenza,
coronavirus, rhinovirus, enterovirus, Epstein-Barr
virus, herpes simplex virus, etc.)
                    ↓
Viruses gain access to the mucosal cells lining the
nasopharynx oropharynx and replicate
in these cells
                    ↓
Infection or inflammation of the mucous membrane
of nasopharynx or oropharynx (Acute pharyngitis)
```

Clinical Features

- Persistent sore throat for more than six weeks which is reddish and enlarged
- Excessive drooling
- Trismus
- Unilateral facial swelling
- Dysphagia
- Dyspnea
- Persistent unilateral tonsillar enlargement
- Neck stiffness
- Photophobia
- Non-blanching rash
- Difficulty in speaking
- Itchiness of the pharynx
- Hoarseness of voice
- Chills
- Fever
- Malaise
- Headache
- Anorexia
- Nausea
- Vomiting
- Tachycardia.

Complications

- Rheumatic fever
- Acute glomerulonephritis
- Peritonsillar abscess
- Epiglottis
- Retropharyngeal abscess
- Otitis media
- Sinusitis.

Diagnostic Tests

- History
- Physical examination
- Blood examination
- Throat culture
- Rapid antigen tests
- Polymerase chain reaction (PCR) test.

Management

Medical

- **Antimicrobial agents:** It helps in preventing secondary infections. For example, penicillin, amoxicillin, benzathine penicillin G, erythromycin, cephalosporin, etc.
- **Nonsteroidal anti-inflammatory drugs:** It helps to relieve pain caused by neck stiffness. For example, ibuprofen, naproxen, etc.
- **Analgesics:** It helps to quickly relieve inflammation and reduce pain. For example, acetaminophen, paracetamol, etc.
- **Corticosteroids:** It helps to relieve inflammation and reduce the severity of the disease. For example, dexamethasone, methylprednisolone, etc.

Nursing

- Encourage the patient to take a bland diet.
- Ask the patient to gargle frequently with warm salt water (1 tsp of salt in 1 cup warm water) throughout the day.
- Ask the patient to drink plenty of fluids.
- Instruct the patient to avoid smoking.
- Apply ice pack to nose and cheeks of the patient to impede bleeding.
- Encourage the patient to take adequate bedrest during febrile phase.
- Instruct the patient to avoid sharing items such as water bottles, utensils, etc.
- Encourage the patient to do handwashing.
- Encourage the patient to eat ice chips or use throat spray or lozenges for sore throats.
- Encourage the patient to use a cool-mist vaporizer and nasal spray for congestion.

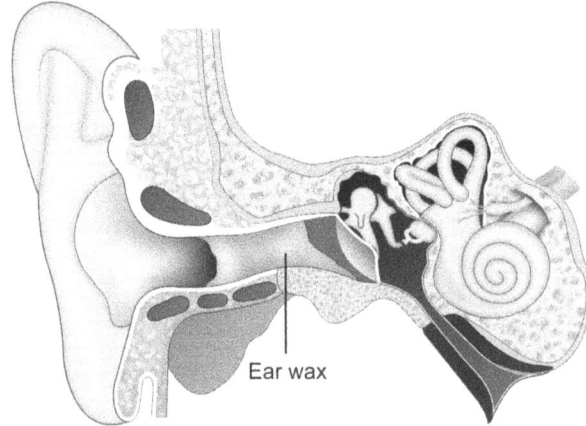

Fig. 4.2: Shows cerumen impaction (ear wax) in a ear.

CERUMEN IMPACTION (EARWAX)

Definition

Cerumen impaction refers to the buildup of layers of earwax within the ear canal to the point of blocking the canal and putting pressure on the eardrum.

Etiology

- Use of a hearing aid
- Anatomic anomalies (stenotic ear canals seen with Down's syndrome)
- Excess cerumen production
- Narrow or abnormally shaped ear canals
- Incorrect use of cotton swabs
- Foreign bodies.

Risk Factors

- Advanced age
- Being children
- People with developmental disabilities
- Conditions that produce too much cerumen, such as keratosis and other skin diseases
- Swimming
- Producing naturally hard or dry earwax
- Bony growths in the outer part of the ear canal
- People with recurring ear infections
- Dense hair growth in the ear canal
- Trying to remove cerumen with a cotton-tipped swab.

Pathophysiology

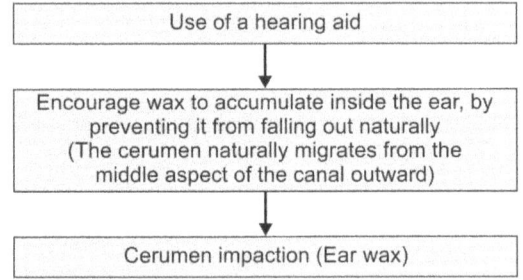

Clinical Features

- Difficulty in hearing, which may continue to worsen
- Dizziness
- Pain in the ear
- Ear discomfort
- A feeling of fullness in the ear
- Tinnitus (ringing in the ears)
- A feeling of itchiness in the ear
- Discharge from the ear
- Odor coming from the ear
- Cough.

Complications

- Conductive hearing loss
- Meningitis
- Recurrent infections
- Formation of cysts
- Enlarged adenoid glands.

Diagnostic Tests

- History
- Physical examination
- Rinne test
- Weber test
- Otoscopic examination.

Management

Medical

- **Cerumenolytic agents:** It helps to dissolve the wax in the ear canal. For example, glycerin, hydrogen peroxide, saline solution, etc.
- **Nonsteroidal anti-inflammatory drugs:** It helps to relieve pain caused by cerumen impaction. For example, ibuprofen, naproxen, etc.
- **Analgesics:** It helps to quickly reduce pain. For example, acetaminophen, paracetamol, etc.
- **Antibiotics:** It helps in treating ear infections. For example, amoxicillin, etc.

Surgical

- **Irrigating or syringing the ear:** It is a procedure in which warm water from a syringe is used to wash the wax out of the ear canal.
- **Microsuction of the ear:** It is a procedure in which a small plastic tube that is connected to a machine is used to suck the impacted wax out of the ear.
- **Removing the wax manually using special instruments (Aural toilet):** It is a procedure in which a curette is used (scoop-like instrument) or forceps to remove the impacted wax.

Nursing

- Instruct the patient to restrict cleaning the ears with anything more than a soapy washcloth on the outer rim of the ear.
- Ask them not to use cotton-tipped swabs to clean anywhere inside the ears.
- Ask the patient not to make an attempt on their own to remove the ear wax but to seek medical opinion for the same.
- Strictly avoid ear candling among patients.
- Encourage the patient to use wax-softening drops or oil twice a week.
- Instruct the patient not to use hair pins and bell pins to remove the wax.
- Ask the patient to limit ear cleaning to the outer ear only.
- Instruct the patient to keep the ears clean and dry.
- Ask the patient to avoid swimming in contaminated water.
- Instruct the patient to avoid scratching the ears.
- Ask the patient to dry the ear completely after exposure to moist conditions.

DEVIATED NASAL SEPTUM

Definition

A deviated nasal septum is a condition where the nasal septum (the bone and cartilage that divide the nasal cavity of the nose into two) is crooked and does not form a straight line.

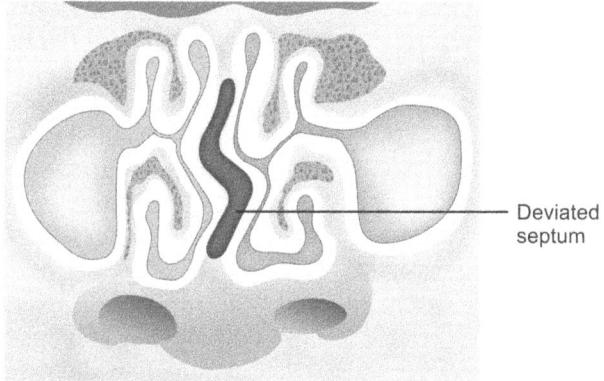

Fig. 4.3: Portrays deviated nasal septum.

Etiology

- Abnormal intrauterine posture during second stage of labor
- Direct trauma
- Birth injury to the nose
- Hereditary
- Developmental error or buckling (the septum grows rapidly on one side)
- Secondary to a tumor.

Risk Factors

- Playing contact sports
- Not wearing seatbelt while riding in a motorized vehicle
- A bump while moving around
- Being children
- Collision of two persons
- Heavy labor works.

Types

- **Spurs:** These are sharp angulations seen in the nasal septum occurring at the junction of the vomer below, with a septal cartilage and ethmoid bone above. This type of deformity is the result of vertical compression forces.
- **Deviations:** It is of C-shaped or S-shaped and occurs in either vertical or horizontal plane and it involves both cartilage and bone.
- **Dislocations:** In this the lower border of the septal cartilage is displaced from its medial position and projects into one of the nostrils.

Pathophysiology

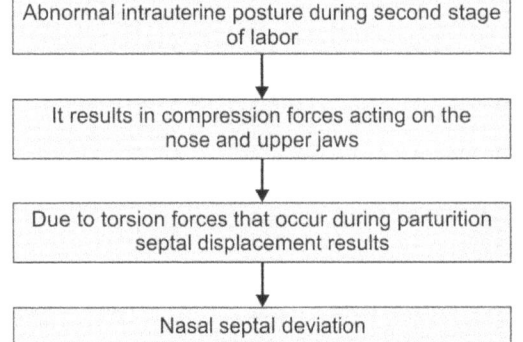

Clinical Features

- Blockage of one or both nostrils
- Facial pain
- Postnasal drip
- Headache
- Frequent nosebleeds
- Anosmia
- External deformity
- Middle ear infections
- Noisy breathing during sleeping.

Complications

- Dry mouth due to chronic mouth breathing
- Nasal congestion
- Difficulty in breathing
- Frequent sinus infections
- Disturbed sleep.

Diagnostic Tests

- History
- Physical examination
- Cottle's test
- Nasal endoscope
- X-ray examination of paranasal sinuses
- Computed tomography (CT) scan for paranasal sinuses.

Management

Medical

- **Antihistamines:** These are drugs that inhibit the action of histamine in the body by blocking the receptors of histamine. For example, phenergan, allegra, diphenhydramine, etc.
- **Nasal decongestant:** It helps to relieve nasal congestion in the upper respiratory tract (blocked nose) by narrowing (constricting) the blood vessels and reducing blood flow to facilitate breathing. For example, ipratropium bromide, oxymetazoline, phenylephrine, etc.
- **Nonsteroidal anti-inflammatory drug:** It helps to relieve facial pain. For example, ibuprofen, naproxen, etc.
- **Analgesic:** It helps to quickly relieve inflammation and reduce pain. For example, acetaminophen, paracetamol, etc.

- **Nasal corticosteroid spray:** It helps to reduce the inflammation in the nasal passage. For example, prednisone, methylprednisolone, etc.

Surgical

- **Septoplasty:** It is a surgical procedure that is done to fix a deviated nasal septum.
- **Rhinoplasty:** It is a surgical procedure done on the nose to change its shape or improve its functions.
- **Submucous resection (SMR):** It is a surgical procedure to correct a deviated nasal septum, in which obstructing septal cartilage or bone is removed after elevation of the investing mucoperichondrial flaps on each side.

Nursing

- Encourage the patient to wear a seat belt while traveling in a car.
- Ask them to wear a helmet when playing contact sports or riding a bike.
- Instruct the patient to keep the head elevated during sleep to reduce the swelling.
- Instruct the patient strictly not to blow the nose.
- Ask them to wear clothes with buttons so that it does not require to be pulled of above the head.
- Instruct the patient to avoid vigorous sports activity.
- Instruct the patient to limit their physical activity to reduce the swelling.

EPISTAXIS

Definition

Epistaxis (nosebleed) is defined as bleeding from the nostril, nasal cavity or nasopharynx due to the rupture of tiny, distended vessels in the mucous membrane of any area of the nose.

Etiology

- Blunt trauma
- Fragile blood vessels that bleed easily, mostly in warm or dry weather
- An infection of the lining of the nostrils, sinuses or adenoids
- Colds, flu, allergy or hay fever
- Bumps or falls
- Nose-picking

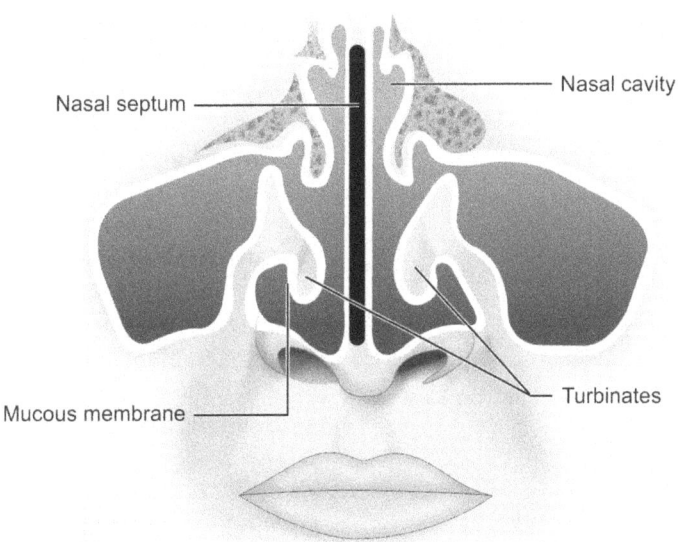

Fig. 4.4: Shows bleeding from the nostril (epistaxis or nosebleed).

- Constipation causing straining
- Certain medication (e.g., Warfarin, aspirin, clopidogrel, etc.)
- Bleeding disorder
- Anatomical deformities (e.g., Septal spurs)
- Inhalation of illicit drugs (e.g., Cocaine)
- Intranasal tumors
- Low relative humidity of inhaled air
- Foreign body in the nose
- Deviated nasal septum
- Otic barotrauma (such as from descent in aircraft or ascent in scuba diving)
- Nasal prong oxygen administration (tends to dry the olfactory mucosa)
- Nasal sprays (particularly prolonged or improper use of nasal steroids)
- Surgery (e.g., Septoplasty).

Risk Factors

- Allergies
- Cardiovascular diseases
- Alcohol (due to vasodilation)
- Anemia
- Connective tissue disorder
- Blood dyscrasias
- Envenomation
- Hematological malignancy
- Hypertension
- Idiopathic thrombocytopenic purpura
- Pregnancy
- Vascular disorders
- Vitamin C or vitamin K deficiency
- Von Willebrand's disease.

Pathophysiology

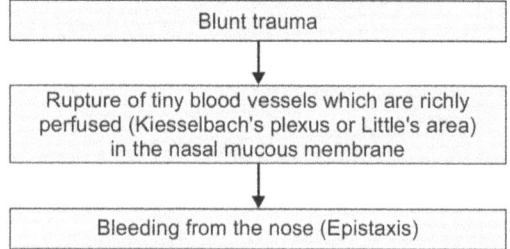

Clinical Features

- Bleeding from one or both the nostrils
- Swelling of the soft tissues
- Deformity
- Frequent swallowing
- Sensation of fluid flow in the back of the nose and throat
- Anxiety
- Shock
- Uncontrolled bleeding.

Complications

- Hypovolemia due to excessive bleeding
- Iron-deficiency anemia
- Anosmia
- Nasal septal perforation
- Toxic shock syndrome.

Diagnostic Tests

- History
- Physical examination
- Blood examination
- Nasal endoscopy
- X-ray examination
- Computed tomography (CT) scan.

Management

Medical

- **Direct pressure:** Applying direct pressure for about 5–20 minutes will stop bleeding to a great extent.
- **Vasoconstrictive agents:** It helps to reduce the bleeding time in epistaxis. For example, oxymetazoline, phenylephrine, adrenaline, etc.
- **Topical antibiotics:** It is effective in the management of recurrent epistaxis. For example, amoxicillin, neomycin, etc.
- **Anti-fibrinolytic drugs:** It is a potent competitive inhibitor of plasminogen activator and thus of the fibrinolytic system and, therefore, prevents clot disintegration and reduces the likelihood of rebleed. For example, tranexamic acid, etc.

Surgical

- **Coagulation mesh:** These are calcium alginate mesh or swabs that are inserted in the nasal cavity to accelerate coagulation. For example, coalgan, NasalCEASE, etc.

- **Anterior nasal packing with chemical cauterization:** It is a procedure in which cauterization of any bleeding vessels or packing of the nose with ribbon gauze or an absorbent dressing is carried out by using local application of silver nitrate compound to any visible bleeding vessels.
- **Arterial embolization:** It is a surgical procedure in which an interventional radiologist injects small particles into each of the nasal arteries and is performed for bleeding that is severe and unresponsive to other therapies.
- **Laser therapy:** It is a surgical procedure done on patients who have moderate nose bleeds. A small beam is directed around the margins of the each telangiectasia and photocoagulation occurs.
- **Arterial ligation:** It is a surgical procedure, in which a ligature consists of a piece of thread (suture) tied around an anatomical structure, usually a blood vessel or another hollow structure (epistaxis) to shut it off.
- **Septoplasty:** It is an operative procedure done to straighten or reconstruct the center divider or septum of the nose
- **Septal dermoplasty:** It is a surgical procedure done to replace the normally fragile lining of the nose with a tougher lining, a split thickness graft of skin removed from the thigh.

Nursing

- Ask the patient to take rest quietly for the next 12–24 hours.
- Apply ice pack to nose and cheeks of the patient to impede bleeding.
- Pinch the nose of the patient firmly and hold it for some time to stop the bleeding.
- Instruct the patient to avoid hot liquids for at least 24 hours after a nosebleed.
- Ask the patient to stay calm and sit upright.
- Instruct the patient not to pick or blow the nose for 12 hours.
- Instruct the patient to avoid strenuous exercise, straining or lifting heavy items for 7 seven days.
- Instruct the patient to avoid smoking.
- Teach the patient regarding the use of saline nasal spray.
- Ask the patient to drink plenty of fluids.

HEARING LOSS

Definition

Hearing is the ability to perceive sound and a person suffering from hearing loss has

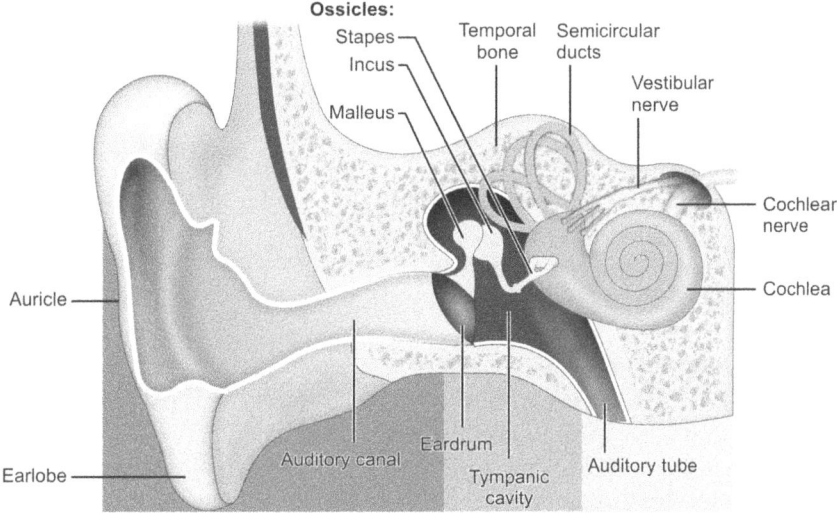

Fig. 4.5: Depicts the picture of the ear with its parts.

difficulty in perceiving or identifying sound clearly due to auditory problems. It may be unilateral or bilateral.

Etiology

- Wax impaction in ear canal (impacted cerumen)
- Fluid in the middle ear from colds or allergies
- Otitis media
- Poor eustachian tube function
- Hole in the eardrum
- Foreign body in the ear canal
- Malformation of the ear
- Head trauma
- Tumors
- Damage to cranial nerve VIII
- Meniere's syndrome
- Atresia of ear canal
- Presbycusis
- Viral infection during pregnancy.

Risk Factors

- Aging
- Drugs that are toxic to hearing
- Hearing loss that runs in the family
- Prolonged exposure to loud noise
- Traumatic brain injury
- Down's syndrome
- Diabetes
- Carpentry workers
- Coal workers
- Plumbing workers.

Types

There are four types of hearing loss as follows:
1. **Conductive hearing loss:** It is caused by any condition or disease that impedes the conveyance of sound in its mechanical form through the middle ear cavity to the inner ear.
2. **Sensorineural hearing loss:** It is a pathological process of the inner ear or of the sensory fibers that lead to the cerebral cortex. It is often permanent and measures must be taken to reduce further damage or to attempt to amplify sound as a means of improving hearing to some degree.
3. **Mixed hearing loss:** It can be thought of as a sensorineural hearing loss with a conductive component overlaying all or part of the audiometric range tested. There is also a dysfunction of the middle ear mechanism that makes the hearing worse than the sensorineural loss alone.
4. **Central hearing loss:** It is caused by a problem with the auditory nerve or sound centers. Sound waves may travel through the ear but this nerve pathway is unable to send electrical impulses to the brain. As a result, the hearing centers do not receive the signals correctly. It can be a result of a head injury or disease. The most common symptom is the ability to detect sound but not being able to understand it.

Degree of Hearing Loss

- *Mild:* Difficult to identify soft sound such as whispering
- *Moderate:* Unable to hear clearly what others are saying during conversation and hearing aids are necessary.
- *Severe:* Unable to clearly hear loud noises such as telephone ring.
- *Very severe:* Can only hear very loud noises and sounds such as shouting or vacuum cleaner noise.
- *Profound:* Difficult to perceive any sound.

Pathophysiology

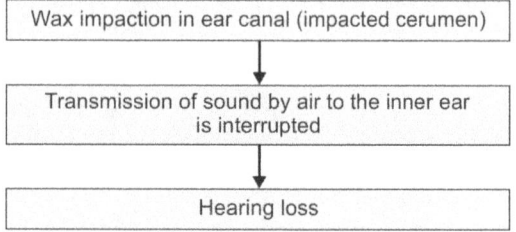

Clinical Features

Early Features

- Tinnitus
- Increasing inability to hear in groups
- Need to turn up the volume of the television
- Frequently asking people to repeat statement

- Withdrawing from social interactions
- Straining to hear
- Turning head to favor one ear (or) leaning forward
- Shouting in conversation
- Failing to respond when not looking in the direction of the sound
- Irritability
- Answering questions incorrectly.

Late Features

- Tendency to dominate the conversation
- Itching
- Hearing loss
- Plugged feeling in ear
- Redness
- Edema
- Pain
- Pressure in ear
- Fatigue
- Insecurity.

Complications

- Depression
- Anxiety
- Permanent deafness.

Diagnostic Tests

- History
- Physical examination
- Blood examination
- Otoscopic examination
- X-ray examination of the ear
- Computed tomography (CT) scan
- Magnetic resonance imaging (MRI) scan
- Ear swab culture examination
- Bone conduction audiometric examination
- Tympanogram
- Electrocochleogram
- Electronystagmography.

Management

Medical

- **Hearing aids:** It is a device that brings sound to the ear more effectively by amplifying the sound and to couple the amplified sound to the ear.
- **Cochlear implant:** It stimulated the auditory system with electrical impulses as compared with a hearing aid.

Nursing

- Face the patient when having a one to one conversation.
- Turn off background noise when having a conversation with the patient.
- Choose a quiet place to have conversation with the patient.
- Encourage others to speak clearly with the patient.
- Educate patient to consider using an assistive listening device.

LABYRINTHITIS

Definition

Labyrinthitis is an inflammation of a structure within the inner ear called the labyrinth.

Etiology

- Viral infection of the inner ear (Herpes simplex virus, Epstein-Barr virus, measles virus, mumps virus, etc.).
- Bacterial infection of the inner ear (*Streptococcus pneumoniae, Streptococcus pyogenes, Staphylococcus aureus, Haemophilus influenzae, Moraxella catarrhalis*, etc.).
- Bronchitis
- Otitis media
- Injury to the ear
- Immune system dysfunction (autoimmune labyrinthitis)
- Allergic rhinitis
- Lyme's disease.

Risk Factors

- Benign positional vertigo
- Meniere's disease
- Smoking
- Fatigue
- Excessive alcohol intake
- Extreme stress
- Over-the-counter (OTC) medications (Aspirin, Phenytoin, Lasix, etc.).

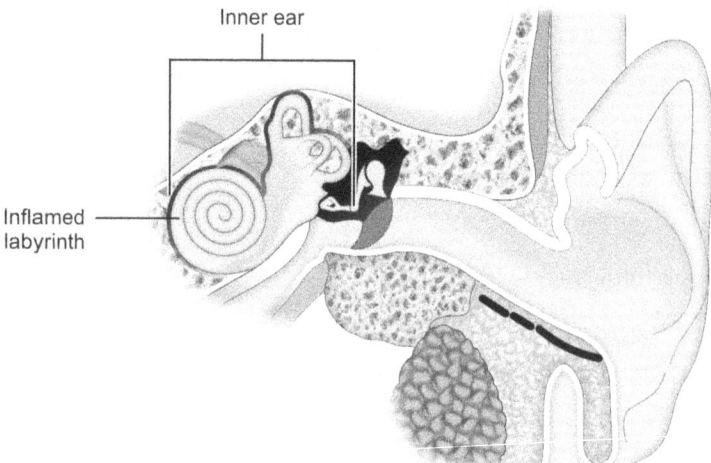

Fig. 4.6: Shows inflamed labyrinth within the inner ear.

Pathophysiology

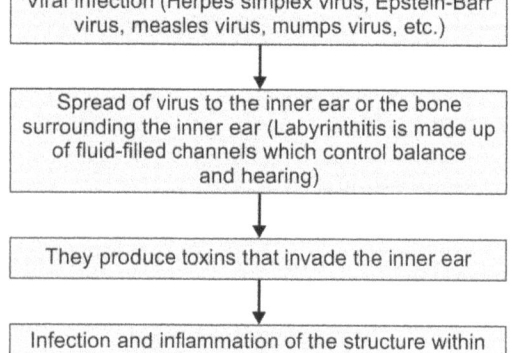

Clinical Features

- Dizziness
- Vertigo
- Loss of balance
- Tinnitus
- Earache
- Nausea
- Vomiting
- Loss of hearing in the high-frequency range in one year
- Irritability
- Fever
- Lethargy
- Difficulty in focusing the eyes.

Complications

- Hearing loss
- Brain infection
- Meningitis
- Recurrent ear infection.

Diagnostic Tests

- History
- Physical examination
- Blood examination
- Vestibular function tests (Balance tests)
- Hearing tests (Audiogram)
- Electronystagmography
- Electroencephalography
- Brainstem auditory evoked response (BAER)
- Electrocochleography
- Magnetic resonance imaging (MRI) scan
- Computerized axial tomography (CAT) scan.

Management

Medical

- **Vestibular suppressants:** It helps to relieve dizziness and loss of balance associated with labyrinthitis. For example, meclizine, glycopyrrolate, lorazepam, diazepam, etc.
- **Anti-emetics:** It works by preventing the actions of histamine (It blocks histamine

receptors in an area of the brain called the vomiting center). For example, phenergan, domperidone, etc.
- **Antiviral agents:** It slows the growth and spread of the herpes virus in the body. For example, acyclovir, zidovudine, rimantadine, etc.
- **Anti-histamine agents:** It is used to prevent and treat nausea, vomiting and dizziness associated with labyrinthitis. For example, benadryl, cetirizine, fexofenadine, etc.
- **Nonsteroidal anti-inflammatory drugs:** It helps to reduce swelling. For example, ibuprofen, naproxen, etc.
- **Analgesics:** It helps to quickly relieve swelling and fever. For example, acetaminophen, paracetamol, etc.
- **Corticosteroids:** It helps to reduce the severity of the disease. For example, dexamethasone, methylprednisolone, etc.
- **Antimicrobial agents:** It helps in preventing secondary infections. For example, penicillin, amoxicillin, benzathine penicillin G, erythromycin, cephalosporin, etc.

Nursing
- Instruct the patient not to drive, operate machinery or carry out any strenuous activity until fully recovered.
- Encourage the patient to follow a healthy diet.
- Instruct the patient to maintain a healthy lifestyle.
- Instruct the patient to reduce the noise and stress from the area around them.
- Encourage the patient to lie down still in a comfortable position mostly in lateral (side) position.
- Ask the patient to avoid bright lights.
- Instruct the patients to avoid stimulants like coffee, alcohol, sugar, salt and smoking.
- Instruct the patient to drink plenty of water to prevent dehydration.
- Instruct the patient to avoid sudden movements or positional changes.

MASTOIDITIS

Definition
Mastoiditis is an infection and inflammation of the mastoid cells inside the bone behind the earlobe, the portion of the temporal lobe of the skull that is behind the ear which contains open air containing spaces.

Etiology
- Bacterial infection (*Streptococcus pneumoniae, Streptococcus pyogenes, Staphylococcus*

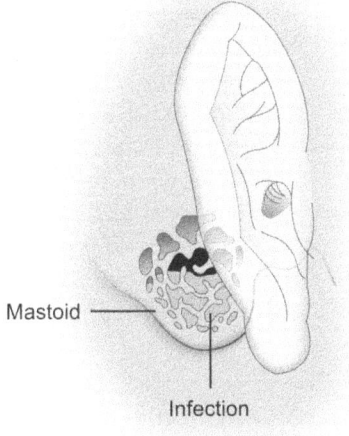 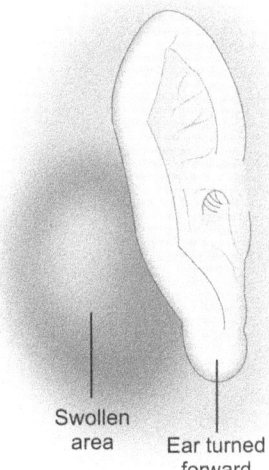

Fig. 4.7: Shows inflammation of the mastoid cells inside the bone behind the earlobe (Mastoiditis).

aureus, Haemophilus influenzae, Moraxella catarrhalis, etc.)
- Untreated acute otitis media
- Cleft palate
- Sudden changes in air pressure
- Blocked eustachian tube.

Risk Factors
- Being young children
- Recent history of ear infection
- Weakened immune system
- Pre-existence of cholesteatoma
- Swimming in polluted water
- Overzealous cleaning of the ears
- Failure to dry the outer ear properly after swimming or bathing
- Kawasaki disease
- Mononucleosis
- Leukemia
- Temporal bone sarcoma.

Pathophysiology

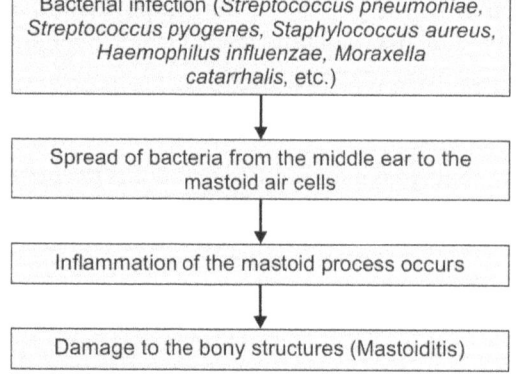

Clinical Features
- Pain and tenderness behind the ear
- Swelling of the earlobe
- Recent ear infection
- Ear pain (Otalgia)
- Fever
- Headache
- Anorexia
- Diarrhea
- Irritability
- Itching of the outer ear
- Mild deafness or the sensation that sound is muffled
- Blisters on the outer ear or along the ear canal
- Redness or swelling of the bone behind the ear
- Drainage from the ear.

Complications
- Meningitis
- Sepsis
- Vertigo
- Brain abscess
- Hearing loss
- Labyrinthitis
- Facial nerve palsy.

Diagnostic Tests
- History
- Physical examination
- Blood examination
- Culture from the infected ear
- Lumbar puncture
- X-ray examination
- Magnetic resonance imaging (MRI) scan
- Computed tomography (CT) scan.

Management

Medical
- **Antibiotics:** It helps to prevent the secondary infections. For example, ceftriaxone, etc.
- **Nonsteroidal anti-inflammatory drugs:** It helps to relieve pain caused by otalgia. For example, ibuprofen, naproxen, etc.
- **Analgesics:** It helps to quickly relieve inflammation and reduce pain. For example, acetaminophen, paracetamol, etc.
- **Corticosteroids:** It helps to relieve inflammation and reduce the severity of the disease. For example, dexamethasone, methylprednisolone, etc.

Surgical
- **Myringotomy:** It is a surgical procedure in which a small incision is made into the tympanic membrane (eardrum) to drain the pus from the middle ear.

- **Mastoidectomy:** It is a surgical procedure in which part of the bone is removed and mastoid process is drained.

Nursing

- Encourage the patient to take timely treatment of acute otitis media.
- Encourage the patient to take protein and vitamin rich diet.
- Instruct the patient to maintain a healthy lifestyle.
- Ask the patient to dry the outer ear properly after swimming or bathing.
- Ensure effective treatment of all kinds of ear infection to help in preventing the spread of the infection to the mastoid bone.

MENIERE'S DISEASE (ENDOLYMPHATIC HYDROPS)

Definition

Meniere's disease is a disorder of the inner ear that causes severe dizziness (vertigo), ringing in the ears (tinnitus), hearing loss and a feeling of fullness or congestion in the ear. It usually affects only one ear.

Etiology

- Labyrinthitis
- Circulation problems
- Viral infection
- Allergies
- An autoimmune reaction
- Genetic predisposition
- Migraine.

Risk Factors

- Intake of caffeine
- Smoking
- Alcohol consumption
- Bright lights
- Stress
- Overwork
- Fatigue
- Pre-morbid conditions
- Pressure changes
- Excessive salt in the diet
- Family history of Meniere's disease.

Stages

- *Stage one: Early stage (Unpredictable attacks of vertigo):* It can last from a few minutes to hours. During the attack, there is a variable amount of hearing loss along with a sensation of fullness in the affected ear. The fullness in the ear and tinnitus may precede the attacks of vertigo, but they will attack without warning. In between the attacks, the hearing and sensation in the ear return to normal.
- *Stage two: Intermediate stage (Attacks of vertigo, tinnitus and hearing loss):* The attacks of vertigo continue with variable remissions however may be less severe. After or perhaps before the

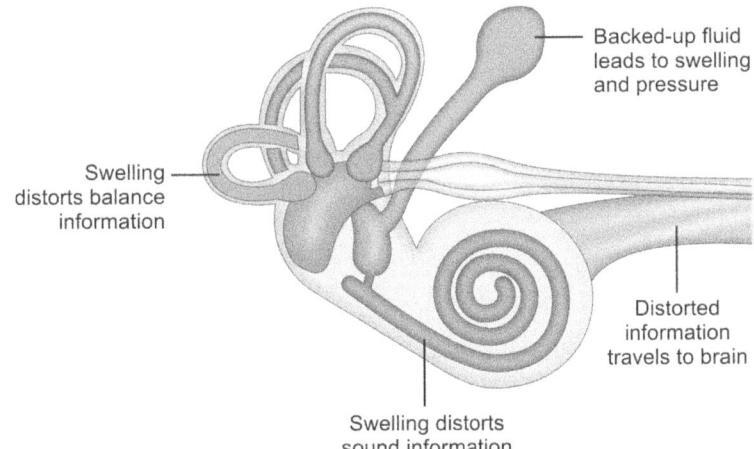

Fig. 4.8: Depicts Meniere's disease with backed-up fluid which leads to swelling and pressure.

attack, the person may experience a period of imbalance and movement, induced giddiness. Permanent hearing loss develops and continues to fluctuate with the vertigo attacks. Tinnitus becomes more prominent often fluctuating or increasing with the attacks.
- **Stage three: Late stage (Hearing loss, balance difficulties and tinnitus):** In this stage, the hearing loss increases and often the attacks of vertigo diminish or stop. There is permanent damage to the balance organ in the ear and significant general balance problems are common, especially in the dark.

Pathophysiology

```
Labyrinthitis (the buildup of fluid in the
compartments of the inner ear)
              ↓
The endolymph buildup in the labyrinth interferes
with the normal balance and hearing signals
between the inner ear and the brain
              ↓
Dizziness (vertigo), ringing in the ears (tinnitus),
hearing loss and a feeling of fullness or
congestion in the ear in one or both ears
(Meniere's disease)
```

Clinical Features

- Two or more episodes of vertigo lasting at least 20 minutes each
- Tinnitus
- Fluctuating hearing loss
- Aural fullness (a feeling of fullness in the ear)
- Loss of balance
- Lightheadedness
- Headache
- Increased ear pressure
- Sound sensitivity
- Nausea
- Vomiting
- Cold sweat palpitations or rapid pulse
- Trembling
- Blurry vision or eye jerking
- Diarrhea
- Vague feeling of uneasiness.

Complications

- Dysfunction in the inner ear
- Frequent falls
- Emotional stress
- Permanent hearing loss
- Anxiety
- Depression.

Diagnostic Tests

- History
- Physical examination
- Blood examination
- Vestibular function tests (Balance tests)
- Hearing tests (Audiogram)
- Electronystagmography
- Brainstem auditory evoked response (BAER)
- Electrocochleography
- Magnetic resonance imaging (MRI) scan
- Computed tomography (CT) scan.

Management

Medical

- **Intermittent anti-vertigo agents:** It helps to relieve dizziness and shorten the attack. For example, meclizine, diazepam, glycopyrrolate, lorazepam, etc.
- **Diuretics:** It helps to control dizziness by reducing the amount of fluid the body retains, which may help lower fluid volume and pressure in the inner ear. For example, aldactone, furosemide, etc.
- **Antibiotics:** It helps to prevent the secondary infections. For example, ceftriaxone, cephalosporin, etc.
- **Histamine analog agents:** It works by acting on histamine receptors that are found in the walls of blood vessels in the inner ear which reduce the pressure of the fluid that fills the labyrinth in the inner ear. For example, betahistine, prochlorperazine, cinnarizine, etc.
- **Corticosteroids:** Dexamethasone, methylprednisolone, etc. It helps to reduce the severity of the disease.

Surgical

- **Selectively destructive surgery:** It is a surgical procedure in which the balance

part of the inner ear is destroyed with the medicine called gentamicin, which is injected through the eardrum and enters the labyrinth.
- **Endolymphatic sac decompression:** It is a surgical procedure that involves opening the mastoid and decompressing to remove the bone over this sac which, in turn, helps to reduce the pressure in the inner ear by increasing the drainage of the fluid of the inner ear.
- **Selective vestibular neurectomy:** It is a procedure in which the balance nerve is cut as it leaves the inner ear and goes to the brain as it permanently prevents vertigo attacks and preserves the hearing function of the ear.
- **Labyrinthectomy and eighth nerve section:** It is a procedure in which the balance and hearing mechanism in the inner ear are destroyed on one side and helps in controlling vertigo attacks to a greater extent.

Nursing

- Ask the patient to avoid the triggers that make the symptoms worse which include sudden movement, bright lights, watching television or reading.
- Instruct the patient to avoid driving as it may lead to an accident and injury.
- Ask the patient to take complete bedrest during vertigo attacks.
- Instruct the patient to reduce the salt (sodium) intake in the diet and it should not be more than 460 mg – 920 mg (i.e., one teaspoon of salt contains 2,300 mg of sodium) per day.
- Instruct the patient to avoid caffeine, chocolate and alcohol intake.
- Instruct the patient to maintain a healthy lifestyle.
- Encourage the patient to quit smoking.
- Encourage the patient to eat meals at regular intervals as it helps to regulate the body fluids.

NASAL POLYPS

Definition

The soft noncancerous (benign) growths that develop on the lining of the nose or sinuses are known as nasal polyps.

Etiology

- Allergic rhinitis (hay fever)
- Asthma
- Aspirin sensitivity
- Chronic sinus infections
- Cystic fibrosis
- Genetic predisposition.

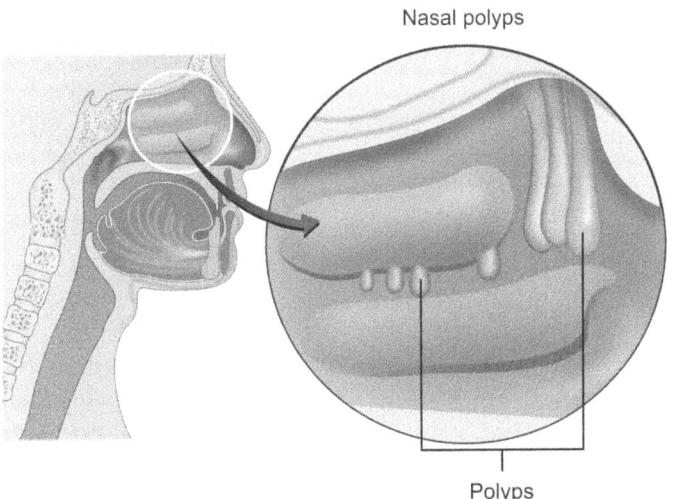

Fig. 4.9: Depicts benign growth over the lining of the nose (Nasal polyps).

Risk Factors

- Condition which leads to chronic inflammation in your nose or sinuses
- People with allergitic fungal sinuses
- Churg-Strauss syndrome (a rare disease which inflames the blood vessels)
- People older than 40 years of age
- Being males.

Types

- *Antrochoanal nasal polyps:* These grow as single large masses and are predominantly found among children, where males are usually affected more than females. They are pedunculated (they lie on top) and originate from the maxillary sinuses.
- *Ethmoidal nasal polyps:* They are bilateral and grow in multiple masses. They are mostly found among adults and affect both males and females. The grape-like appearance commonly attributed to nasal polyps are found in ethmoidal polyps.
- *Allergic nasal polyps:* They are usually the most common type of polyp, and can be triggered by any type of allergies that affect the nasal cavity.
- *Nonallergic nasal polyps:* They are similar in appearance and characteristic to allergic polyps, but develop without the allergen stimulus.

Pathophysiology

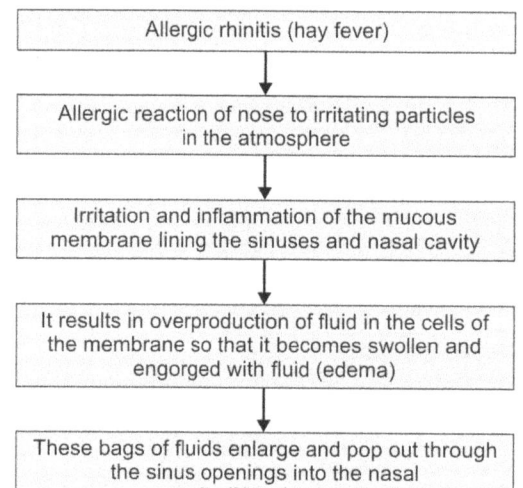

Clinical Features

- Nasal obstruction
- Running nose (Rhinorrhea)
- Nasal congestion
- Persistent stuffiness
- Chronic sinus infections
- Postnasal drip
- Difficulty in breathing through the nose
- Dulled sense of smell and taste
- Pain/pressure over the face
- Dull headache
- Snoring.

Complications

- Acute or chronic sinus infections
- Obstructive sleep apnea (a potentially serious condition in which a client stops and starts breathing a number of times during sleep)
- Altered facial structure
- Double vision
- Meningitis (infection of the tissues around the brain and spinal cord)
- Orbital cellulitis (infection around the tissues of the eye)
- Osteitis (infection of the sinus bones).

Diagnostic Tests

- History
- Physical examination
- Blood examination
- Allergic testing
- Nasal endoscopy
- Polyp biopsy
- Computed tomography (CT) scan
- Magnetic resonance imaging (MRI) scan.

Management

Medical

- **Corticosteroid nasal spray:** It helps to relieve inflammation, increases nasal airflow and helps to shrink polyps. For example, fluticasone, triamcinolone, budesonide, flunisolide, mometasone, etc.
- **Oral corticosteroids:** It helps to relieve inflammation and reduce the severity of the

disease. For example, methylprednisolone, etc.
- **Antihistamine:** It helps to relieve allergic reactions. For example, pheniramine maleate, etc.
- **Antibiotics:** It helps to prevent any secondary infection. For example, ciprofloxacin, metronidazole, etc.

Surgical
- **Polypectomy:** It is a surgical procedure in which the small or isolated polyps will be removed completely using a small mechanical suction device or a microdebrider (an instrument that cuts and extracts soft tissue.
- **Endoscopic sinus surgery:** It is a surgical procedure in which the polyps are removed and also open the part of the sinus cavity where polyps usually form.

Nursing
- Irrigate the nose of patient with salt water to relieve mild nasal congestion.
- Avoid saline sprays containing additives such as benzalkonium which inflames the mucus lining of the nose on patients.
- Encourage the use of preservative free saline spray among patients.
- Instruct the patient to avoid nasal irritants.

OTITIS MEDIA

Definition
Otitis media is an infection and inflammation of the middle ear, usually the area between the eardrum and the inner ear including a duct known as the eustachian tube.

Etiology
- Viral or bacterial upper respiratory tract infection
- Food and airborne allergies
- Ruptured eardrum
- Infected or overgrown adenoids (tonsils)
- Being around someone who smokes
- Blockage of the eustachian tube
- Nutritional deficiency (Vitamin-A, zinc and iron deficiencies)
- Being fed by lying down on the back (bottle-fed).

Risk Factors
- Being children
- Craniofacial abnormalities

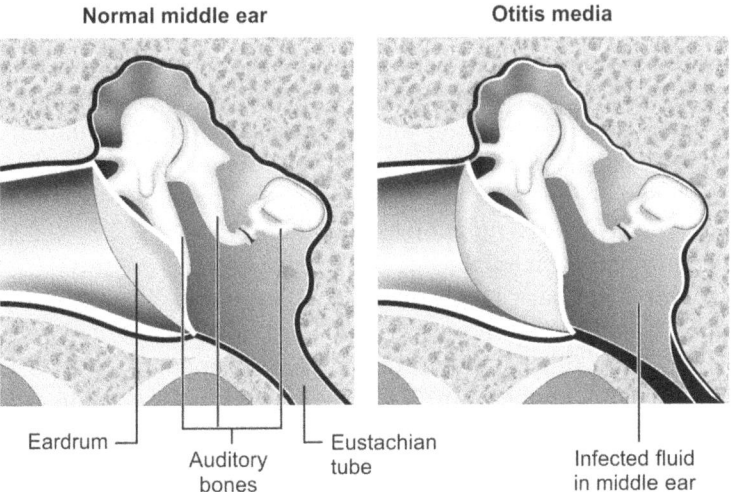

Fig. 4.10: Shows the comparison of normal middle ear with that of otitis media.

- Exposure to environmental smoke
- Exposure to group daycare
- Having a cold
- Family history of recurrent otitis media
- Having a history of gastroesophageal reflux disease (GERD)
- Immunodeficiency
- Overcrowded homes
- Winter
- Pacifier use (dummy)
- Absence of breastfeeding
- Premature birth.

Types

- *Acute suppurative otitis media (ASOM):* It is usually due to a viral infection of upper respiratory tract infection. There is congestion and mild discomfort in this type. Viral otitis media can very easily lead to bacterial otitis media in a very short time. The individual with bacterial acute otitis media has the classic "earache" which is accompanied by mild-grade fever.
- *Otitis media with effusion (OME):* It is also known as serous or secretory otitis media. There is a collection of fluid within the middle ear as a result of the negative pressure produced by altered eustachian tube function. This type is purely a viral infection with no pain or bacterial infection. Fluid in the middle ear sometimes causes conductive hearing impairment. Its early onset is associated with feeding while lying down and too short period of breastfeeding.
- *Chronic suppurative otitis media (CSOM):* This type involves perforation in the eardrum and active bacterial infection within the middle ear space for several weeks or more. It is common in persons with poor eustachian tube function. In this type there may be enough pus that it drains to the outside of the ear or the purulence may be minimal enough to only be seen on examination using a binocular microscope. It is accompanied with hearing impairment.

Pathophysiology

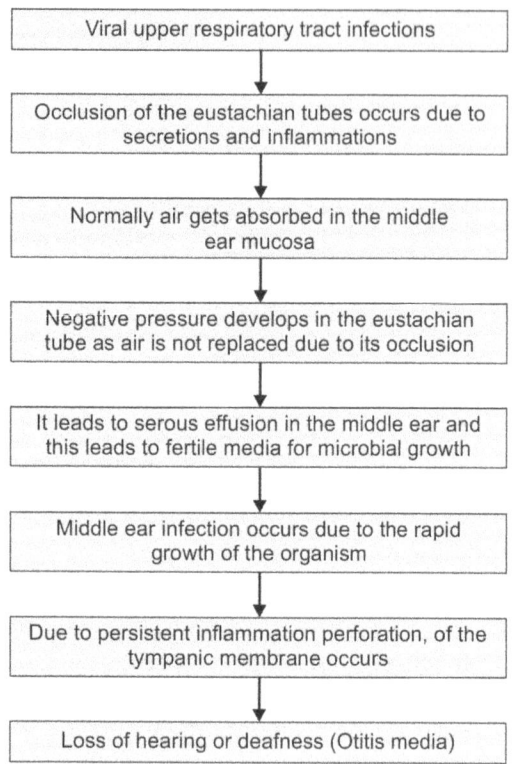

Clinical Features

- Hearing difficulties
- Sudden and severe earache (Otalgia)
- Tinnitus (ringing or buzzing in the ear)
- Sense of fullness in the ear
- Irritability
- Scratching or holding the ear
- Fever
- Headache
- Dizziness
- Loss of balance
- Loss of appetite
- Change in the sleeping pattern
- Fluid leaking from the ear
- Nausea
- Burst of eardrum.

Complications

- Post-auricular abscess
- Facial nerve palsy
- Labyrinthitis
- Mastoiditis
- Brain abscess
- Otitic hydrocephalus
- Petrositis
- Meningitis
- Total deafness
- Cholesteatoma.

Diagnostic Tests

- History
- Physical examination
- Blood examination
- Pneumatic otoscope
- Tympanometry
- Acoustic reflectometry
- Tympanocentesis
- Audiogram.

Management

Medical

- **Antibiotics:** It helps to prevent the secondary infections. For example, amoxicillin, ampicillin, cefaclor, erythromycin, clarithromycin, bactrim, etc.
- **Analgesics:** It helps to relieve the pain in ears. For example, acetaminophen, ibuprofen, etc.

Surgical

- **Myringotomy:** It is a surgical procedure in which a small incision is made in the eardrum and inserts a tiny ventilation tube called a tympanostomy tube to promote drainage of fluid from the middle ear and keeps it from recurring.
- **Tympanoplasty:** It is a surgical procedure in which through plastic operation procedure the damaged eardrum is repaired.
- **Myringoplasty:** It is a surgical procedure in which perforation in the eardrum is closed by means of a tissue graft.
- **Adenoidectomy:** It is a surgical procedure in which the adenoids are removed surgically and it is performed in children's older than 4 years of age and with serous otitis media in which the adenoids are repeatedly inflamed.
- **Tonsillectomy:** It is a surgical procedure in which tonsils are removed surgically and is performed in children's older than 4 years of age and with serous otitis media in which the tonsils are repeatedly inflamed.
- **Stapedectomy:** It is a surgical procedure in which the stapes (stirrup) are replaced with prosthesis and is performed in case of hearing loss.

Nursing

- Instruct the mothers to vaccinate all infants and children against viral respiratory infections.
- Instruct the parents to avoid smoking in front of the infants and children.
- Educate the mother to safeguard the child against environmental tobacco smoke.
- Encourage the mothers to breastfeed their child rather than bottle-feeding.
- Instruct the mothers not to use a pacifier.
- Keep the child away from other children who are sick.
- Instruct the patient to raise the head-end of the bed while sleeping to help drain fluids from the middle ear.

OTOSCLEROSIS

Definition

Otosclerosis is an abnormal growth of bone of the middle ear which prevents structures within the ear from working properly and causes hearing loss.

Etiology

- Hereditary (Temporal bone abnormalities)
- Viral infections such as measles
- Metabolic disorders
- Immune disorders

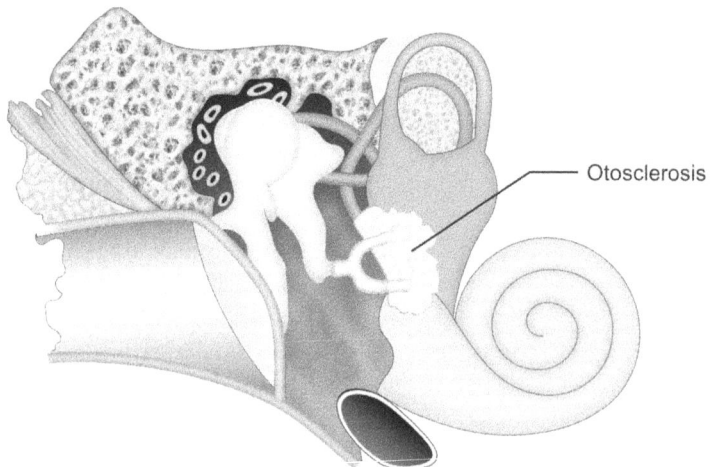

Fig. 4.11: Depicts abnormal bony overgrowth in the middle ear.

- Vascular disorders
- Idiopathic.

Risk Factors

- Being white middle-aged women
- Family history of otosclerosis
- Pregnancy
- Stress
- Menopause.

Types

- ***Early focal otosclerosis:*** In this type, the abnormalities are localized to one or two small areas of the normal footplate section.
- ***Diffuse active otosclerosis:*** In this type, there is abnormal vascularity with a great increase in size and number of marrow spaces and most of these spaces are lined by osteoblasts.
- ***Quiescent otosclerosis:*** In this stage, there in increase in the size and number of marrow spaces, there is no evidence of bone formation and destruction. Osteoblasts and osteoclasts are only occasionally seen.
- ***Cochlear otosclerosis:*** In this stage, the condition causes pure sensorineural deafness without stapes fixation and otosclerotic foci may occur in the otic capsule without the involvement of stapedial footplate.

Pathophysiology

Hereditary (Temporal bone abnormalities)
↓
Stapes, the last bone in the chain which rests in the entrance to the inner ear (the oval window) gets affected
↓
The abnormal bone fixates the stapes in the oval window and interferes with sound passing waves to the inner ear
↓
Gradual onset of hearing loss (Otosclerosis)

Clinical Features

- Gradual loss of hearing
- Not able to hear low-pitched sounds or whispering
- Dizziness
- Tinnitus (Sensation of ringing, roaring, buzzing or hissing in the ears or head)
- Vertigo
- Frequently asking people to repeat statement
- Straining to hear
- Turning head to favor one ear (or) leaning forward
- Failing to respond when not looking in the direction of the sound

- Irritability
- Answering questions incorrectly.

Complications
- Anxiety
- Depression
- Permanent deafness.

Diagnostic Tests
- History
- Physical examination
- Blood examination
- Otoscopic examination
- X-ray examination of the ear
- Computed tomography (CT) scan
- Magnetic resonance imaging (MRI) scan
- Ear swab culture examination
- Bone conduction audiometric examination
- Tympanogram
- Electrocochleogram
- Electronystagmography.

Management

Medical
- **Hearing aids:** It is a device that brings sound to the ear more effectively by amplifying the sound and to couple the amplified sound to the ear.
- **Cochlear implant:** It stimulated the auditory system with electrical impulses as compared with a hearing aid.
- **Fluoride therapy:** It inhibits the rapid progression of the disease by formation of hydroxylapatite crystals which lead to stapes fixation. The presumed action of the fluoride is to convert the active bone-destroying otospongiotic lesions into inactive otosclerotic lesions.

Surgical
- **Total stapedectomy:** It is a surgical procedure in which the entire diseased stapes bone is bypassed with a prosthetic device that allows sound waves to be passed to the inner ear.
- **Partial stapedectomy:** It is a surgical procedure in which only the inhibited portion of the footplate is removed and is replaced with a prosthesis.

Nursing
- Face the patient when having a one-to-one conversation.
- Turn off background noise when having a conversation with the patient.
- Choose a quiet place to have conversation with the patient.
- Encourage others to speak clearly with the patient.
- Educate the patient to consider using an assistive listening device.
- Encourage the patient to take fluoride intake between 460 mg and 920 mg per day to inhibit the rapid progression of the disease.

PERITONSILLAR ABSCESS (QUINSY)

Definition
Peritonsillar abscess (Quinsy) is a pus-producing bacterial infection occurring in the cavity at the back of the throat, near the tonsils.

Etiology
- Malfunction of Weber's glands
- Bacterial infection (e.g., Group A beta-hemolytic streptococci, etc.) of the tonsils

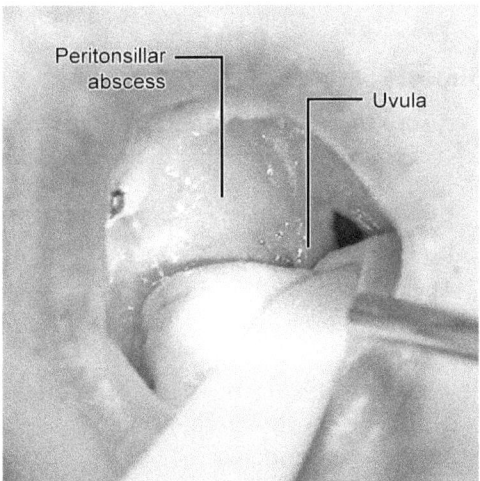

Fig. 4.12: Shows collection of pus at the back of the throat near the tonsils.

- Infectious mononucleosis
- Chronic lymphocytic leukemia (CLL).

Risk Factors

- Being males
- Those who are between 20 years and 40 years of age
- Recent throat or dental infection
- Periodontal disease
- Smoking
- Diabetes mellitus
- Weakened immune system
- Tonsilloliths (calcium deposits in the tonsils).

Pathophysiology

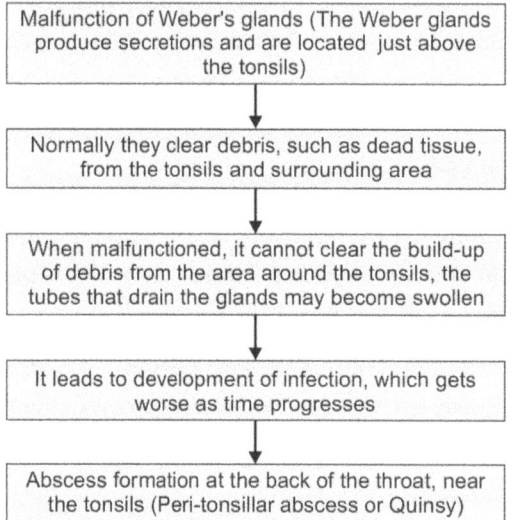

Clinical Features

- A sore throat that suddenly intensifies in severity, often spreading to the soft palate
- Ipsilateral ear pain
- Fever
- Chills
- Malaise
- Odynophagia (difficulty in swallowing even liquids)
- Trismus (difficulty in opening the mouth)
- Muffled voice (hot potato voice)
- Swollen face and neck
- Headache
- Drooling
- Bad breath
- Enlarged lymph nodes (swollen glands) in the neck
- Discomfort in the uvula and soft palate (tissue at the roof of the mouth).

Complications

- Airway obstruction
- Aspiration pneumonia
- Necrotizing fasciitis
- Pleural effusion
- Septicemia
- Death.

Diagnostic Tests

- History
- Physical examination
- Blood examination
- Needle aspiration test
- Ultrasound examination
- Computed tomography (CT) scan
- Magnetic resonance imaging (MRI) scan.

Management

Medical

- **Antimicrobial agents:** It helps in preventing secondary infections. For example, penicillin, amoxicillin, benzathine penicillin G, erythromycin, cephalosporin, etc.
- **Nonsteroidal anti-inflammatory drugs:** It helps to relieve swelling caused by swollen face and neck. For example, ibuprofen, naproxen, etc.
- **Analgesics:** It helps to quickly reduce pain. For example, acetaminophen, paracetamol, etc.
- **Corticosteroids:** It helps to relieve swelling and reduce the severity of the disease. For example, dexamethasone, methylprednisolone, etc.

Surgical

- **Needle aspiration:** It is a surgical procedure in which long, fine needle is used to draw

out the pus that is build-up at the back of the throat, near the tonsils.
- **Incision and drainage:** It is a surgical procedure in which a cut is made in the affected area to drain the fluid from the abscess.
- **Tonsillectomy:** It is a surgical procedure in which the tonsils found at the back of the throat, behind the tongue are removed.

Nursing

- Ask the patient to gargle frequently with warm salt water (1 tsp of salt in 1 cup warm water) throughout the day
- Encourage the patient to take adequate bedrest during febrile phase.
- Instruct the patient to avoid sharing items such as water bottles, utensils, etc.
- Ask the patient to drink plenty of fluids.
- Instruct the patient to avoid smoking.
- Encourage the patient to take a bland diet.
- Encourage the patient to do hand washing.
- Encourage the patient to eat ice chips or use throat spray or lozenges for sore throats.
- Encourage the patient to use a cool-mist vaporizer and nasal spray for congestion.

RHINITIS

Definition

Rhinitis refers to the presence of inflammation of the mucosa of the nasal cavity (i.e., the lining of the nasal cavity).

Etiology

- Pollen given off by trees, grass and weeds
- Dust mites
- Mold
- Cockroach waste
- Animal dander
- Fumes and odors
- Overuse of topical nose sprays.

Risk Factors

- Family history of asthma
- Having atopic dermatitis (eczema)
- Smoking
- Living or working in an environment that constantly exposes to allergens
- Food allergies
- Cold weather
- Hormonal changes.

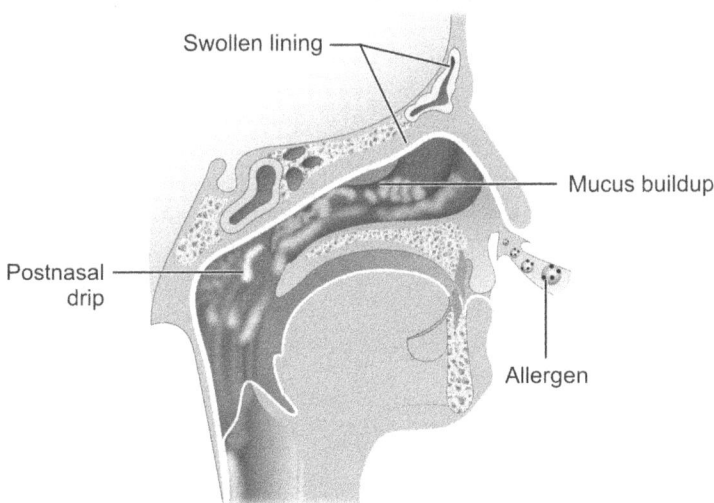

Fig. 4.13: Shows inflamed and swollen lining of the mucosa of the nasal cavity.

Types

- *Allergic rhinitis (Hay fever):* It is an inflammation of the nasal passages caused by an allergic reaction to breathing air containing an allergen.
- *Nonallergic rhinitis:* It refers to rhinitis that is not due to an allergy
- *Infectious rhinitis:* It refers to rhinitis that is commonly caused by a viral or bacterial infection.

Pathophysiology

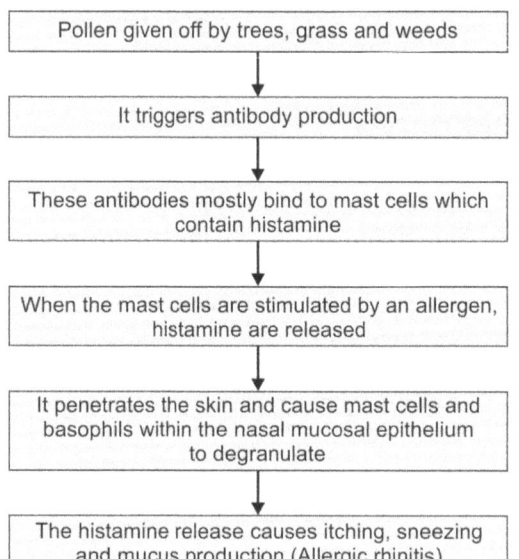

Clinical Features

- Stuffy nose
- Runny nose
- Sneezing
- Itchy nose, throat, eyes and ears
- Nosebleeds
- Clear drainage from the nose
- Ear infections that keep coming back
- Snoring
- Breathing through the mouth
- Tiredness
- Dark circles under the eyes
- Puffiness under the eyes
- Watery eyes
- Headache
- Irritability.

Complications

- Otitis media
- Eustachian tube dysfunction
- Sinusitis
- Poor sleep
- Nasal polyps.

Diagnostic Tests

- History
- Physical examination
- Blood examination
- Skin prick allergy test
- X-ray examination
- Nasal endoscope
- Ultrasound examination
- Computed tomography (CT) scan
- Magnetic resonance imaging (MRI) scan.

Management

Medical

- **Antihistamines:** These are drugs that inhibit the action of histamine in the body by blocking the receptors of histamine. For example, phenergan, allegra, diphenhydramine, etc.
- **Nasal decongestants:** It helps to relieve nasal congestion in the upper respiratory tract (blocked nose) by narrowing (constricting) the blood vessels and reducing blood flow to facilitate breathing. For example, ipratropium bromide, oxymetazoline, phenylephrine, etc.
- **Antimicrobial agents:** It helps in preventing secondary infections. For example, penicillin, amoxicillin, benzathine penicillin G, erythromycin, cephalosporin, etc.
- **Corticosteroids:** It helps to reduce the severity of the disease. For example, dexamethasone, methylprednisolone, etc.

Surgical

- **Allergen immunotherapy (allergy shots):** It is a procedure in which an injection is given of the particular allergen in gradually increasing doses to develop immunity or tolerance to the allergen.

- **Coblation turbinoplasty:** It is a surgical procedure in which enlarged turbinates are brought to an optimum size without removing any of the bone or tissue.
- **Turbinectomy:** It is a partial or complete resection of the inferior turbinate with or without the guidance of an endoscope.
- **Functional endoscopic sinus surgery (FESS):** It is a surgical procedure that involves the insertion of the endoscope, a very thin fiber-optic tube into the nose for a direct visual examination of the openings into the sinuses with the purpose of removing abnormal and obstructive tissues from the nose.
- **Cryotherapy (tissue-freezing):** It is a technique that uses an extremely cold liquid or instrument to freeze and destroy abnormal skin cells that require removal.
- **Submucous diathermy:** It involves passing a probe just below the mucosal surface lining of the turbinate bones and cauterizing using heat energy to shrink the size of these structures. This preserves most of the mucosal lining and allows for preservation of normal function.
- **Septoplasty:** It is a surgical procedure that's done to fix a deviated nasal septum.

Nursing

- Instruct the patient to avoid areas where there is heavy dust, mites or molds.
- Ask the patient to avoid pet animals.
- Encourage the patient to wash the floors frequently with a wet mop.
- Instruct the patient to reduce air humidity with a dehumidifier to maintain indoor humidity around 40–45%.
- Instruct the patient to put special dust mite covers on mattresses.
- Ask the patient to remove houseplants.
- Ask the patient to stay indoors during high pollen times.
- Encourage the patient to remove furniture that collects dust.
- Instruct the patient to avoid tobacco smoking.
- Instruct the patient to avoid using window fans that can draw pollens and molds into the house.

SINUSITIS

Definition

Sinusitis is an inflammation of the sinuses that can be caused by viruses, bacteria, fungi, allergies or even an autoimmune reaction.

Etiology

- Viral infection (Common cold)
- Bacterial infection (e.g., Group A beta-hemolytic streptococci, etc.)
- Cystic fibrosis
- Dental infection
- Nasal polyps
- Deviated nasal septum
- Lack of cilia motility
- Enlarged or infected adenoids
- Lack of sufficient humidity
- Pollen given off by trees, grass and weeds
- Head injury.

Risk Factors

- Being young children or elderly
- Having a history of allergies
- Recent upper respiratory infection
- History of asthma
- Breathing aided by mechanical ventilator
- Weakened immune system
- Smoking
- Cocaine use
- Diabetes

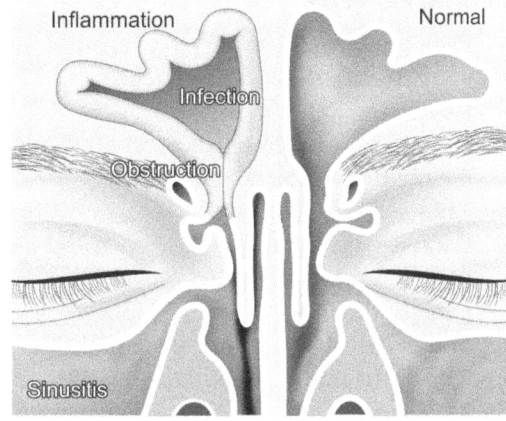

Fig. 4.14: Shows the comparison of inflamed sinus cavity with that of normal one.

- Gastroesophageal reflux disease
- Oral or intravenous steroid treatment
- Hypothyroidism
- Kartagener's syndrome
- Changes in atmospheric pressure.

Types

- ***Acute sinusitis:*** It comes on suddenly and brings about symptoms similar to that of a cold. Usually, it lasts for 1–4 weeks period
- ***Subacute sinusitis:*** It produces the symptoms and usually it lasts for 1 to 2 months.
- ***Chronic sinusitis:*** It produces the symptoms and usually it lasts for more than 2 months.
- ***Recurrent sinusitis:*** It produces the symptoms and occurs several times a year.

Pathophysiology

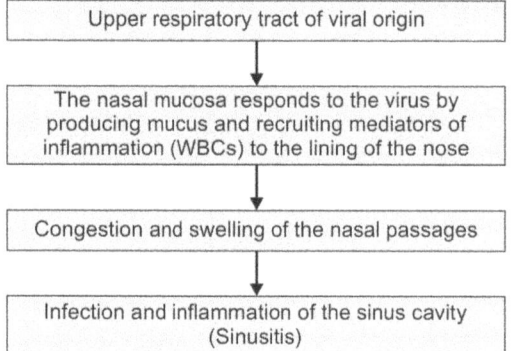

Clinical Features

- Pain, tenderness and swelling around the eyes, cheeks, nose and forehead
- Headache
- Thick yellow or greenish discharge from the nose
- Fatigue
- Decreased sense of smell
- Reduced sense of taste
- Sore throat
- Cough that is heavy during the night
- Pain in the upper jaw and teeth
- Bad breath
- Fever
- Nose congestion or stuffiness
- Itching eyes
- Sneezing
- Bodyache
- Ear pain.

Complications

- Periorbital cellulitis
- Cavernous sinus thrombosis
- Brain abscess
- Meningitis
- Status asthmaticus.

Diagnostic Tests

- History
- Physical examination
- Nasal endoscopy
- Nasal and sinus culture
- Skin allergy test
- Computed tomography (CT) scan
- Magnetic resonance imaging (MRI) scan.

Management

Medical

- **Antibiotics:** It helps to eliminate the sinusitis by attacking the bacteria that cause it. For example, amoxicillin, penicillin, etc.
- **Nasal decongestants:** These medications shrink swollen nasal passages, facilitating the flow of drainage from the sinuses. For example, ipratropium bromide, oxymetazoline, phenylephrine, etc.
- **Topical nasal corticosteroids:** They are effective in shrinking and preventing the return of nasal polyps. For example, dexamethasone, methylprednisolone, etc.
- **Antihistamines:** It block inflammation caused by an allergic reaction so they can help to fight against allergies that can lead to swollen nasal and sinus passages. For example, phenergan, allegra, diphenhydramine, etc.
- **Nonsteroidal anti-inflammatory drugs:** It helps to relieve pain caused by sinusitis. For example, ibuprofen, naproxen, etc.
- **Analgesics:** It helps to quickly relieve inflammation and reduce pain. For example, acetaminophen, paracetamol, etc.

- **Antiviral agents:** It slows the growth and spread of the influenza virus in the body. For example, acyclovir, zidovudine, rimantadine, etc.

Surgical

- **Functional endoscopic surgery:** It is a surgical procedure in which through an endoscope the diseased tissues are removed to enlarge the sinus openings for drainage.
- **Balloon sinuplasty:** It is a surgical procedure in which a catheter with an inflatable balloon is inserted into the sinus and the balloon is then inflated to widen sinus openings.
- **Open sinus surgery:** It is a surgical procedure in which an incision is made directly over the sinus to remove the diseased tissue and the sinus is reconstructed.

Nursing

- Instruct the patient to avoid close contact with individuals who suffer from cold.
- Recommend the patient to wash the hands with soap and water at frequent intervals.
- Instruct the patient to avoid smoking and cocaine use.
- Encourage the patient to use modifier at home to add moisture to the indoor spaces.
- Ask the patient to avoid going to places which are polluted and overcrowded.

TONSILLITIS

Definition

Tonsillitis is an infection of the tonsils, which are glands on either side of the back of the throat.

Etiology

- Viral infection (e.g., Herpes simplex virus, *Streptococcus pyogenes*, adenovirus, cytomegalovirus, enterovirus, Epstein-Barr virus, measles virus, etc.)
- Bacterial infection (e.g., *Streptococcus pyogenes*, etc.)

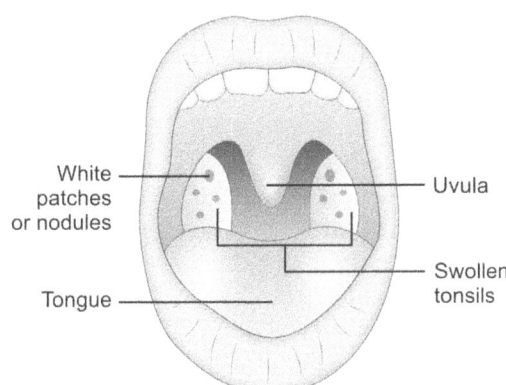

Fig. 4.15: Depicts swollen tonsils on either side at the back of the throat.

- Infectious mononucleosis
- Chronic lymphocytic leukemia (CLL).

Risk Factors

- Being children and young adults
- Overcrowding
- Exposure to other in public places
- Smoking
- Being males
- Recent throat or dental infection
- Weakened immune system.

Pathophysiology

Viral infection (e.g., Herpes simplex virus, *Streptococcus pyogenes*, adenovirus, cytomegalovirus, enterovirus, Epstein-Barr virus, measles virus, etc.)

↓

Viruses gain access to the mucosal cells lining the tonsils and replicate in these cells

↓

Infection or inflammation of the tonsils (Tonsillitis)

Clinical Features

- Throat pain, either mild or severe
- Sore throat
- Drooling
- Pain when swallowing
- Neck stiffness
- Fever
- Chills
- Swollen lymph glands on either side of the jaw

- Headache
- Bad breath
- Ear pain
- Cough
- Vomiting
- Red and swollen tonsils (with pus)
- Refusal to eat
- Stomach upset or pain
- General malaise
- Hoarseness of voice
- Snoring at night.

Complications

- Otitis media
- Obstructive sleep apnea
- Scarlet fever
- Acute rheumatic fever
- Post-streptococcal glomerulonephritis
- Peritonsillar abscess
- Retropharyngeal abscess.

Diagnostic Tests

- History
- Physical examination
- Blood examination
- Needle aspiration test
- Ultrasound examination
- Computed tomography (CT) scan
- Magnetic resonance imaging (MRI) scan.

Management

Medical

- **Antimicrobial agents:** It helps in preventing secondary infections. For example, penicillin, amoxicillin, benzathine penicillin G, erythromycin, cephalosporin, etc.
- **Nonsteroidal anti-inflammatory drugs:** It helps to relieve swelling caused by swollen face and neck. For example, ibuprofen, naproxen, etc.
- **Analgesics:** It helps to quickly reduce pain. For example, acetaminophen, paracetamol, etc.
- **Antiviral agents:** It slows the growth and spread of the herpes virus in the body. For example, acyclovir, zidovudine, rimantadine, etc.
- **Corticosteroids:** It helps to relieve swelling and reduce the severity of the disease. For example, dexamethasone, methylprednisolone, etc.

Surgical

- **Needle aspiration:** It is a surgical procedure in which long, fine needle is used to draw out the pus that builds-up at the back of the throat, near the tonsils.
- **Tonsillectomy:** It is a surgical procedure in which the tonsils found at the back of the throat, behind the tongue are removed.

Nursing

- Ask the patient to gargle frequently with warm salt water (1 tsp of salt in 1 cup warm water) throughout the day.
- Ask the patient to drink plenty of fluids.
- Instruct the patient to avoid smoking.
- Encourage the patient to eat ice chips or use throat spray or lozenges for sore throats.
- Encourage the patient to use a cool-mist vaporizer and nasal spray for congestion.
- Encourage the patient to take a bland diet.
- Encourage the patient to do handwashing.
- Encourage the patient to take adequate bedrest during febrile phase.
- Instruct the patient to avoid sharing items such as water bottles, utensils, etc.

5

CHAPTER

Disorders of Gastrointestinal System

CHAPTER OUTLINE

- Amoebic dysentery
- Anal fissure
- Anal fistula
- Appendicitis
- Bacillary dysentery
- Cholecystitis
- Cholelithiasis
- Constipation
- Crohn's disease
- Deficiency diseases
- Diarrhea
- Gastritis
- Gastroesophageal reflux disease (GERD) with esophagitis
- Hemorrhoids
- Hepatic encephalopathy
- Hepatitis
- Hernia
- Intestinal obstruction
- Liver abscess
- Liver cirrhosis
- Malabsorption syndrome
- Pancreatitis
- Parasitic infestations
- Peptic ulcer disease
- Peritonitis
- Pharyngitis
- Ulcerative colitis

AMOEBIC DYSENTERY (AMOEBIASIS)

Definition

Amoebic dysentery is an infection of the intestines caused by the parasite *Entamoeba histolytica*.

Etiology

Parasitic infection (*Entamoeba histolytica*).

Risk Factors

- Alcoholism
- Cancer
- Malnutrition
- Advanced age
- Pregnancy
- Recent travel to a tropical region
- Use of corticosteroid medication to suppress the immune system.

Diarrhea may be caused by bacteria or parasites found in food and water

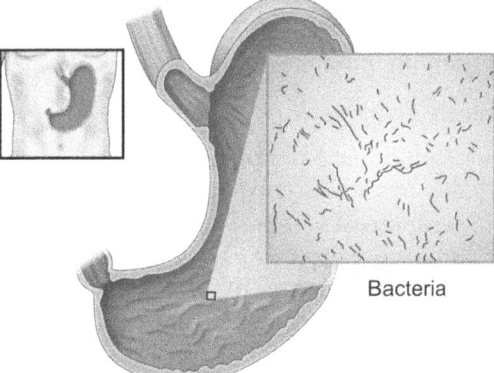

Fig. 5.1: Shows infection of the intestines.

Pathophysiology

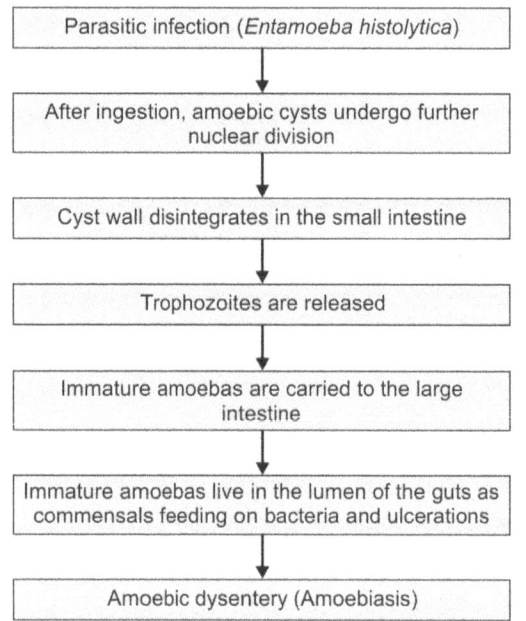

Clinical Features

Mild Symptoms

- Abdominal cramps
- Intermittent diarrhea consisting of three to eight foul-smelling loose or watery stools daily containing mucus and blood.
- Fatigue
- Flatulence
- Abdominal cramping
- Slight pain
- Tenesmus (rectal pain while having a bowel movement)
- Unintentional weight loss.

Severe Symptoms

- Abdominal tenderness
- Bloody stools consisting of liquid stools with streaks of blood, passage of 10–20 stools per day
- High fever (104°F–105°F)
- Hepatomegaly
- Vomiting.

Complications

- Hepatic abscess
- Peritonitis
- Peptic ulcer
- Intestinal perforation.

Diagnostic Tests

- History
- Physical examination
- Stool examination
- Blood examination
- Sigmoidoscopic examination.

Management

Medical

- **Antibiotics:** It helps to prevent secondary infections. For example, metronidazole, etc.
- **Tissue amoebicides:** It acts by destroying trophozoites in tissue including those in the wall of the intestine. For example, iodoquinol, diphosphate, emetine, etc.
- **Luminal amoebicides:** It acts by direct contact with trophozoites dwelling in the bowel lumen. For example, furamide, di-iodohydroxyquin, etc.

Nursing

- Instruct the client to avoid contaminated food and water.
- Encourage the patient to maintain general sanitation.
- Educate to avoid scalding of vegetables and the use of iodine-releasing tablet in drinking water.
- Ask them not to eat any foods cooked in unhygienic circumstances such as from street vendors.
- Ask them to eat only cooked foods that have been heated to a high temperature
- Consider traveling with an alcohol-based hand sanitizer.

ANAL FISSURE

Definition

An anal fissure is a longitudinal tear or ulceration in the lining of the anal canal.

Etiology

- Passing hard stools
- Chronic constipation

Disorders of Gastrointestinal System

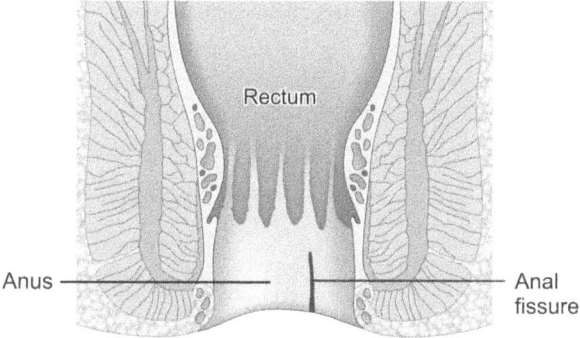

Fig. 5.2: Depicts a cut of tear in the thin and delicate lining of the anus.

- Child birth (Straining of perineum)
- Decreased blood flow to the anorectal area
- Overly tight or spastic anal sphincter muscles
- Anal cancer
- Tuberculosis
- Syphilis.

Risk Factors

- Infancy
- Older adults
- Pregnancy
- Overuse of laxatives
- Crohn's disease.

Pathophysiology

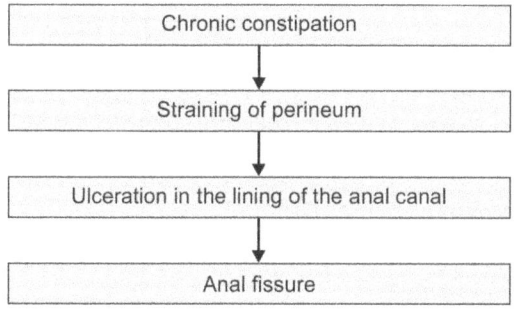

Clinical Features

- Sharp pain in the anal area during bowel movements
- Burning sensation in the anal area
- A visible tear in the skin around the anus
- Bright red blood from the anus
- Presence of blood in stools
- Spasm of the anal canal.

Complications

- Anal fistulas
- Anal stenosis
- Recurrence.

Diagnostic Tests

- History
- Physical examination
- Blood examination
- Blood culture
- Flexible sigmoidoscopic examination
- Colonoscopic examination.

Management

Medical

- **Stool softeners:** It helps to prevent constipation. For example, Naturolax, etc.
- **Emollient suppositories:** It helps to prevent constipation. For example, dulcolax, etc.
- **Antibiotics:** It helps to prevent secondary infections For example, ciprofloxacin, etc.
- **Topical corticosteroids:** It helps to promote blood flow to the area and promote healing in the anal area. For example, prednisone, cortisone, etc.
- **Topical analgesic agents:** I helps to ease any discomfort. For example, anusol, lidocaine, etc.

Surgical

- **Fissurectomy with lateral internal sphincterectomy:** It is a surgical procedure through which surgical removal of the anal

fissure is done with an opening made into the sphincter guarding the anus.
- **Sitz bath with potassium permanganate:** It involves sitting in a shallow bath of warm water mixed with potassium permanganate for around 20 minutes.

Nursing

- Instruct to change diapers frequently in infants.
- Instruct them to keep the anal area dry.
- Ask them to cleanse the area gently with mild soap and warm water.
- Instruct them to avoid constipation by drinking 6-8 glasses of everyday water, eating fibrous foods and exercising regularly.
- Ask them to take regular sitz baths.

ANAL FISTULA

Definition

An anal fistula is a tiny, tubular abnormal opening on the cutaneous surface near the anus usually resulting from a local crypt abscess.

Etiology

- Anal abscess
- A growth or ulcer (Painful sore)
- A complication of surgery
- Tuberculosis
- Chlamydia
- Syphilis
- Local crypt abscess
- Congenital defects
- Trauma during child birth
- Regional enteritis.

Risk Factors

- Diabetes mellitus
- Crohn's disease
- Colitis
- Immunocompromised persons
- Radiotherapy for rectal cancer
- Chronic diarrhea.

Types

- *Intersphincteric fistula:* The tract begins in the space between the internal and external sphincter muscles and opens very close to the anal opening.
- *Transsphincteric fistula:* The tract begins in the space between the internal and external sphincter muscles or in the space behind the anus. It then crosses the external sphincter and opens an inch or two outside the anal opening. These can wrap around the body in a U shape, with external openings on both sides of the anus (also known as horseshoe fistula).
- *Suprasphincteric fistula:* The tract begins in the space between the internal and external sphincter muscles and turns upward to a point above the puborectal muscle, crosses this muscle, then extends

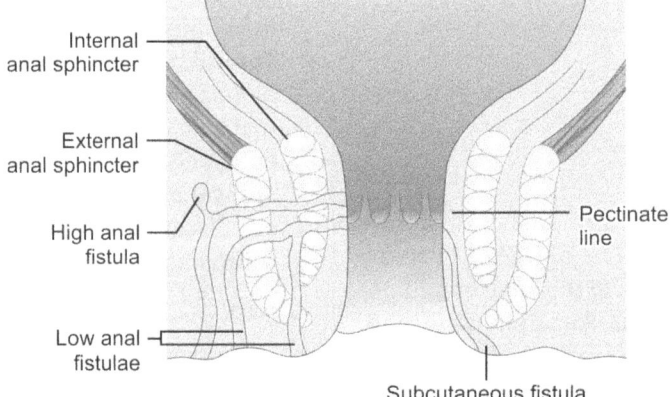

Fig. 5.3: Shows tiny tubular abnormal opening on the cutaneous surface near the anus.

downward between the puborectal and levator ani muscle and opens an inch or two outside the anus.
- **Extrasphincteric fistula:** The tract begins at the rectum or sigmoid colon and extends downward, passes through the levator ani muscle and opens around the anus.

Pathophysiology

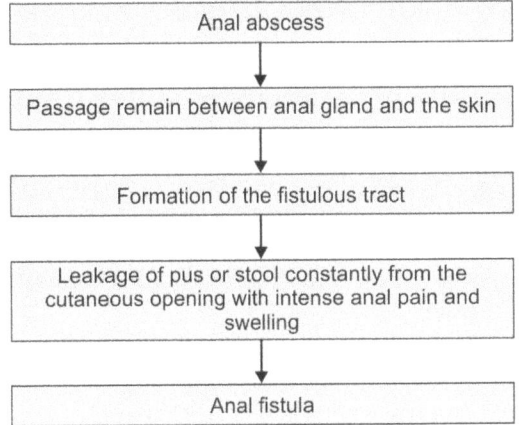

Clinical Features

- Intense anal pain and swelling that may be worse when sitting down, moveing around or during bowel movement.
- Leakage of pus or stool constantly from the cutaneous opening
- Skin irritation around the anus
- Passage of flatus or feces from the vagina or bladder
- Discharge of pus or blood when having a bowel movement
- Constipation
- Fever and chills
- Feeling tired and sick.

Complications

- Infection
- Incontinence
- Recurrence.

Diagnostic Tests

- History
- Physical examination
- Blood culture
- Blood examination
- Fistula probe examination
- Anoscopic examination
- Fistulographic examination
- Magnetic resonance imaging (MRI) scan
- Computed tomography (CT) scan
- Flexible sigmoidoscopic examination
- Colonoscopic examination.

Management

Medical

- **Laxatives:** It helps to prevent constipation. For example, dulcolax, etc.
- **Antibiotics:** It helps to reduce the risk of infections. For example, ciprofloxacin, etc.
- **Analgesic agents:** It helps to relieve pain. For example, paracetamol, ibuprofen, buscopan, tramadol, etc.
- **Topical corticosteroids:** It helps to promote blood flow to the area and promotes healing in the anal area. For example, prednisone, cortisone, etc.

Surgical

- **Fistulotomy:** It is the surgical procedure in which fistula is dissected out or laid open by an incision from its rectal opening to its outlet.
- **Fistulectomy:** It is the surgical removal of the fistula.
- **Advancement rectal flap:** It is a surgical procedure in which a surgeon cores out the tract and then cuts a flap into the rectal wall to access and remove the fistula's internal opening, then stitches the flap back down. This is often done to reduce the amount of sphincter muscle to be cut.
- **Seton placement:** It is a surgical procedure in which a seton (silk string or rubber band) is used to create a scar tissue around part of the sphincter muscle before cutting it with a knife.

Nursing

- Ask them to wear a pad over the anal area until the healing is complete.

- Instruct them to keep the anal area dry and clean.
- Instruct them to resume normal activities only when they are asked to do so.
- Instruct them to avoid constipation by drinking 6-8 glasses of water everyday, eating fibrous foods and exercising regularly.
- Ask them to do soaking in a warm bath 3-4 times a day.

APPENDICITIS

Definition

It is swelling (inflammation) of the appendix, which is a small pouch attached to the large intestine.

Etiology

- Food or fecal matter getting lodged in the appendix
- Obstruction (foreign object, or tumor).
- Infection.

Risk Factors

- Having a family history of appendicitis
- Being a male
- Being between the ages of 10 and 19 years old
- Having a long-lasting inflammatory or bowel disease.

Pathophysiology

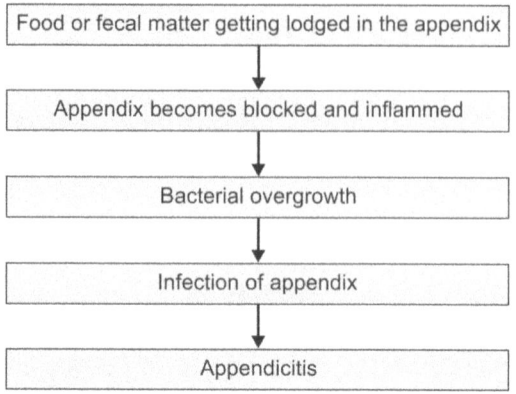

Clinical Features

- Sharp and severe pain around the belly button and tends to focus at a spot directly above the appendix called McBurney's point
- Pain may be worse when they walk, cough or make sudden movements
- Progressively worsening pain
- Nausea
- Vomiting
- Loss of appetite
- Lowgrade fever and chills
- Constipation or diarrhea
- Gas and bloating
- Rebound tenderness.

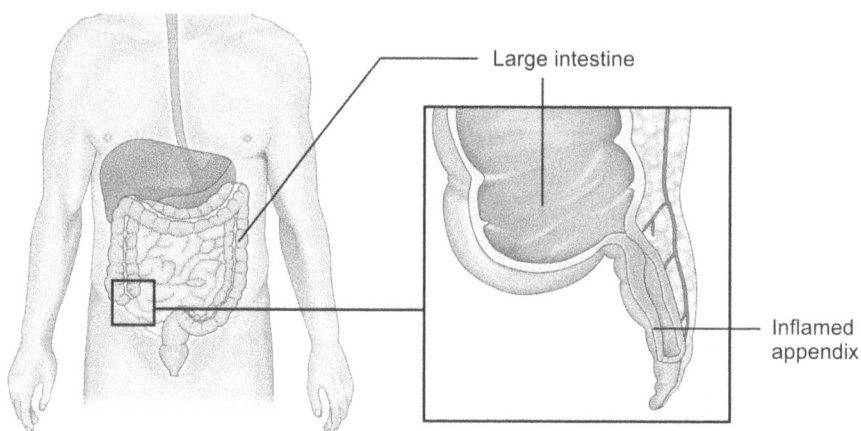

Fig. 5.4: Shows the inflamed appendix which is a small pouch like projection attached to the large intestine.

Complications
- Necrosis
- Gangrene
- Rupture or perforation of appendix.

Diagnostic Tests
- History
- Physical examination
- Blood examination
- Urine examination (a protein detectable in urine serve as a biomarker for appendicitis)
- Magnetic resonance imaging (MRI)
- CT scan.

Management

Medical

Antibiotics: It helps to prevent secondary infections. For example, ciprofloxacin, gentamicin, cephalosporin, etc.

Surgical

Surgery is the only treatment for acute appendicitis.
- **Open appendectomy:** It is a traditional surgical procedure through which the appendix is removed within hours of diagnosis and the incision is then closed with stitches.
- **Laparoscopic appendectomy:** It is a less invasive surgical procedure in which the appendix is removed through a small tube, leaving a very tiny scar.

Nursing
- Instruct them to refrain from strenuous activities (heavy lifting, sports, gym activities, etc.) for few weeks.
- Encourage them to keep the surgical area clean and watch for signs of infection.
- Encourage the patient to maintain general sanitation.
- Encourage the patient to eat soft and bland diet.

BACILLARY DYSENTERY OR SHIGELLOSIS

Definition
It is an acute, self-limited infection of the intestinal tract which is caused by the bacteria (*Shigella dysenteriae*) and characterized by diarrhea, fever and abdominal pain.

Etiology
Bacterial infection (*Shigella dysenteriae*).

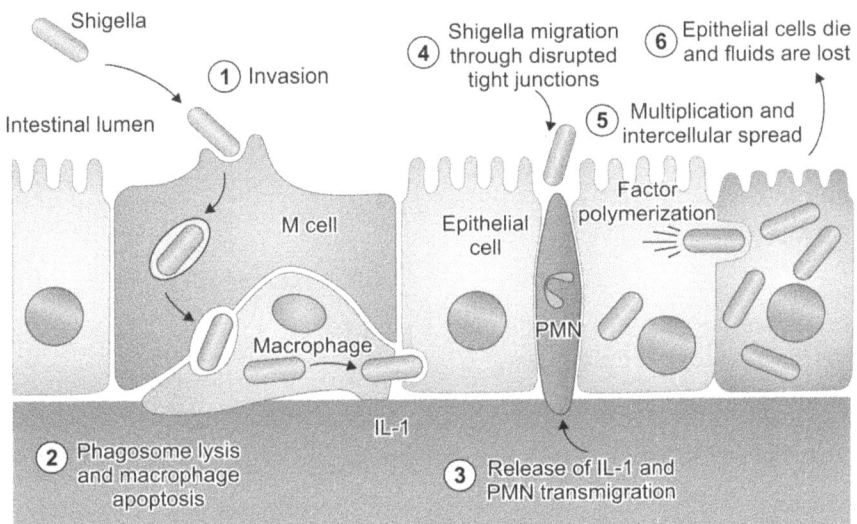

Fig. 5.5: Shows the acute infection of the intestinal tract caused by the bacteria Shigella.

Risk Factors

- Young children
- HIV infected persons
- Travellers to developing countries
- Traditionally observant Jewish communities.

Pathophysiology

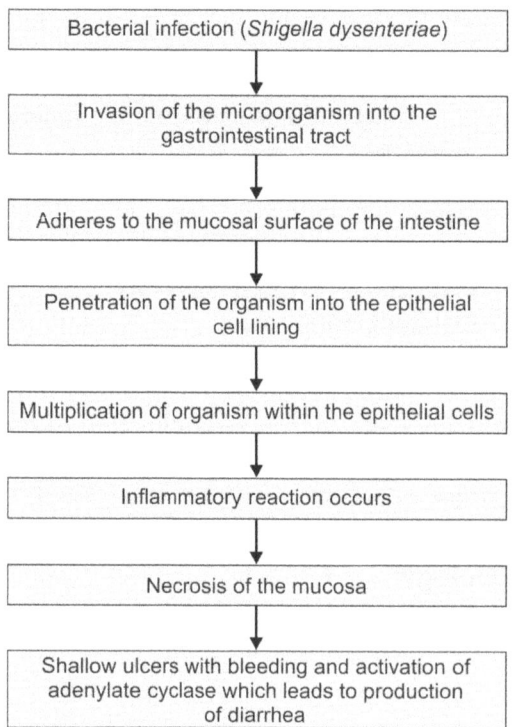

Clinical Features

- Fever
- Abdominal pain
- Diarrhea
- Tenesmus
- Headache
- Nausea
- Vomiting
- Myalgia
- Greenish liquid stools containing mucus
- Abdominal tenderness
- Splenomegaly
- Hyperactive bowel sounds.

Complications

- Post-infectious arthritis
- Seizures
- Perforation of the colon
- Bacteremia
- Reiter's syndrome
- Hemolytic uremia syndrome
- Peripheral neuropathy.

Diagnostic Tests

- History
- Physical examination
- Blood examination
- Blood culture
- Stool examination
- Stool culture.

Management

Medical

- **Antibiotics:** It helps to prevent any secondary infections For example, ampicillin, bismuth subsalicylate, tetracycline, etc.
- **Analgesics:** It helps to relieve pain. For example, voveran, tramadol, etc.

Nursing

- Ask them to follow food and water precautions strictly when traveling internationally.
- Instruct them to wash hands with soap frequently.
- Instruct the client to maintain proper sanitation.
- Encourage to maintain adequate sewage disposal.
- Instruct them not to prepare food for others when they are sick.
- Instruct them to avoid swimming until they are fully recovered.

CHOLECYSTITIS

Definition

The infection and inflammation of the gallbladder is known as cholecystitis.

Etiology

- Cholelithiasis
- Infection
- Tumors of the gallbladder.

Disorders of Gastrointestinal System

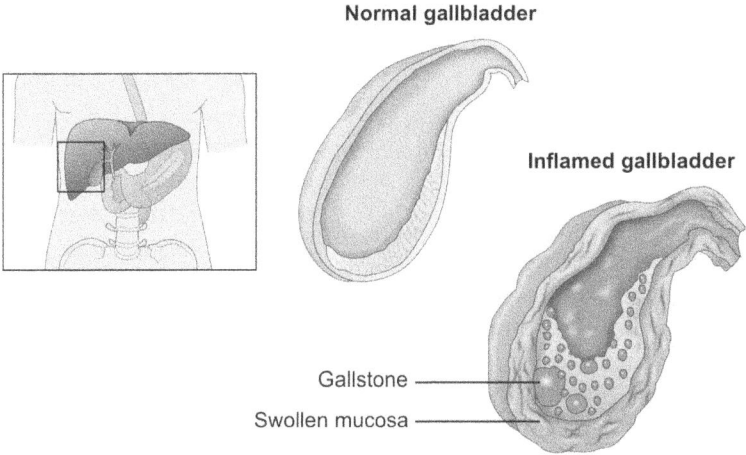

Fig. 5.6: Shows the comparison of normal and inflamed gallbladder.

Risk Factors

- Being females
- Pregnancy
- Estrogen therapy
- Old age
- Obesity
- Losing or gaining weight rapidly
- Diabetes.

Pathophysiology

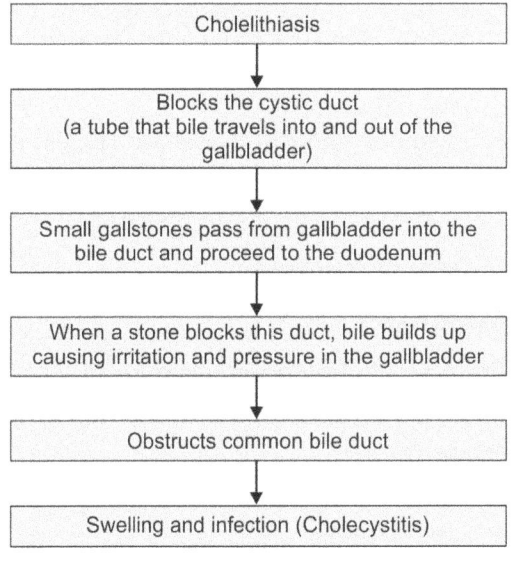

Clinical Features

- Fever
- Abdominal pain that lasts for several hours
- Episodic colicky pain in epigastric area which radiates to back and shoulder
- Chest pain after eating fatty or fried foods
- Nausea
- Vomiting
- Indigestion
- Jaundice
- Murphy's sign (inability to take a deep inspiration when examiner's fingers are pressed below the hepatic margin)
- Flatulence
- Belching
- Clay-colored stools
- Dark amber-colored urine
- Steatorrhea
- Pruritus (itching)
- Mild hepatomegaly.

Complications

- Gangrene
- Hemorrhage
- Cirrhosis
- Intestinal perforation
- Pancreatitis
- Peritonitis.

Diagnostic Tests

- History
- Physical examination
- Oral cholecystography—to know the presence of stones or inflammation
- Ultrasonography—to detect gallstones
- Percutaneous transhepatic cholangiography—to distinguish obstructive jaundice
- Endoscopic retrograde cholangiopancreatography—to visualize the common bile, pancreatic and hepatic ducts
- Hepatobiliary iminodiacetic scan (HIDA scan)—to diagnose hepatobiliary disorders
- Blood examination
- Liver function tests
- Cholangiogram—to visualize gallbladder and bile duct.

Management

Medical

- **Antibiotics:** It helps to prevent any secondary infections. For example, ampicillin, cephalothin, bismuth subsalicylate, tetracycline, etc.
- **Antilithic agents:** It solubilizes the gallstones. For example, chenodiol, ursodiol, etc.
- **Analgesics:** It helps to relieve pain. For example, meperidine, morphine, etc.
- **Anticholinergics:** It helps in reducing the secretions. For example, propantheline, dicyclomine, etc.
- **Antiemetics:** It helps in preventing vomiting. For example, Prochlorperazine, etc.
- **Vitamin supplements:** It helps in providing vitamins for body regulation. For example, cyanocobalamine, Phytonadione, etc.

Surgical

- **Extracorporeal shock wave lithotripsy:** It is a surgical procedure in which gallstones are fragmented into small pieces.
- **Choledochostomy:** It is a surgical procedure in which an incision is made into the common bile duct usually for the removal of stones.
- **Cholecystostomy:** It is a surgical procedure where a stoma is created in the gallbladder to remove the gallstones and also to facilitate placement of a tube for drainage of bile or the purulent drainage.
- **Laparoscopic laser cholecystectomy:** It is the surgical removal of gallbladder through a small incision or puncture made through the abdominal wall in the umbilicus.
- **Cholecystectomy:** In this surgical procedure, in which the gallbladder is removed through an abdominal incision (Usually through right subcostal area).
- **Endoscopic sphincterotomy:** It is a relatively new endoscopic technique developed to examine and treat abnormalities of the bile ducts, pancreas and gallbladder.

Nursing

- Ask them to follow food and water precautions strictly when traveling internationally.
- Encourage them to take low-fat, high-protein, high fiber and high carbohydrate diet.
- Instruct them to take complete bedrest.
- Facilitate them with calm and quiet environment.
- Encourage them to do exercise 5 times per week for at least 30 minutes each time.
- Instruct them not to lose weight so rapidly.

CHOLELITHIASIS

Definition

The presence of one or more calculi (gallstones) in the gallbladder is known as cholelithiasis.

Etiology

- Sickle cell anemia
- Liver cirrhosis

Disorders of Gastrointestinal System

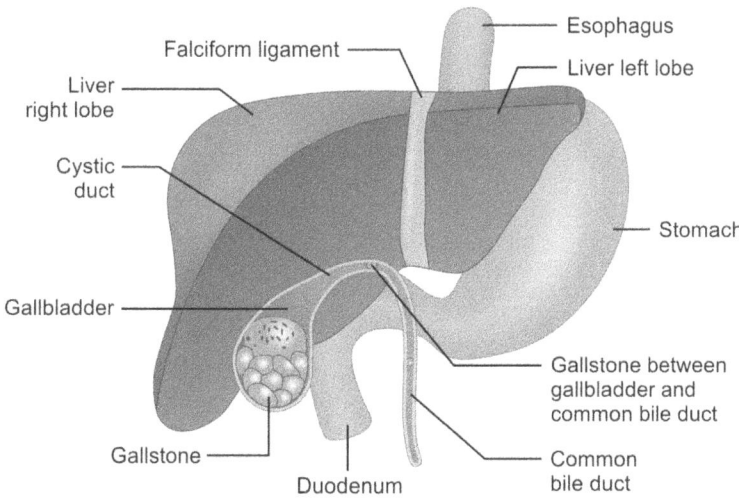

Fig. 5.7: Shows the presence of one or more calculi (gallstones) in the gallbladder.

- Gallbladder abnormalities
- Intake of high fatty diet
- Obesity
- Diabetes mellitus
- Losing or gaining weight rapidly
- Intake of high fiber diet
- Biliary tract infections.

Risk Factors

- Being females
- Increased age
- American Indian ethnicity
- Increased triglycerides
- Dehydration
- Family history of cholelithiasis
- Pregnancy
- Hormone replacement therapy.

Types

There are several types of gallstones as follows:
- **Cholesterol stones:** It accounts for more than 85% of gallstones in the world.
- **Black pigment stones:** These are small, hard gallstones composed of Ca bilirubinate and inorganic calcium salts.
- **Brown pigment stones:** These are soft and greasy consisting of bilirubinate and fatty acids.

Pathophysiology

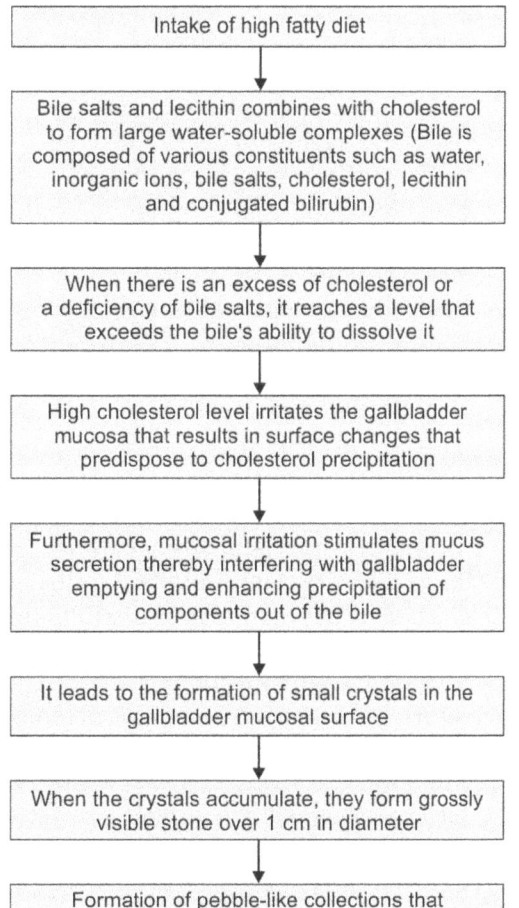

Clinical Features

- Anorexia
- Nausea
- Vomiting
- Weight loss
- Diarrhea
- Fat intolerance
- Tea-colored urine
- Clay-colored stool
- Jaundice
- Biliary colic.

Complications

- Cholecystitis
- Cholangitis
- Choledocholithiasis
- Pancreatitis.

Diagnostic Tests

- History
- Physical examination
- Computed tomography (CT) scan
- Ultrasonography—to detect gallstones
- Percutaneous transhepatic cholangiography (PTCA)
- Endoscopic retrograde cholangiopancreatography (ERCP)
- Gallbladder radionuclide scan
- Endoscopic ultrasound
- Blood examination
- Liver function tests.

Management

Medical

- **Antibiotics:** It helps to prevent any secondary infections. For example, ampicillin, cephalothin, bismuth subsalicylate, tetracycline, etc.
- **Antilithic agents:** It solubilizes the gallstones. For example, chemodiol, ursodiol, etc.
- **Analgesics:** It helps to relieve pain. For example, meperidine, morphine, etc.
- **Antiemetics:** It helps in preventing vomiting. For example, prochlorperazine, etc.

Surgical

- **Cholecystostomy:** It is a surgical procedure where a stoma is created in the gallbladder to remove the gallstones and also to facilitate placement of a tube for drainage of bile or the purulent drainage.
- **Laparoscopic laser cholecystectomy:** It is the surgical removal of gallbladder through a small incision or puncture made through the abdominal wall in the umbilicus.
- **Cholecystectomy:** In this surgical procedure, in which the gallbladder is removed through an abdominal incision (Usually through right subcostal area).
- **Oral dissolution therapy:** It is a procedure in which drugs (Ursodiol and Chenodiol) made from bile acid are used to dissolve gallstones.
- **Contact dissolution therapy:** It is a surgical procedure in which a drug is injected directly into the gallbladder to dissolve cholesterol stones.

Nursing

- Encourage them to take small and frequent diet.
- Encourage them eat a diet low in saturated fat.
- Encourage them to eat plenty of fruits, vegetables and whole grain foods.
- Instruct them to take complete bedrest.
- Facilitate them with calm and quiet environment.
- Encourage them to do exercise 5 times per week for at least 30 minutes each time.
- Instruct them not to lose weight so rapidly.

CONSTIPATION (DYSCHEZIA)

Definition

Constipation is a condition in which one has fewer than three bowel movements a week, or hard, dry and small bowel movements that are painful or difficult to pass.

Disorders of Gastrointestinal System

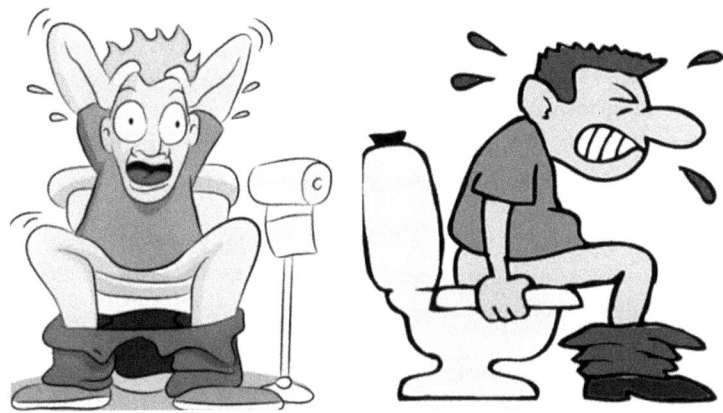

Fig. 5.8: Depicts hard, dry and small bowel movements that are painful or difficult to pass.

Etiology

- Anal fissure
- Bowel obstruction
- Colon cancer
- Narrowing of the colon (bowel stricture)
- Rectal cancer
- Rectocele
- Autonomic neuropathy
- Multiple sclerosis
- Parkinson's disease
- Spinal cord injury
- Diabetes
- Hyperparathyroidism
- Pregnancy.

Risk Factors

- Being females
- Being an older adult
- Being dehydrated
- Eating a diet that is low in fiber
- Getting little or no physical activity.

Pathophysiology

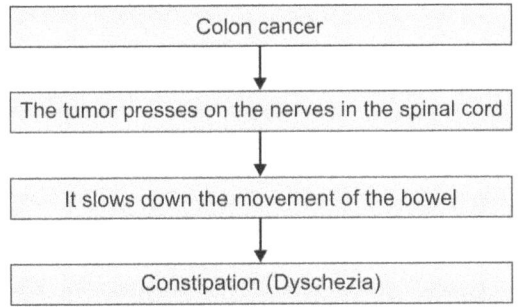

Clinical Features

- Inability to have a bowel movement for several days
- Hard compacted stools that are difficult or painful to pass
- Straining during bowel movements
- Stomach aches that are relieved by bowel movements
- Abdominal bloating, cramps or pain
- Decreased appetite
- Lethargy.

Complications

- Hemorrhoids
- Anal fissure
- Fecal impaction
- Rectal prolapse.

Diagnostic Tests

- History
- Physical examination
- Sigmoidoscopy
- Colonoscopy
- Anorectal manometry
- Colonic transit study
- Defecography.

Management

Medical

- **Bulk-forming agents:** It helps trigger the bowel to contract and push stool out. For example, citrucel, metamucil, serutan, etc.

- **Osmotic agents:** It helps stool retain fluid and increases the number of bowel movements and softens stool. For example, cephulac, milk of magnesia, sorbitol, etc.
- **Stool softeners:** It helps mix fluid into stools to soften them. For example, colace, docusate, etc.
- **Lubricants:** It works by coating the surface of stool, which helps the stool hold in fluid and pass more easily. For example, fleet, zymenol, etc.
- **Stimulants:** It causes the intestines to contract, which moves stool. For example, correctol, dulcolax, purge, senokot, etc.
- **Chloride channel activator:** It increases fluid in the gastrointestinal tract to make the stool softer. For example, lubiprostone, etc.
- **Guanylate cyclase C-agonist:** It eases pain in the abdomen and speeds up the bowel movements. For example, Linaclotide, etc.

Nursing

- Ask them to limit stress in life.
- Encourage them to gradually increase the high fiber diet.
- Instruct them to drink 6–8 glasses of water each day.
- Encourage them to take more raw fruits and vegetables.
- Ask them to go for a short walk when they feel anxious or stressful.
- Instruct them to limit refined and processed foods.
- Encourage them to do exercise 5 times per week for at least 30 minutes each time.

CROHN'S DISEASE

Definition

Crohn's disease is a chronic or a long-lasting disease that causes inflammation, irritation or swelling in the gastrointestinal tract.

Etiology

- Autoimmune reaction
- Inherited genes
- Environmental factors
- Stress
- Idiopathic.

Risk Factors

- Smoking
- Certain medications (Aspirin, Ibuprofen, etc.)

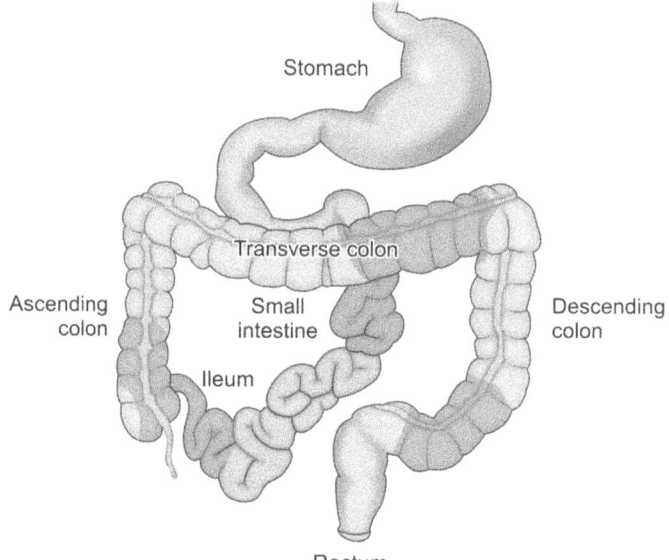

Fig. 5.9: Depicts inflamed and swollen gastrointestinal tract due to Crohn's disease.

- Seasonal changes
- Those between 20 and 29 years
- Family history of Crohn's disease
- Ethnicity
- Use of oral contraceptives
- Tobacco chewing.

Pathophysiology

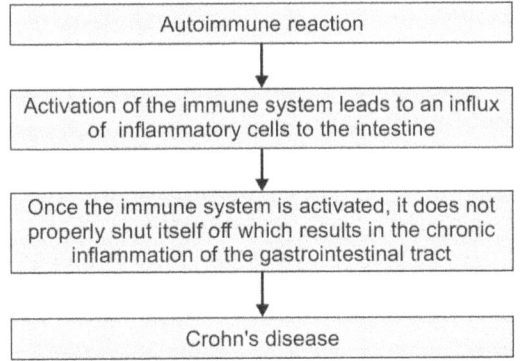

Clinical Features

- Crampy abdominal pain
- Fever
- Fatigue
- Anemia
- Joint pain or soreness
- Eye irritation
- Mouth ulcers
- Loss of appetite
- Tenesmus (Pain while passing stools)
- Persistent watery diarrhea
- Urgent need to move bowels
- Night sweats
- Weight loss
- Rectal bleeding
- Sensation of incomplete evacuation
- Malnutrition and vitamin deficiencies
- Bone loss (osteoporosis).

Complications

- Abscesses
- Bowel obstructions
- Erythema nodosum
- Swollen joints
- Pyoderma gangrenosum.

Diagnostic Tests

- History
- Physical examination
- Sigmoidoscopy
- Barium enema
- Computed tomography (CT) scan
- Capsule endoscopy
- Magnetic resonance imaging (MRI) scan
- Enteroscopy
- Blood examination.

Management

Medical

- **Aminosalicylates:** It works at the level of the lining of the gastrointestinal tract to decrease inflammation. They are effective in treating mild to moderate episodes of Crohn's disease and useful as a maintenance treatment in preventing relapses of the disease. For example, sulfasalazine, mesalamine, olsalazine, balsalazide, etc.
- **Corticosteroids:** It is used to treat moderate to severely active Crohn's disease. For example, prednisone, methylprednisolone, etc.
- **Immunomodulators:** It suppresses the body's immune system response so it cannot cause ongoing inflammation. For example, azathioprine, 6-mercaptopurine, etc.
- **Antibiotics:** It helps to prevent secondary infections. For example, ciprofloxacin, metronidazole, ampicillin, etc.
- **Biologic therapies:** These are antibodies grown in the laboratory that stop certain proteins in the body from causing inflammation. For example, infliximab, adalimumab, certolizumab, natalizumab, etc.

Surgical

- **Total proctocolectomy with ileostomy:** It is the surgical removal of the entire colon (colon, rectum and anus with anal closure) and rectum and a stoma or opening is

made in the abdomen in the last section of the small intestine to allow drainage of fiscal matter from the ileum to the outside of the body.
- **Ileostomy:** It is a surgical procedure in which a hole is created in the abdomen for the elimination of waste.
- **Subtotal colectomy (Large bowel resection):** It is a surgical procedure in which the diseased portion of the colon is removed and the healthy intestine on either side of the removed area is sewn together.
- **Small bowel resection:** It is a surgical procedure in which a segment of the small intestine is removed and the two ends of healthy intestine are joined together (anastomosis).
- **Total abdominal colectomy:** It is the surgical removal of the large intestine from the lowest part of the small intestine (ileum) to the rectum. After it is removed, the end of the small intestine is sewn to the rectum.

Nursing

- Ask them to eat a well-balanced diet including enough calories, proteins, and nutrients from a variety of groups.
- Encourage them to eat small amount of food throughout the day.
- Instruct them to avoid high fiber foods (beans, nuts, seeds and popcorn).
- Instruct them to avoid dairy products.
- Encourage them to take more raw fruits and vegetables.
- Instruct them to limit refined and processed foods.

DEFICIENCY DISEASES

Definition

The deficiency of organic compounds (vitamins) and inorganic compounds which are essential for growth, reproduction, good health and resistance to infection and also to serve variety of physiologic functions are known as deficiency diseases.

Components

The following are the organic and inorganic compounds which are very essential.

Organic

- Vitamin A (Retinol)
- Vitamin B1 (Thiamine)
- Vitamin B2 (Riboflavin)
- Vitamin B6 (Pyridoxine)

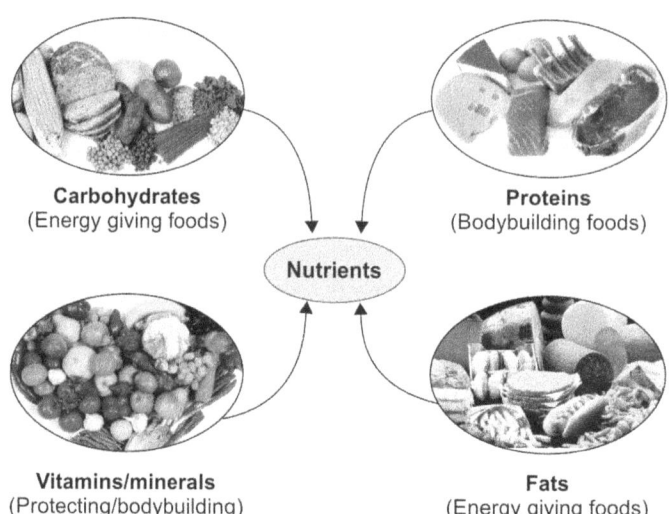

Fig. 5.10: Depicts organic and inorganic compounds essential for growth, reproduction, good health and resistance to infection.

- Vitamin B12 (Cyanocobalamine)
- Folate (Folic acid)
- Niacin
- Vitamin C (Ascorbic acid)
- Vitamin D (Calciferol)
- Vitamin E (Tocopherol)
- Vitamin K.

Inorganic
- Calcium
- Iodine
- Iron
- Phosphorus
- Potassium
- Sodium.

Sl. No.	Vitamin	Clinical features	Diagnostic test findings	RDA	Management
1.	Vitamin A (Retinol)	• Night blindness • Xerophthalmia • Dryness of mucosa • Dry skin • Soreness of mouth • Vomiting • Diarrhea • Urinary and vaginal infections	• History • Physical examination • Blood examination	700–900 mg	• Good dietary sources of vitamin A as green leafy vegetables, fruits and liver • Vitamin A supplements of 30,000 IU
2.	Vitamin B1 (Thiamine)	• Beriberi • Irritability • Nervousness • Memory loss • Muscle pain • Loss of appetite • Dyspnea • Constipation	• History • Physical examination • Erythrocyte transketolase activity less than 15%–20%	1.1 mg	• High-protein diet • Supplementary B complex vitamins • Thiamine-rich foods such as meat, wheat gram, enriched grains and beans
3.	Vitamin B2 (Riboflavin)	• Sore throat • Cheilosis • Dermatitis • Burning and itching of eyes • Tearing and vascularization of corneas • Neuropathy • Growth retardation	• History • Physical examination • Erythrocyte glutathione activity greater than 1.2–1.3	1.1 mg	• Vitamin B2-rich foods such as dairy products, vegetables, eggs, liver, nuts, enriched grains, etc. • Oral supplements of 5–15 mg/day
4.	Vitamin B6 (Pyridoxine)	• Anemia • Weakness • Glossitis • Cheilosis • Irritability • Seizures	• History • Physical examination • Pyridoxal phosphate levels less than 50 mg/ml	1.2–1.5 mg	• Oral supplements of 10–20 mg • Good dietary sources of B12 vitamin such as banana, fish, meat, whole grains, liver etc.
5.	Vitamin B12 (Cyanacobalamine)	• Megaloblastic anemia • Memory impairment • Confusion • Depression	• History • Physical examination • Decreased hematocrit • Schilling test	2.4 µg	• Vitamin B12 rich sources such as eggs, fish, organ meats, dairy products, etc. • Vitamin B12 supplements orally 200 mg/day

Contd...

Contd...

Sl. No.	Vitamin	Clinical features	Diagnostic test findings	RDA	Management
		• Fatigue • Nervousness • Speech difficulties • Decreased reflex response • Anorexia • Vomiting • Weight loss • Abdominal pain • Glossitis			
6.	Folate (Folic acid)	• Glossitis • Diarrhea • Megaloblastic anemia • Digestive problems	• History • Physical examination	400 µg	• Rich sources of folic acid such as citrus fruits, eggs, milk, green leafy vegetables, dairy products, meats, etc.
7.	Niacin	• Apathy • Fatigue • Appetite loss • Headache • Indigestion • Muscle weakness • Insomnia • Confusion • Memory impairment • Pellagra	• History • Physical examination	14–16 mg	• Oral supplementation of 10–150 mg • Niacin-rich foods such as eggs, organ meats, poultry, seafood, fish, dairy products, nuts and enriched grains
8.	Vitamin C (Ascorbic acid)	• Bleeding gums • Tooth decay • Low-infection resistance • Bruising • Anemia • Delayed wound healing • Joint pain • Nose bleeds	• History • Physical examination	65–90 mg	• Vitamin rich foods such as citrus fruits, green leafy vegetables, tomatoes, peppers, potatoes, strawberries • Oral supplementation of 100–1000 mg/day
9.	Vitamin D (Calciferol)	• Rickets • Osteomalacia	• History • Physical examination • Low levels of vitamin D and calcium • Radiographic bone deformities	50–15 mg	Good sources of vitamin D such as egg yolks, milk, fish, liver oils, etc.
10.	Vitamin E (Tocopherol)	• Neuromuscular disturbances • Decreased reflexes • Ataxia	• History • Physical examination • Low serum levels less than 0.5 mg/dL	15 mg	Vitamin E supplements such as 100–400 IU/day. Good sources of vitamin E are vegetable oils, milk, eggs, meat, fish, green leafy vegetables, etc.

Contd...

Contd...

Sl. No.	Vitamin	Clinical features	Diagnostic test findings	RDA	Management
11.	Vitamin K	• Abnormal bleeding • Epistaxis • Hematemesis • Bleeding at any orifice	• History • Physical examination	75–120 mg	Good sources of vitamin K such as green leafy vegetables, liver, wheat, gram, cheese, egg yolk, soyabean
12.	Calcium	• Tooth decay • Tetany • Nervousness • Muscle cramps • Heart failure • Paresthesia	• History • Physical examination		Calcium-rich sources such as milk products, green leafy vegetables, legumes, etc. Calcium supplementation of 1–2 g/day
13.	Iodine	• Hypothyroidism • Nervousness • Irritability • Obesity • Cold hands and feet • Brittle hair • Thick tongue • Poor memory	• History • Physical examination • Low T3 and T4 levels • Thyroid scan	150 µg	Oral supplementation of 50–100 mg/day Good sources of iodine such as iodized salt, sea food, etc.
14.	Iron	• Iron deficiency • Dyspnea • Fatigue • Susceptibility to infection • Brittle nails • Tachycardia	• History • Physical examination • Blood examination	8–18 mg	Good sources of iron such as egg yolk, fish, organ meat, wheat gram, beans, beef, potatoes, peas, Interferon: 250 mg/day
15.	Phosphorus	• Osteomalacia • Paresthesia • Mental status change • Hypoxia • Tremor • Weakness	• History • Physical examination • Serum levels greater than 405 mg/dL	700–1250 mg	• Good sources of phosphate such as dairy products, eggs, fish, grains, meat, poultry, cheese, beans, liver, milk, peas, nuts, etc.
16.	Potassium	• Muscle weakness • Flaccidity • Mental confusion • Irritability • Dysrhythmia • Metabolic alkalosis	• History • Physical examination	4700 mg	• Good sources of potassium are bananas, oranges, beef, beans, seafoods, etc.
17.	Sodium	• Muscle weakness • Irritability • Headache • Seizures • Hypotension • Abdominal cramping • Tachycardia	• History • Physical examination • Serum levels greater than 145 mEq/h	1200–1500 mg	• Low-sodium diet • Restrict water intake

*RDA, Recommended dietary allowance.

Disorders of Gastrointestinal System

DIARRHEA

Definition
Diarrhea is defined as the passage of three or more loose or liquid stools per day which is often associated with an urgency to go to the toilet.

Etiology
- Infections (Bacterial, viral or parasitic)
- Malnutrition
- Contaminated water
- Anxiety
- Stress
- Using too many laxatives
- Eating too much fiber
- Caffeine intake
- Sweets containing sorbitol
- Long-lasting constipation
- Radiotherapy.

Risk Factors
- Undercooked meat or fish
- People with weakened immune system
- People who take antacids frequently
- People who travel during certain seasons
- Under-five children
- Excessive alcohol
- Poor personal hygiene
- Foods stored in unhygienic conditions
- Fish and seafood from polluted water.

Types
There are three clinical types of diarrhea:
1. ***Acute watery diarrhea:*** It is a type of diarrhea that lasts for several hours or days and includes cholera.
2. ***Acute bloody diarrhea:*** It is a type of diarrhea in which traces of blood is visible in the stools and it is due to invasion of the bowel tissue.
3. ***Persistent diarrhea:*** It is a type of diarrhea that lasts for 14 days or longer.

Pathophysiology

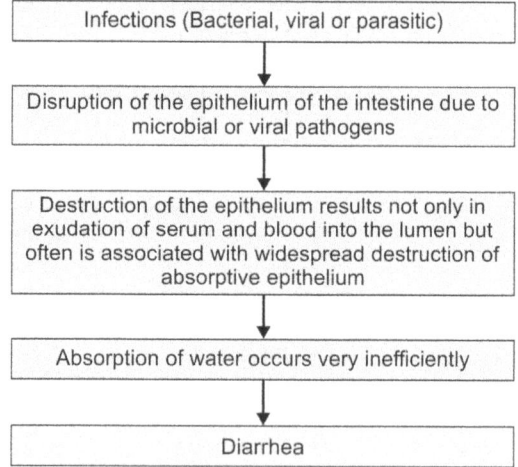

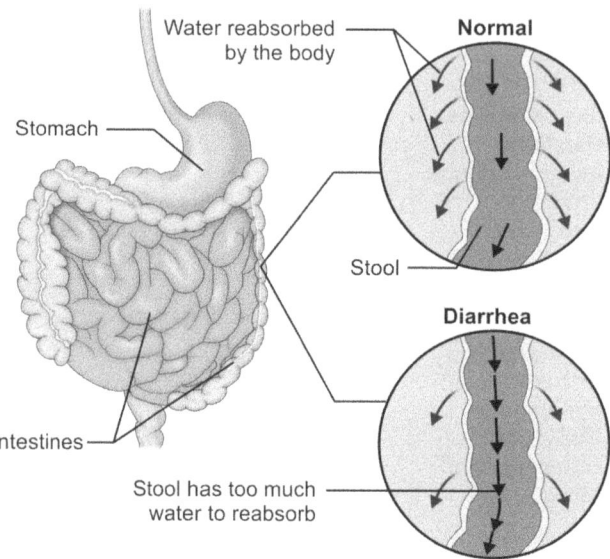

Fig. 5.11: Shows water reabsorbed by the body normally and with that of diarrhea.

Clinical Features

- Frequent, loose watery stools
- Abdominal cramps
- Abdominal pain
- Fever
- Bleeding
- Lightheadedness or dizziness
- Bloating
- Urgent need to go to the toilet
- Change in color of the stools
- Mucus, pus, blood or fat in the stools
- Vomiting
- Rapid heart rate
- Dry, flushed skin
- Irritability or confusion.

Complications

- Dehydration
- Low blood pressure
- Seizures
- Kidney failure
- Shock
- Coma
- Death.

Diagnostic Tests

- History
- Physical examination
- Stool culture
- Blood examination
- Fasting tests to reveal food intolerance
- Sigmoidoscopic examination
- Colonoscopic examination.

Management

Medical

- **Antidiarrheal agents:** It slows down muscle movements in the gut, which leads to more water being absorbed from the feces and the feces then become firmer and are passed less frequently. For example, loperamide, etc.
- **Bismuth subsalicylate:** It helps to shorten the frequency of stools and decreases the duration of illness. For example, pepto-bismol, etc.
- **Antibiotics:** It helps to prevent secondary infections. For example, ciprofloxacin, metronidazole, ampicillin, etc.

Nursing

- Provide access to safe drinking water.
- Encourage handwashing with soap before meals.
- Ask them to follow good personal and food hygiene.
- Provide health education about how infections spread.
- Instruct them to opt for rotavirus vaccination.
- Instruct use of improved sanitation.
- Encourage exclusive breastfeeding for the first six months of life among infants.
- Never place cooked meat on surfaces or plates that have held raw meat.
- Ensure that meat is cooked thoroughly.

GASTRITIS

Definition

Gastritis is an inflammation of the gastric mucosa. It may be acute (lasting several hours to few days) or chronic (lasting for many days).

Etiology

- Highly seasoned or spicy foods
- Excessive alcohol intake
- Radiation therapy
- Ingestion of strong acid or alkali
- Any acute illness
- Burns
- Severe infection
- Hepatic, renal or respiratory failure
- Any autoimmune diseases
- Benign or malignant ulcers of the stomach
- *Helicobacter pylori*
- Overuse of caffeine
- Chronic smoking
- Extreme stress
- Eating or drinking causative or corrosive substances
- Cocaine abuse.

Risk Factors

- Overuse of aspirin
- Overuse of nonsteroidal anti-inflammatory drugs
- Recent heavy alcohol use
- Major surgery

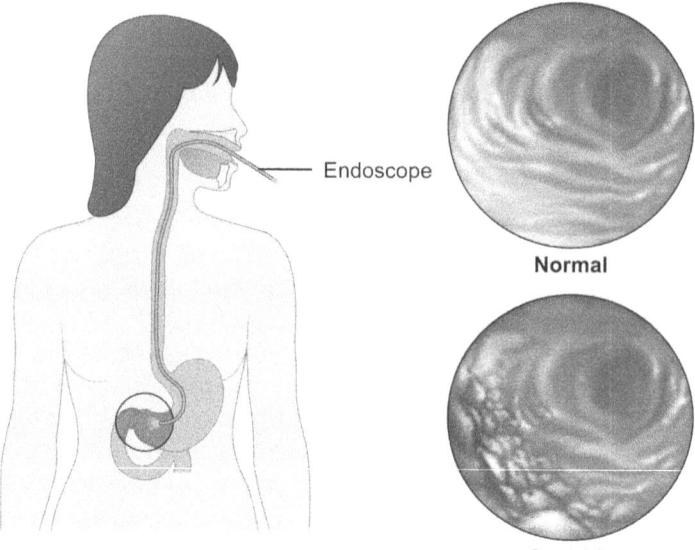

Fig. 5.12: Depicts normal and inflamed gastric mucosa (Gastritis).

- Kidney failure
- Liver failure
- Respiratory failure
- Bile reflux
- Food poisoning
- Too many processed foods
- Low-fiber diet.

Pathophysiology

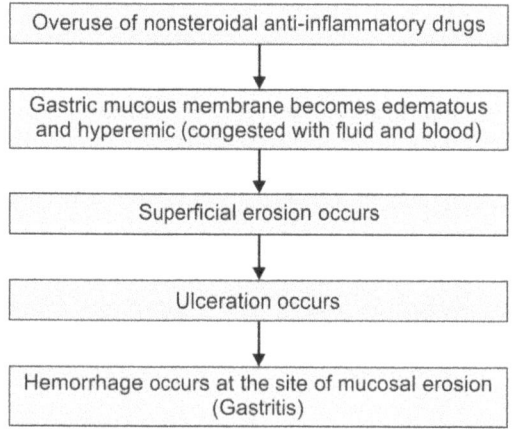

Clinical Features

- Loss of appetite
- Nausea
- Vomiting
- Indigestion
- Abdominal bloating
- Hiccups
- Pain in the upper part of the belly or abdomen
- Black tarry stools
- Blood vomiting appearance similar to coffee ground like material.

Complications

- Severe bleeding
- Peptic ulcer
- Atrophic gastritis
- Vitamin B12 deficiency
- Anemia.

Diagnostic Tests

- History
- Physical examination
- Blood examination
- Gastroscopy
- Stool examination
- Upper GI endoscopic examination
- Urea breath test.

Management

Medical

- **Antacids:** It provides protection for the stomach lining and helps with healing. For example, gelusil, etc.

- **H2-receptor antagonists:** They work to inhibit acid production in the stomach, inhibiting histamine from switching on acid production and also they help to heal the irritation and damage to the stomach lining. For example, cimetidine, ranitidine, famotidine, etc.
- **Proton pump inhibitors:** They work to inhibit acid production in the stomach, to help enable healing of the irritation of the lining more quickly. For example, omeprazole, lanzoprazole, pontoprazole, etc.

Surgical

- **Gastrectomy:** It is the surgical removal of the stomach due to chronic ulcer or gastritis.
- **Vagotomy:** It is a surgical procedure in which the the vagus nerve is cut to interrupt messages from the brain that stimulate acid secretion in the stomach.
- **Antrectomy:** It is a surgical procedure in which lower part of the stomach is removed as this part of the stomach manufactures the hormone responsible for stimulating digestive juices..
- **Pyloroplasty:** It is a surgical procedure in which the opening of the small intestine is enlarged so that the stomach contents can pass into it more easily.

Nursing

- Ask them to engage in stress reduction strategies to control their emotions and feel calmer.
- Ensure adequate amount of natural, unprocessed foods and have proper fiber intake.
- Instruct them not to lie down 3–4 hours after eating.
- Ask them to avoid spicy foods.
- Instruct them to avoid smoking and alcohol.
- Instruct them to limit their intake of caffeine.

GASTROESOPHAGEAL REFLUX DISEASE WITH ESOPHAGITIS

Definition

Gastroesophageal reflux disease (GERD) is a disorder in which gastric contents flow back into the esophagus due to incomplete lower esophageal sphincter (LES) which may lead to inflammation of the esophageal mucosa.

Etiology

- Incomplete lower esophageal sphincter
- Achalasia (great difficulty in swallowing)
- Impaired gastric emptying from gastroparesis or partial gastric outlet obstruction
- Scleroderma
- Esophageal spasm.

Risk Factors

- High fatty foods
- High levels of estrogen and progesterone
- Ganglionic stimulants
- Xanthine derivatives (theophylline and caffeine drinks)

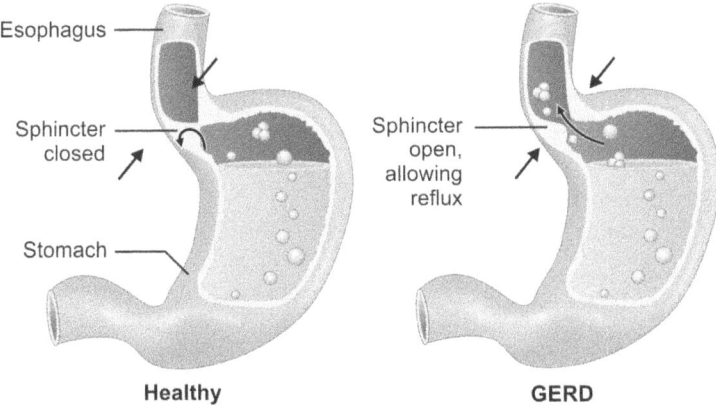

Fig. 5.13: Shows the comparison of healthy and refluxed contents from the stomach (GERD).

- Beta adrenergic agents
- Gastroparesis
- Pregnancy
- Obesity
- Hiatal hernia.

Pathophysiology

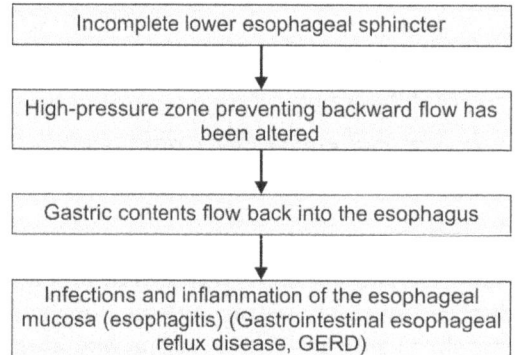

Clinical Features

- Heart burn (pyrosis) typically occurring 20–60 minutes after meals
- Globus (sensation of something in throat)
- Mild epigastric pain
- Dyspepsia
- Nausea
- Vomiting
- Dysphagia
- Chest pain
- Shortness of breath
- Hoarseness
- Recurrent sore throat
- Chronic cough
- Dental enamel loss
- Bronchospasm
- Odynophagia (sharp substernal pain on swallowing)
- GI bleeding
- Weight loss.

Complications

- Esophageal stricture formation
- Ulceration of the esophagus
- Aspiration
- Pneumonia.

Diagnostic Tests

- History
- Physical examination
- Endoscopic examination
- Esophageal manometry—to determine whether esophageal peristalsis is adequate or not
- Barium esophagography—to diagnose mechanical and motility disorders
- Esophageal biopsy
- Cytologic examination
- Analysis of gastric secretions.

Management

Medical

- **Antacids:** It helps in reducing the gastric acidity. For example, gelusil, etc.
- **H2-receptor antagonists:** It helps in reducing gastric acid secretions. For example, cimetidine, ranitidine, famotidine, etc.
- **Proton pump inhibitors:** It helps in blocking gastric acid secretions. For example, omeprazole, lansoprazole, pantoprazole, etc.
- **Calcium channel blockers:** It decreases lower esophageal contractility. For example, verapamil, amlodipine, diltiazem, etc.

Surgical

- **Antireflux surgery (nissen fundoplication):** It is a surgical procedure in which upper portion of the stomach is wrapped around the distal esophagus and sutured, creating a tight lower esophageal sphincter.
- **Transoral incisionless fundoplication:** It is a surgical procedure in which a barrier is created between the stomach and the esophagus.
- **Implanted device (Linx)** It is a procedure in which an implanted device (Linx) is permanently placed in the esophagus to prevent reflux of gastric acid into the throat.

Nursing

- Elevate the head-end of the bed to 6–8 inches.
- Instruct them not to lie down 3–4 hours after eating.
- Encourage them to take bland diet.
- Instruct them to avoid overeating.
- Instruct them not to wear tight-fitted clothes.

- Instruct them to avoid smoking and alcohol.
- Encourage them to participate in weight reduction program.

HEMORRHOIDS

Definition

Hemorrhoids are dilated portions of veins in the anal canal or a varicosity in the lower rectum or anus caused by congestion in the veins of the hemorrhoid plexus.

Etiology

- Abnormal dilation of veins of internal hemorrhoidal venous plexus
- Abnormal distension of the arteriovenous anastomoses
- Downward displacement or prolapse of anal cushions
- Destruction of the anchoring connective tissue system.

Risk Factors

- Pregnancy
- Prolonged sitting
- Straining at stools
- Anal infection
- Rectal surgery
- Episiotomy
- Heredity
- Exercise
- Coughing, sneezing, vomiting
- Loss of muscle tone due to age
- Anal intercourse
- Increased intra-abdominal pressure
- Loosening of vessels from surrounding connective tissue.

Types

There are two types of hemorrhoids as follows:
1. **Internal hemorrhoids:** Hemorrhoids above the internal sphincter are called internal hemorrhoids.
2. **External hemorrhoids:** Hemorrhoids appearing outside the external sphincter are called external hemorrhoids.

Pathophysiology

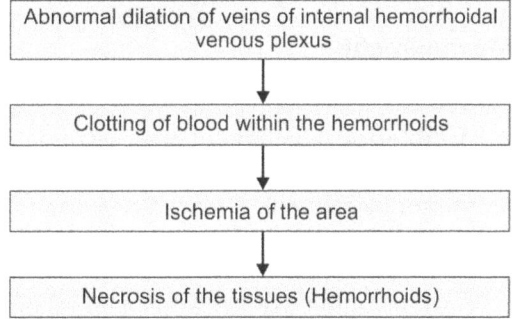

Clinical Features

- Bright red bleeding with defecation
- Pain
- Itching at the anus
- Constipation

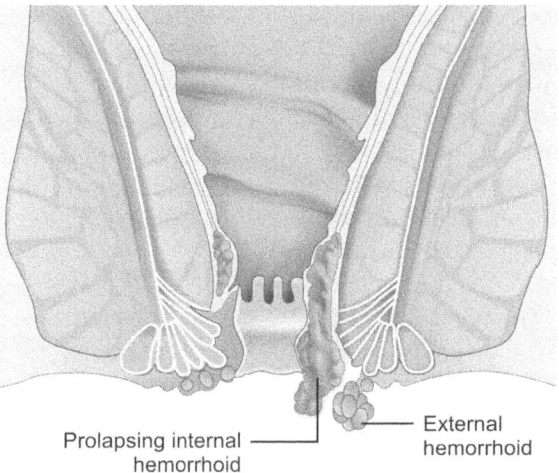

Fig. 5.14: Shows prolapsed internal and external hemorrhoids.

- Rectal prolapse
- Sensation of incomplete fecal evacuation
- Sudden rectal pain due to thrombosis.

Complications
- Hemorrhage
- Anemia
- Incontinence
- Strangulation.

Diagnostic Tests
- History
- Physical examination
- Anoscopic examination
- Digital palpation
- Proctoscopic examination
- Colonoscopic examination.

Management
Medical
- **Antibiotics:** It helps to prevent secondary infections. For example, ciprofloxacin, metronidazole, etc.
- **Analgesics:** It helps to relieve pain. For example, tramadol, buscopan, etc.
- **Antihistamine agents:** It helps to relieve itching. For example, pheniramine maleate, etc.
- **Rectal suppositories:** It helps in preventing constipation. For example, Dulcolax, etc.

Surgical
- **Hemorrhoidectomy:** It is the procedure in which the hemorrhoids are removed through surgical incision.
- **Cryosurgical hemorrhoidectomy:** It is the freezing of the hemorrhoid for a sufficient time to cause necrosis.
- **Infrared photocoagulation (Infrared radiation):** It is the surgical procedure in which the heat is used to shrink the hemorrhoid tissue.
- **Bipolar diathermy (heat):** It is a surgical procedure in which high frequency electric current is delivered via shortwave, microwave or ultrasound to generate deep heat in body tissues to shrink the hemorrhoid.
- **Laser therapy (YAG laser):** It is a surgical procedure in which laser therapy is used to excise hemorrhoids.
- **Sclerotherapy:** It is a surgical procedure in which chemical solution is injected into the blood vessel to shrink the hemorrhoid.
- **Rubber band ligation:** It is a surgical procedure in which a special rubber band is placed around the base of the hemorrhoid. The band cuts of circulation causing the hemorrhoid to shrink.

Nursing
- Encourage them to take high-fiber diet.
- Instruct them to drink 6–8 glasses of water each day.
- Encourage them to take more raw fruits and vegetables.
- Instruct them to avoid sedentary lifestyle the maximum.
- Encourage them to do exercise 5 times per week for at least 30 minutes each time.
- Instruct them not to ignore the "urge" to have a bowel movement.

HEPATIC ENCEPHALOPATHY

Definition
Hepatic encephalopathy is a worsening of brain function that occurs when the liver is no longer able to remove toxic substances in the blood.

Etiology
- Cirrhosis of liver
- Hepatitis
- Infections (Pneumonia)
- Kidney problems
- Bleeding from the stomach, intestine or esophagus.

Risk Factors
- Dehydration
- Low oxygen levels (hypoxia) in the body
- Recent surgery or trauma
- Use of medications to suppress the immune system
- Eating too much proteins

- Certain medications use (Barbiturates)
- Electrolyte imbalance
- Diuretics
- Hypoglycemia
- Hypokalemia.

Pathophysiology

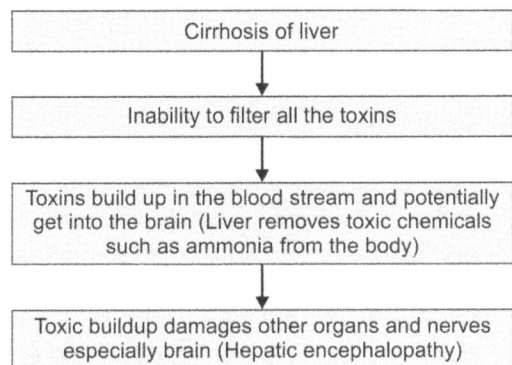

Clinical Features

- Breath with a musty or sweet odor
- Change in sleep patterns
- Difficulty in thinking
- Confusion
- Drowsiness or lethargy
- Anxiety
- Mental fogginess
- Seizures
- Severe personality changes
- Fatigue
- Confused speech
- Shaky hands
- Slow movements
- Poor concentration
- Problems with handwriting
- Forgetfulness
- Poor judgment.

Complications

- Brain herniation
- Brain swelling
- Organ failure
- Progressive, irreversible coma.

Diagnostic Tests

- History
- Physical examination
- Blood examination
- Liver function tests
- Computed tomography (CT) scan
- Magnetic resonance imaging (MRI)
- Electroencephalogram (EEG).

Management

Medical

- **Antibiotics:** It helps to lower amino acid production by decreasing the concentration of ammonia-forming colonic bacteria. For example, neomycin, rifaximin, etc.
- **Cathartics:** It helps in reducing the nitrogen load from the gut. For example, lactulose, etc.

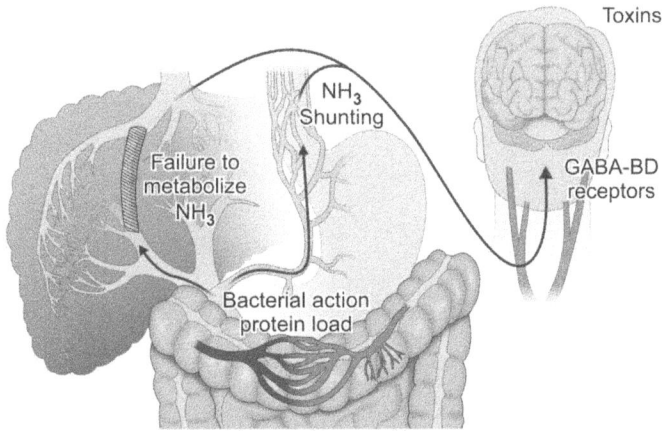

Fig. 5.15: Depicts failure of liver to metabolize and remove toxic substances in the blood.

Nursing

- Instruct them to avoid fatty foods.
- Encourage them to maintain a healthy weight.
- Ask them to avoid sedatives and narcotics.
- Encourage them to use diet containing vegetable proteins.
- Enforce them to avoid prolonged periods of fasting.
- Ensure patient safety and monitor the mental status of the patient at frequent intervals.

HEPATITIS

Definition

Hepatitis is any injury to the liver characterized by presence of inflammatory cells in the liver tissue.

Etiology

- Viral infection (HBV virus)
- Toxic substances (alcohol, certain medications, etc.)
- Autoimmune diseases
- Unprotected sexual contact
- Infants of HBV carrier mothers.

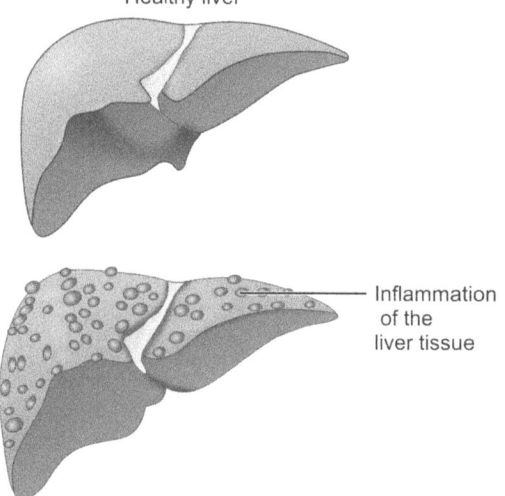

Fig. 5.16: Shows the comparison of healthy and inflamed liver tissue.

Risk Factors

- Healthcare workers
- Recipients of blood transfusion
- Homosexuals
- IV drug abusers
- Immunocompromised people
- Overcrowding.

Types

There are five types of hepatitis as follows:
1. **Hepatitis A:** It is spread by either direct contact with an infected person's feces or by indirect fecal contamination of food or water. The symptoms include: fever, dark urine, light stool and jaundice. Most people in areas of the world with poor sanitation have been infected with this virus. Proper handwashing is a good way to prevent hepatitis.
2. **Hepatitis B:** Hepatitis B virus (HBV) can spread through body fluids, urine, semen and from mother to infant soon or right after birth. The symptoms include: abdominal pain, jaundice, nausea, vomiting fever and joint pain. A blood test is needed to diagnose HBV and vaccinations are available to protect people at high risk for infection. It also poses a risk to healthcare workers who sustain accidental needle stick injuries while caring for infected HBV patients. Safe and effective vaccines are available to prevent HBV.
3. **Hepatitis C:** Hepatitis C (HCV) most commonly spreads by exposure to contaminated blood or needles. It increases a person's risk for liver cancer. There is no vaccine for HCV.
4. **Hepatitis D:** People with HBV often develop hepatitis D (HPD), which spreads through contaminated blood products and unprotected sex with an infected person. The dual infection of HDV and HBV can result in a more serious disease and worse outcome. Hepatitis B vaccines provide protection from HDV infection.
5. **Hepatitis E:** Hepatitis E virus (HEV) is found in underdeveloped areas of the world

and is spread by the feco-oral route. HEV is a common cause of hepatitis outbreaks in developing parts of the world and is increasingly recognized as an important cause of disease in developed countries. Safe and effective vaccines to prevent HEV infection have been developed but are not widely available.

Pathophysiology

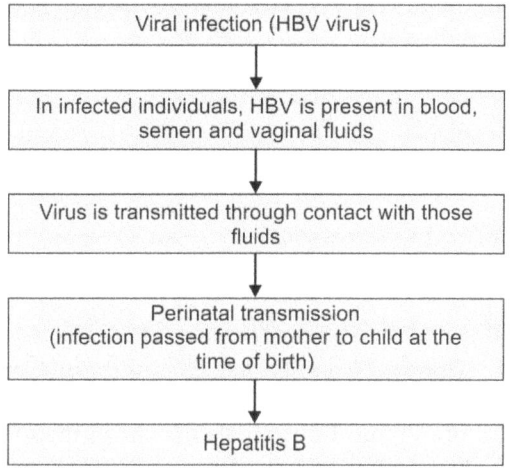

Clinical Features

- Fever
- Weakness
- Nausea
- Vomiting
- Headache
- Loss of appetite
- Muscle aches
- A constant discomfort in the upper right portion of the belly
- Joint pains
- Drowsiness
- Skin rash along with itching.

Complications

- Fibrosis
- Cirrhosis of liver
- Liver cancer
- Liver failure
- Glomerulonephritis
- Cryoglobulinemia
- Hepatic encephalopathy
- Portal hypertension
- Porphyria.

Diagnostic Tests

- History
- Physical examination
- Liver biopsy
- Liver function test
- Blood examination
- Viral antibody testing
- Ultrasonogram.

Management

Medical

- **Antiviral drugs:** It blocks a protein needed by the hepatitis virus to multiply. For example, adefovir dipivoxil, interferon, lamivudine, tenofovir, etc.

Nursing

- Ask them not to share the needles or sharp objects.
- Instruct them not to share shaving razors or toothbrushes with others.
- Instruct them to avoid unprotected sex.
- Encourage them to ensure proper screening of blood before transfusion.
- Instruct them to dispose the needles after use.
- Encourage them to sterilize objects after use.
- Instruct them to avoid alcohol as it can speed up liver damage.
- Ask them to absolutely abstain from drugs and unnecessary medicines.
- Ask them to stay hydrated as much as possible.
- Encourage them to eat a balanced diet.
- Instruct them to avoid strenuous exercise and ask them to take rest as much as possible to help boost the natural immunity of the body.

■ HERNIA

Definition

A hernia refers to when an internal body part pushes through a weak area of muscle or the

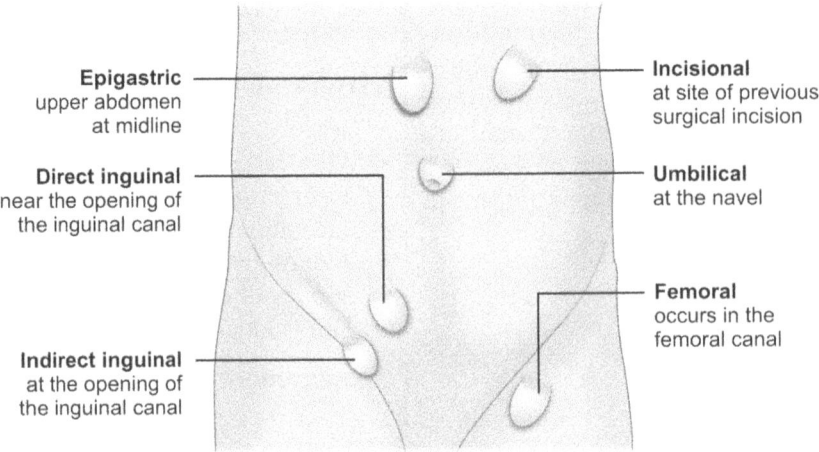

Fig. 5.17: Portrays different types of hernia.

surrounding tissue wall. Hernias often do not cause any symptoms, although a swelling may appear in the abdomen or groin.

Etiology

- Obesity
- Pregnancy
- Muscle atrophy
- Chronic cough
- Incorrect posture or blows to the organ
- Heavy lifting
- Straining during bowel movements or urination
- Surgical incision
- Trauma.

Risk Factors

- Abdominal wall defects
- Advanced age
- Ascites
- Connective tissue disorders
- Cystic fibrosis
- Prematurity
- Positive family history
- Shunt for hydrocephalus
- Undescended testis
- Stress
- Peritoneal dialysis
- Poor nutrition
- Smoking.

Types

There are five types of hernias as follows:

1. **Femoral hernia:** They are more common in women who have been pregnant or are obese but they can also occur in men. A femoral hernia develops when fat or part of our intestine pushes through a weak spot in the muscles or tissue and enters the femoral canal. The femoral canal is a passageway that carries large blood vessels in and out of our leg.
2. **Incisional hernia:** An incisional hernia is caused by weakening in the scar tissue that develops after we have had an operation on our abdomen. If we gain a lot of weight after an operation, we are at higher risk of developing an incisional hernia. Forceful activities, such as coughing, sneezing or lifting heavy weights, may also lead to this type of hernia.
3. **Epigastric hernia:** It can develop in both women and men. This type of hernia appears as a bulge in the area below the ribcage and above the belly button. At first, the bulge may be small but epigastric hernias can become quite large over time. Epigastric hernias usually develop in people who are born with a weak spot in their abdominal muscles. If one has this type

of weakness, any forceful activity, such as sneezing, coughing or lifting heavy objects, could be all it takes to push abdominal fat through the opening.
4. **Umbilical hernia:** An umbilical hernia develops in the area of the belly button. This type of hernia is seen most often in babies and young children. It can also develop in pregnant women and in people who are overweight or obese.
5. **Inguinal hernia:** This is the most common form of hernia and refers to when bowel or fatty tissue protrudes into the groin. This type of hernia mainly occurs in men. It can occur on one or both sides of the groin or scrotum. About 70% of inguinal hernias are indirect. This type of hernia occurs in a natural weak spot of the groin around the spermatic cord. About 30% of inguinal hernias are direct. This type of hernia occurs from weak tissue being aggravated by straining or lifting over time.

Pathophysiology

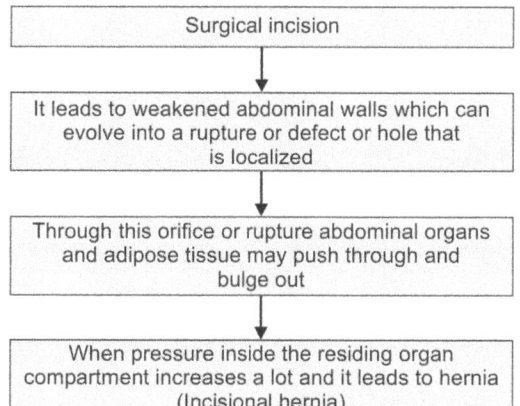

Clinical Features

- A visible lump or a swollen area
- A heavy or uncomfortable feeling in the gut, particularly when bending over
- Pain or aching particularly on exertion (such as lifting or carrying heavy objects)
- Digestive upsets, such as constipation
- The lump disappears when the person is lying down.
- The lump enlarges upon coughing, straining or standing up.

Complications

- Strangulation
- Intestinal obstruction
- Infection (after surgery)
- Inflammation
- Irreducibility.

Diagnostic Tests

- History
- Physical examination
- Abdominal X rays
- Computed tomography (CT) scan
- Ultrasonogram.

Management

Surgical

- **Herniorrhaphy (Open hernia repair):** It is a surgical procedure in which the surgeon makes an incision in the groin, moves the hernia back into the abdomen and reinforces the muscle wall with stitches.
- **Hernioplasty:** It is a surgical procedure in which the area of muscle weakness is reinforced with a synthetic mesh or screen to provide additional support
- **Laparoscopy:** It is a surgical procedure in which the surgeon inserts a laparoscope in the lower abdomen and repairs the hernia using synthetic mesh.

Nursing

- Ask them to take frequent short walks to improve blood circulation and to minimize the risk of blood clots in the legs.
- Encourage them to use an ice pack 3–5 times a day for 15–20 minutes at a time.
- Instruct the patient to avoid heavy lifting for a minimum of a week.
- Encourage them to eat a healthy diet and to drink plenty of water.
- Instruct them to wear loose clothing when at home.
- Strictly ask them not to smoke.
- Instruct them to have a proper follow-up care.

INTESTINAL OBSTRUCTION

Definition

Intestinal obstruction results when normal peristaltic movement of intestinal contents is interfered due to neurologic or mechanical impairment.

Etiology

- Carcinoma of the bowel
- Hernias
- Adhesions or scar tissue (that forms abnormal connections after surgery or inflammation)
- Volvulus (twisting of the intestines)
- Intussusception (telescoping of the bowel on itself)
- Paralytic ileus (interference with neural innervation of the intestines resulting in a decrease or absence of peristalsis)
- Fecal impaction
- Mesenteric ischemia (decreased blood supply to the intestines)
- Diverticulitis
- Foreign bodies (eaten materials that block the intestines).

Risk Factors

- Abdominal or pelvic surgery
- Crohn's disease
- Tumors blocking the intestines.

Types

There are two types of intestinal obstruction as follows:
1. ***Mechanical obstruction:*** It this blockage occurs without vascular compromise. Ingested fluid and food, digestive secretions and gas accumulate above the obstruction. The proximal bowel distends and the distal segment collapses. The normal secretory and absorptive functions of the mucosa are depressed and the bowel wall becomes edematous and congested.
2. ***Functional obstruction:*** In this, the intestinal musculature cannot propel the contents along the bowel.

Pathophysiology

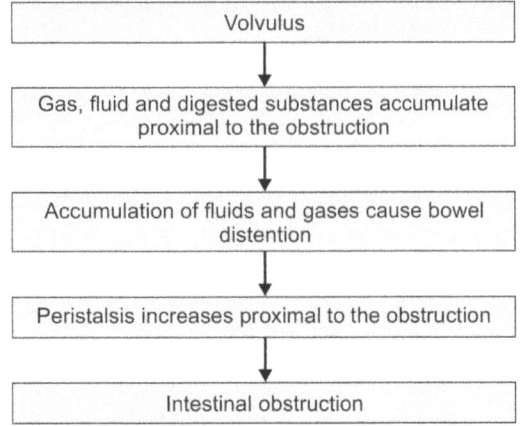

Clinical Features

- Colicky abdominal pain
- Severe abdominal cramps
- Constipation
- Severe bloating
- Loss of appetite
- Abdominal distention
- Decreased or absent bowel sounds
- Vomiting
- Fever
- Breath odor

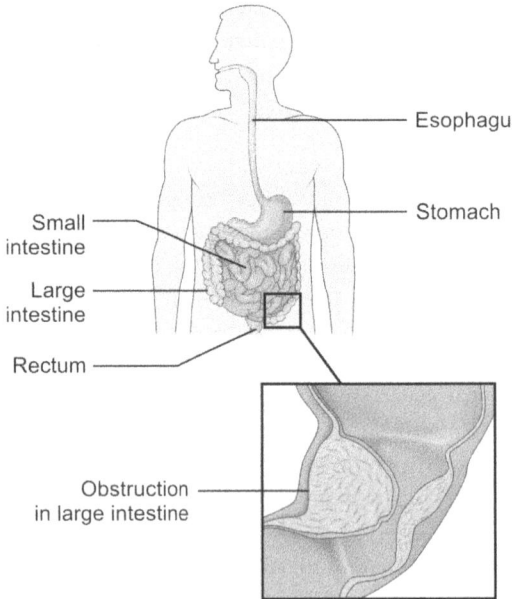

Fig. 5.18: Depicts obstruction in large intestine.

- Peritoneal irritation
- Increased WBC count.

Complications
- Electrolyte imbalance
- Dehydration
- Intestinal perforation
- Infections
- Jaundice (Yellowing of the skin and eyes).

Diagnostic Tests
- History
- Physical examination
- Abdominal CT scan
- Abdominal X-ray
- Barium enema
- Colonoscopic examination
- Blood examination.

Management

Medical

- **Antibiotics:** It helps to reduce the risk of infections. For example, ciprofloxacin, amoxicillin, metronidazole, neomycin, etc.
- **Antiemetics:** It helps to prevent vomiting. For example, prochlorperazine, etc.
- **Analgesic agents:** It helps to relieve pain. For example, meperidine, tramadol, etc.
- **Cholinesterase inhibitor:** It enhances cholinergic action by facilitating the transmission of impulses across neuromuscular junctions. For example, neostigmine, etc.

Surgical

- **Colostomy:** It is a surgical procedure in which an opening is made in the colon of the large intestine.
- **Caecostomy:** It is a surgical procedure in which an opening is made in the cecum of the large intestine.
- **Ileostomy:** It is a surgical procedure in which an opening is made in the ileum of the large intestine.
- **Gastric decompression:** It is a surgical procedure used to relieve pressure on an organ or part such as the abdomen.

Nursing

- Instruct them to avoid heavy lifting which increases pressure inside the abdomen.
- Ask them not to do anything that takes extra effort until they are back to normal activities.
- Initiate prompt treatment of abdominal and other infections.
- Encourage them to eat a balanced diet low in fat with plenty of vegetables and fruits.
- Strictly ask them not to smoke.

LIVER ABSCESS

Definition
An abscess formation in the liver cells usually caused by an amoebic infection, bacterial infection or trauma is known as liver abscess.

Etiology
- Abdominal infections (appendicitis, diverticulitis or a perforated bowel, etc.)
- Parasitic infection (*Entamoeba histolytica*)
- Bacterial infections (*Escherichia coli, Streptococcus milleri,* etc.)
- Infections in the blood
- Infection of the bile draining tubes
- Recent endoscopy of the bile draining tubes
- Trauma to the liver.

Risk Factors
- Malignancy
- Poor hygiene and sanitation
- Hypoalbuminemia
- Multiple abscesses
- Alcoholism
- HIV infection
- Malnutrition
- Corticosteroid use
- Disorders of cell mediated immunity.

Types
There are two types of liver abscess as follows:
1. ***Amoebic liver abscess:*** It is most commonly caused by *Entamoeba histolytica* and occurs in developing countries.
2. ***Pyogenic liver abscess:*** It is caused by bacterial infection and mostly seen in the developed countries.

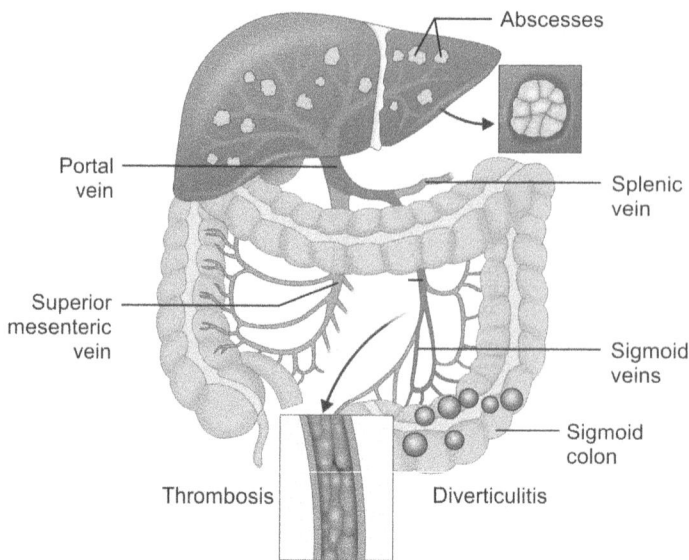

Fig. 5.19: Shows abscess formation in the liver cells.

Pathophysiology

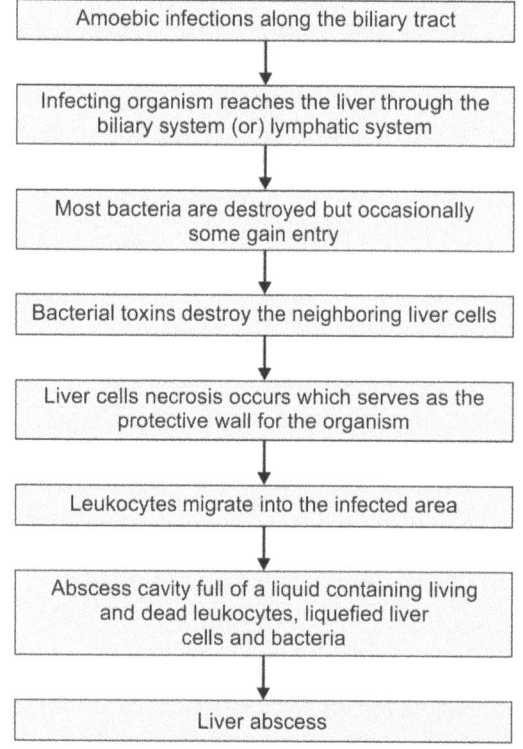

Clinical Features

- Painful hepatomegaly
- Fever
- Chills
- Dull abdominal pain
- Tenderness in the right upper quadrant of the abdomen
- Diaphoresis
- Malaise
- Anorexia
- Nausea
- Vomiting
- Clay-colored stools
- Dark-colored urine
- Unintentional weight loss
- Jaundice
- Anemia.

Complications

- Sepsis
- Shock.

Diagnostic Tests

- History
- Physical examination
- Liver function test
- Liver biopsy
- Blood examination
- Ultrasound examination
- Computed tomography (CT) scan
- Magnetic resonance imaging (MRI) scan.

Management

Medical

- **Antibiotics:** It helps to reduce the risk of infections. For example, ciprofloxacin, amoxicillin, metronidazole, etc.
- **Amoebicidal agents:** It helps to fight against the infected parasites. For example, tinidazole, chloroquine, etc.
- **Antiemetics:** It helps to prevent vomiting. For example, prochlorperazine, etc.
- **Luminal agents:** It eradicates intestinal colonization of parasites. For example, paromomycin, iodoquinol, etc.
- **Analgesic agents:** It helps to relieve pain. For example, meperidine, tramadol, etc.
- **Anticholinergics:** It helps to reduce the secretions. For example, propantheline, dicyclomine, etc.

Surgical

- **Percutaneous needle aspiration (PNA):** It is a surgical procedure in which removal and examination, usually microscopic, of tissue from the living body, often to determine whether a tumor is malignant or benign.
- **Percutaneous catheter drainage (PCD):** It is a surgical procedure that uses imaging guidance to place a thin needle through the skin into the abscess to remove or drain the infected fluid and to promote healing.

Nursing

- Initiate prompt treatment of abdominal and other infections.
- Instruct them to avoid heavy lifting.
- Ask them not to do anything that takes extra effort until they are back to normal activities.
- Encourage high carbohydrate diet.
- Provide complete bedrest.
- Provide calm and quiet environment.

LIVER CIRRHOSIS

Definition

Cirrhosis is a chronic progressive disease of the liver characterized by extensive degeneration and destruction of the liver parenchymal cells.

Etiology

- Hepatitis B or C infection
- Alcohol abuse
- Rightsided heart failure
- Viral, toxic or idiopathic hepatitis
- Bile duct disorders
- Tricuspid insufficiency
- Nonalcoholic fatty liver disease (NAFLD)
- Nonalcoholic steatohepatitis (NASH).

Risk Factors

- Malignancy
- Poor hygiene and sanitation
- Hypoalbuminemia
- Multiple abscesses
- Alcoholism
- HIV infection
- Malnutrition
- Corticosteroid use
- Disorders of cell-mediated immunity
- Being male

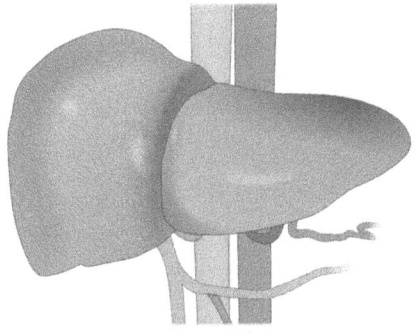
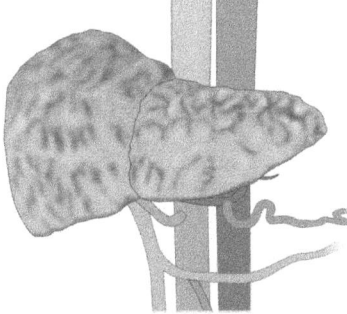

Fig. 5.20: Shows the comparison of normal and degenerative and destructed liver (Cirrhosis of liver).

- Obesity
- Inherited diseases (Hemochromatosis, Wilson's disease, etc).

Types

There are four types of liver cirrhosis as follows:
1. **Alcoholic cirrhosis:** It is also known as Laennec's or portal cirrhosis. It occurs due to alcoholism and scar formation occurs throughout the liver.
2. **Post-necrotic cirrhosis:** It results due to acute viral hepatitis or exposure to hepatotoxins. It occurs after massive liver necrosis and scar tissue causes destruction of liver lobules and the entire lobes.
3. **Biliary cirrhosis:** It is associated with chronic biliary obstruction and infection and scarring occurs in the liver around the bile ducts.
4. **Cardiac cirrhosis:** It is associated with severe right-sided heart failure and it results in an enlarged, edematous, congested liver. The liver becomes anoxic resulting in liver cell necrosis and fibrosis.

Pathophysiology

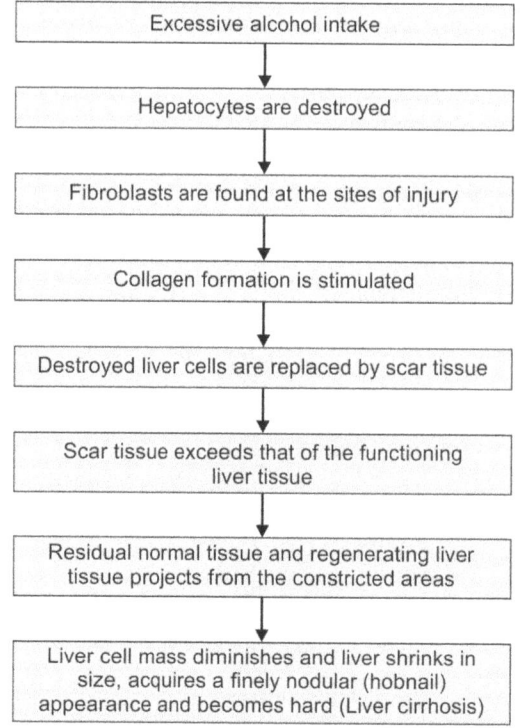

Clinical Features

- Malaise
- Loss of energy
- Anorexia
- Weight loss
- Nausea
- Vomiting
- Abdominal distress
- Spider angiomas on the nose, cheeks, upper thorax and shoulders
- Hepatomegaly
- Splenomegaly
- Liver tenderness
- Protruding umbilicus
- Dilated abdominal veins
- Flatulent dyspepsia
- Palmar erythema (reddened palms)
- Intermittent mild fever
- Purpura (due to decreased platelet count)
- Clubbing of fingers
- Delirium
- Fluid buildup on the legs (edema) and in the abdomen (ascites)
- Jaundice
- Pale or clay-colored stools.

Complications

- Portal hypertension
- Coagulopathy
- Asterixis (liver flap): A coarse tremor characterized by rapid, non-rhythmic flexions in the wrists and fingers
- Bacterial peritonitis
- Fetor hepaticus (fruity breath odor of chronic renal failure)
- Esophageal varices (rupturing of esophageal veins)
- Hepatorenal syndrome (functional renal failure)
- Hepatocellular carcinoma
- Hepatic encepahlopathy.

Diagnostic Tests

- History
- Physical examination
- Liver function test
- Liver biopsy
- Blood examination

- Ultrasound examination
- Endoscopic examination
- Radioisotope liver scan
- Computed tomography (CT) scan
- Magnetic resonance imaging (MRI) scan.

Management

Medical

- **Potassium-sparing diuretics:** It helps to reduce the fluid accumulated in the abdomen. For example, spironolactone, triamterene, etc.
- **Antibiotics:** It inhibits protein synthesis in the bacteria and decreases the production of ammonia. For example, neomycin, etc.
- **Antiemetics:** It helps to prevent vomiting. For example, prochlorperazine, etc.
- **Anti-inflammatory agents:** It is used to increase the length of survival in patients with mild to moderate cirrhosis. For example, colchicine, etc.
- **Vitamin and nutritional supplements:** It helps to promote healing of damaged liver cells. For example, betaine, milk thistle, etc.
- **Antacids:** It decreases gastric distress and minimizes the possibility of GI bleeding. For example, Gelusil, etc.

Surgical

- **Paracentesis:** It is a surgical procedure in which fluid is drained from the abdomen.
- **Peritoneovenous shunt:** It is a surgical procedure in which a shunt is placed to reroute the blood from the liver and to achieve the continuous emptying of ascitic fluid from the peritoneal cavity and thereby lowering the portal hypertension.
- **Endoscopic sphincterotomy:** It is a surgical procedure in which the endoscopic technique was used to examine and treat abnormalities of the bile ducts, pancreas and gallbladder.

Nursing

- Instruct them to avoid alcohol intake.
- Encourage them to eat a healthy diet that is low in salt.
- Provide complete bedrest to the patient.
- Encourage low-fat, high-protein, high-fiber and high-carbohydrate diet.
- Provide calm and quiet environment.
- Safeguard the patient against any injuries.

MALABSORPTION SYNDROME

Definition

Malabsorption syndrome refers to a number of disorders in which the intestine can't adequately absorb certain nutrients into the blood stream. It can impede the absorption of macronutrients (proteins, carbohydrates and fats), micronutrients (vitamins and minerals) or both.

Etiology

- Abnormal physical processes
- Bile acid disorders
- Liver dysfunction
- Whipple's disease
- Cow's milk protein intolerance
- Crohn's disease
- Damage from radiation treatments
- Parasitic infections (*Giardia lamblia*)
- Soy milk protein intolerance
- Pancreatic insufficiency
- Zollinger-Ellison syndrome
- Disaccharidase deficiency
- Bacterial overgrowth.

Risk Factors

- Excessive alcohol consumption
- Premature birth
- Family history of cystic fibrosis
- Recent intestinal surgery
- Travel to countries with high incidence of intestinal parasites
- Certain medications (cholestyramine, tetracycline, etc.)
- Excessive use of antibiotics
- Use of laxatives.

Types

- ***Primary:*** In this type, disturbance is within the intestinal lumen due to various reasons like insufficiency of digestive enzymes or bile ducts or damaged intestinal mucosa.

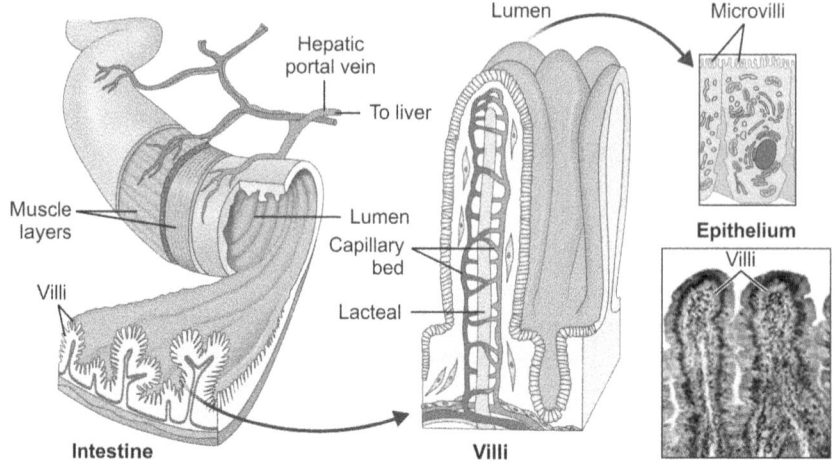

Fig. 5.21: Depicts failure of intestine to absorb certain nutrients into the blood stream.

- *Secondary:* In this type, the intestinal change is secondary to other factors (failure of digestion, failure of absorption and failure of transport).

Pathophysiology

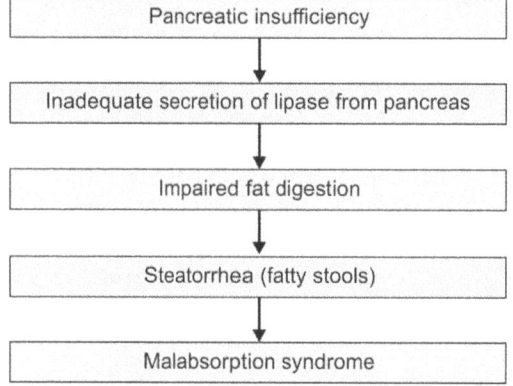

Clinical Features

- Bulky, foul-smelling stools
- Steatorrhea (fatty stools)
- Failure to thrive
- Muscle wasting
- Weight loss
- Abdominal distension and bloating
- Flatulence
- Chronic diarrhea
- Muscle cramping
- Weakness
- Fatigue
- Swelling or fluid retention.

Complications

- Refractory anemia
- Gallstones
- Kidney stones
- Osteoporosis
- Vitamin deficiencies
- Growth failure
- Autoimmune disorders
- Small bowel malignancy.

Diagnostic Tests

- History
- Physical examination
- Blood examination
- Urine examination
- Pancreatic function test
- Xylose absorption test
- Hydrogen breath test
- Schilling test
- Secretin stimulation test
- Small bowel biopsy
- Stool culture
- Culture of small intestine aspirate
- Stool fat testing
- X-rays of the small bowel
- Computed tomography (CT) scan of the abdomen.

Management

Medical

- **Correction of nutritional deficiencies:** It involves supplementing various minerals such as calcium, magnesium, iron and vitamins that are deficient in the condition.
- **Protease supplements:** Protease breaks down the proteins and helps to keep the intestines free of parasites. For example, papain (a protease enzyme from papaya), etc.
- **Lipase supplements:** It works with bile from the liver to break down fat molecules so that they can be absorbed and used by the body. For example, VeganZyme, etc.
- **Antibiotics:** It helps to reduce the risk of infections. For example, neomycin, chloramphenicol, etc.
- **Corticosteroids:** It helps to facilitate absorption of nutrients properly in the small intestine. For example, prednisone, etc.
- **Anti-inflammatory agents:** It diffuses freely across the mucous barrier into gastric epithelial cells and widens blood vessels by relaxing smooth muscle cells in vessel walls. For example, ibuprofen, etc.

Nursing

- Instruct them to minimize the use of certain medications such as antibiotics that can adversely affect the function of the intestines.
- Instruct them to strictly prohibit the intake of alcohol.
- When on travel, ask them to consume only bottled water, eat only cooked foods and avoid fresh salads.
- Ask them to limit or avoid intake of laxatives.
- Instruct the patient to adhere to the gluten-free diet.
- Educate the patient to avoid lactose-containing foods until restitution of a normal mucosa as it can worsen gastrointestinal symptoms.

PANCREATITIS

Definition

An acute or chronic inflammation of the pancreas associated with escape of pancreatic enzymes into the surrounding tissue is known as pancreatitis.

Etiology

- Autoimmune conditions
- Trauma to the pancreas
- Genetic mutations due to cystic fibrosis
- Blocked pancreatic duct or common bile duct
- Long-term heavy alcohol consumption
- Cholelithiasis
- Viral or bacterial infections
- Hypercalcemia
- Hyperparathyroidism
- Idiopathic.

Risk Factors

- Familial pancreatitis
- Ischemic vascular disease
- Peptic ulcer disease
- Postoperative gastrointestinal surgery
- Ingested medicines
- High triglyceride levels in the blood
- High calcium levels in the blood.

Types

There are two types of pancreatitis as follows:
1. *Acute pancreatitis:* It usually begins with gradual or sudden pain in the upper abdomen that sometimes extends to the back. The pain may be mild at first and become worse after eating. The pain is often severe, constant and commonly lasts for several days in the absence of treatment. A person with acute pancreatitis usually looks and feels very ill and needs immediate medical attention. Most of them require hospitalization for 3–5 days for close monitoring, pain control and intravenous hydration.
2. *Chronic pancreatitis:* It is inflammation of the pancreas that does not heal or improve

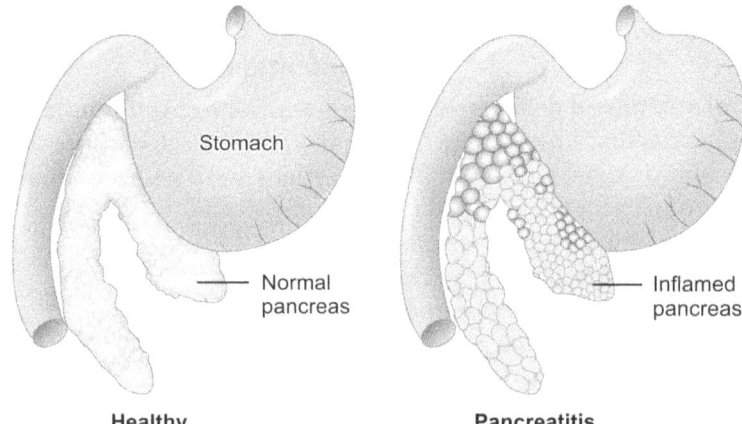

Fig. 5.22: Shows the comparison of healthy and inflamed pancreas (Pancreatitis).

and it gets worse over time and leads to permanent damage. It eventually impairs a patient's ability to digest food and make pancreatic hormones.

Pathophysiology

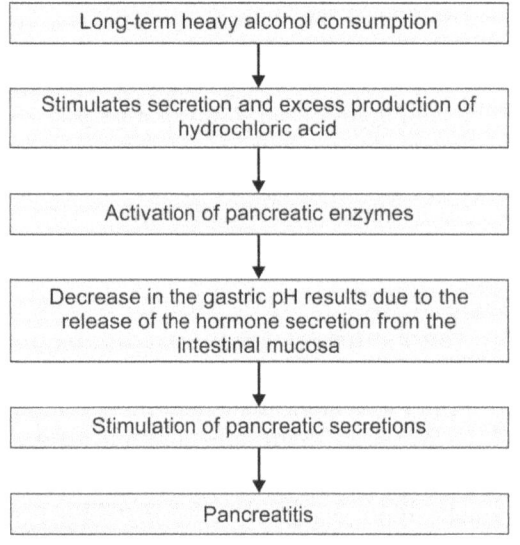

Clinical Features

- Nausea
- Vomiting
- Weight loss
- Diarrhea
- Clay-colored stools
- Swollen and tender abdomen
- Low-grade fever
- Tachycardia
- Abdominal pain
- Hypotension
- Steatorrhea (stools with high fat content)
- Cullen's sign (discoloration of the abdomen and periumbilical area)
- Turner's sign (bluish discoloration of the flanks)
- Absent or decreased bowel sounds
- Elevated lipase and amylase levels
- Elevated WBC, glucose, bilirubin and alkaline phosphatase.

Complications

- Pancreatic cancer
- Acute renal failure
- Diabetes
- Malnutrition
- Pancreatic infection
- Hemorrhage
- Biliary tract obstruction.

Diagnostic Tests

- History
- Physical examination
- Liver function test
- X-ray studies of the abdomen
- Blood examination
- Transabdominal ultrasound
- Endoscopic ultrasound (EUS)
- Radioisotope liver scan
- Computed tomography (CT) scan

- Magnetic resonance cholangiopancreatography (MRCP)
- Stool examination
- Elevated serum lipase and serum amylase.

Management

Medical

- **H2-receptor antagonists:** It helps to decrease pancreatic activity by inhibiting hydrochloric acid secretion accumulated in the abdomen. For example, cimetidine, ranitidine, etc.
- **Antibiotics:** It helps to prevent any secondary infections. For example, ciprofloxacin, amoxicillin, etc.
- **Antiemetics:** It helps to prevent vomiting. For example, prochlorperazine, Perinorm, Stemetil, etc.
- **Analgesics:** It helps to alleviate any pain. Meperidine, etc.
- **Carbonic anhydrase inhibitors:** It reduces the concentration of bicarbonate. For example, acetazolamide, etc.
- **Antacids:** It neutralizes gastric hydrochloric acid secretion. For example, Gelusil, etc.

Surgical

- **Pancreaticojejunostomy:** It is a surgical procedure in which side-to-side anastamosis or joining of the pancreatic duct to the jejunum allows drainage of pancreatic secretions into jejunum.
- **Choledochojejunostomy:** It is a surgical procedure in which bile is diverted around the ampulla of vater where there may be spasm or hypertrophy of the sphincter. In this procedure, the common bile duct is anastamosed with the jejunum.
- **Pancreaticoduodenectomy (Whipple's procedure):** It is a surgical procedure in which the surgeon removes the head of the pancreas, the gallbladder, part of the duodenum which is the upper most portion of the small intestine, a small portion of the stomach called the pylorus and the lymph nodes near the head of the pancreas.

Nursing

- Instruct them to avoid alcohol intake.
- Teach the importance of taking medications containing pancreatic enzymes.
- Encourage deep breathing exercise.
- Provide complete bedrest to the patient.
- Encourage high protein and carbohydrate diet.
- Provide calm and quiet environment.
- Encourage small feedings with low fat and nongas-producing liquids.

PARASITIC INFESTATIONS

Definition

A living organism which gets nourishment from another living organism where it lives is called parasites. The infections caused by such organism are known as parasitic infestations.

Etiology

- *Entamoeba histolytica*
- *Leishmania trypanosomea*
- *Plasmodium toxoplasma*
- *Schistosoma fasciola*
- *Taenia echinococcus*
- *Ascaris lumbricoides.*

Risk Factors

- Undercooked meat
- Insect bites
- Walking barefoot
- Eating contaminated raw fruits and vegetables
- Eating foods prepared by infected handlers
- Drinking contaminated water
- Contact with infected persons
- Inhaling dusts that contain parasitic eggs or cysts
- Prolonged antibiotic use
- Malabsorption syndrome
- Obesity
- Weakened immune system
- Diet high in fat and low in fiber.

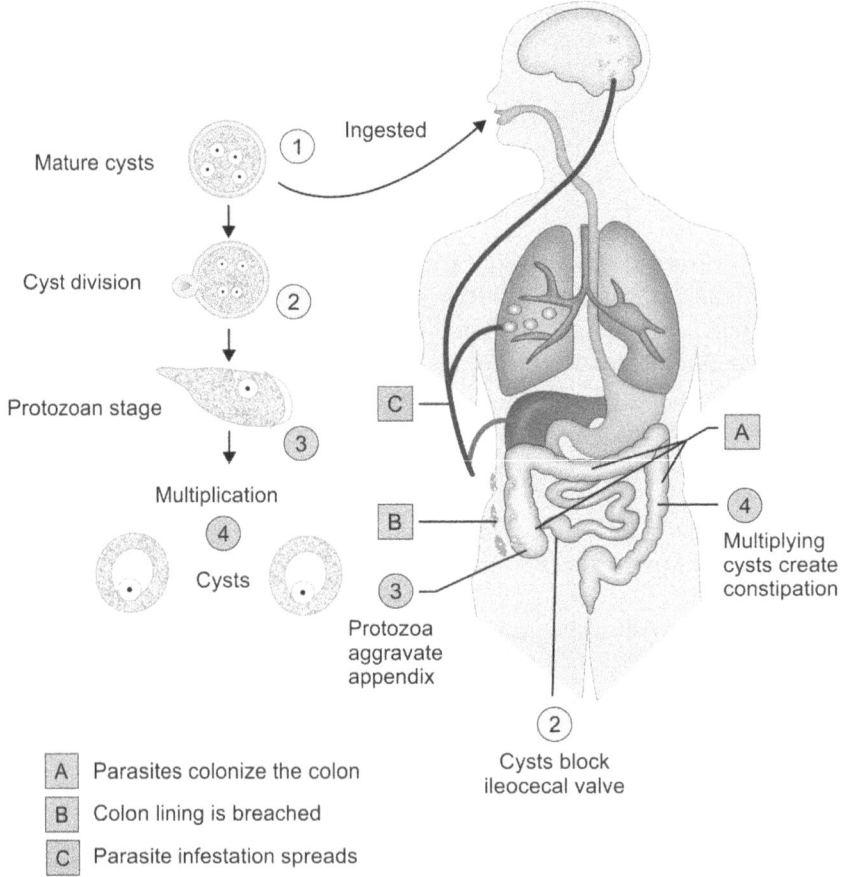

Fig. 5.23: Shows the development of intestinal ulcers due to amoebic infection (Parasitic infestations).

Types

The parasitic infestations are classified into two types as follows:
1. **Protozoa**
   - **Amoebae:** For example, *Entamoeba histolytica*
   - **Flagellates:** For example, *Leishmania trypanosomea*
   - **Sporozoa:** For example, *Plasmodium toxoplasma*.
2. **Helminthes**
   - **Trematodes:** For example, *Schistosoma fasciola*
   - **Cestodes:** For example, *Taenia echinococcus*
   - **Nematodes:** For example, *Ascaris lumbricoides*.

Pathophysiology

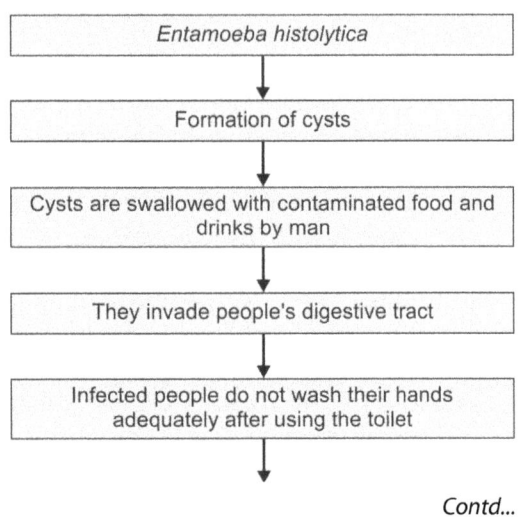

Contd...

Contd...

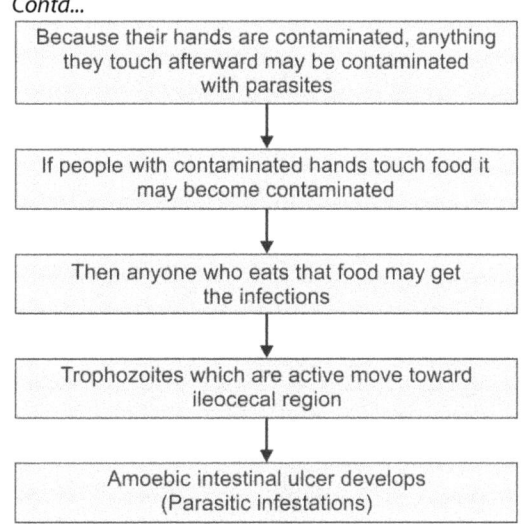

Clinical Features

- Frequent passage of stools mixed with mucus and blood
- Flatulence
- Malabsorption
- Nausea
- Anorexia
- Diarrhea with foul smelling stools
- Losing weight with constant hunger
- Intestinal ulceration
- Distended abdomen
- Malaise
- Fever
- Abdominal cramps.

Complications

- Infection
- Fluid and electrolyte imbalance
- Eosinophilia
- Hepatomegaly
- Splenomegaly.

Diagnostic Tests

- History
- Physical examination
- Blood examination
- Stool examination
- Proctosigmoidoscopic examination

- Computed tomography (CT) scan
- Magnetic resonance imaging (MRI) scan
- X-rays.

Management

Medical

- **Antimalarial agents:** It helps to treat extraintestinal amoebiasis. For example, chloroquine, etc.
- **Antibiotics:** It helps to prevent any secondary infections. For example, metronidazole, tinidazole, etc.
- **Antiemetics:** It helps to prevent vomiting. For example, prochlorperazine, Perinorm, Stemetil, etc.

Nursing

- Instruct them to wash all fruits and vegetables in clean water before eating.
- Ask them to wear shoes or slippers to prevent hookworm infection.
- Encourage them to wash hands after using toilet.
- Ask them to periodically consume curry meals.
- Ensure that all meat and fish are properly cooked.
- Instruct them not to use microwave to cook food as they don't heat foods completely.
- Encourage them to eat high-fiber foods.

PEPTIC ULCER DISEASE

Definition

A peptic ulcer is a defect in the lining of the stomach or the first part of the small intestine, an area called the duodenum. A peptic ulcer in the stomach is called a gastric ulcer. An ulcer in the duodenum is called a duodenal ulcer.

Etiology

- Bacterial infection of the stomach (*Helicobacter pylori*)

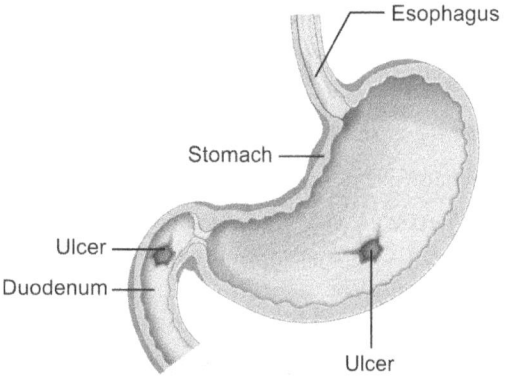

Fig. 5.24: Shows the defective lining of the stomach and duodenum due to peptic ulcer disease.

- Zollinger-Ellison syndrome (Gastrinoma)
- Drinking too much alcohol
- Regular use of certain medications (Aspirin, Ibuprofen, etc)
- Stress
- Genetic factors.

Risk Factors

- Advancement in age
- Use of corticosteroids
- Smoking cigarettes or chewing tobacco
- A history of ulcer disease
- Being critically ill (Being on a breathing machine)
- Having radiation treatments
- Hypercalcemia.

Types

There are two types of peptic ulcer disease as follows:

1. **Gastric ulcer:** Its symptoms often do not follow a consistent pattern (e.g., eating sometimes exacerbates rather than relieves pain). This is especially true for pyloric channel ulcers, which are often associated with symptoms of obstruction (e.g., bloating, nausea, vomiting) caused by edema and scarring.
2. **Duodenal ulcer:** It tends to cause more consistent pain. Pain is absent when the patient awakens but appears in mid-morning, and is relieved by food, but recurs 2–3 hours after a meal. Pain that awakens a patient at night is common and is highly suggestive of duodenal ulcer.

Pathophysiology

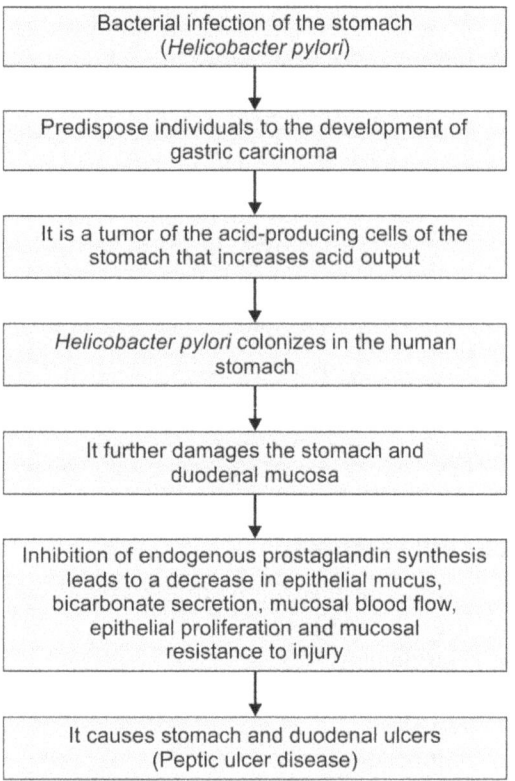

Clinical Features

- A gnawing or burning pain in the middle or upper stomach between meals or at night
- Severe pain in the mid to upper abdomen
- Bloating
- Heartburn
- Feeling of fullness
- Hunger and an empty feeling in the stomach, often 1–3 hours after a meal
- Mild nausea
- Bloody or dark tarry stools (melena)
- Fatigue
- Vomiting, possibly blood
- Indigestion
- Unexplained weight loss.

Complications

- Bleeding inside the body (internal bleeding)
- Gastric outlet obstructions
- Peritonitis (inflammation of the tissue that lines the wall of the abdomen)
- Perforation of the stomach and intestines.

Diagnostic Tests

- History
- Physical examination
- Blood examination
- Stool examination
- Endoscopic examination
- Biopsy examination
- Barium X-ray examination
- Esophagogastroduodenoscopy (EGD) examination.

Management

Medical

- **Proton pump inhibitors:** It helps to decrease acid secretion and allows the ulcer to heal. For example, prevacid, aciphex, protonix, etc.
- **H2-receptor antagonists:** It helps to decrease pancreatic activity by inhibiting hydrochloric acid. For example, cimetidine, ranitidine, etc.
- **Antibiotics:** It helps to treat Helicobacter pylori infections. For example, Ciprofloxacin, Amoxicillin, etc.
- **Antiemetics:** It helps to prevent vomiting. For example, Prochlorperazine, Perinorm, Stemetil, etc.
- **Analgesics:** It helps to alleviate any pain in the gastric or intestinal mucosa. Meperidine, etc.
- **Antacids:** It neutralizes gastric hydrochloric acid secretion. For example, Gelusil, etc.
- **Prostaglandin E1 analog:** It increases mucosal resistance and inhibits acid secretion to a minor degree. For example, misoprostol, etc.

Surgical

- **Billroth I procedure:** It is a surgical procedure that involves the partial gastrectomy or removal of the antrum and pylorus of the stomach with anastomosis of the gastric stump to the duodenum. It is also known as gastroduodenostomy.
- **Billroth II procedure:** It is a surgical procedure that involves the partial gastrectomy or removal of the antrum and pylorus of the stomach with anastomosis of the gastric stump to the jejunum. It is also known as gastrojejunostomy.

Nursing

- Instruct them to avoid alcohol intake.
- Ask them to avoid tobacco products.
- Encourage consumption of foods that are cooked thoroughly.
- Instruct them to use regular medications with caution.
- Ask them to wash the hands regularly to protect themselves from infections.
- Encourage to take bland diet.
- Instruct them to avoid spicy foods.

PERITONITIS

Definition

Peritonitis is an inflammation of the peritoneum, the thin tissue that lines the inner wall of the abdomen and covers most of the abdominal organs.

Etiology

- Pancreatitis
- Burst appendix
- Stomach ulcer
- Crohn's disease
- Diverticulitis

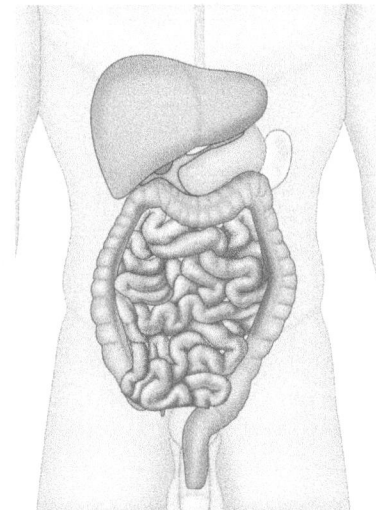

Fig. 5.25: Depicts inflamed peritoneum lining the inner wall of the abdomen.

- Peritoneal dialysis
- Excess fluid in the abdomen
- Stab wound.

Risk Factors

- Cirrhosis of liver
- Weakened immune system
- Pelvic inflammatory disease
- Torn or twisted intestine
- Blood infection
- Ectopic pregnancy
- Salpingitis
- Abdominal surgery
- Necrotizing enterocolitis
- Perforated gallbladder
- Family history of peritonitis.

Types

Peritonitis is classified as follows:
- *Spontaneous or primary peritonitis:* It can occur in patients with severe liver disease, heart disease or kidney disease. Often these diseases cause the accumulation of fluid within the abdominal cavity. This is called ascites.
- *Secondary peritonitis:* It is the escape of pus from an infected abdominal organ.

Pathophysiology

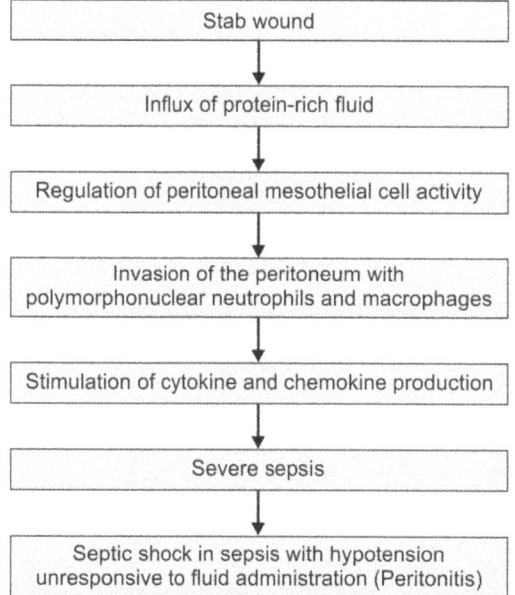

Clinical Features

- Severe and constant abdominal pain ranging from dull aches to severe, sharp pain
- Fever
- Chills
- Inability to break wind or pass stools
- Nausea
- Vomiting
- Diarrhea
- Fatigue
- Sore or swollen belly
- Loss of appetite
- Excessive thirst
- Minimal urine output
- Trouble breathing
- Low blood pressure and shock.

Complications

- Sepsis
- Hepatic encephalopathy
- Hepatorenal syndrome
- Abnormal clotting of the blood
- Scar tissue in the peritoneum
- Acute respiratory distress syndrome.

Diagnostic Tests

- History
- Physical examination
- X-ray studies of the abdomen
- Blood examination
- Peritoneal fluid culture
- Laparoscopic examination
- Transabdominal ultrasound
- Computed tomography (CT) scan
- Magnetic resonance imaging (MRI) scan.

Management

Medical

- **Antibiotics:** It helps to prevent any secondary infections. For example, cephalosporin, metronidazole, ciprofloxacin, amoxicillin, etc.
- **Antiemetics:** It helps to prevent vomiting. For example, prochlorperazine, Perinorm, Stemetil, etc.
- **Analgesics:** It helps to alleviate any pain. Meperidine, etc.

Surgical

- **Laparotomy:** It is a surgical procedure in which full exploration and lavage of the peritoneum is performed to correct any gross anatomical damage that may have caused the disease.

Nursing

- Instruct them to avoid refined foods, such as white bread and sugar.
- Encourage them to drink 6–8 glasses of water daily.
- Teach the importance of avoiding caffeine, alcohol and tobacco.
- Encourage them to take antioxidant-rich foods.
- Encourage foods high in vitamin B and calcium.
- Ask them to use healthy oils in foods such as olive or vegetable oil.

PHARYNGITIS

Definition

The infection and inflammation of the pharynx is known as pharyngitis. It usually causes symptom of a sore throat.

Etiology

- *Group A beta-hemolytic streptococcus*
- Measles
- Adenovirus
- Chickenpox
- Croup
- Whooping cough.

Risk Factors

- Adults who work in dusty surroundings
- Habitual users of alcohol based
- Those who suffer from chronic cough
- Cold and flu seasons
- Frequent sinus infections
- Allergies.

Pathophysiology

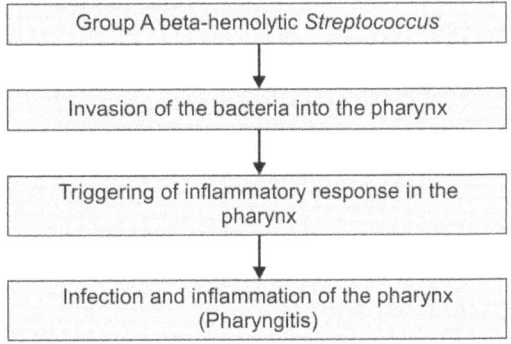

Clinical Features

- Sore throat
- Low-grade fever
- Edema
- Headache
- Joint pain and muscle aches
- Skin rashes
- Enlarged cervical lymph nodes
- Swollen lymphoid follicles
- Fatigue
- Cough
- Chills
- Sneezing
- Running nose

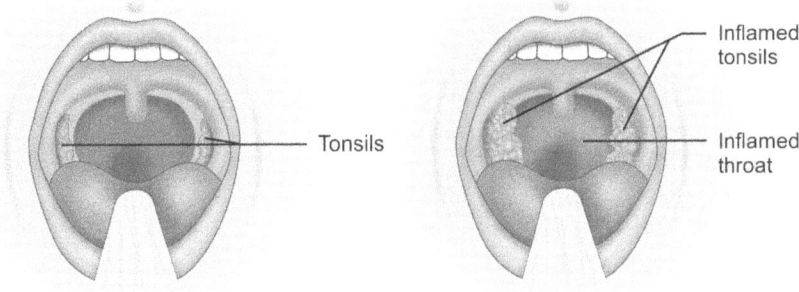

Fig. 5.26: Shows the comparison of normal throat and throat with inflamed pharynx (Pharyngitis).

- Swelling in the uvula and soft palate
- General malaise
- Loss of appetite
- Unusual taste in the mouth
- Nausea
- Difficulty in swallowing.

Complications

- Mastoiditis
- Sinusitis
- Otitis media
- Peritonsillar abscess
- Abscess near the tonsils
- Cervical adenoiditis
- Pneumonia
- Meningitis
- Rheumatic fever
- Nephritis.

Diagnostic Tests

- History
- Physical examination
- Throat swab culture
- Nasal swab examination
- Blood examination
- Latex agglutination test.

Management

Medical

- **Antibiotics:** It helps to reduce the risk of infections. For example, penicillin, erythromycin, neomycin, etc.
- **Analgesics:** It helps to alleviate any pain. For example, Aspirin, Paracetamol, etc.
- **Antitussives:** It suppresses coughing, possibly by reducing the activity of the cough center in the brain. For example, Tessalon, Bronchophan, Benylin, etc.

Nursing

- Instruct them to avoid sharing food, drinks and eating utensils.
- Ask them to avoid individuals who are sick.
- Instruct them to avoid smoking and inhaling second-hand smoke.
- Encourage alcohol-based hand sanitizers when soap and water are not available.
- Encourage them to drink plenty of fluids.
- Instruct them to gargle with warm salt water.
- Ensure complete bed rest until they feel better.

ULCERATIVE COLITIS

Definition

Ulcerative colitis is a recurrent ulcerative and inflammatory disease of the mucosal and submucosal layers of the colon and rectum.

Etiology

- Emotional stress
- Overactive intestinal immune system
- Genetic predisposition
- Allergies
- Infections
- Idiopathic.

Risk Factors

- It occurs between 15 and 30 years of age.
- Older than 60 years of age
- Intake of high fat diet
- Previous history of inflammatory bowel disease (IBD)
- Jewish descent
- Oral contraceptives
- Nonsteroidal anti-inflammatory drugs.

Pathophysiology

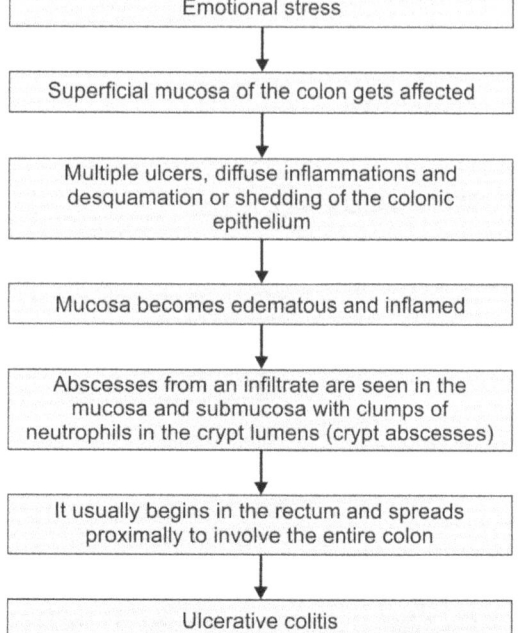

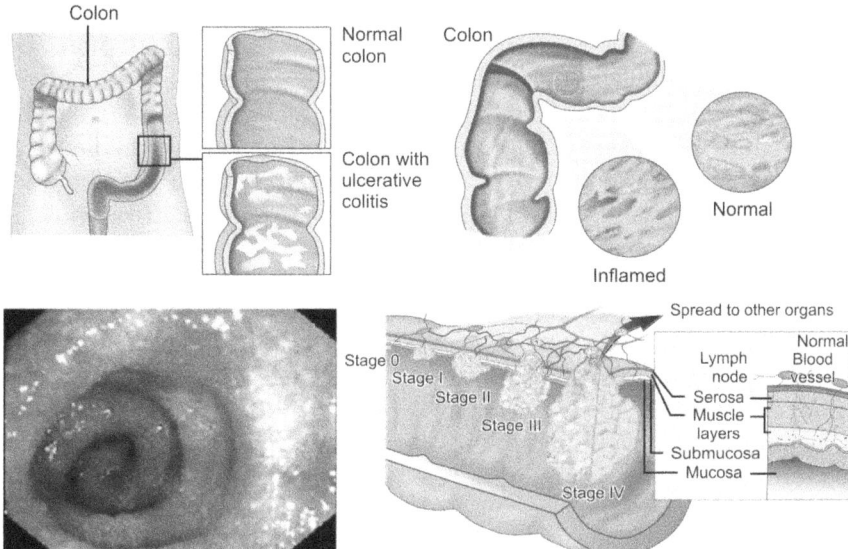

Fig. 5.27: Depicts inflammatory and disease of the mucosal and submucosal layers of the colon and rectum (Ulcerative colitis).

Clinical Features

- Lower left quadrant abdominal pain
- Intermittent tenesmus
- Rebound tenderness in the right lower quadrant
- Malaise
- Anorexia
- Weight loss
- Severe diarrhea containing blood and mucus
- Fever
- Feeling of an urgent need to defecate
- Passage of 10–20 liquid stools each day
- Vomiting
- Anemia
- Rectal bleeding
- Hypocalcemia
- Deficiency of vitamin-K.

Complications

- Toxic megacolon
- Perforation
- Massive bleeding in the colon
- Dehydration
- Malabsorption.

Diagnostic Tests

- History
- Physical examination
- Stool examination
- Blood examination
- Sigmoidoscopic examination
- Abdominal X-ray studies
- CT scan
- Magnetic resonance imaging
- Ultrasound.

Management

Medical

- **Corticosteroids:** It helps to reduce the activity of the immune system and decreases inflammation and also brings down the remission rate. For example, prednisone, budesonide, methylprednisone, hydrocortisone, etc.
- **Immunomodulators:** It acts by reducing the immune system activity, resulting in less inflammation in the colon. For example, 6 - mercaptopurine, azothioprine, cyclosporine, etc.
- **Aminosalicylates:** It helps in controlling the inflammation of the colon. For example, balsalazide, mesalamine, olsalazine, etc.
- **Antibiotics:** It helps in preventing secondary infections. For example, ampicillin, etc.

- **Biologic agents:** These are designed to stimulate the immune system and interfere with specific proteins (cytokines called tumor necrosis factor [TNF]) involved with the inflammatory response. For example, infliximab (Remicade), etc.
- **Antidiarrheal agents:** It helps in controlling diarrhea. For example, loperamide (Imodium), etc.

Surgical

- **Total proctocolectomy with ileostomy:** It is the surgical removal of the entire colon (colon, rectum and anus with anal closure) and rectum and a stoma or opening is made in the abdomen in the last section of the small intestine to allow drainage of fecal matter from the ileum to the outside of the body.
- **Total proctocolectomy with ileal pouch anal anastomosis (IPAA):** It is the surgical removal of the entire colon and creation of the permanent ileoanal reservoir (J-pouch) to connect the ileum to the anus to facilitate waste gets stored in the pouch and passes through the anus.

Nursing

- Instruct the client to eat small amounts of diet throughout the day.
- Ask them to stay hydrated by drinking lots of water (frequent consumption of small amounts throughout the day).
- Educate to avoid high-fiber and spicy foods.
- Encourage the patient to eat soft and bland diet.
- Educate to avoid or limit caffeine consumption.

6
CHAPTER

Disorders of Respiratory System

CHAPTER OUTLINE

- Atelectasis
- Bronchial asthma
- Bronchiectasis
- Bronchitis
- Chest trauma
- Chronic obstructive pulmonary disease
- Cor pulmonale
- Cystic fibrosis
- Hypoxia
- Lung abscess
- Pleural effusion
- Pleurisy
- Pneumonia
- Pneumothorax
- Pulmonary embolism
- Pulmonary hypertension
- Pulmonary tuberculosis
- Respiratory failure
- Sarcoidosis
- Tracheal obstruction

ATELECTASIS

Definition

The collapse or airless condition of the alveoli caused by hypoventilation, obstruction to the airways or compression is known as atelectasis.

Etiology

- Hypoventilation
- Obstruction to the airways
- Aspiration
- Reduced amount of surfactant (a liquid that keeps the lung expanded).

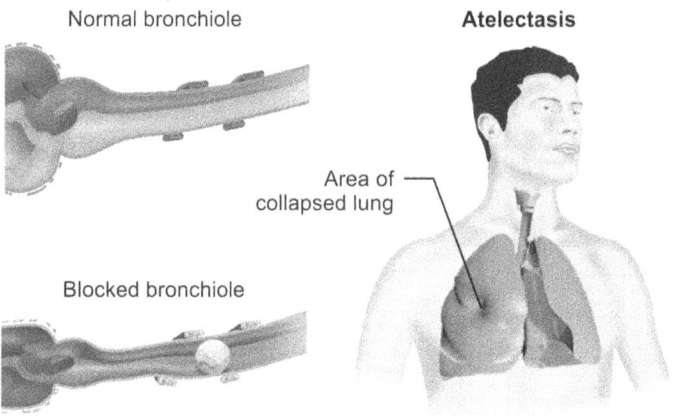

Fig. 6.1: Depicts lung with normal bronchiole and blocked bronchiole.

Risk Factors

- Chronic obstructive pulmonary disease
- Immobility
- Smoking
- Weakened respiratory muscles
- Premature birth in which lungs are not fully developed
- Increased duration of anesthesia
- Pain
- Decreased level of consciousness
- Mechanical ventilation
- Anesthesia.

Types

- *Acute atelectasis:* It occurs frequently in the postoperative setting or in people who are immobilized.
- *Chronic atelectasis:* It occurs frequently in patients with a chronic airway obstruction that blocks airflow to an area of the lung.

Pathophysiology

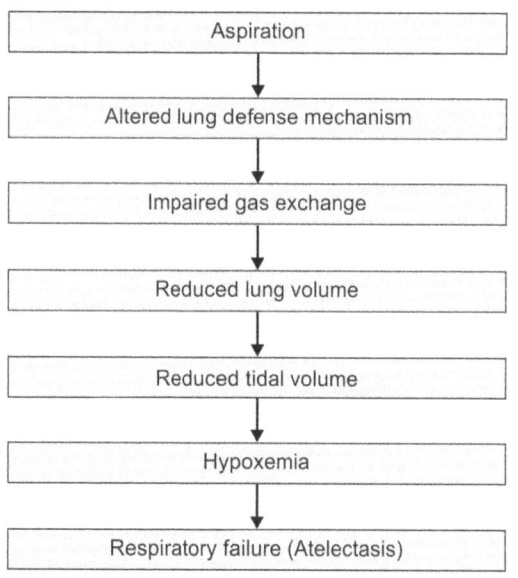

Clinical Features

- Dyspnea
- Tachycardia
- Tachypnea
- Pleural pain
- Central cyanosis (bluish skin)
- Cough
- Sputum production
- Low-grade fever
- Decreased chest movement during breathing.

Complications

- Shock
- Death
- Respiratory failure
- Pneumonia.

Diagnostic Tests

- History
- Physical examination
- Blood examination
- Chest X-ray
- CT scan of the chest
- Pulmonary function test
- Sputum culture examination
- Pulse oximetric examination
- Bronchoscopic examination.

Management

Medical

- **Oxygen therapy:** One of the most important methods of treating atelectasis is to administer oxygen. This increases the concentration of oxygen being inhaled which increases the partial pressure of oxygen in the blood and corrects hypoxia.
- **Chest physiotherapy:** It helps in mobilizing the secretions from the lungs.
- **Bronchodilators:** It helps to dilate the bronchial smooth muscles. For example, theophylline, Theo-Dur, etc.
- **Corticosteroids:** It helps to reduce the severity of the disease. For example, beclomethasone, budesonide, prednisone, etc.

Surgical

Thoracentesis: It is a procedure to remove fluid from the space between the lining of the outside of the lungs (pleura) and the wall of the chest.

Nursing

- Encourage frequent change of positions to promote ventilation and prevent secretions from accumulating.
- Teach deep breathing and coughing exercise to mobilize secretions and prevent them from accumulating.
- Perform suctioning to remove tracheobronchial secretions.
- Teach the technique of incentive spirometry.
- Encourage early mobilization from bed to chair followed by early ambulation.
- Instruct the patient to stop smoking.

BRONCHIAL ASTHMA

Definition

Bronchial asthma is an intermittent, reversible, obstructive airway in which the trachea and bronchi respond in a hyperactive way to certain stimuli.

Etiology

- Exposure to indoor and outdoor allergens
- Occupational sensitizers
- Viral respiratory tract infections
- Certain medication
- Sinusitis
- Gastroesophageal reflux
- Air pollution.

Risk Factors

- Atopy
- Female gender
- Smoking
- Exercise
- Stress or emotional upsets
- Exposure to sulphur dioxide
- Weather changes.

Types

- ***Allergic asthma:*** It is caused by known allergens such as dust, pollens, etc.
- ***Nonallergic asthma:*** It is not related to a specific allergens such as respiratory tract infections.
- ***Mixed asthma:*** It is the most common form of asthma resembling both allergic and nonallergic forms.

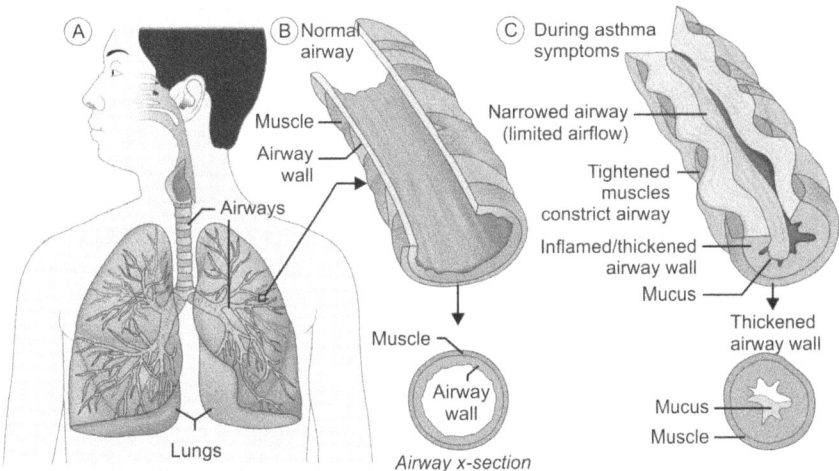

Fig. 6.2: Shows the comparison of lungs with normal airway and narrowed airway (Bronchial asthma).

Pathophysiology

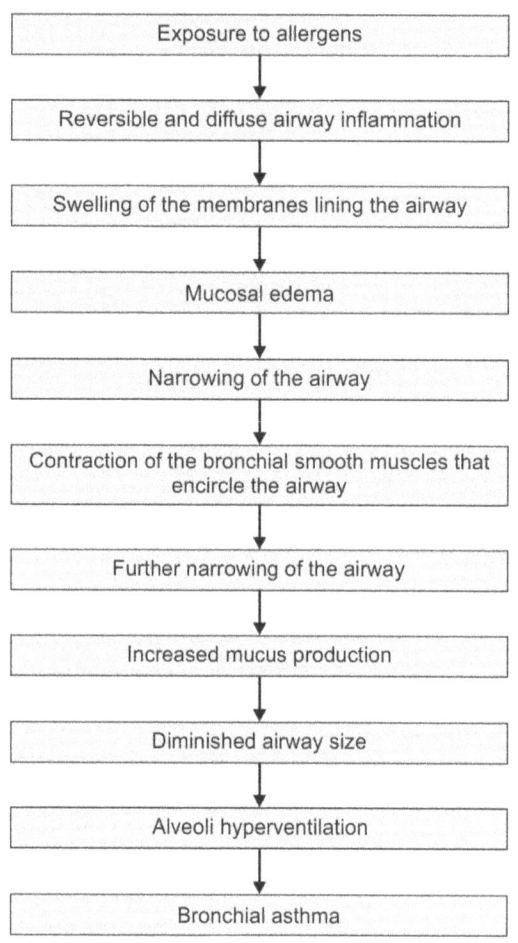

Clinical Features

- Dyspnea
- Wheezing
- Cough
- Chest tightness
- Diaphoresis
- Tachycardia
- Widened pulse pressure
- Hypoxemia
- Cyanosis
- Palpitations.

Complications

- Status asthmaticus
- Respiratory failure
- Pneumonia
- Atelectasis
- Fracture.

Diagnostic Tests

- History
- Physical examination
- Sputum examination
- Blood examination
- Chest X-ray
- CT scan of the chest
- Pulmonary function test
- Sputum culture examination.

Management

Medical

- **Methylxanthines:** It helps to relax bronchial smooth muscles and increases the movement of mucus in the airways. For example, theophylline, Theo-Dur, etc.
- **Corticosteroids:** It helps to reduce infection, inflammation and bronchoconstriction. For example, beclomethasone, budesonide, etc.
- **Leukotriene inhibitors:** It helps to dilate blood vessels and to other permeability. For example, accolate, montelukast, etc.
- **Anticholinergic agents:** It helps to relieve airway obstruction through dilating the bronchioles. For example, ipratropium bromide, etc.
- **Beta-adrenergic agents:** It helps to dilate bronchial smooth muscles. For example, salmeterol, albuterol, etc.
- **Mast cell inhibitors:** It helps to dilate the bronchioles and decreases airway inflammation. For example, cromolyn sodium, nedocromil sodium, etc.

Nursing

- Instruct the patient to avoid dairy products.
- Encourage the patient to take more fluids.
- Teach deep breathing and coughing exercise.
- Ask the patient to avoid work involving risk of exposure.

- Ask the patient to cover the mouth when coughing or sneezing.
- Instruct the patient to stop smoking and avoidance of other airborne irritants.
- Teach the method of using inhalers.
- Ensure them to take medications properly.

BRONCHIECTASIS

Definition

Bronchiectasis is a chronic dilatation of the bronchi and bronchioles due to inflammation and destruction of their walls.

Etiology

- Airway obstruction
- Diffuse airway injury
- Cystic fibrosis
- Pulmonary infections
- Obstruction of the bronchus
- Aspiration of foreign bodies
- Idiopathic.

Risk Factors

- Recurrent respiratory infections in early childhood
- Measles
- Influenza
- Tuberculosis
- Immune deficiency.

Pathophysiology

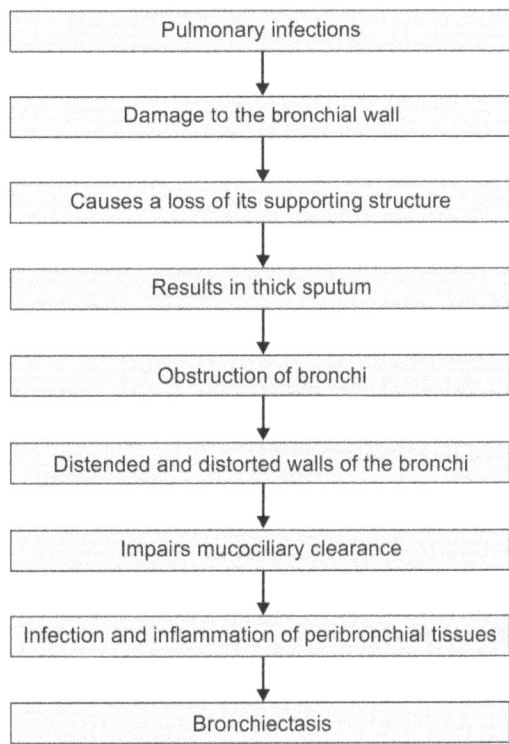

Clinical Features

- Persistent cough with production of copious amounts of purulent sputum
- Recurrent fever
- Hemoptysis

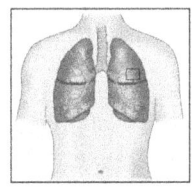

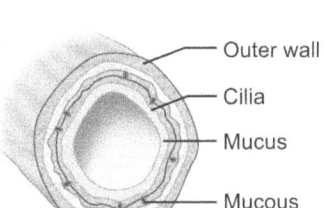

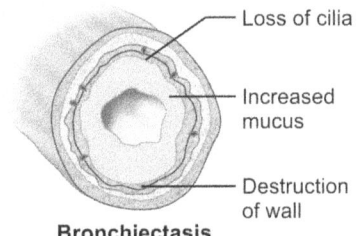

Fig. 6.3: Shows the comparison of lungs with normal bronchus and inflamed bronchus (Bronchiectasis).

- Shortness of breath
- Clubbing of fingers
- Crackles and rhonchi heard on auscultation.

Complications
- Progressive suppuration
- Chronic obstructive pulmonary disease (COPD)
- Emphysema
- Chronic respiratory insufficiency.

Diagnostic Tests
- History
- Physical examination
- Sputum examination
- Blood examination
- Chest X-ray
- CT scan of the chest
- Pulmonary function test
- Sputum culture examination.

Management
Medical
- **Antibiotics:** It helps to prevent secondary infections. For example, amoxicillin, ampicillin, gentamicin, etc.
- **Bronchodilators:** It helps to prevent vasospasm. For example, theophylline, aminophylline, etc.

Surgical
- **Segmental resection:** It is the surgical procedure in which a segment of the lobe is removed.
- **Lobectomy:** It is the surgical procedure in which lobe of the lung is removed.
- **Pneumonectomy:** It is the surgical procedure in which the entire lung is removed.

Nursing
- Encourage increased intake of fluids to reduce viscosity of sputum and make expectoration easier.
- Encourage chest physiotherapy techniques.
- Encourage patient to engage in physical activity throughout the day to help mobilize mucus.
- Encourage regular dental care because copious sputum production may affect the dentition.
- Encourage use of face masks during short-term tasks involving exposure to dust.
- Instruct the patient to avoid smoking.
- Ask the patient to cover the mouth when coughing or sneezing.

BRONCHITIS

Definition
Bronchitis is an inflammation of the bronchial tubes, the airways that carry air to the lungs.

Etiology
- Viral infection (90% of cases caused by influenza virus)
- Bacterial infection (*Bordetella pertussis*)
- Environmental irritants
- Upper respiratory tract infection.

Risk Factors
- Tobacco smoking (including secondhand smoke)
- Dust
- Fumes (from an explosion)
- Vapors
- Air pollution
- Poverty
- Alcohol consumption
- Alpha antitrypsin deficiency
- Childhood respiratory infection
- Family history of bronchitis
- Bronchial hyperresponsiveness
- Low birth weight.

Types
- *Acute bronchitis:* It may get better within several days but the cough can last for several weeks after the infection is gone and can be treated.
- *Chronic bronchitis:* It is a long-term condition that keeps coming back or never goes away completely.

Disorders of Respiratory System

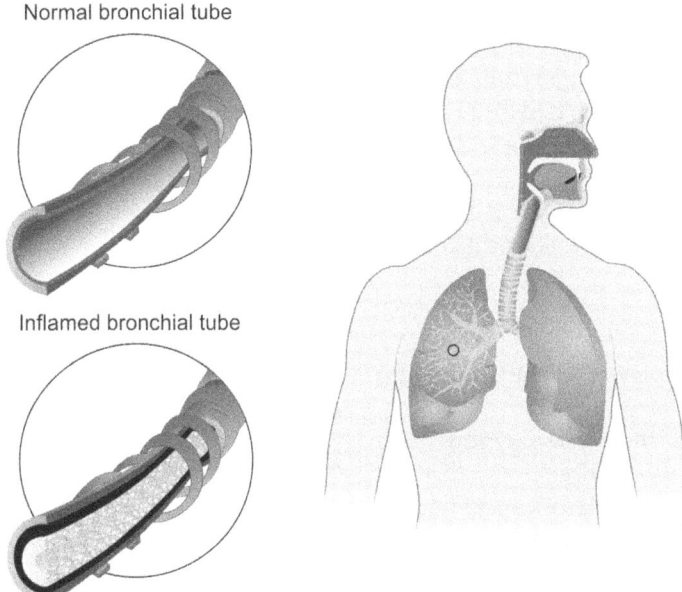

Fig. 6.4: Shows the comparison of normal and inflamed bronchial tube (Bronchitis).

Pathophysiology

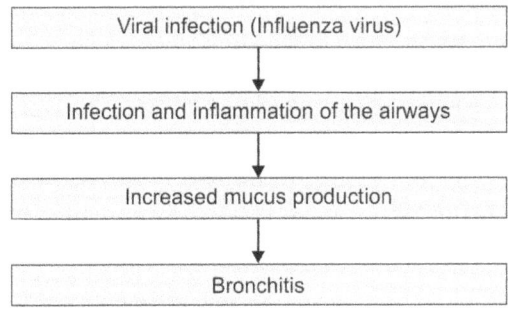

Clinical Features

- Dyspnea
- Shortness of breath
- Chest tightness
- Fever
- Tachypnea
- Productive cough with purulent sputum
- Pleuritic chest pain
- Rhonchi and crackles heard on auscultation.

Complications

- Pneumonia
- Sinusitis
- Respiratory failure
- Dysrhythmias
- Atelectasis.

Diagnostic Tests

- History
- Physical examination
- Blood examination
- Chest X-ray
- Sputum culture examination
- Bronchial dilation test
- Spirometric examination
- Pulmonary function studies
- Arterial blood gas analysis.

Management

Medical

- **Bronchodilators:** It helps to open obstructed airways to make breathing easier. For example, theophylline, salbutamol, etc.
- **Corticosteroids:** It helps to acute exacerbations of chronic bronchitis. For example, methylprednisolone, beclomethasone, fluticasone, etc.

- **Antibiotics:** It helps to prevent acute exacerbations of chronic bronchitis. For example, amoxicillin, augmentin, etc.
- **Anticholinergic agents:** It helps to relieve airway obstruction. For example, ipratropium bromide, etc.
- **Beta-adrenergic agonists:** It helps to reduce airway obstruction. For example, terbutaline, etc.

Nursing

- Limit patient exposure to cold and damp environments.
- Provide good initial treatment and guidance.
- Ask the patient to avoid work involving risk of exposure.
- Ask the patient to cover the mouth when coughing or sneezing.
- Instruct the patient to stop smoking and avoidance of other airborne irritants.
- Encourage use of face masks during short-term tasks involving exposure to dust.
- Teach and supervise breathing exercises to strengthen diaphragmatic muscles.
- Encourage them to take more fluids (2–2.5 liters per day).
- Encourage improvement of the quality of outdoor air and indoor air, at home and in places of work.

CHEST TRAUMA

Definition

A chest trauma can occur as the result of an accident or deliberate penetration of a foreign object into the chest.

Etiology

- Motor vehicle accidents
- Crush injuries
- Sports-related injuries
- Falls
- Assault.

Risk Factors

- Being elders
- Smoking
- Alcohol consumption
- Sportsman
- Driving vehicles
- Violent acts.

Types

- **Blunt chest trauma:** It occurs when the chest is directly hit and causes injuries to the rib cage.
- **Flail chest trauma:** It occurs when three or more ribs are broken in at least two places, front and back. This will only happen if there has been a great deal of

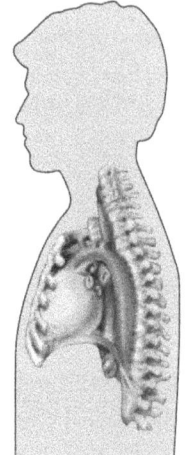 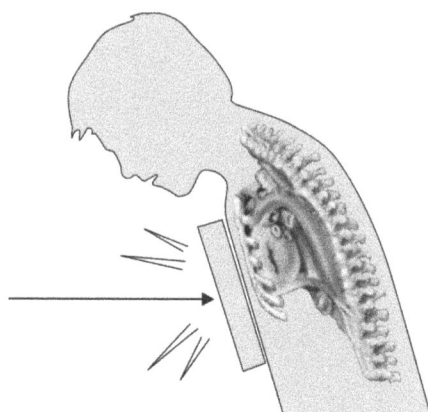

Fig. 6.5: Depicts the occurrence of chest trauma as a result of an accident or deliberate penetration of a foreign object into the chest.

blunt force. The key sign of flail chest is 'paradoxical movement', which means the natural movement of the rib cage during breathing is in reverse. For example, the injured area of rib cage sinks in when the person inhales, instead of lifting outwards.

Pathophysiology

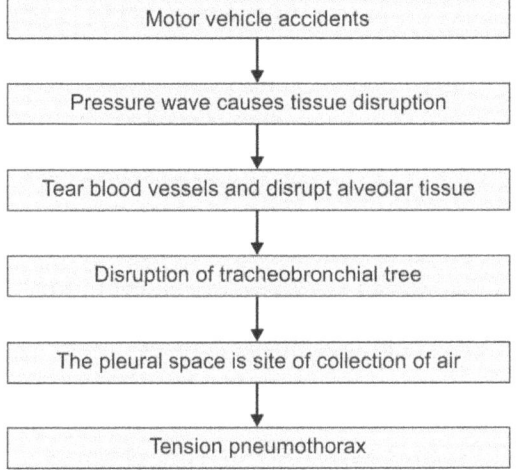

Clinical Features

- Pain at the injury site
- Pain when the ribcage flexes
- Crunching or grinding sounds (crepitus) when the injury site is touched or moved.
- Muscle spasm of the ribcage
- Dyspnea
- Abdominal injuries.

Complications

- Pneumothorax
- Hemothorax
- Splenic rupture
- Chest infections
- Rib fracture.

Diagnostic Tests

- History
- Physical examination
- Blood examination
- Chest X-ray
- Computed tomography (CT) scan
- Angiography
- Bronchoscopic examination
- Echocardiography
- Electrocardiogram.

Management

Medical

- **Oxygen therapy:** One of the most important methods of flail chest trauma is to administer oxygen.
- **Mechanical ventilation:** It helps to provide short-term support of ventilation.
- **Rib fracture fixation:** It is a procedure in which metal is used to stabilize the 'flail' segment of the chest wall.
- **Chest tube insertion:** It is a surgical procedure in which a hollow plastic tube is inserted between the ribs and into the pleural space.
- **Bronchodilators:** It helps to open obstructed airways to make breathing easier. For example, theophylline, salbutamol, etc.
- **Antibiotics:** It helps to prevent secondary infections on patients with perforated viscus. For example, cefuroxime, metronidazole, etc.
- **Analgesics:** It is widely used for acute and short-term pain relief. For example, entonox, etc.

Nursing

- Provide adequate bedrest to the patient.
- Instruct the patient to avoid activities that may aggravate the injury.
- Provide ice-packs as it may help to reduce inflammation in the early stages.
- Provide good initial treatment and guidance.
- Instruct the patient to stop smoking.
- Teach the patient to cough with the help of a pillow support in the painful area.
- Teach and supervise breathing exercises to strengthen diaphragmatic muscles.
- Instruct the patient not to lie down or still for long periods of time.
- Instruct them not to lift, pull or push anything that makes the pain worse.

CHRONIC OBSTRUCTIVE PULMONARY DISEASE

Definition

Chronic obstructive pulmonary disease (COPD) is a disease state characterized by airflow limitation that is not fully reversible. It includes chronic bronchitis and pulmonary emphysema.

- **Chronic bronchitis:** It is a chronic inflammation of the lower respiratory tract characterized by excessive mucus secretion, cough and dyspnea associated with recurring infections of the lower respiratory tract.
- **Pulmonary emphysema:** It is a complex lung disease characterized by destruction of the alveoli, enlargement of distal airspaces and a breakdown of alveolar walls.

Etiology

- Air pollution
- Cigarette smoking
- Occupational exposure to dusts and fumes
- Infection
- Exposure to tobacco smoke
- Genetic predisposition.

Risk Factors

- Allergy
- Alpha, antitrypsin deficiency
- Environmental factors
- Aging
- Previous tuberculosis
- Childhood asthma.

Stages of COPD

- **Stage 0: At risk**-Normal spirometry
- **Stage 1: Mild COPD**-Mild airflow limitation (FEV1/FVC < 70%; FEV1 > 80% predicted) and sometimes, but not always, chronic cough and sputum production. At this stage, the individual may not be aware that his or her lung function is abnormal.
- **Stage 2: Moderate COPD**-Worsening airflow limitation (FEV1/FVC < 70%; 50% < FEV1 < 80% predicted), with shortness of breath typically developing during exertion. This is the stage at which patients typically seek medical attention because of chronic respiratory symptoms or an exacerbation of their disease.
- **Stage 3: Severe COPD**-Further worsening of airflow limitation (FEV1/FVC < 70%; 30% < FEV1 < 50% predicted), greater shortness of breath, reduced exercise capacity and repeated exacerbations which have an impact on patients' quality of life.
- **Stage 4: Very severe COPD**-Severe airflow limitation (FEV1/FVC < 70%; FEV1 < 30% predicted) or FEV1 < 50% predicted plus chronic respiratory failure. Patients may

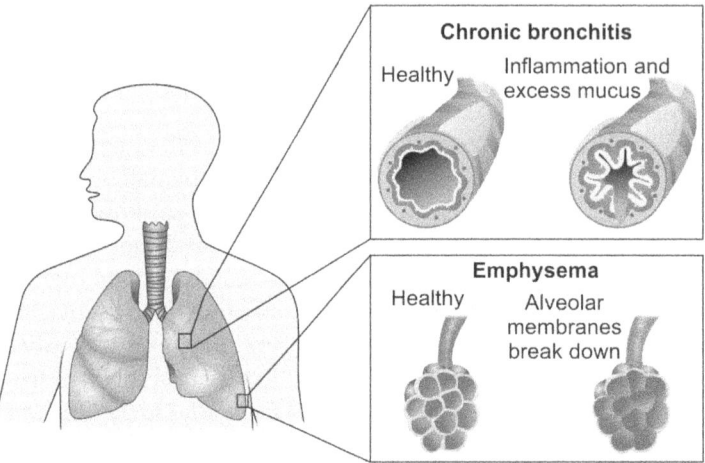

Fig. 6.6: Shows the comparison of healthy and inflamed bronchial tube (Chronic bronchitis) and shows the comparison of healthy alveoli with that of alveolar membranes breakdown.

have very severe (Stage IV) COPD even if the FEV1 is > 30% predicted, whenever this complication is present. At this stage, quality of life is very appreciably impaired and exacerbations may be life-threatening.

Pathophysiology

Chronic Bronchitis

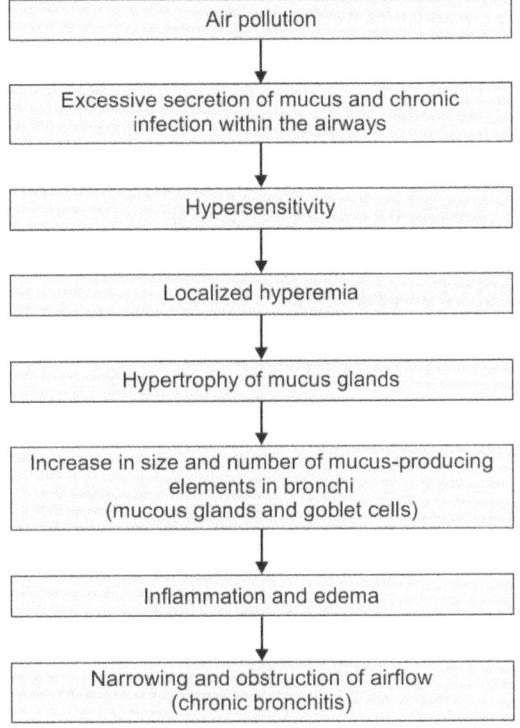

Pulmonary Emphysema

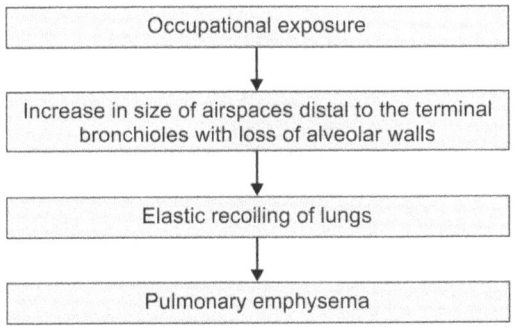

Clinical Features

Chronic Bronchitis

- Presence of productive cough lasting at least 3 months a year for 2 successive years
- Production of thick, gelatinous sputum
- Dyspnea
- Wheezing.

Pulmonary Emphysema

- Dyspnea
- Decreased exercise tolerance
- Mild sputum expectoration
- Increased anteroposterior diameter of chest (barrel chest).

Complications

- Respiratory failure
- Pneumonia
- Right-sided heart failure
- Depression
- Dysrhythmias
- Skeletal muscle dysfunction
- Atelectasis
- Pneumothorax.

Diagnostic Tests

- History
- Physical examination
- Pulmonary function studies
- Spirometric examination
- Arterial blood gas analysis
- Chest X-ray
- Alpha, antitrypsin assay.

Management

Medical

- **Methylxanthines:** It helps to relieve bronchospasm and reduce airway obstruction by allowing increased oxygen distribution throughout the lungs. For example, deriphylline, theophylline, etc.
- **Corticosteroids:** It helps to remove the severity of the disease. For example, beclomethasone, budesonide, fluticasone, etc.
- **Antichlolinergic agents:** It helps to relieve bronchospasm. For example, ipratropium bromide, etc.
- **Beta-adrenergic agonists:** It helps to remove airway obstruction. For example, salbutamol, terbutaline, etc.

Nursing

- Instruct the patient to stop smoking.
- Administer oxygen as prescribed.
- Encourage high level of fluid intake (2–2.5 liters per day).
- Teach and supervise breathing exercise to strengthen diaphragmatic muscles.
- Ask the patient to avoid work involving risk of exposure.
- Ask the patient to cover the mouth when coughing or sneezing.
- Encourage use of face masks during short-term tasks involving exposure to dust.

COR PULMONALE

Definition

Cor pulmonale is defined as enlargement of the right ventricle secondary to abnormality of the lung, thorax, pulmonary vasculature or circulation.

Etiology

- Alveolar hypoxia
- Blood acidosis
- Emphysema
- Bronchial asthma
- Pulmonary tuberculosis
- Cystic fibrosis
- Bronchiectasis
- Pulmonary emboli
- Erythrocytosis
- Sickle cell disease
- DILD (Diffuse infiltrative lung disease)
- Filariasis
- Schistosomiasis.

Risk Factors

- Living at high altitude
- Mechanical ventilation
- Obstructive sleep apnea
- Kyphoscoliosis
- Obesity
- Chronic obstructive pulmonary disease (COPD)
- Acute lung disease (ARDS)
- Cardiomyopathy.

Pathophysiology

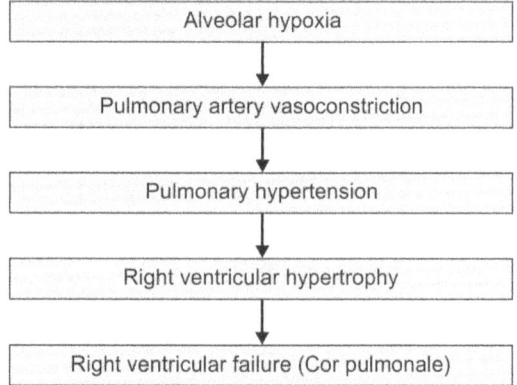

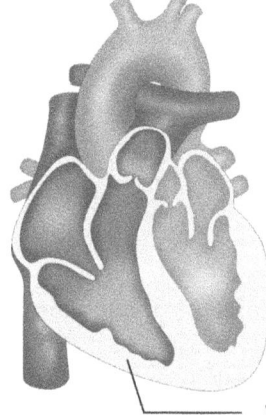
Normal heart

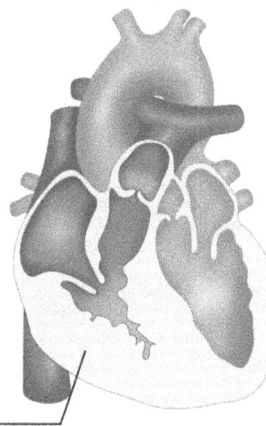
Right ventricular hypertrophy

Ventricle wall

Fig. 6.7: Shows the comparison of normal heart with that of right ventricular hypertrophy and failure (Cor pulmonale).

Clinical Features

- Shortness of breath
- Excessive fatigue
- Lightheadedness
- Syncope
- Chest discomfort, usually in the front of the chest
- Chest pain
- Tachycardia
- Wheezing
- Excessive coughing
- Loss of appetite
- Swelling of the feet or ankles.

Complications

- Exertional syncope
- Peripheral edema
- Peripheral venous insufficiency
- Tricuspid regurgitation
- Death.

Diagnostic Tests

- History
- Physical examination
- Chest radiography
- Electrocardiography
- Doppler echocardiography
- Radionuclide ventriculography
- Magnetic resonance imaging (MRI) scan
- Lung biopsy
- Right heart catheterization
- Blood examination
- Pulmonary function test.

Management

Medical

- **Oxygen therapy:** One of the most important methods of treating cor pulmonale is to administer oxygen. This increases the concentration of oxygen being inhaled which increases the partial pressure of oxygen in the blood and corrects alveolar hypoxia.
- **Anticoagulants (blood thinners):** These medications prevent new clots from forming and existing clots from growing larger. For example, heparin, warfarin, etc.
- **Bronchodilators:** It helps to dilate the bronchial smooth muscles. For example, theophylline, Theo-Dur, etc.
- **Corticosteroids:** It helps to reduce the severity of the disease. For example, beclomethasone, budesonide, prednisone, etc.
- **Diuretics:** It induces a hypokalemic metabolic alkalosis which can lessen respiratory drive through reducing the hypercapnic stimulus to breath and also reduces peripheral edema. For example, furosemide, bumetanide, etc.

Surgical

- **Atrial septostomy:** It is a surgical procedure in which a catheter with a balloon on one end is moved into the atria and the balloon is inflated to make an opening between the right and left atria for blood to flow through and the blood is full of oxygen for the left ventricle to pump into the body.
- **Phlebotomy:** It is a procedure performed on patients with pulmonary edema to decrease their total blood volume.
- **Lung transplantation:** It is a therapeutic measure of last resort for patients with end-stage lung disease who have exhausted all other available treatments without improvement.

Nursing

- Instruct the patient to avoid traveling to high altitude.
- Instruct the patient to avoid strenuous activities and heavy lifting.
- Instruct the patient to quit smoking.
- Educate the patients to limit their intake of liquids as there is risk for swelling which can worsen the condition.
- Ask them to consume foods that are low in sodium.
- Encourage the patient to participate in weight reduction program.

- Instruct the patient to avoid consumption of alcohol.
- Ask the patient to avoid pregnancy, as the heart needs to work harder than usual and may be life-threatening to both the mother and the baby.

CYSTIC FIBROSIS (CYSTIC LUNGS)

Definition

Cystic fibrosis is an inherited autosomal-recessive disorder of the exocrine glands, causing those glands to produce abnormally thick secretions of mucus, elevation of sweat electrolytes, increased organic and enzymatic constituents of saliva and overactivity of the autonomic nervous system. The glands mostly affected are those in the pancreas and respiratory system and the sweat glands.

Etiology

- Gene mutations
- Idiopathic.

Risk Factors

- Caucasian population
- Latinos and American Indians
- Advanced age
- Family history of cystic fibrosis
- Being physically inactive
- Secondhand smoke
- Alcohol consumption
- Neonates.

Pathophysiology

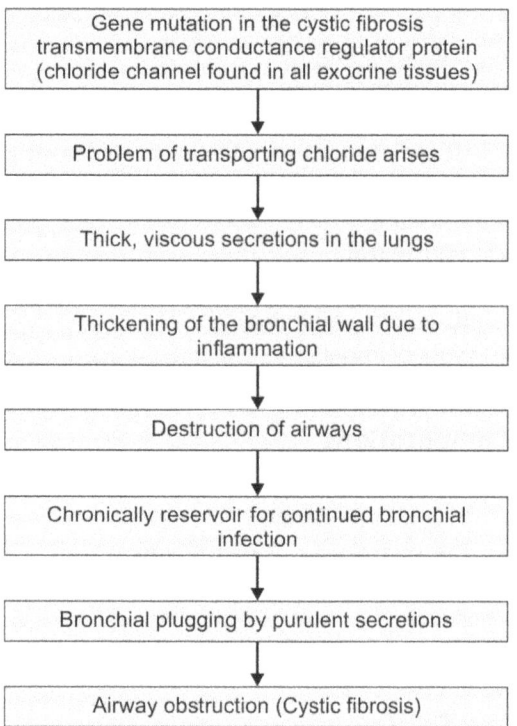

Clinical Features

- Persistent cough with productive thick mucus
- Dyspnea
- Hypoxia
- Myalgias
- Fever
- Weight loss or failure to gain weight despite increased appetite

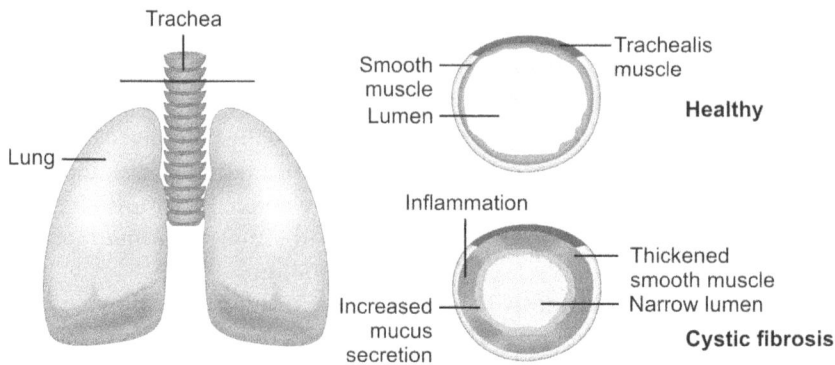

Fig. 6.8: Shows the comparison of healthy trachea with that of inflamed trachea (Cystic fibrosis).

- Clubbing of fingers
- Crackles heard on auscultation
- Wheezing
- Persistent upper respiratory tract infections
- Foul-smelling stools
- Pancreatic insufficiency
- Recurrent abdominal pain
- Genitourinary problems
- Salty tasting sweat.

Complications

- Cystic fibrosis-related diabetes (CFRD)
- Liver disease
- Distal intestinal obstruction syndrome (DIOS)
- Osteoporosis
- Nasal polyps
- Meconium ileus (an obstruction of the small bowel by viscid stool)
- Infertility.

Diagnostic Tests

- History
- Physical examination
- Pulmonary function test
- Arterial blood gas analysis
- Chest X-ray
- Sweat chloride test
- Molecular test
- Sputum examination
- Immunoreactive trypsinogen (IRT) test.

Management

Medical

- **Oxygen therapy:** One of the most important methods of treating cystic fibrosis is to administer oxygen. This increases the concentration of oxygen being inhaled which increases the partial pressure of oxygen in the blood and corrects alveolar hypoxia.
- **Bronchodilators:** It helps to dilate the bronchial smooth muscles. For example, theophylline, Theo-Dur, etc.
- **Mucolytic agents:** It helps to liquify the thick, tenacious mucus. For example, salmeterol, etc.
- **Corticosteroids:** It helps to reduce the severity of the disease. For example, beclomethasone, budesonide, prednisone, etc.
- **Antibiotics:** It helps to prevent lung infections. For example, tobramycin, azithromycin, etc.

Surgical

Lung transplantation: It is a therapeutic measure of last resort for patients with end-stage lung disease who have exhausted all other available treatments without improvement.

Nursing

- Encourage the patient to drink plenty of fluids as it can help in thinning of mucus secretions.
- Ask them to avoid smoke, pollen and mold as it can worsen the condition.
- Encourage regular exercise as it can liquefy the mucus secretions.
- Provide frequent mouthwash to the patient.
- Encourage high-calorie, high-protein and moderate-fat diet.
- Ensure the room temperature is always below 72 degree Fahrenheit to prevent excessive perspiration.

HYPOXIA

Definition

The decrease in oxygen supply to the tissues and cells is known as hypoxia.

Etiology

- Cardiac arrest
- Severe asthmatic attack
- Drug overdose or poisoning
- Seizures
- Attempted suicide (hanging) of near-drowning
- Severe blood loss
- Anesthesia accidents
- Electrocution.

Risk Factors

- Smoking
- Alcohol consumption

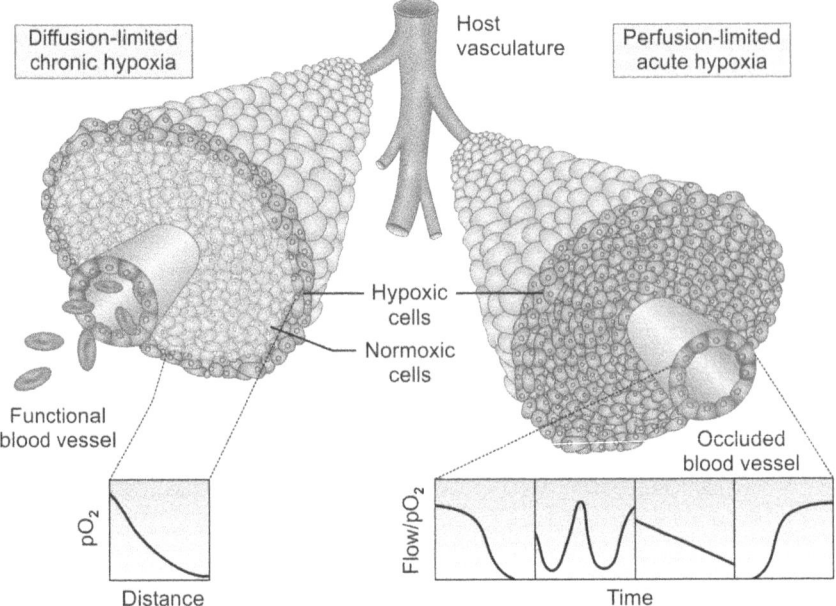

Fig. 6.9: Shows the diffusion-limited chronic hypoxia with that of perfusion-limited acute hypoxia.

- Intake of coffee
- Anemia
- Living in high altitude
- Impaired diffusion
- Hypoventilation
- Ventilation/perfusion ratio inequality
- Right to left shunt.

Types

- ***Hypoxic hypoxia:*** It is decreased oxygen level in the blood resulting in decreased oxygen diffusion into the tissues. It is caused by hypoventilation, high altitudes and pulmonary diffusion defects. It is corrected by providing supplemental oxygen.
- ***Stagnant hypoxia:*** It results from inadequate capillary circulation. It is caused by decreased cardiac arrest. It is corrected by treating the underlying cause.
- ***Anemic hypoxia:*** It results due to decreased effective hemoglobin concentration, which causes a decrease in the oxygen-carrying capacity of the blood. It leads to carbon monoxide poisoning, because it reduces the oxygen-carrying capacity of hemoglobin.
- ***Histotoxic hypoxia:*** It occurs when a toxic substance such as cyanide, interferes with the ability of tissues to use available oxygen.

Stages

- ***Asymptomatic stage:*** People are not generally aware of the effects of hypoxia at this stage. The primary symptoms are loss of night vision and a loss of color vision. These changes can occur at relatively modest altitudes (as low as 4,000 feet) and are probably most significant to pilots operating at night. Arterial oxygen saturations are typically between 90 and 95%
- ***Compensatory stage:*** In healthy people, this stage may occur at altitudes between 10,000 and 15,000 feet. The body generally has the ability to stay off further effects of hypoxia by increasing the rate and depth of ventilation and cardiac output. Arterial oxygen saturations during this phase are typically between 80 and 90%.
- ***Deterioration stage:*** In this stage, people are unable to compensate for the lack of oxygen. Unfortunately, not everyone recognizes or experiences the signs and symptoms associated with this stage. If they

do not, they cannot take steps to correct the problem. Arterial oxygen saturations during this phase typically are between 70 and 80%.
- **Critical stage:** This is the terminal stage leading up to death. People are almost completely incapacitated physically and mentally. People in this stage will lose consciousness, have convulsions, stop breathing and finally die. Arterial oxygen saturations are less than 70%.

Pathophysiology

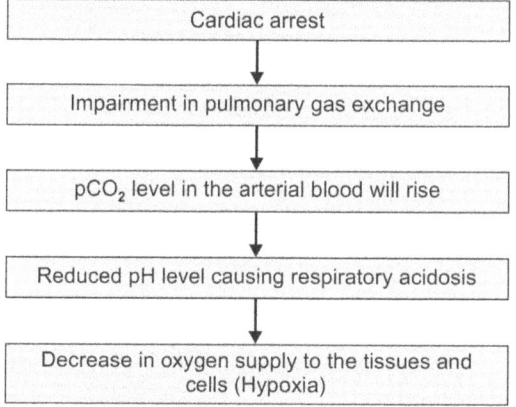

Clinical Features

- Apprehension
- Restlessness
- Irritability
- Lethargy
- Dyspnea on exertion
- Tachypnea
- Tachycardia
- Mild hypertension
- Arrhythmia
- Diaphoresis
- Decreased urinary output
- Use of accessory muscles
- Cool, clammy skin.

Complications

- Loss of consciousness
- Coma
- Seizures
- Priapism
- Secondary polycythemia

- Cyanosis
- Death.

Diagnostic Tests

- History
- Physical examination
- Blood examination
- Magnetic resonance imaging (MRI) scan
- Angiogram of the brain
- Computed tomography (CT) scan
- Electroencephalogram (EEG)
- Brainstem auditory evoked response (BAER) test.

MANAGEMENT

Medical

- **Oxygen therapy:** One of the most important methods of treating hypoxia is to administer oxygen. This increases the concentration of oxygen being inhaled which increases the partial pressure of oxygen in the blood and corrects hypoxia. Some of the devices for delivering oxygen via inhalation include: nasal cannula (delivers oxygen at a flow rate of 1–6 liters per minute, at concentrations of 24–44%), simple oxygen face mask (delivers oxygen at 6–8 liters per minute, at concentrations of 40–60%), non-rebreather mask (delivers oxygen at 8–15 liters per minute, at concentrations of 60–80%), bag valve mask (delivers oxygen at least 15 liters per minute, at concentrations of 60–90%), and transport ventilator (delivers oxygen at various ranges and at concentrations of 21–100%)
- **Mechanical ventilation:** It helps to provide short-term support to ventilation.
- **Bronchodilators:** For example, theophylline, aminophylline, etc. It helps to control the growth of the microorganism.
- **Corticosteroids:** For example, Prednisone, etc. It helps to reduce the severity of the disease
- **Anticonvulsant agents:** For example, phenytoin, phenobarbital, valproic acid, etc. It helps in preventing the episode of seizure occurrence.

Nursing

- Provide oxygen therapy to increase the partial pressure of oxygen in blood.
- Encourage the patients to do regular exercise when have trouble breathing as they can improve the overall strength and endurance.
- Instruct the patient to avoid smoking as secondhand smoke can cause further lung damage
- Encourage them to pack medications in carry-on luggage when traveling in a flight
- Instruct them to avoid high altitude to a certain extent
- Instruct them to avoid deep sea diving.

LUNG ABSCESS

Definition

Lung abscess is defined as necrosis of the pulmonary tissue and formation of cavities containing necrotic debris or fluid caused by microbial infection.

Etiology

- Bacterial infections (*Staphylococcus aureus*)
- Fungal infections (*Aspergillus*)
- Parasitic infections (*Entamoeba histolytica*)
- Aspiration of vomitus
- Aspiration of foreign body into the lungs
- Pulmonary embolus
- Trauma
- Tuberculosis
- Necrotizing pneumonia
- Bronchial obstruction.

Risk Factors

- Following general anesthesia
- Alcohol consumption
- Drug addiction
- Diabetes mellitus
- Esophageal immune function
- Severe periodontal disease
- Central nervous system disorders
- Compromised immune function
- Congenital heart disease
- Cystic fibrosis.

Types

- ***Primary lung abscess:*** It is the necrosis of lung parenchyma due to an existing disease like aspiration pneumonia and it is more common.
- ***Secondary lung abscess:*** It is secondary to septic embolization or bronchial obstruction (lung cancer) and it is less common.

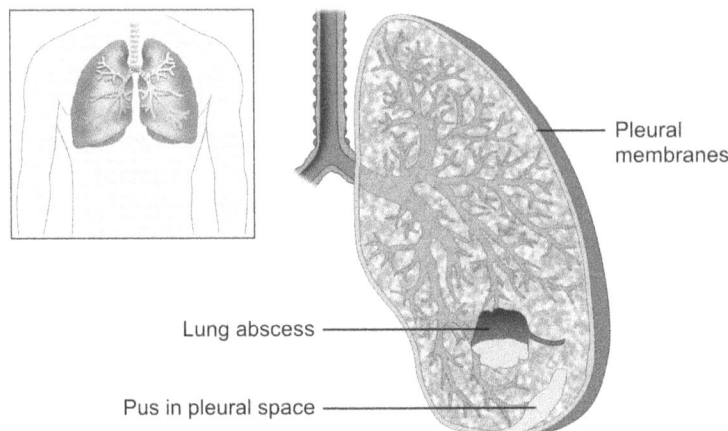

Fig. 6.10: Portrays necrosis of the pulmonary tissue (Lung abscess).

Pathophysiology

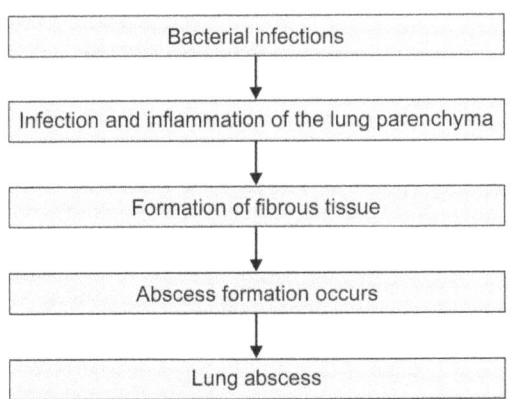

Clinical Features

- Production of mucopurulent sputum
- Pleuritic chest pain
- Deep cough that may produce foul-tasting or bloody sputum
- Spiking temperature with rigors and night sweats
- Malaise
- Dyspnea
- Tachypnea
- Tachycardia
- Headache
- Weakness
- Leukocytosis
- Decreased or absent breath sounds
- Intermittent pleural friction rub
- Anemia
- Bluish discoloration of the skin
- Loss of appetite and weight loss
- Digital clubbing (late features).

Complications

- Hemoptysis from erosion of a vessel
- Empyema
- Pneumatocele
- Bronchopleural fistula.

Diagnostic Tests

- History
- Physical examination
- Blood examination
- Liver function test
- Renal function test
- Blood culture examination
- Sputum culture examination
- Chest X-ray
- Computed tomography (CT) scan
- Fiberoptic bronchoscopic examination.

Management

Medical

- **Oxygen therapy:** One of the most important methods of treating lung abscess is to administer oxygen. This increases the concentration of oxygen being inhaled which increases the partial pressure of oxygen in the blood and corrects hypoxia.
- **Chest physiotherapy:** It helps in mobilizing the secretions from the lungs.
- **Antibiotics:** It helps to prevent secondary infections. For example, penicillin G, clindamycin, amoxicillin, bleomycin, etc.
- **Antifungal agents:** It helps to treat an underlying fungal infection. For example, amphotericin B, fluconazole, ketoconazole, etc.

Surgical

- **Pleurodesis:** It is a procedure in which a special chemical (a sclerosant) is injected into the pleural space. This causes inflammation of the pleural membranes and helps them to 'stick' together. This helps to prevent fluid building up again into the pleural space.
- **Percutaneous transthoracic tube drainage (PTTD):** It is the percutaneous drainage of the abscess through the chest wall.
- **Lobectomy:** It is the surgical removal of lobes of the lungs.

Nursing

- Recommend the patient to take high-calorie and high-protein diet.
- Provide postural chest drainage to the patient.
- Encourage patient to perform deep breathing exercises to promote ventilation.

- Ensure that the information given is at a level of comprehension that is tailored to the patients and their health education.
- Educate the patients to continue the medications as prescribed.

PLEURAL EFFUSION

Definition

A pleural effusion is an abnormal collection of fluid in the pleural space resulting from excess fluid production or decreased absorption or both.

Etiology

- Injury to the lungs
- Adverse drug reaction
- Peritoneal dialysis
- Rheumatoid arthritis
- Pneumonia
- Nephritic syndrome
- Pulmonary embolism
- Systemic lupus erythematosus.

Risk Factors

- Preexisting lung disease
- Smoking
- Having occupational exposure to asbestos
- Radiation therapy
- Liver cirrhosis
- Heart failure
- Alcohol consumption.

Pathophysiology

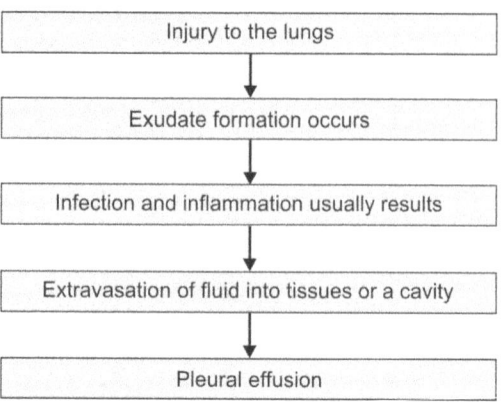

Clinical Features

- Prior infection of the upper respiratory tract
- Dyspnea
- Tachycardia
- Pleuritic chest pain
- Pain in the muscles of the chest
- Pain is exacerbated by deep breathing or coughing
- Persistent cough
- Fever
- Chills
- Hiccups
- General malaise
- Dullness or flatness to percussion with decreased or absent breath sounds.

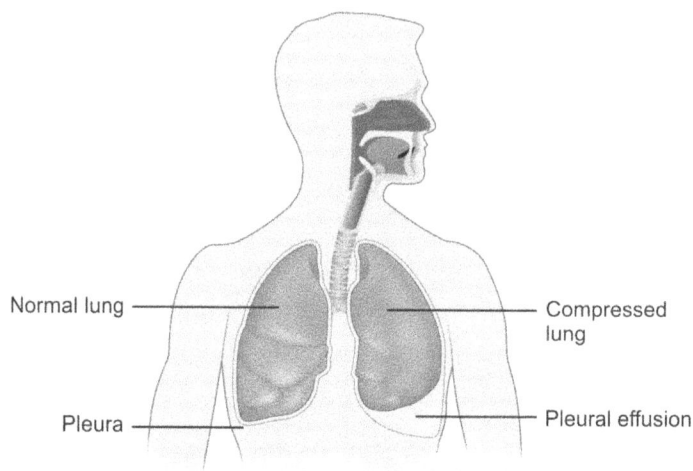

Fig. 6.11: Shows the comparison of normal lungs with that of fluid-filled lungs (Pleural effusion).

Complications

- Empyema
- Pneumothorax
- Respiratory failure
- Death.

Diagnostic Tests

- History
- Physical examination
- Chest X-ray
- Computed tomography (CT) scan
- Thoracoscopic examination
- Pleural biopsy
- Blood examination.

Management

Medical

- **Oxygen therapy:** One of the most important methods of treating pleural effusion is to administer oxygen. This increases the concentration of oxygen being inhaled which increases the partial pressure of oxygen in the blood and corrects alveolar hypoxia.
- **Antibiotics:** It helps to prevent secondary infections. For example, amoxicillin, bleomycin, etc.
- **Bronchodilators:** It helps in preventing bronchospasm. For example, theophylline, etc.

Surgical

- **Thoracentesis:** It is a surgical procedure in which excess pleural fluid is removed.
- **Tube thoracostomy:** It is a surgical procedure in which a tube is placed in the side of the chest to allow fluid to drain.
- **Thoracotomy:** It is an incision into the pleural space of the chest to remove the excess pleural fluid.
- **Pleurectomy:** It is the surgical removal of the pleura to facilitate fluid drain out of the lungs.

Nursing

- Elevate the head of the patient in Fowler's position to promote lung expansion.
- Administer supplemental oxygen as prescribed to maximize oxygen available for cellular uptake.
- Ensure that the information given is at a level of comprehension that is tailored to the patients and their health education.
- Educate the patients to continue the medications as prescribed.
- Encourage adequate rest periods between activities to limit fatigue.
- Discontinue activities that cause undesired psychological changes to conserve energy and promote safety.
- Encourage patient to perform deep breathing exercises to promote ventilation.

PLEURISY (PLEURITIS OR PLEURODYNIA)

Definition

Pleurisy is the inflammation and irritation of the pleura, a thin, two-layered membrane that lines the lung and chest cavity that typically results in characteristic pleuritic pain and has a variety of possible causes for it.

Etiology

- Pneumonia
- Bacterial infection (*Mycobacterium tuberculi*)
- Viral infection (e.g., *Coxsackie virus*)
- Bronchiectasis
- Collapse of part of the lung
- Pulmonary embolus
- Trauma to the chest
- Cancer
- Collagen vascular disease (Systemic lupus erythematosus or rheumatoid arthritis)
- Congestive cardiac failure
- Kidney and liver diseases.

Risk Factors

- Obesity
- Smoking
- Use of immunosuppressive drugs
- Inhaling asbestos
- Smoking
- Certain medication (e.g., Nitrofurantoin).

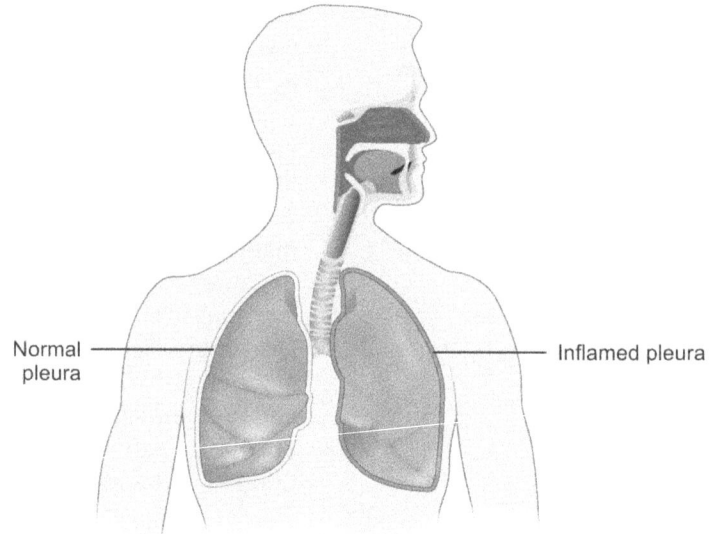

Fig. 6.12: Shows the comparison of normal and inflamed pleura (Pleurisy).

Pathophysiology

```
Pneumonia
    ↓
Inflammation that occurs at the periphery of the
lung parenchyma can extend into the pleural
space and involve the parietal pleura
    ↓
As the parietal pleura is innervated by somatic
nerves that sense pain when the parietal pleura is
inflamed whereas the visceral pleura does not
contain any nociceptors or pain receptors
    ↓
Activates the somatic pain receptors
    ↓
Pleuritic pain (Pleurisy)
```

Clinical Features

- Sudden chest pain that worsens with breathing and coughing.
- Pain in the chest
- Pain in the muscles of the chest
- Stabbing sensation
- Persistent cough
- Fever
- Discomfort on moving the affected side
- Rapid, shallow breathing
- General malaise.

Complications

- Pleural effusion
- Atelectasis
- Lung compression
- Scarring and adhesions at the site of inflammation, restricting lung expansion
- Death.

Diagnostic Tests

- History
- Physical examination
- Blood examination
- Chest X-ray
- Computed tomography (CT) scan
- Bronchoscopic examination
- Thoracentesis.

Management

Medical

- **Oxygen therapy:** One of the most important methods of treating pleurisy is to administer oxygen.
- **Chest physiotherapy:** It helps in mobilizing the secretions from the lungs.
- **Nonsteroidal anti-inflammatory drugs:** It helps to relieve chest pain or discomfort. For example, ibuprofen, aspirin, etc.

- **Antibiotics:** It helps to prevent secondary infections. For example, amoxicillin, bleomycin, tetracycline, etc.
- **Narcotic analgesics:** It helps to relieve severe pleuritic chest pain. For example, indomethacin, etc.

Surgical

- **Thoracentesis:** It is a surgical procedure in which excess pleural fluid is removed.
- **Thoracotomy:** It is an incision into the pleural space of the chest to remove the excess pleural fluid.
- **Open decortication:** It is a surgical procedure that removes a restrictive layer of fibrous tissue overlying the lungs to remove the excess pleural fluid.

Nursing

- Administer supplemental oxygen as prescribed to maximize oxygen available for cellular uptake.
- Elevate the head of the patient in Fowler's position to promote lung expansion.
- Educate the patients to continue the medications as prescribed.
- Encourage patient to perform deep breathing exercises to promote ventilation.
- Instruct the patient to avoid strenuous activities and heavy lifting.
- Instruct the patient to quit smoking.
- Ask the patient to cover the mouth when coughing or sneezing.

PNEUMONIA

Definition

Pneumonia is an infection of one or both lungs that can cause mild to severe in people of all ages.

Etiology

- Bacterial infection (e.g., *Steptococcus pneumoniae*)
- Viral infection (e.g., Human metapneumovirus)
- Mycoplasmas (e.g., *Mycoplasma pneumoniae*)
- Fungal infections
- Various chemicals.

Risk Factors

- Cigarette smoking
- Recent viral respiratory infection (cold, laryngitis, influenza, etc.)
- Difficulty in swallowing
- Chronic lung disease (COPD, cystic fibrosis, bronchiectasis, etc.)
- Cerebral palsy
- Liver cirrhosis
- Diabetes
- Hospitalization
- Impaired consciousness

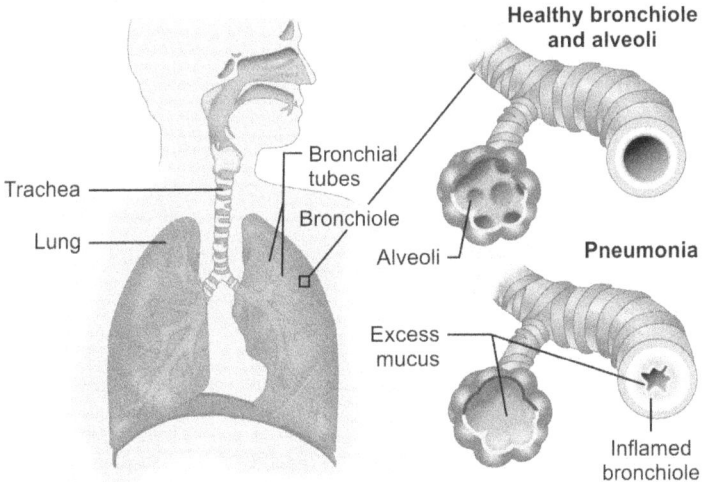

Fig. 6.13: Shows the comparison of healthy bronchiole and alveoli with that of inflamed and mucus-filled bronchiole (Pneumonia).

- Recent surgery or trauma
- Having a weakened immune system
- Infants from birth to age two
- Drug abusers.

Types

- ***Community-acquired pneumonia:*** It is the most common form of pneumonia because one can catch it in public places such as at school or work.
- ***Hospital-acquired pneumonia:*** It develops during a hospital stay for a different health problem.
- ***Aspiration pneumonia:*** It can develop after a person inhales food, liquid, gases or dust.
- ***Opportunistic pneumonia:*** It develops in people with a weakened immune system.

Stages

Pneumonia has four stages, namely consolidation, red hepatization, grey hepatization and resolution:

- ***Stage of consolidation:*** It occurs in the first 24 hours. The cellular exudate containing neutrophils, lymphocytes and fibrin replaces the alveolar air. The capillaries in the surrounding alveolar walls become congested. The infection spreads to the hilum and pleura rapidly. Pleurisy occurs and it was marked by coughing and deep breathing.
- ***Stage of red hepatization:*** It occurs in the 2–3 days after consolidation. At this point the consistency of the lungs resembles that of the liver. The lungs become hyperemic and the alveolar capillaries are engorged with blood. The fibrinous exudates fill the alveoli and this stage is characterized by the presence of many erythrocytes, neutrophils, desquamated epithelial cells and fibrin within the alveoli.
- ***Stage of grey hepatization:*** It occurs in the 2–3 days after red hepatization. This is an avascular stage and the lung appears grey-brown to yellow because of fibrinopurulent exudates, disintegration of red cells and hemosiderin. The pressure of the exudates in the alveoli causes compression of the capillaries and the leukocytes migrate into the congested alveoli.
- ***Stage of resolution:*** This stage is characterized by the resorption and restoration of the pulmonary architecture. A large number of macrophages enter the alveolar spaces and phagocytosis of the bacteria-laden leukocytes occurs. Consolidation tissue re-aerates and the fluid infiltrate causes sputum and fibrinous inflammation may extend to and across the pleural space, causing a rub heard by auscultation and it may lead to resolution or to organization and pleural adhesions.

Pathophysiology

Bacterial infection (e.g., *Steptococcus pneumoniae*)

↓

Acute inflammation occurs that causes excess water and plasma proteins to go to the dependent areas of the lower lobes

↓

RBCs, fibrin and polymorphonuclear leukocytes infiltrate the alveoli

↓

Containment of the bacteria within the segments of pulmonary lobes by cellular recruitment

↓

Consolidation of leukocytes and fibrin within the affected area

↓

Engorgement of alveolar spaces within fluid and hemorrhagic exudate (stage of congestion)

↓

Proliferation and rapid spread of organism through the lobe

↓

Coagulation of exudates occurs resulting to the red appearance of the affected lung (stage of red hepatization)

↓

The decrease in number of RBC in the exudates is replaced by neutrophils which infiltrate the alveoli making the lung tissue to be solid and greyish in color (stage of gray hepatization)

↓

Pneumonia

Clinical Features

- Worsening cough
- Fever, which may be mild or high
- Shaking chills
- Shortness of breath
- Wheezing
- Stuffy nose
- Tachycardia
- Tachypnea
- Sharp or stabbing chest pain that gets worse when they breathe deeply or cough
- Bluish discoloration of skin
- Blood in sputum
- Headache
- Excessive sweating and clammy skin
- Loss of appetite
- Low energy
- Fatigue
- Confusion, especially in older people.

Complications

- Pleural effusion
- Empyema
- Delayed resolution
- Lung abscess
- Bacteremia
- Septicemia
- Meningitis
- Septic arthritis
- Endocarditis
- Pericarditis.

Diagnostic Tests

- History
- Physical examination
- Blood examination
- Chest X-ray
- Pulse oximetric examination
- Computed tomography (CT) scan
- Sputum examination.

Management

Medical

- **Oxygen therapy:** One of the most important methods of treating pneumonia is to administer oxygen.
- **Chest physiotherapy:** It helps in mobilizing the secretions from the lungs.
- **Bronchodilators:** It helps to dilate the bronchial smooth muscles. For example, theophylline, etc.
- **Antibiotics:** It helps to prevent secondary infections. For example, amoxicillin, bleomycin, etc.
- **Analgesics:** It helps to reduce pain and fever. For example, Aspirin, ibuprofen, acetaminophen, codeine, etc.

Surgical

- **Thoracotomy:** It is a procedure in which an incision is made into the lungs to remove the dead or damaged lung tissue.
- **Lobectomy:** It is the surgical procedure in which the entire lobe of the lung is removed in severe cases.
- **Chest tube drainage:** It is the surgical procedure that allows escape of air or fluid out of the lungs.
- **Lung transplantation:** It is a therapeutic measure of last resort for patients with end-stage lung disease who have exhausted all other available treatments without improvement.

Nursing

- Encourage the patient to take adequate bedrest.
- Instruct the patient to avoid the intake of alcohol.
- Instruct the patient to quit smoking.
- Encourage the patient to do regular exercise when have trouble breathing as they can improve the overall strength and endurance.
- Give high concentrations of oxygen to patients to reduce their respiratory drive.
- Encourage the patients to eat a balanced diet.
- Encourage the patients to perform deep breathing exercises to promote ventilation.

■ PNEUMOTHORAX

Definition

A pneumothorax is defined as the presence of air between visceral and parietal pleura that leads to lung collapse.

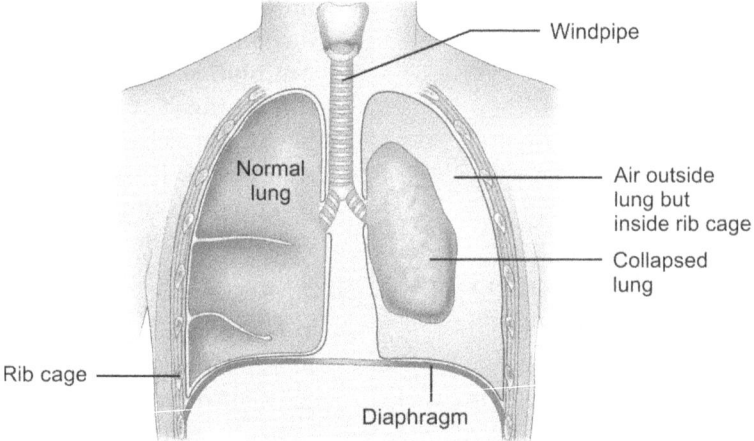

Fig. 6.14: Shows the comparison of normal lungs with that of collapsed lung (Pneumothorax).

Etiology

- Penetrating chest trauma
- Interstitial lung disease
- Emphysema
- Rib fractures
- Abdominal trauma
- Thoracentesis or pleural biopsy
- CVP insertion
- Idiopathic
- Chronic lung disease
- Positive pressure ventilation.

Risk Factors

- Being male
- Smoking
- Advanced age
- Previous history of pneumothorax
- Mechanical ventilation
- Genetic predisposition
- Occupational asbestos exposure
- Marfan's syndrome
- Having a history of violent fighting
- Playing hard contact sports.

Types

- ***Simple pneumothorax:*** It occurs when air enters the pleural space through a breach of either the parietal or visceral pleura. It occurs in the absence of any trauma.
- ***Traumatic pneumothorax:*** It occurs when air escapes from a laceration in the lung and enters the plural space through a wound in the chest wall.
- ***Tension pneumothorax:*** It occurs when air is drawn into the pleural space from a lacerated lung or through a small hole in the chest wall. It interferes with filling of both the heart and lungs.

Pathophysiology

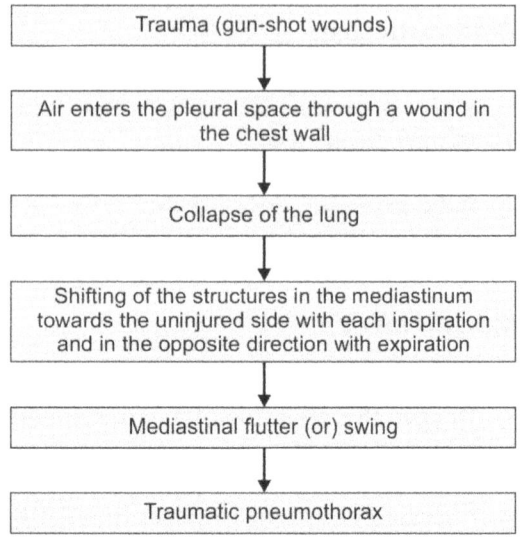

Clinical Features
- Sudden pain
- Pleuritic chest pain
- Respiratory distress
- Slight chest discomfort
- Tachypnea
- Dyspnea
- Air hunger
- Increased use of accessory muscles
- Central cyanosis
- Severe hypoxemia
- Diminished breath sounds
- Agitation
- Hypotension.

Complications
- Acute respiratory failure
- Cardiovascular collapse
- Infection
- Pneumomediastinum (air in the mediastinal space)
- Shock
- Death.

Diagnostic Tests
- History
- Physical examination
- Chest X-ray
- Blood examination
- Arterial blood gas analysis
- Pulse oximetric examination
- Upright posteroanterior chest radiograph
- Computed tomography (CT) scan
- Lung sonography
- Thoracic ultrasonogram
- Electrocardiogram.

Management

Medical
- **Oxygen therapy:** One of the most important methods of treating pneumothorax is to administer oxygen. This increases the concentration of oxygen being inhaled which increases the partial pressure of oxygen in the blood and corrects hypoxia.

Surgical
- **Thoracotomy (or) pleurodesis:** It is the surgical resection of apical blebs (large air-filled blisters that exists on the surface of the the lungs).
- **Chest tube drainage (or) thoracentesis:** It is the surgical procedure that allows escape of air out of the lungs.

Nursing
- Provide adequate rest to the patient to limit fatigue.
- Elevate the head of the patient in Fowler's position to promote lung expansion.
- Administer supplemental oxygen as prescribed to maximize oxygen available for cellular uptake.
- Prepare for chest tube placement until the lung has expanded fully.
- Ensure that the information given is at a level of comprehension that is tailored to the patient and their health education.
- Encourage patient to perform deep breathing exercises to promote ventilation.

PULMONARY EMBOLISM

Definition
Pulmonary embolism refers to the obstruction of the pulmonary artery or one of its branches by a thrombus (or thrombi) that originates somewhere in the venous system and travels through the bloodstream and lodges in the lung.

Etiology
- Hospitalization
- Postoperative state
- Trauma (fracture of the leg or hip)
- Congenital/acquired coagulation defect
- Injury to the vein.

Risk Factors
- Cancer and chemotherapy
- Family history of embolism
- Previous history of heart attack or stroke
- Pregnancy
- Thrombophilia
- Major surgery
- Varicose veins
- Obesity
- Sedentary lifestyle
- Advancement in age
- Hormone replacement therapy.

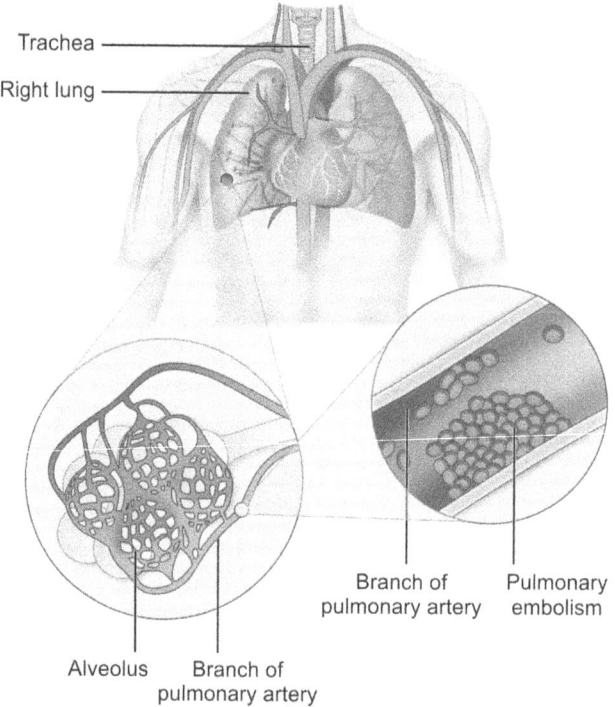

Fig. 6.15: Depicts obstruction of the pulmonary artery by a thrombus.

Pathophysiology

Trauma (fracture of the leg or hip)
↓
Impairs the efficient transfer of oxygen and carbon dioxide across the lung
↓
Decreased arterial PO_2 (hypoxemia)
↓
Increase in the alveolar-arterial oxygen-tension gradient
↓
Total dead space increases
↓
Ventilation and perfusion becomes mismatched
↓
Shunting of venous blood into the systemic circulation (Pulmonary embolism)

Clinical Features

- Shortness of breath that is sudden or gradual
- Clammy or bluish skin
- Irregular heartbeat
- Anxiety
- Anterior chest pain
- Pleuritic pain
- Syncope
- Rales
- Lightheadedness
- Tachycardia
- Tachypnea
- Hypoxemia
- Hypotension
- Distended jugular veins
- Restlessness
- Weak pulse
- Spitting up blood.

Complications
- Post-thrombotic syndrome (PTS)
- Pulmonary hypertension
- Respiratory failure
- Death.

Diagnostic Tests
- History
- Physical examination
- Blood examination
- D-dimer test
- CT scan of the chest
- Pulmonary angiography
- Ventilation/perfusion lung scan
- Magnetic resonance imaging (MRI) scan
- Contrast venogram.

Management

Medical
- **Anticoagulants (blood thinners):** For example, heparin, warfarin, etc. These medications increase the time it takes for the blood to clot. They prevent new clots from forming and existing clots from growing larger. Overtime, the body absorbs the clot, more or less successfully getting rid of them.
- **Thrombolytic agents (clot busters or dissolvers):** These drugs speed up the breakdown of a clot. For example, streptokinase, tissue plasminogen activator (t-PA), etc.

Surgical
- **Thrombectomy:** It is a procedure done by a vascular surgeon or radiologist, where a catheter is advanced into the clot and clot buster medication is injected into the clot to soften it up
- **Inferior vena cava (IVC) filters (Vein filters and stents):** It is also known as Greenfield filters. It is a surgical procedure in which an umbrella-shaped device is placed into the large vein in the abdomen. The IVC filter traps blood clots that have broken loose from a deep vein thrombosis and prevents them from reaching the lungs, where they could become a pulmonary embolism. These stents can be removed weeks to months after placement and are referred to as removable or transient IVC filters.
- **Open-heart surgery:** It is a surgical procedure performed when there is a very large clot to be floating inside the heart in which the chest is opened and the clot is extracted and is used only in emergency situations when a person is in shock or medications are not working to break up the clot.
- **Clot removal through catheterization:** It is a surgical procedure in which small tubes are inserted through the veins of the leg.
- **Extracorporeal membrane oxygen (ECMO):** It is a surgical procedure that allows restoration of the circulation if the heart stops or is severely dysfunctional and ensures the organs receive the blood they need. Also it allows the blood to be oxygenated in those cases where the lungs are not able to function properly. It is used in the treatment of unstable pulmonary embolism.

Nursing
- Encourage them to wear mechanical compression stockings to regularly squeeze the veins in the calf muscles who are not able to walk.
- Encourage the patient to get out of bed as soon as possible.
- Instruct them to avoid situations where blood clots might form, such as while staying in a fixed seated position for a long duration in a plane or car.
- Instruct the patient to participate in weight management program.
- Keep the patient in Fowler's position to enhance ventilation.

- Ensure that the information given is at a level of comprehension that is tailored to the patients and their health education.
- Educate the patients to continue the medications as prescribed.

PULMONARY HYPERTENSION

Definition

Pulmonary hypertension is raised blood pressure within the pulmonary arteries, which are the blood vessels that supply the lungs.

Etiology

- Interstitial lung diseases
- Left ventricular pump failure
- Left ventricular stiffness
- Valve disease
- Chronic bronchitis and emphysema
- Hypoxia
- Portal hypertension
- Connective tissue diseases
- Pulmonary thromboembolism
- Schistosomiasis
- Sickle cell anemia.

Risk Factors

- Family history of pulmonary hypertension
- Obesity
- Being women
- Pregnancy
- High-altitude dwelling
- Smoking
- Alcohol consumption
- Sleep apnea
- Certain medications (For example, methamphetamine, etc).

Types

- ***Pulmonary arterial hypertension:*** It originates at the pulmonary arteries. This can be idiopathic, heritable or associated with an underlying disease or condition.
- ***Pulmonary venous hypertension:*** It occurs due to the result of left heart disease like heart failure or heart valve disease.
- ***Chronic thromboembolic pulmonary hypertension (CTEPH):*** It is caused by unresolved clots in the pulmonary arteries.

Pathophysiology

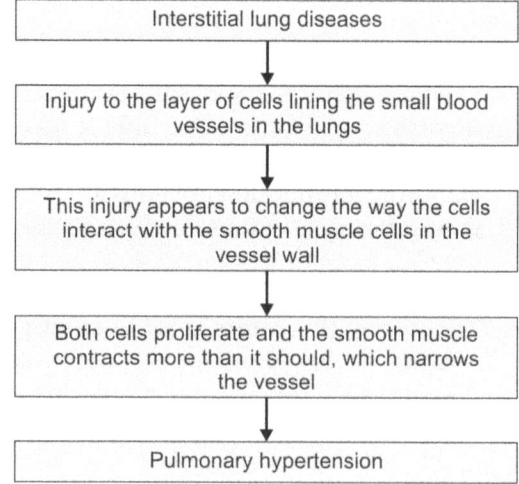

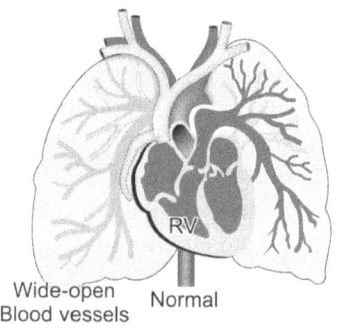
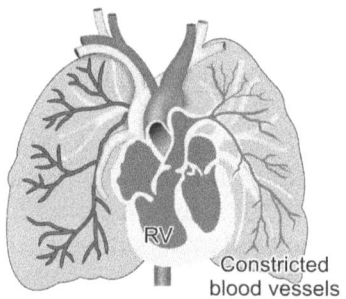

Fig. 6.16: Shows the comparison of normal and raised blood pressure pulmonary arteries which supply the lungs.

Clinical Features

- Shortness of breath during day-to-day activities
- Extreme fatigue
- Dizziness
- Swelling in the ankles, abdomen or legs
- Bluish discoloration of skin
- Chest pain
- Tachycardia
- Trouble breathing at rest.

Complications

- Cor pulmonale
- Hemoptysis
- Arrhythmias
- Blood clots.

Diagnostic Tests

- History
- Physical examination
- Blood examination
- Echocardiogram
- Chest X-ray
- Walk test
- Pulmonary function tests
- Polysomnogram or overnight oximetric examination
- Right heart catheterization
- Ventilation perfusion scan (V/Q scan)
- Computed tomography (CT) scan of the chest
- Pulmonary angiogram.

Management

Medical

- **Oxygen therapy:** One of the most important methods of treating pulmonary hypertension is to administer oxygen.
- **Anticoagulants (Blood thinners):** It decreases blood clot formation so that blood can flow more easily through blood vessels. For example, warfarin sodium (Coumadin), etc.
- **Bronchodilators:** It helps to dilate the bronchial smooth muscles. For example, theophylline, etc.
- **Diuretics (Water pills):** It reduces swelling and ease breathing by helping to eliminate extra fluids in the tissues and bloodstream. For example, furosemide, etc.
- **Vasodilators:** For example, epoprostenol, treprostinil sodium, etc. It lowers pulmonary vessel pressure and improves the pumping ability of the right side of the heart.
- **Endothelin receptor antagonists:** For example, bosentan (Tracleer), ambrisentan, etc. It helps in blocking the action of endothelin, which constricts blood vessels and raises blood pressure in the lungs.
- **Phosphodiesterase inhibitors:** For example, sildenafil, tadalafil, etc. It relaxes pulmonary smooth muscle cells, leading to the dilation of the pulmonary arteries.

Surgical

- **Pulmonary thromboendarterectomy:** It is a surgical procedure that can remove a large clot or clots in pulmonary arteries.
- **Lung transplantation:** It is a therapeutic measure of last resort for patients with end-stage lung disease who have exhausted all other available treatments without improvement.

Nursing

- Instruct the patient to reduce the intake of sodium-rich diet.
- Ask the patient to cut down the intake of fluids to prevent the severity of the condition.
- Encourage the patient to take low-calorie, low-fat and high-fiber foods.
- Monitor the weight of the patient at regular intervals.
- Encourage the patient to participate in weight reduction program.

- Give high concentrations of oxygen to patients to reduce their respiratory drive.
- Instruct the patient to avoid the intake of alcohol.
- Instruct the patient to quit smoking.
- Ask the patient to avoid pregnancy, as the heart needs to work harder than usual and may be life-threatening to both the mother and the baby.
- Restrict the patient from lifting, pushing or pulling to more than 20 pounds to avoid increasing the pressure in the arteries and lungs.
- Encourage the patient to do regular exercise when have trouble in breathing as they can improve the overall strength and endurance.

PULMONARY TUBERCULOSIS

Definition

Pulmonary tuberculosis is an infectious disease caused by *Mycobacterium tuberculi* that primarily affected the lung parenchyma.

Etiology

Bacterial infection (*Mycobacterium tuberculi*).

Risk Factors

- Close contact with someone who has active TB.
- Immunocompromised status
- Preexisting medical conditions (e.g., diabetes, chronic renal failure, malignancies, etc.)
- Being a healthcare worker performing high-risk activities
- Substance abuse
- Child younger than 5 years of age
- People recently infected with TB bacteria
- Poverty
- Overcrowding
- Substandard housing
- Inadequate health care
- Malnutrition
- Those who have been in prison.

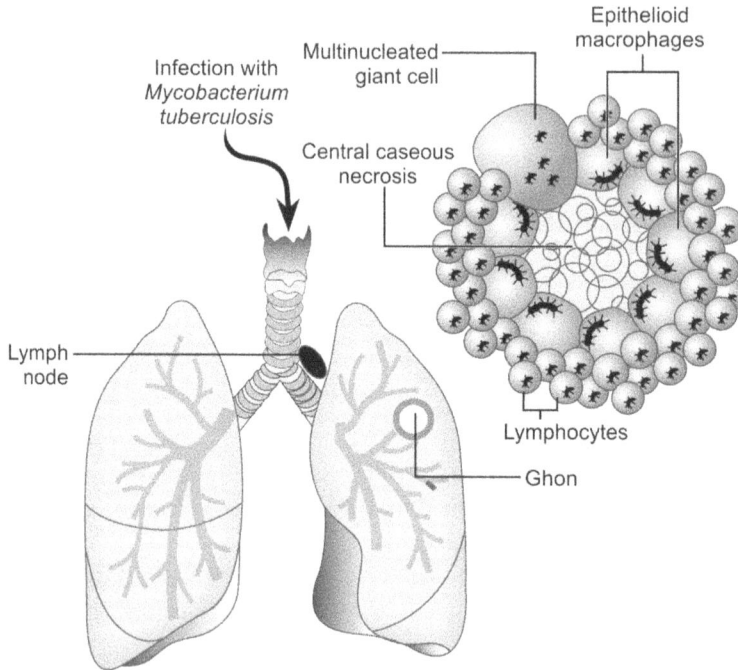

Fig. 6.17: Depicts lungs infected with *Mycobacterium tuberculosis* (Pulmonary tuberculosis).

Pathophysiology

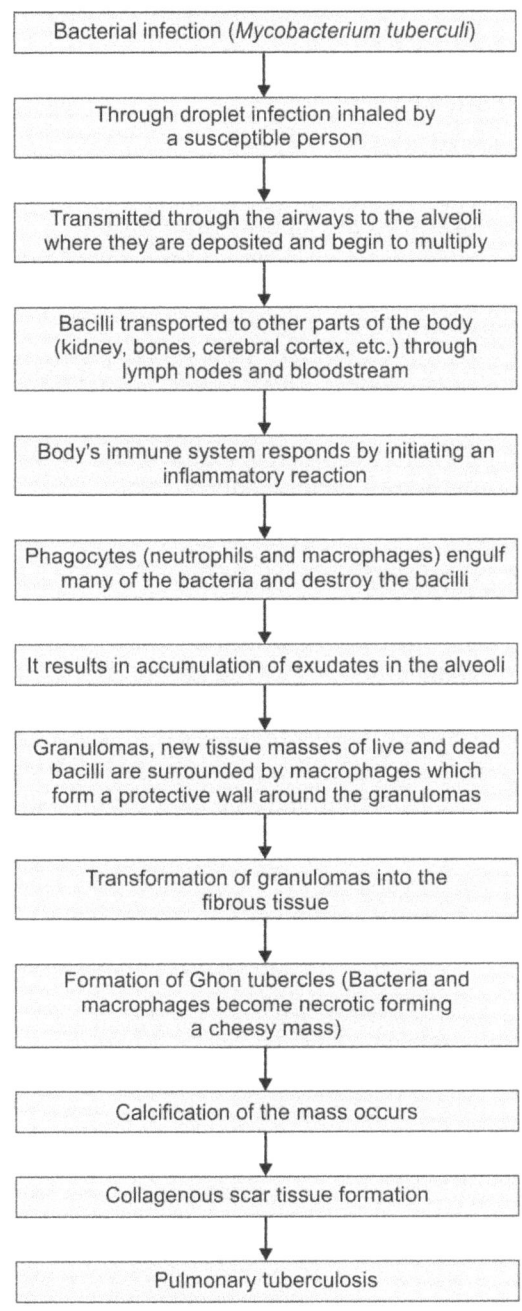

Clinical Features

- Low-grade fever
- Severe cough that lasts for 3 weeks or longer and gets progressively worse
- Fatigue
- Anorexia
- Night sweats
- Loss of weight for no obvious reason
- Indigestion
- Chills
- Dyspnea
- Chest pain
- Hemoptysis (coughing up blood).

Complications

- Pleural effusion
- Pneumonia
- Malnutrition
- Multidrug resistance
- Miliary tuberculosis.

Diagnostic Tests

- History
- Physical examination
- Sputum smear examination
- Sputum culture examination
- Tuberculin skin test (Mantoux test)
- Blood examination.

Management

Medical

- **Bactericidal agents:** It helps to reduce the risk of secondary infections. For example, isoniazid, rifampin, pyrazinamide, streptomycin, etc.
- **Bacteriostatic agents:** It helps to control the growth of the microorganism. For example, ethambutol, etc.
- **Vitamin supplements:** It helps to prevent INH-associated peripheral neuropathy. For example, pyridoxine, etc.

Nursing

- Encourage the importance of nutritious diet to the patient.
- Encourage them to take high-protein diet.
- Provide complete bedrest to avoid exertion.
- Educate the patient to control spread of infection.
- Participate in observation of medication taking.
- Restrict visitors in the ward.

- Encourage them to drink plenty of oral fluids.
- Instruct them to take their medication every day at the right time of the day.
- Instruct them to carry spare medications while at work or in travel.
- Make sure the patients have a full course of correct treatment as soon as the diagnosis is made.

RESPIRATORY FAILURE

Definition

Respiratory failure is an alteration in the function of the respiratory system that causes the partial pressure of arterial oxygen (PaO_2) to fall below 50 mm Hg (hypoxemia) and the partial pressure of arterial carbon dioxide ($PaCO_2$) to raise above 50 mm Hg (hypercapnia), with an arterial pH of less than 7.35.

Etiology

- Aspiration
- Drug ingestion and overdose (sedatives)
- Infections
- Trauma
- Major surgery (thoracic or abdominal)
- Systemic sepsis
- Air embolism metabolic disorders (hypothyroidism)
- Decreased respiratory drive (brain injury)
- Shock.

Risk Factors

- Excessive alcohol consumption
- Family history of respiratory disease
- Sustaining an injury to the spine, brain and chest
- Tobacco consumption
- History of long-term respiratory problems
- Dysfunctions of the chest wall (poliomyelitis, Guillain-Barre syndrome)
- Dysfunction of lung parenchyma (pneumothorax, pleural effusion, etc).

Types

- **Acute respiratory failure:** It is characterized by hypoxemia (PaO_2 less than 50 mm Hg) and hypercapnia ($PaCO_2$ greater than 50 mm Hg) and an arterial pH of less than 7.35.
- **Chronic respiratory failure:** It is characterized by hypoxemia (decreased PaO_2) and hypercapnia (increased $PaCO_2$) with

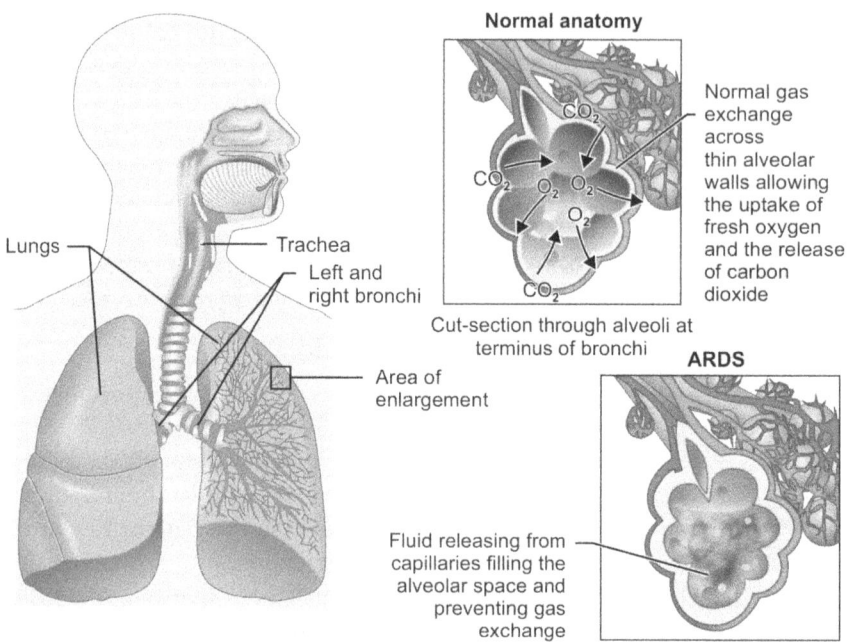

Fig. 6.18: Shows the comparison of normal gas exchange with that of fluid-filled capillaries that prevents gas exchange.

a normal pH (7.35 to 7.45). It occurs over a period of months to years.

Pathophysiology

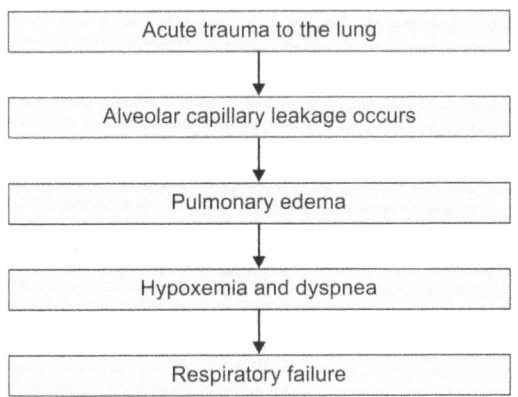

Clinical Features

- Hypoxemia
- Hypercapnia
- Restlessness
- Agitation
- Dyspnea
- Disorientation
- Confusion
- Delirium
- Loss of consciousness
- Headache
- Dizziness
- Tachypnea
- Usage of accessory muscles
- Fatigue
- Increased blood pressure
- Diaphoresis
- Cyanosis
- Respiratory arrest.

Complications

- Oxygen toxicity
- Barotrauma
- Dysrhythmias
- Renal failure
- Pulmonary fibrosis
- Infections
- Pulmonary emboli
- Disseminated intravascular coagulation.

Diagnostic Tests

- History
- Physical examination
- Arterial blood gas analysis
- Blood examination
- Chest X-ray
- Pulse oximetric examination
- Electrocardiogram
- Blood culture examination
- Sputum culture examination.

Management

Medical

- **Mechanical ventilation:** It helps in providing short-term support of ventilation.
- **Oxygen therapy:** One of the most important methods of treating hypoxia is to administer oxygen. This increases the concentration of oxygen being inhaled which increases the partial pressure of oxygen in the blood and corrects hypoxia.
- **Chest physiotherapy:** It helps in mobilizing the secretions from the lungs.
- **Bronchodilators:** It helps to dilate the bronchial smooth muscles. For example, theophylline, etc.
- **Diuretics:** It helps in preventing pulmonary congestion. For example, furosemide, etc.
- **Corticosteroids:** It helps to reduce the severity of the disease. For example, prednisone, etc.

Nursing

- Observe the respiratory function of the patients for rate, depth, pattern and breath sounds.
- Ensure the patients are sitting upright rather than lying down which enables gravity to assist breathing thereby helping lung expansion.
- Provide a calm, controlled environment to reduce the fear of the patient.
- Provide adequate rest to the patient because increased work consumes more oxygen as a result the oxygen demand of respiratory muscle is increased.

- Encourage them to take at least six deep breaths every hour with those at risk of developing an infection.
- Give high concentrations of oxygen to patients to reduce their respiratory drive.

SARCOIDOSIS

Definition

Sarcoidosis is a disorder resulting in non-caseating granulomas in one or more organs and tissues. The lungs and lymphatic system are most often affected, but sarcoidosis may affect any organ.

Etiology

- Abnormal immune response
- Infective agent or an allergy combined with susceptible genes
- Idiopathic.

Risk Factors

- People of African and Scandinavian descent
- Irish immigrants in London
- Natives of Martinique living in France
- More common in cooler climates
- Family history of sarcoidosis
- Being women
- Exposure to dusty or moldy environments
- People between 20 to 40 years of age
- Smoking.

Pathophysiology

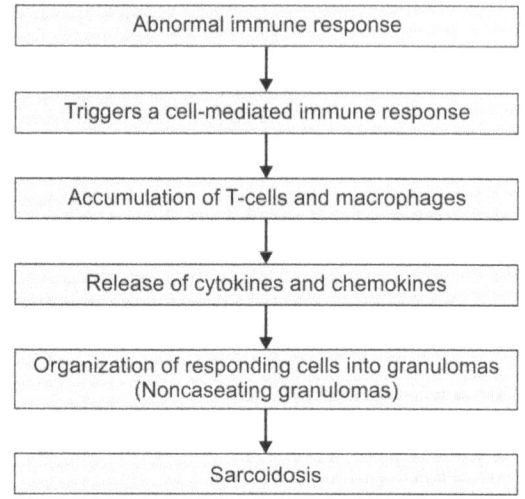

Clinical Features

- Dyspnea
- Dry cough
- Low-grade fever
- Anorexia
- Chest pain or discomfort

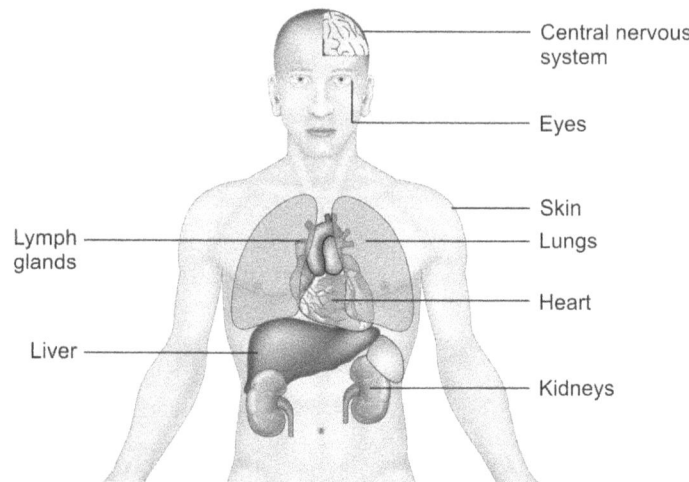

Fig. 6.19: Depicts occurrence of noncaseating in one or more organs and tissues.

- Wheezing
- Nasal stuffiness and hoarse voice
- Night sweats
- Unexplained weight loss
- Fatigue
- Facial swelling
- General feeling of ill health
- Red or sore eyes
- Painful red lumps called erythema nodosum on the front of the legs
- Swollen lymph glands in the face, neck or armpits
- Rashes on the upper part of the body
- Painful joints or bones
- Arrhythmias
- Sensitivity to light
- Blurred vision.

Complications

- Pulmonary fibrosis
- Pulmonary arterial hypertension
- Cor pulmonale
- Hemoptysis
- Hypercalcemia
- Blindness
- Peripheral neuropathy
- Meningitis
- Kidney failure.

Diagnostic Tests

- History
- Physical examination
- Blood examination
- Urine examination
- Breathing tests
- Chest X-ray of the lungs
- Computed tomography (CT) scan of the lungs
- Bronchoscopic examination
- Mediastinoscopic examination
- Skin biopsy
- Eye tests
- Neurological tests
- Electrocardiogram (ECG)
- Echocardiogram.

Management

Medical

- **Oxygen therapy:** One of the most important methods of treating sarcoidosis in severe cases is to administer oxygen.
- **Corticosteroids:** It helps to turn down the immune system's activity and reduces the severity of the disease. For example, prednisone, etc.
- **Immunomodifying agents:** It may ease symptoms and prevent further organ damage. For example, methotrexate, azathioprine, thalidomide, etc.
- **Antimalarial agents:** It may help with sarcoidosis that involves the skin or joints and prevent further organ damage. For example, hydroxychloroquine, chloroquine, etc.
- **Nonsteroidal anti-inflammatory drugs:** They are used to treat musculoskeletal discomfort with sarcoidosis that involves the joints. For example, ibuprofen, Aspirin, etc.

Surgical

Lung transplantation: It is a therapeutic measure of last resort for patients with end-stage lung disease who have exhausted all other available treatments without improvement.

Nursing

- Encourage the patient to eat a well-balanced diet with a variety of fresh fruits and vegetables.
- Encourage the patient to take plenty of fluids.
- Encourage the patient to participate in weight reduction program.
- Instruct the patient to avoid smoking.
- Encourage the patients to do regular exercise when have trouble in breathing as they can improve the overall strength and endurance.
- Instruct the patient to avoid exposure to dust, chemicals, fumes, gases, toxic

inhalants and other substances that can harm the lungs.
- Ensure 6-8 hours of sleep for the patient at each night.
- Instruct the patients to avoid the intake of excessive amounts of calcium and vitamin-D rich foods.

TRACHEAL OBSTRUCTION

Definition
Any foreign body lodged in the trachea that obstructs respiration is known as tracheal obstruction.

Etiology
- Aspiration of foreign bodies
- Vegetables like peas and beans
- Anaphylaxis (severe allergic reactions)
- Infections (Bacterial and viral) of the epiglottis
- Tracheomalacia (tracheal collapse)
- Trauma
- Aspiration of a bolus of meat
- Peritonsillar abscess.

Risk Factors
- Inhalation of smoke
- Vocal cord damage
- Throat cancer
- Children below the age of 10 years
- Retropharyngeal abscess.

Pathophysiology

Aspiration of foreign bodies
↓
Foreign bodies get arrested in the trachea
↓
Prevents entry of air into the lungs
↓
Obstructs respiration
↓
Oxygen saturation of the blood decreases rapidly
↓
Oxygen deficit occurs in the brain
↓
Within 3–5 minutes
↓
Unconsciousness
↓
Death due to tracheal obstruction

Clinical Features
- Dyspnea with stridor
- Increased rate of breathing
- Choking
- Coughing
- Palpatory thud
- Wheezing

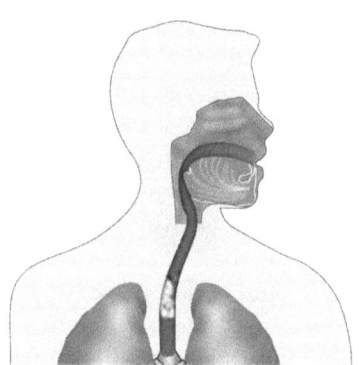
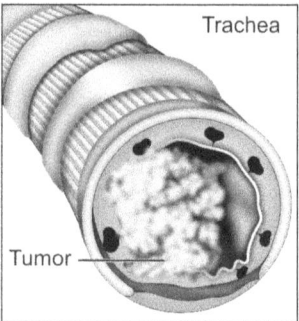

Fig. 6.20: Portrays tracheal obstruction that obstructs respiration.

- Audible slap
- Unable to speak or talk
- Confusion
- Unconsciousness
- Fatigue
- Cyanosis (blue-purple discoloration of the skin due to lack of oxygen)
- Drooling (dribbling of saliva outside the mouth)
- Flaring nostrils
- Refusing to lie flat.

Complications

- Severe respiratory distress
- Brain damage
- Empyema
- Lung abscess
- Bronchiectasis.

Diagnostic Tests

- History
- Physical examination
- Chest X-ray
- Bronchoscopic examination
- Laryngoscopic examination.

Management

Surgical

- **Tracheostomy:** It is a surgical procedure to create an opening through the neck into the trachea (windpipe).
- **Oropharyngeal airway insertion:** It is a surgical procedure in which a semicircular tube or tube-like plastic device that is inserted over the back of the tongue into the lower posterior pharynx in a patient who is breathing spontaneously but who is unconscious.
- **Endotracheal intubation:** It is a surgical procedure in which an airway is established for a patient who cannot be adequately ventilated with an oropharyngeal airway.
- **Cricothyroidotomy:** It is the surgical procedure in which cricothyroid membrane is opened to establish an airway and this procedure is used in emergency situations in which endotracheal intubation is either not possible or contraindicated.

Nursing

- Ensure that ventilation is adequate by checking for equal bilateral breath sounds.
- Quickly assess for absent or diminished breath sounds.
- Monitor pulse oximetry, capnography and arterial blood gases to check whether the patient requires airway or ventilatory assistance.
- Encourage the victim to cough forcefully and to persist with spontaneous coughing and breathing efforts as long as good air exchange exists.
- Initiate rescue breathing once the obstruction is removed.
- Instruct the patient to eat food slowly and chew food completely.
- Instruct the patient to keep the small objects away from children.

7

CHAPTER

Disorders of Cardiac System

CHAPTER OUTLINE

- Angina pectoris
- Aortic aneurysm
- Atherosclerosis
- Cardiac arrest
- Cardiac dysrhythmias
- Cardiomyopathy
- Congestive cardiac failure
- Coronary artery disease (Ischemic heart disease)
- Endocarditis
- Hypertension
- Hypotension
- Myocardial infarction
- Myocarditis
- Pericarditis
- Rheumatic fever
- Valvular heart disease

ANGINA PECTORIS

Definition

Angina pectoris is a syndrome characterized by chest pain resulting from an imbalance between oxygen supply and demand, and is most commonly caused by the inability of atherosclerotic coronary arteries to perfuse the heart under conditions of increased myocardial oxygen consumption.

Etiology

- Coronary atherosclerosis
- Coronary artery spasm
- Severe anemia
- Aortic insufficiency

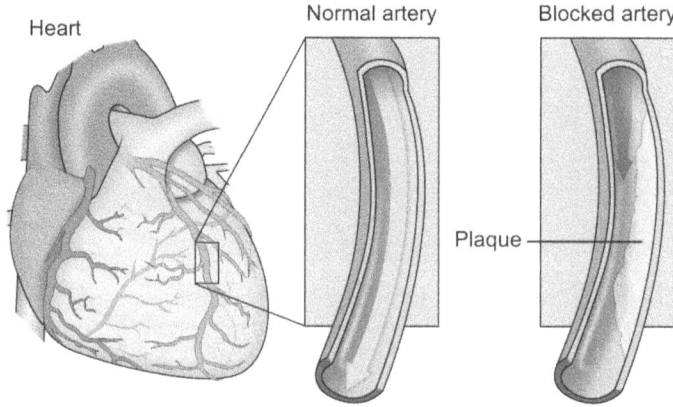

Fig. 7.1: Shows the comparison of normal artery with that of blocked artery (Angina pectoris).

- Hypertrophic obstructive cardiomyopathy
- Arrhythmias
- Arteritis.

Risk Factors

- Advancement in age
- Being males
- High blood pressure
- Metabolic syndrome
- Lack of regular exercise
- Smoking
- Uncontrolled diabetes
- Obesity
- Stress
- Hyperlipidemia.

Types

It is of five types as follows:
1. **Stable angina:** It is the most common type of angina. It occurs when the heart is working harder than usual. It has a regular pattern and is predictable. Increased physical activity and stress may develop mid-sternal chest pain in a patient which can be managed with nitroglycerin and rest. Pain subsides when the activity is stopped.
2. **Unstable angina:** It doesn't follow a pattern. It occurs more often and more severe than stable angina in patients with worsening coronary artery disease. The episode of chest pain is increased by severity and frequency and is not relieved by rest. It is very dangerous and requires emergency treatment.
3. **Variant (Prinzmetal's) angina:** It is a very rare type or angina and usually occurs due to any spasm in the coronary artery when an individual is at rest and the pain can be severe and long-lasting. It usually happens between midnight and early morning. It is more common in women and pain is relieved by medications.
4. **Microvascular angina:** It is more severe and lasts longer than other types of angina. The patients with this condition experience chest pain but have no apparent coronary artery blockages. Medication can not relieve this type of angina.
5. **Silent ischemia:** It occurs without chest pain or symptoms of angina mostly among older adults with hypertension or diabetes.

Pathophysiology

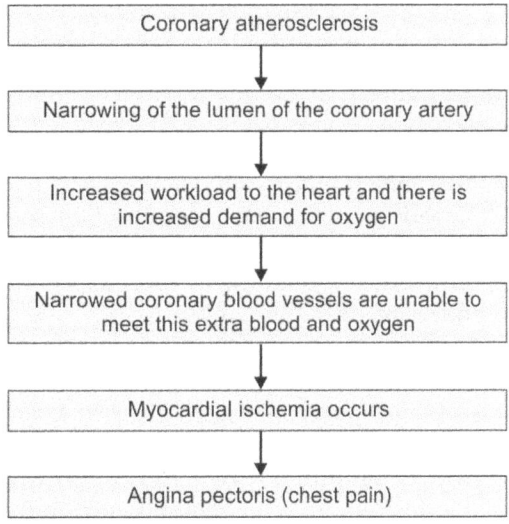

Clinical Features

- Pain which is of squeezing, burning and tightness in the chest
- Chest discomfort
- Pain duration lasting for 1–5 minutes, no more than 30 minutes
- Dyspnea on exertion which subsides on rest
- Shortness of breath
- Palpitations
- Dizziness
- Diaphoresis
- Fatigue
- Nausea.

Complications

- Myocardial infarction
- Stroke
- Depression.

Diagnostic Tests

- History
- Physical examination
- Resting ECG

- Myocardial perfusion scintigraphy
- Echocardiogram (an ultrasound of the heart)
- Exercise stress testing
- Electrocardiogram
- Ambulatory Holter monitoring
- Radioisotope studies
- Coronary arteriography
- Cardiac catheterization.

Management

Medical

- **Nitrates:** It relaxes and widens the blood vessels allowing more blood to flow into the heart muscle and prevents triggering angina. For example, nitroglycerin, nitrostat, nitroquick, etc.
- **Aspirin:** It reduces the ability of the blood to clot, making it easier for blood to flow through narrowed heart arteries. For example, astrix, aspro, etc.
- **Anticoagulants:** It helps in preventing blood clots from forming by making the blood platelets less likely to stick together. For example, clopidogrel, prasugrel, ticagrelor, etc.
- **Beta blockers:** It helps blood vessels relax and open up to improve blood flow, thus reducing or preventing angina. It works by blocking the effects of the hormone epinephrine, also known as adrenaline. As a result, the heart beats more slowly and with less force, thereby reducing blood pressure and angina. For example, propranolol, metoprolol, atenolol, etc.
- **Statins or HMG-CoA reductase inhibitors:** These are drugs used to lower blood cholesterol by inhibiting the enzyme HMG-CoA reductase. It also helps the body to reabsorb cholesterol that has accumulated in plaques in the artery walls, helps in preventing further blockage in the blood vessels. For example, atorvastatin, lovastatin, simvastatin, etc.
- **Calcium channel blockers:** It relaxes and widens blood vessels by affecting the muscle cells in the arterial walls and thus increases blood flow into the heart, reducing or preventing angina. For example, diltiazem, verapamil, nicardipine, etc.

Surgical

- **Angioplasty and stenting (Percutaneous coronary intervention):** It is a procedure in which a tiny balloon is inserted into the narrowed artery. The balloon is inflated to widen the artery and then a small wire mesh coil (stent) is inserted to keep the artery open. It improves blood flow into the heart, reducing or eliminating angina.
- **Coronary artery bypass surgery:** It is a surgical procedure in which a vein or artery from elsewhere in the body is used to bypass a blocked or narrowed heart artery. It increases blood flow into the heart and reduces or eliminates angina.

Nursing

- Encourage proper bedrest.
- Encourage the patient to take a diet low in cholesterol and saturated fats to reduce the risk of atherosclerosis.
- Instruct the patient not to smoke.
- Motivate the patient to have their blood pressure and cholesterol checked regularly
- Instruct the patient to maintain a healthy weight
- Encourage the patient to do regular exercise.

AORTIC ANEURYSM

Definition

A swelling of the wall of an artery, vein of the heart due to weakening of its wall by disease, injury, or an abnormality present at birth is called an aneurysm.

Etiology

- Atherosclerosis
- Genetic conditions (Marfan syndrome, Loeys-Dietz syndrome, Ehlers-Danlos syndrome and Turner syndrome)
- Poststenotic dilatation

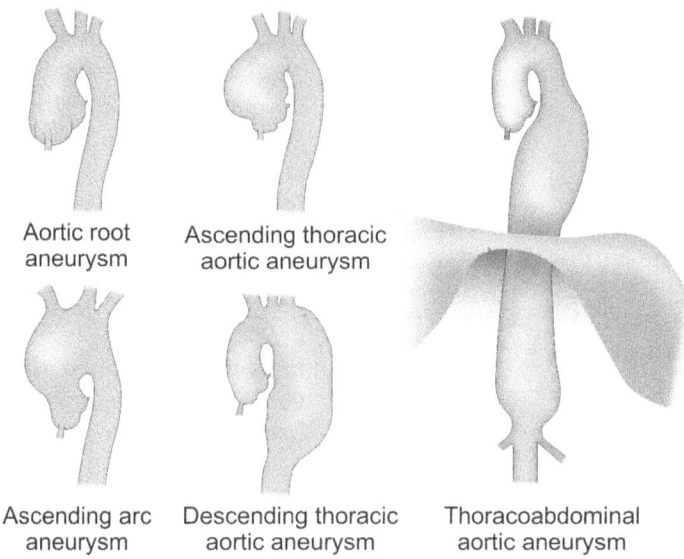

Fig. 7.2: Depicts aortic aneurysm at different sites.

- Cystic medial necrosis
- Untreated syphilis
- Traumatic injury
- Vasculitis
- Aortic dissection
- Aortic arteritis (Takayasu's arteritis).

Risk Factors

- Advancement in age
- Being male
- Overweight
- Limited physical activity
- Tobacco use
- Prolonged hypertension
- Cocaine use
- Family history.

Types

It is of two types as follows:
1. **Abdominal aortic aneurysm**: It occurs in the abdominal portion of the aorta and is most commonly seen type of aneurysm.
2. **Thoracic aortic aneurysm**: It occurs in the chest portion of the aorta and it is less commonly seen type of aneurysm.

Pathophysiology

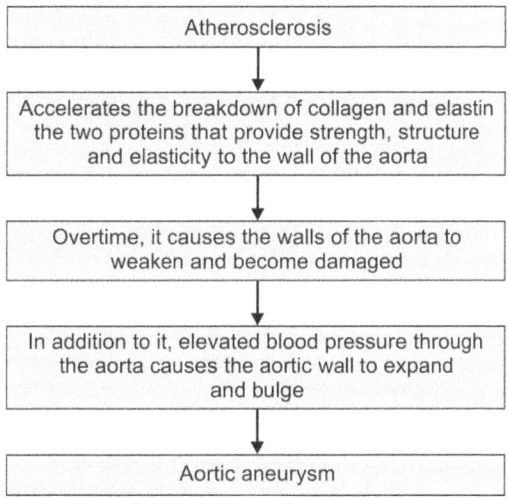

Clinical Features

- Tenderness or pain in the chest
- Back pain
- Hoarseness
- Cough
- Shortness of breath
- Difficulty in swallowing.

Complications
- Heart failure
- Aortic dissection.

Diagnostic Tests
- History
- Physical examination
- Angiography (an X-ray of the blood vessels)
- Echocardiogram (an ultrasound of the heart)
- Computed tomography (CT) scan
- Magnetic resonance imaging (MRI) scan.

Management

Medical
Beta blockers: It decreases blood pressure and the force of the heart's contractions, thus reducing pressure against the walls of the aorta. For example, propranolol, metoprolol, atenolol, etc.

Surgical
- **Open-abdominal or open-chest repair:** It is a surgery which involves a major incision (cut) in the abdomen or chest and incised part of the aorta is replaced with a graft made of materials such as Dacron or Teflon.
- **Endovascular repair:** It is a surgical procedure in which a graft is inserted into the aorta to strengthen it. Then a catheter is inserted into an artery in the groin (upper thigh) and threads it to the aneurysm. Then, using an X-ray, the surgeon threads the graft into the aorta to the aneurysm. The graft is then expanded inside the aorta and fastened in place to form a stable channel for blood flow. The graft reinforces the weakened section of the aorta and prevents it from rupturing.

Nursing
- Encourage the patient to take a diet low in cholesterol and saturated fats to reduce the risk of atherosclerosis.
- Instruct the patient not to smoke.
- Motivate the patients to have their blood pressure and cholesterol checked regularly.
- Instruct the patient to maintain a healthy weight.
- Encourage the patient to do regular exercise.

ATHEROSCLEROSIS

Definition
Atherosclerosis is a disease in which plaque (which is made up of fat, cholesterol, calcium and other substances) builds up inside the arteries that carry oxygen-rich blood to the heart and other parts of the body.

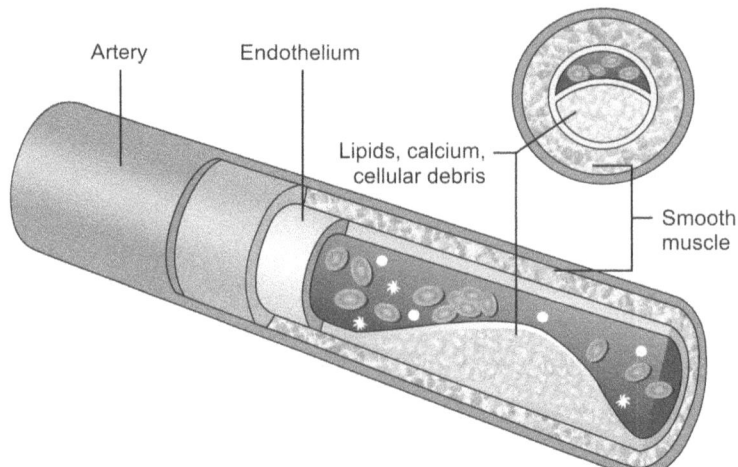

Fig. 7.3: Depicts plaque formation within the arteries that carries oxygen-rich blood to the heart and other parts of the body (Atherosclerosis).

Etiology

- Elevated cholesterol and triglyceride levels
- Deposition of fat containing substances along the intima of blood vessels
- Smooth muscle cell proliferation.

Risk Factors

- Advancement in age
- High blood pressure
- Lack of regular exercise
- Smoking
- Stress
- Alcohol
- Uncontrolled diabetes
- Obesity
- Family history of heart disease
- Consumption of fatty rich foods.

Pathophysiology

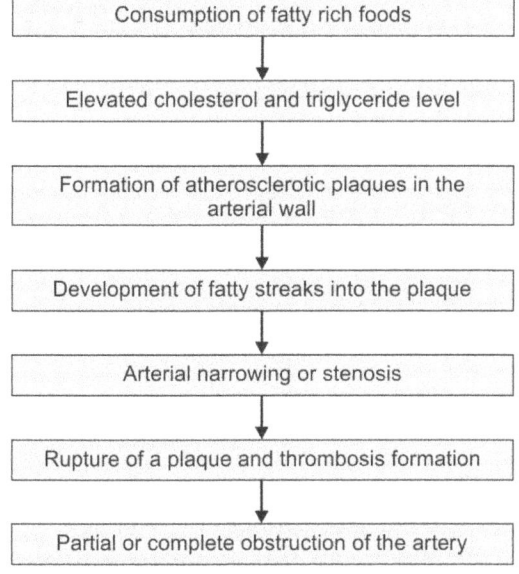

Clinical Features

It usually does not cause any symptoms until blood supply to an organ is reduced:
- Substernal pain in the chest
- Shortness of breath
- Dyspnea
- Palpitations
- Syncope
- Light-headedness
- Diaphoresis
- Nausea.

Complications

- Coronary artery disease
- Carotid artery disease
- Peripheral artery disease
- Aortic aneurysm
- Atheroembolic disease
- Visceral ischemia.

Diagnostic Tests

- History
- Physical examination
- Blood tests
- Chest X-ray
- Duplex scanning
- Ankle/Brachial index
- Echocardiogram (an ultrasound of the heart)
- Exercise stress testing
- Electrocardiogram
- Computed tomography (CT) scan
- Magnetic resonance imaging (MRI) scan
- Positron emission tomography (PET) scan
- Coronary arteriography
- Pharmacologic stress testing.

Management

Medical

- **Nitrates:** It relaxes and widens the blood vessels allowing more blood to flow into the heart muscle. For example, nitroglycerine, nitrostat, nitroquick, etc.
- **Aspirin:** It reduces the ability of the blood to clot, making it easier for blood to flow through narrowed heart arteries. For example, Astrix, Aspro, etc.
- **Anticoagulants:** It helps in preventing blood clots from forming by making the blood platelets less likely to stick together. For example, clopidogrel, prasugrel, ticagrelor, etc.
- **Beta blockers:** It helps blood vessels relax and open up to improve blood flow into the coronary artery. It works by blocking the effects of the hormone epinephrine,

also known as adrenaline. As a result, the heart beats more slowly and with less force, thereby reducing blood pressure. For example, propranolol, metoprolol, atenolol, etc.
- **Bile acid sequestrants:** It binds bile acids in the intestine and increases the excretion of bile acids in the stool. This reduces the amount of bile acids returning to the liver and forces the liver to produce more bile acids to replace the bile acids lost in the stool. In order to produce more bile acids, the liver converts more cholesterol into bile acids, which lowers the level of cholesterol in the blood. For example, colestipol, cholestyramine, colesevelam, etc.
- **Fibrates (fibric acid derivatives):** It lowers blood triglyceride levels by reducing the livers production of VLDL (the triglyceride-carrying particle that circulates in the blood) and by speeding up the removal of triglycerides from the blood. For example, gemfibrozil, fenofibrate, etc.
- **Glycoprotein receptor inhibitors:** It works by preventing platelet aggregation and thrombus formation in the blood vessels facilitating blood into the narrowed heart arteries. For example, abciximab, eptifibatide, tirofiban, etc.
- **Niacin:** It helps in lowering cholesterol and triglycerides. For example, niaspan, niacor, etc.
- **Ezetimibe:** It reduces blood cholesterol by inhibiting the absorption of cholesterol in the small intestine. For example, ezetrol, Zetia, etc.
- **Statins or HMG-CoA reductase inhibitors:** These are drugs used to lower blood cholesterol by inhibiting the enzyme HMG-CoA reductase. It also helps the body to reabsorb cholesterol that has accumulated in plaques in the artery walls, helps in preventing further blockage in the blood vessels. For example, atorvastatin, lovastatin, simvastatin, etc.
- **Calcium channel blockers:** It relaxes and widens blood vessels by affecting the muscle cells in the arterial walls and thus increases blood flow into the heart. For example, diltiazem, verapamil, nicardipine, etc.
- **Thrombolytics:** They dissolve blood clots by activating plasminogen, which forms a cleaved product called plasmin. Plasmin is a proteolytic enzyme that is capable of breaking cross-links between fibrin molecules, which provide the structural integrity of blood clots. For example, tissue plasminogen activator (t-PA), streptokinase, anistreplase, urokinase, etc.

Surgical

- **Balloon angioplasty:** It is a procedure in which a tiny balloon is inserted into the narrowed artery to keep the artery open to improve the blood flow into the heart.
- **Atherectomy:** It is a surgical procedure in which the blocked area inside the artery is "shaved" away by a tiny device on the end of a catheter.
- **Laser angioplasty:** It is a procedure in which laser is used to "vaporize" the blockage in the artery.
- **Coronary artery stenting:** It is a procedure in which a tiny coil (stent) is expanded inside the blocked artery to open the blocked area and is left in place to keep the artery open.
- **Brachytherapy:** It reduces the incidence of lesion recurrence (restenosis) after percutaneous coronary intervention.
- **Percutaneous transluminous coronary angioplasty (PTCA):** It helps in compressing the plaque against the walls of the artery and dilutes the vessel.
- **Coronary artery bypass grafting (CABG):** It helps in improving blood flow to the myocardial tissue that is at risk for ischemia or infarction because of the occluded artery.

Nursing

- Encourage the patient to take a diet low in cholesterol and saturated fats to reduce the risk of atherosclerosis.
- Instruct the patient not to smoke.
- Motivate the patients to have their blood pressure and cholesterol checked regularly.
- Instruct the patient to maintain a healthy weight.
- Encourage the patient to do regular exercise.

CARDIAC ARREST

Definition

Cardiac arrest is the failure of the heart to pump blood adequately to meet the oxygenation needs of the body.

Etiology

- Impairment in the contractile property of the heart
- Myocardial infarction
- Coronary artery disease
- End-stage cardiomyopathy
- Severe valvular dysfunction
- Congenital heart disease
- Electrical problems in the heart
- Ventricular aneurysm.

Risk Factors

- Family history of coronary artery disease
- High blood pressure
- Smoking
- Uncontrolled diabetes
- Obesity
- Hyperlipidemia
- Sedentary lifestyle
- Drinking too much alcohol
- Previous episode of cardiac arrest
- Previous heart attack
- Advancement in age
- Nutritional imbalance
- Being male
- Using illicit drugs like cocaine, amphetamines, etc.

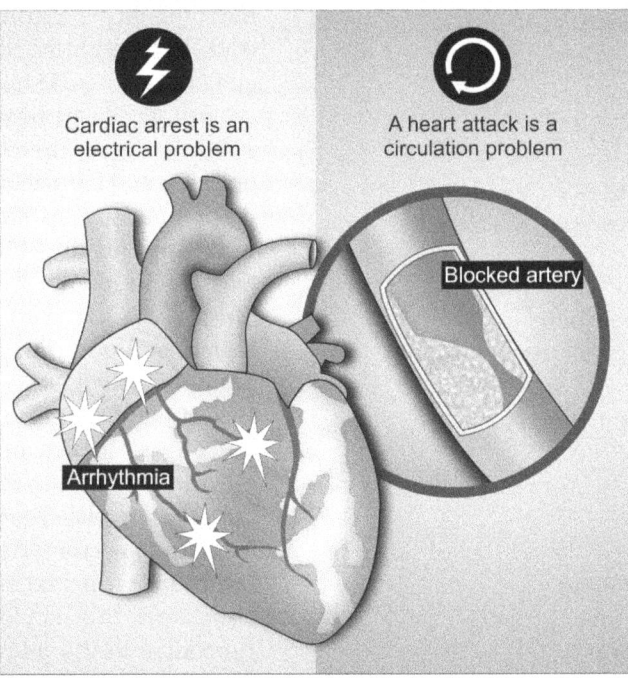

Fig. 7.4: Depicts failure of the heart to pump blood adequately to meet the demands of the body (Cardiac arrest).

Pathophysiology

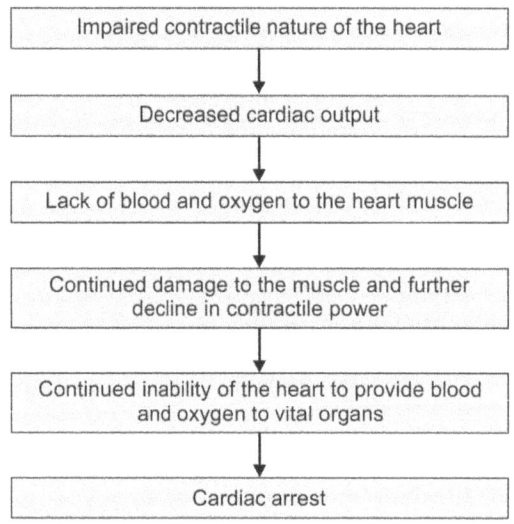

Clinical Features

- Fatigue
- Fainting
- Blackouts
- Dizziness
- Chest pain
- Shortness of breath
- Weakness
- Palpitations
- No pulse
- No breathing
- Sudden collapse
- Loss of consciousness.

Complications

- Neurologic impairment
- Acute respiratory distress syndrome
- Renal failure
- Multiorgan dysfunction syndrome
- Death.

Diagnostic Tests

- History
- Physical examination
- Chest X-ray
- Electrocardiogram
- Increased pulmonary capillary wedge pressure
- Cardiac enzyme test
- Elevated blood urea nitrogen creatinine
- Elevated serum lactate
- Hormone test
- Ejection fraction testing
- Echocardiogram (an ultrasound of the heart)
- Nuclear scan
- Coronary catheterization (angiogram)
- Electrophysiological testing and mapping.

Management

Medical

- **Nitrates:** It relaxes and widens the blood vessels allowing more blood to flow into the heart muscle and decreases the workload of the heart by reducing venous return and lessening the resistance against which the heart pumps. For example, nitroglycerin, nitroprusside, nitrostat, nitroquick, etc.
- **Cardiac glycosides:** It improves contractile property of the heart. For example, digoxin, dopamine, etc.
- **Beta blockers:** It helps blood vessels relax and open up to improve blood flow, thus reducing or preventing cardiac arrest. It works by blocking the effects of the hormone epinephrine, also known as adrenaline. As a result, the heart beats more slowly and with less force, thereby reducing blood pressure and cardiac arrest. For example, propranolol, metoprolol, atenolol, etc.
- **Calcium channel blockers:** It relaxes and widens blood vessels by affecting the muscle cells in the arterial walls and thus increases blood flow into the heart. For example, amiodarone, cordarone, etc.
- **Diuretics:** It mobilizes edematous fluid, thereby reducing pulmonary venous pressure and in turn reduces preload. For example, metolazone, furosemide, etc.
- **Angiotensin-converting enzyme (ACE) inhibitors:** It prevents an enzyme in the body from producing angiotensin II, a substance in the body that narrows the blood vessels and releases hormones that raises the blood pressure. For example, captopril, enalapril, fosinopril, etc.

Surgical

- **Defibrillation:** It is a procedure in which electrical shock is delivered through the chest wall to the heart in order to restore the normal heart rhythm that has momentarily stopped functioning.
- **Coronary artery bypass grafting:** It is a surgical procedure in which a vein or artery from elsewhere in the body is used to bypass a blocked or narrowed heart artery. It increases blood flow into the heart and reduces or eliminates cardiac arrest.
- **Implantable cardioverter defibrillator (ICD):** It is a sophisticated device used primarily to treat ventricular tachycardia and ventricular fibrillation, two life-threatening heart rhythms. They constantly monitor the heart rhythm. When it detects a very fast, abnormal heart rhythm, it delivers energy to the heart muscle to cause the heart to beat in a normal rhythm again.
- **Radiofrequency catheter ablation:** During this procedure, high-frequency electrical energy is delivered through a catheter to a small area of tissue inside the heart that causes the abnormal heart rhythm. This energy "disconnects" the pathway of the abnormal rhythm.
- **Heart transplantation:** It is a surgical transplant procedure performed on patients with end-stage heart failure or severe coronary artery disease.

Nursing

- Elevate the head-end of the bed to 20–30 degree.
- Reposition the patient frequently to maintain skin integrity.
- Encourage the patient to verbalize fears about diagnosis and prognosis.
- Instruct the patient not to smoke.
- Motivate the patient to have their blood pressure and cholesterol checked regularly.
- Offer reassurance and encouragement.

CARDIAC DYSRHYTHMIAS

Definition

Any alteration in the automaticity and conductivity property of the heart is known as arrhythmias or dysrhythmias.

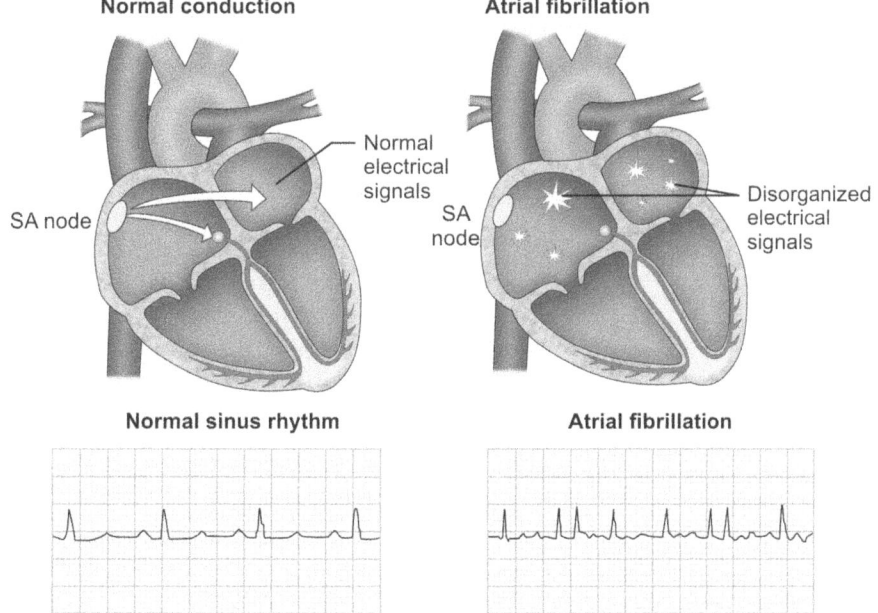

Fig. 7.5: Shows the comparison of normal sinus rhythm heart with that of the altered automaticity and conductive property of the heart (Atrial fibrillation).

Etiology

- Hypertrophy of cardiac muscle
- Congestive cardiac failure
- Conduction defects
- Hypertension
- Myocardial infarction
- Myocardial cell degeneration
- Acid-base imbalance
- Alcohol
- Electrolyte imbalance
- Connective tissue disorders
- Drug toxicity
- Electric shock
- Hypoxia
- Thyroid dysfunction
- Poisoning.

Risk Factors

- Previous heart surgery
- Smoking
- Uncontrolled diabetes
- Congenital heart disease
- Obstructive sleep apnea
- Caffeine or nicotine use
- Drinking too much alcohol.

Types

The classification of cardiac arrhythmias may be considered under the following categories:
1. Arrhythmias in relation to the sinoatrial node
2. Arrhythmias of atrial origin
3. Arrhythmias arising in and around the AV junction
4. Arrhythmias originating in the ventricles.

Arrhythmias in relation to the sinoatrial node:

- *Sinus arrhythmia*
    - It is commonly seen in children between 3 years and 12 years.
    - The heart rate goes up and down in phases during inspiration and expiration respectively.
    - During inspiration due to inhibition of the vagus nerve, the heart rate goes up and the opposite happens during expiration.
- *Sinus tachycardia*
    - The sinus node generates impulses at a rate of more than 100/min.
    - It is either physiological or secondary to fever, anemia, thyrotoxicosis, etc.
- *Sinus bradycardia*
    - The sinus node generates impulses at a rate of less than 60/min.
    - It does not require any treatment except in certain circumstances.

Arrhythmias in relation to the atria:

- *Atrial ectopic beat*
    - This is a premature beat characterized by an abnormal P wave and a normal QRS complex.
    - It may occur in isolation or as a series of consecutive beats.
- *Atrial tachycardia*
    - This originates in one of the atria and is therefore recognized by abnormal P waves occurring at a higher atrial rate (of about 150 - 250/min) with normal QRS complexes following them.
- *Atrial flutter*
    - In this the atrial rate is about 250–350/min.
    - It gives rise to undulating, abnormal P waves called flutter waves or F waves which have a characteristic saw-tooth appearance.
- *Atrial fibrillation*
    - It is caused by rheumatic heart disease in the younger age group and ischemic heart disease in the older age group. The atrial rate in fibrillation is above 350/min.
    - P waves are either totally absent or show variable sizes.
    - The pulse is irregularly irregular.

Junctional rhythms:

- *AV nodal rhythms*
    - It has a negative P wave preceding, following or lost in a QRS complex.
    - It is divided into upper, middle or lower nodal rhythms based on the site of impulse formation.

- *Junctional tachycardia*
  - It occurs at a rate of more than 100/min.
  - Digitalis toxicity commonly leads to junctional tachycardia.

Arrhythmias in relation to the ventricles:
- *Premature ventricular contraction*
  - It is most commonly seen in older age group in various diseases of the heart.
  - The characteristic feature is wide QRS complexes with abnormal ST-T changes.
- *Ventricular flutter*
  It is characterized by large, wide, monophasis but similar QRS complexes without any identifiable P or T waves.
- *Ventricular fibrillation*
  - The abnormal QRS complexes are seen in difficult sizes and shapes.
  - The patient will be usually unconscious without any significant cardiac output.
  - These serious ventricular arrhythmias may end in cardiac arrest which is represented on the ECG as a straight line without any electric activity at all.

Pathophysiology

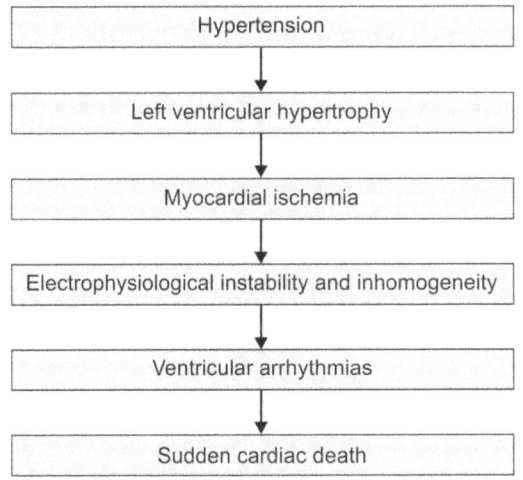

Clinical Features
- Palpitations
- Pounding in the chest
- Dizziness of feeling light-headed
- Fainting
- Chest discomfort
- Shortness of breath
- Weakness or fatigue.

Complications
- Stroke
- Congestive heart failure
- Sudden death.

Diagnostic Tests
- History
- Physical examination
- Electrocardiogram
- Holter monitoring
- Stress test
- Electrophysiology study (EPS)
- Head-up tilt table test
- Echocardiogram (an ultrasound of the heart)
- Coronary catheterization (angiogram).

Management

Medical

- **Beta blockers:** It helps blood vessels relax and open up to improve blood flow, thus reducing or preventing cardiac arrest. It works by blocking the effects of the hormone epinephrine, also known as adrenaline. As a result, the heart beats more slowly and with less force, thereby reducing blood pressure and cardiac arrest. For example, propranolol, metoprolol, atenolol, etc.
- **Anticoagulants:** It helps in preventing blood clots from forming by making the blood platelets less likely to stick together. For example, clopidogrel, prasugrel, ticagrelor, etc.
- **Cardiac glycosides:** It improves contractile property of the heart. For example, digoxin, dopamine, etc.
- **Calcium channel blockers:** It relaxes and widens blood vessels by affecting the muscle cells in the arterial walls and thus increases blood flow into the heart. For example, diltiazem, verapamil, etc.

Surgical

- **Electrical cardioversion:** It is a procedure in which electrical shock is delivered to the chest wall that synchronizes the heart and allows the normal rhythm to restart.
- **Cardiac pacemaker:** It is a device that sends small electrical impulses to the heart muscle to maintain a suitable heart rate. It primarily prevents the heart from beating too slowly. The pacemaker has a pulse generator (which houses the battery and a tiny computer) and leads (wires) that send impulses from the pulse generator to the heart muscle. They have many sophisticated features that are designed to help manage arrhythmias and optimize heart rate-related function as much as possible.
- **Implantable cardioverter defibrillator (ICD):** It is a sophisticated device used primarily to treat ventricular tachycardia and ventricular fibrillation, two life-threatening heart rhythms. They constantly monitor the heart rhythm. When it detects a very fast, abnormal heart rhythm, it delivers energy to the heart muscle to cause the heart to beat in a normal rhythm again.
- **Radiofrequency catheter ablation:** During this procedure, high-frequency electrical energy is delivered through a catheter to a small area of tissue inside the heart that causes the abnormal heart rhythm. This energy "disconnects" the pathway of the abnormal rhythm.
- **Defibrillation:** It is a procedure in which electrical shock is delivered through the chest wall to the heart in order to restore the normal heart rhythm that has momentarily stopped functioning.

Nursing

- Instruct the patient to stay away from caffeine products.
- Instruct the patient not to smoke or consume alcohol.
- Educate the patient to avoid cold and cough medications as they contain ingredients that promote irregular heartbeats.
- Offer reassurance and encouragement.

CARDIOMYOPATHY

Definition

Cardiomyopathy is a chronic disease of the heart muscle (myocardium), in which the muscle is abnormally enlarged, thickened and stiffened. The weakened heart muscle loses the ability to pump blood effectively, resulting in

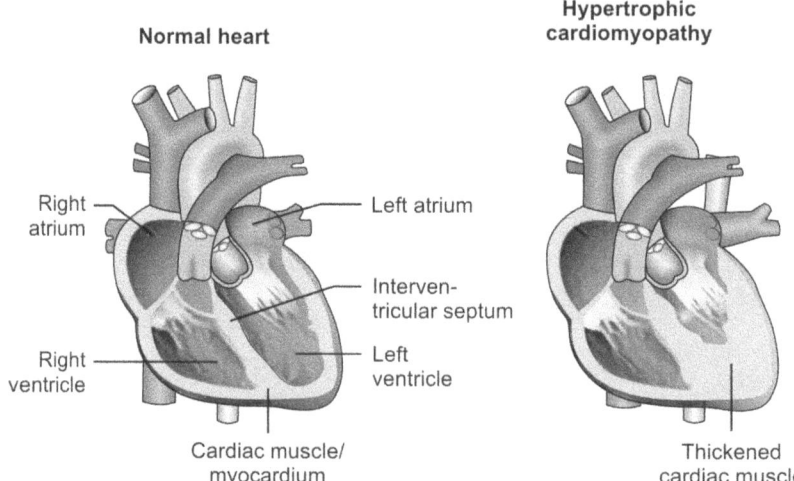

Fig. 7.6: Shows the comparison of normal heart with that of the thickened and stiffened cardiac muscle (Cardiomyopathy).

irregular heartbeats and possibly even heart failure.

Etiology

- Genetic conditions
- Chronic rapid heart rate
- Heart valve problems
- Nutritional deficiencies of essential vitamins or minerals
- Pregnancy complications
- Connective tissue disorders.

Risk Factors

- Family history
- Long-term high blood pressure
- Heart tissue damage from a previous heart attack
- Obesity
- Drinking too much alcohol over many years
- Illicit drug use
- Metabolic disorders
- Use of chemotherapy drugs
- Hemochromatosis
- Sarcoidosis
- Amyloidosis.

Types

It is of three types as follows:
1. ***Dilated cardiomyopathy:*** It is the most common type of cardiomyopathy. In this disorder, the pumping ability of the heart's main pumping chamber, the left ventricle becomes less forceful. The left ventricle becomes enlarged (dilated) and cannot effectively pump blood out of the heart. It occurs most often in middle-aged people and is more likely to affect men. Mostly people with this type have a family history of the condition. The cause may also be unknown (idiopathic).
2. ***Hypertrophic cardiomyopathy:*** It is a genetically transmitted form of cardiomyopathy. It is characterized by impaired diastolic ventricular function and hypertrophy of ventricular muscle mass. This type involves abnormal thickening of the heart muscle, particularly affecting the muscle of heart's main pumping chamber, left ventricle. The thickened heart muscle will make it harder for the heart to pump blood. It can develop at any age, but the condition tends to be more severe if it becomes apparent during childhood. Most affected people will have a family history of the disease and some genetic mutations have been linked to hypertrophic cardiomyopathy.
3. ***Restrictive cardiomyopathy:*** It is characterized by diffuse ventricular hypertrophy and impaired diastolic function with loss of compliance. It often occurs secondary to infiltration of the myocardium with an abnormal substance. The heart muscle becomes rigid and less elastic so that the heart cannot properly expand and fill with blood between heartbeats. It can occur at any age, it most often tends to affect older people. It is the least common type of cardiomyopathy and can occur for no known reason (idiopathic).

Pathophysiology

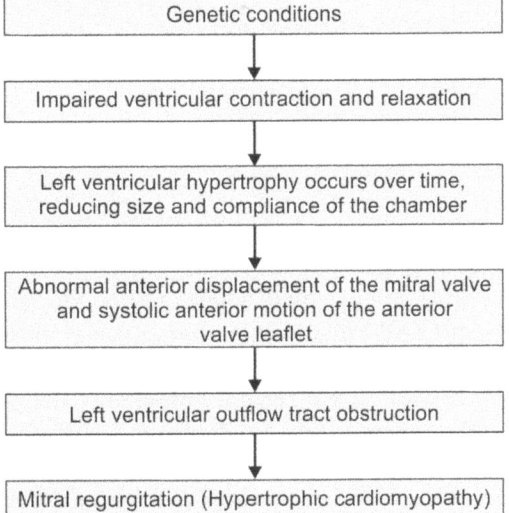

Clinical Features

- Breathlessness with exertion or even at rest
- Swelling of the legs, ankles and feet

- Bloating of the abdomen due to fluid buildup
- Cough while lying down
- Fatigue
- Irregular heartbeats that feel rapid, pounding or fluttering
- Chest pain
- Dizziness, lightheadedness and fainting
- Fatigue
- Nausea.

Complications

- Heart failure
- Blood clots
- Valve problems
- Cardiac arrest
- Sudden death.

Diagnostic Tests

- History
- Physical examination
- Blood tests
- Chest X-ray
- Cardiac magnetic resonance imaging (MRI)
- Echocardiogram (an ultrasound of the heart)
- Exercise stress testing
- Cardiac computed tomography (CT) scan
- Genetic testing or screening
- Cardiac catheterization.

Management

Medical

- **ACE inhibitors:** It promotes vasodilatation and diuresis by decreasing afterload and preload. For example, enalapril, captopril, etc.
- **Angiotensin II receptor blockers (ARBs):** It lowers blood pressure and systemic vascular resistance. For example, losartan.
- **Beta blockers:** It helps blood vessels relax and open up to improve blood flow, thus reducing blood pressure. It works by blocking the effects of the hormone epinephrine, also known as adrenaline. As a result, the heartbeats more slowly and with less force, thereby reducing blood pressure. For example, propranolol, metoprolol, atenolol, etc.
- **Aldosterone antagonists:** It inhibits sodium resorption in the collecting duct of the nephron in the kidneys. This interferes with sodium/potassium exchange, reducing urinary potassium excretion and increases water excretion (diuresis). For example, spironolactone, mexrenone, etc.
- **Diuretics:** It mobilizes edematous fluid, thereby reducing pulmonary venous pressure and in turn reduces preload. For example, metolazone, furosemide, etc.
- **Vasodilators:** It reduces the workload of the heart. For example, hydralazine, isosorbide dinitrate, etc.
- **Human B-type natriuretic peptide:** It helps to restore the body's salt and water balance and thereby increasing cardiac function. For example, nesiritide, etc.
- **Cardiac glycosides:** It improves contractile property of the heart. For example, digoxin, dopamine, etc.
- **Anticoagulants:** It helps in preventing blood clots from forming by making the blood platelets less likely to stick together. For example, clopidogrel, prasugrel, ticagrelor, etc.
- **Calcium channel blockers:** It relaxes and widens blood vessels by affecting the muscle cells in the arterial walls and thus increases blood flow into the heart, thereby reducing systemic vascular resistance. For example, diltiazem, verapamil, nicardipine, etc.

Surgical

- **Implantable cardioverter-defibrillator (ICD):** It is a device that monitors the heart rhythm and delivers electric shocks when needed to control abnormal heart rhythms.
- **Septal myectomy:** It is a surgical procedure in which a surgeon removes part of the thickened heart muscle wall (septum) that separates the two bottom heart chambers.

Removing part of the heart muscle improves blood flow through the heart and reduces mitral valve regurgitation.
- **Septal ablation:** It is a surgical procedure in which a small portion of the thickened heart muscle is destroyed by injecting alcohol thorough a long thin tube (catheter) into the artery supplying blood to that area.
- **Radiofrequency ablation:** It is a surgical procedure in which doctors guide long flexible tubes (catheters) through the blood vessels into the heart. Electrodes at the catheter tips transmit energy to damage a small spot of abnormal heart tissue that is causing the abnormal heart rhythm.

Nursing
- Encourage the patient to have good sleep.
- Encourage the patient to take a healthy diet including a variety of fruits and vegetables and whole grains.
- Instruct the patient to quit smoking.
- Motivate the patient to have their blood pressure and cholesterol checked regularly.
- Instruct the patient to maintain a healthy weight.
- Encourage the patient to do regular exercise.
- Eliminate or minimize the amount of alcohol they drink.
- Teach proper stress management techniques.
- Instruct them to restrict salt in their diet.

CONGESTIVE CARDIAC FAILURE

Definition
Congestive heart failure is the inability of the heart to pump sufficient blood to meet the metabolic demands of the body.

Etiology
- Genetic conditions
- Coronary heart disease
- Rheumatic heart disease
- Congenital heart disease
- Cardiomyopathy
- Valvular disorders
- Myocardial infarction
- Arrhythmias
- Pulmonary emboli
- Thyrotoxicosis
- Rupture of papillary muscles
- Chronic lung disease
- Excessive sodium intake
- Physical and emotional stress.

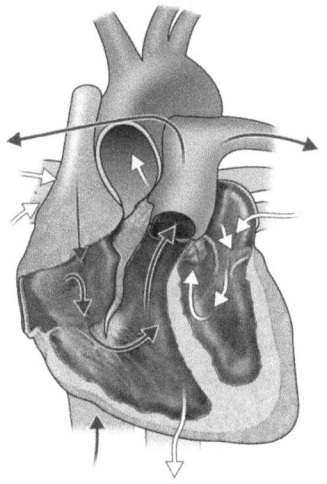
Healthy heart

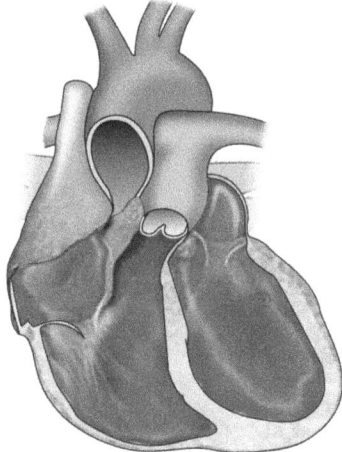
Congested heart

Fig. 7.7: Shows the comparison of healthy heart with that of congested heart (Congestive cardiac failure).

Risk Factors

- Family history
- Anemia
- Infection
- Hypothyroidism
- Paget's disease
- Nutritional deficiencies
- Hypervolemia
- Hypertension
- Hyperlipidemia
- Diabetes
- Alcohol consumption
- Smoking
- Family history
- Use of cardiotoxic drugs.

Types

The New York Heart Association has developed functional guidelines for classifying people with congestive heart failure. The classification is based on the person's tolerance to physical activity.

Class I

- No limitation of physical activity
- Ordinary physical activity does not cause fatigue, dyspnea, palpitations or anginal pain.

Class II

- Slight limitation of physical activity
- No symptoms at rest
- Ordinary physical activity results in fatigue, dyspnea, palpitations or anginal pain.

Class III

- Marked limitation of physical activity
- Usually comfortable at rest
- Ordinary physical activity results in fatigue, dyspnea, palpitations or anginal pain.

Class IV

- Inability to carry on any physical activity without discomfort
- Symptoms of cardiac insufficiency or of angina may be present even at rest.
- If any physical activity is undertaken, discomfort is increased.

Pathophysiology

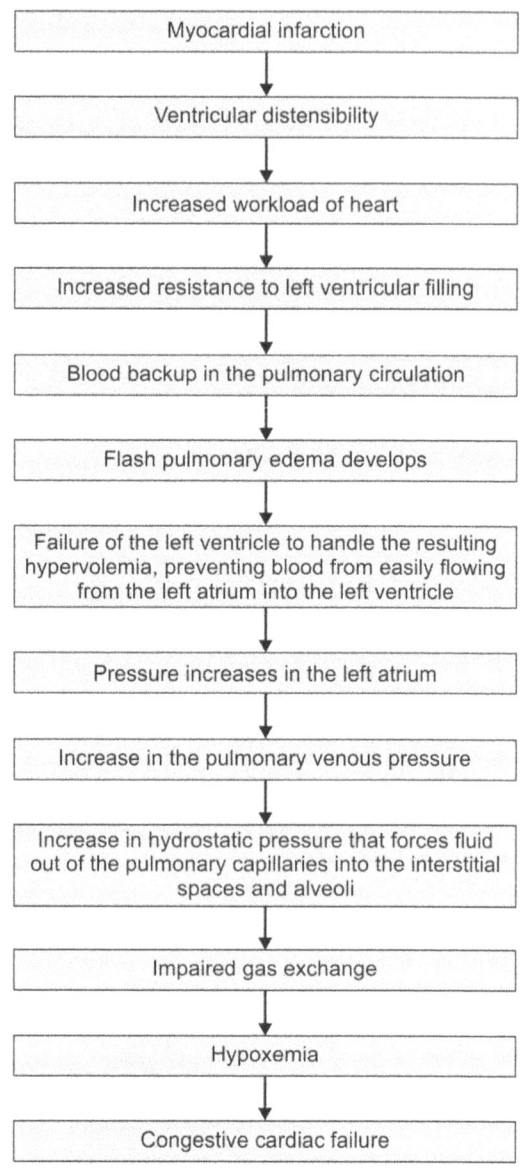

Clinical Features

Left-sided Heart Failure

- Dyspnea on exertion
- Paroxysmal nocturnal dyspnea
- Cough which is productive with frothy sputum
- Pulsus alternans
- Fatigue
- Pallor
- Cyanosis

- Orthopnea
- Presence of rales or crackles on auscultation
- Tachycardia
- Confusion
- Disorientation.

Right-sided Heart Failure

- Distended neck veins
- Dependent edema
- Hepatomegaly
- Ascites
- Weakness
- Nausea
- Anorexia
- Weight gain
- Pitting, dependent edema in the feet, legs, sacrum and buttocks
- Increased abdominal girth
- Nocturnal diuresis
- Abdominal pain.

Complications

- Pleural effusion
- Cardiogenic shock
- Dysrhythmias
- Cardiac tamponade
- Thromboembolism.

Diagnostic Tests

- History
- Physical examination
- Blood examination
- Chest X-ray
- Electrocardiogram
- Echocardiogram
- Cardiac catheterization
- Computed tomography (CT) scan
- Nuclear imaging studies
- Coronary angiogram
- Myocardial biopsy
- Magnetic resonance imaging
- Stress test.

Management

Medical

- **ACE inhibitors:** It promotes vasodilatation and diuresis by decreasing afterload and preload. For example, enalapril, captopril, etc.
- **Angiotensin II receptor blockers (ARBs):** It lowers blood pressure and systemic vascular resistance. For example, losartan.
- **Beta blockers:** It helps blood vessels relax and open up to improve blood flow, thus reducing blood pressure. It works by blocking the effects of the hormone epinephrine, also known as adrenaline. As a result, the heart beats more slowly and with less force, thereby reducing blood pressure. For example, propranolol, metoprolol, atenolol, etc.
- **Aldosterone antagonists:** It inhibits sodium resorption in the collecting duct of the nephron in the kidneys. This interferes with sodium/potassium exchange, reducing urinary potassium excretion and increases water excretion (diuresis). For example, spironolactone, mexrenone, etc.
- **Diuretics:** It mobilizes oedematous fluid, thereby reducing pulmonary venous pressure and inturn reduces preload. For example, metolazone, Furosemide, etc.
- **Vasodilators:** It reduces the workload of the heart. For example, hydralazine, isosorbide dinitrate, etc.
- **Cardiac glycosides:** It improves contractile property of the heart. For example, digoxin, dopamine, etc.
- **Calcium channel blockers:** It relaxes and widens blood vessels by affecting the muscle cells in the arterial walls and thus increases blood flow into the heart, thereby reducing systemic vascular resistance. For example, diltiazem, verapamil, nicardipine, etc.

Surgical

- **Implantable cardioverter-defibrillator (ICD):** It is a device that monitors the heart rhythm and delivers electric shocks when needed to control abnormal heart rhythms.
- **Coronary artery bypass grafting:** It is a surgical procedure in which a vein or artery from elsewhere in the body is used to bypass a blocked or narrowed heart artery. It increases blood flow into the heart and reduces or eliminates cardiac arrest.

- **Heart valve repair or replacement:** It is a surgical procedure in which the original valve is repaired or replaced by an artificial (prosthetic) valve to eliminate backward blood flow.
- **Cardiac resynchronization therapy (CRT) or biventricular pacing:** It is a procedure in which biventricular pacemaker sends timed electrical impulses to both of the heart's lower chambers (the left and right ventricles) so that they pump in a more efficient and coordinated manner.
- **Heart pumps:** These are mechanical devices that are implanted into the abdomen or chest and attached to a weakened heart to help it pump blood to the rest of the body.
- **Heart transplantation:** It is a surgical procedure in which patients with severe heart failure have their diseased heart replaced with a healthy donor heart.

Nursing

- Instruct the patients to restrict salt in their diet.
- Instruct the patient to quit smoking.
- Motivate the patients to have their blood pressure and cholesterol checked regularly.
- Instruct the patient to maintain a healthy weight.
- Encourage the patient to do regular exercise.
- Teach proper stress management techniques.
- Instruct them to restrict salt in their diet.

CORONARY ARTERY DISEASE (ISCHEMIC HEART DISEASE)

Definition
Coronary artery disease is a disease characterized by the accumulation of plaque within the layers of the coronary arteries.

Etiology
- Atherosclerosis
- Coronary vasospasm
- Infection.

Risk Factors

Non-modifiable Factors

- Older age group
- Being male
- Race
- Family history.

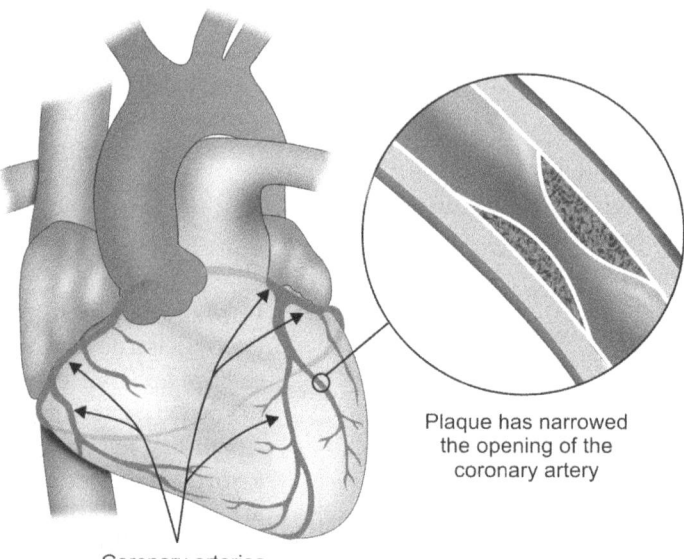

Fig. 7.8: Depicts accumulation of plaque within the layers of the coronary arteries (Coronary artery disease).

Modifiable Factors

- Elevated lipid levels
- Hypertension
- Obesity
- Cigarette smoking
- Sedentary lifestyle
- Diabetes mellitus.

Other Factors

- Stress
- Lack of exercise
- After menopause for women
- Increased levels of lipoprotein
- Left ventricular hypertrophy.

Pathophysiology

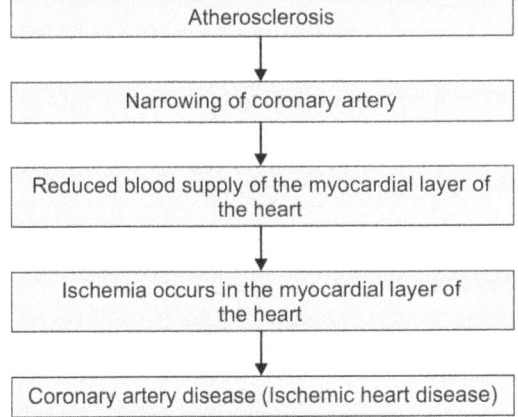

Clinical Features

- Substernal pain that radiates to the left shoulders and down the inner side of the left arm.
- Squeezing, burning, aching or bursting type of pain
- Dyspnea
- Fainting
- Sweating
- Pallor
- Palpitations
- Dizziness
- Nausea
- Vomiting.

Complications

- Sudden death due to lethal dysrhythmias
- Heart failure
- Myocardial infarction
- Vasospasm of the coronary artery.

Diagnostic Tests

- History
- Physical examination
- Blood examination
- Chest X-ray
- Electrocardiogram
- Echocardiogram
- Cardiac catheterization
- Computed tomography (CT) scan
- Positron emission tomography (PET) scan
- Radionuclide imaging
- Electron beam CT scan
- Nuclear imaging studies
- Coronary angiogram
- Myocardial biopsy
- Magnetic resonance imaging
- Stress test.

Management

Medical

- **Nitrates:** It relaxes and widens the blood vessels allowing more blood to flow into the heart muscle. For example, nitroglycerin, Nitrostat, Nitroquick, etc.
- **Aspirin:** It reduces the ability of the blood to clot, making it easier for blood to flow through narrowed heart arteries. For example, Astrix, Aspro, etc.
- **Beta blockers:** It helps blood vessels relax and open up to improve blood flow into the coronary artery. It works by blocking the effects of the hormone epinephrine, also known as adrenaline. As a result, the heart beats more slowly and with less force, thereby reducing blood pressure. For example, propranolol, metoprolol, atenolol, etc.
- **Bile acid sequestrants:** It binds bile acids in the intestine and increases the excretion of bile acids in the stool. This reduces the amount of bile acids returning to the liver and forces the liver to produce more bile acids to replace the bile acids lost in the stool. In order to produce more bile acids, the liver converts more cholesterol into bile

acids, which lowers the level of cholesterol in the blood. For example, colestipol, cholestyramine, colesevelam, etc.
- **Fibrates (fibric acid derivatives):** It lowers blood triglyceride levels by reducing the liver's production of VLDL (the triglyceride-carrying particle that circulates in the blood) and by speeding up the removal of triglycerides from the blood. For example, gemfibrozil, fenofibrate, etc.
- **Glycoprotein receptor inhibitors:** It works by preventing platelet aggregation and thrombus formation in the blood vessels facilitating blood into the narrowed heart arteries. For example, abciximab, eptifibatide, tirofiban, etc.
- **Niacin:** It helps in lowering cholesterol and triglycerides. For example, Niaspan, Niacor, etc.
- **Ezetimibe:** It reduces blood cholesterol by inhibiting the absorption of cholesterol in the small intestine. For example, ezetrol, zetia, etc.
- **Statins or HMG-CoA reductase inhibitors:** These are drugs used to lower blood cholesterol by inhibiting the enzyme HMG-CoA reductase. It also helps the body to reabsorb cholesterol that has accumulated in plaques in the artery walls, helps in preventing further blockage in the blood vessels. For example, atorvastatin, lovastatin, simvastatin, etc.
- **Calcium channel blockers:** It relaxes and widens blood vessels by affecting the muscle cells in the arterial walls and thus increases blood flow into the heart. For example, diltiazem, verapamil, nicardipine, etc.

Surgical

- **Percutaneous coronary revascularization:** It is a procedure in which a long, thin tube (catheter) is inserted into the narrowed part of the artery and a wire with a deflated balloon is then inflated, compressing the deposits against the artery walls. A stent is often left in the artery to help keep the artery open.
- **Intracoronary stent:** It is a surgical procedure in which a diamond mesh tubular device is placed in the coronary vessel to prevent restenosis by providing a skeletal support.
- **Transmyocardial revascularization:** It is a surgical procedure in which by means of a laser beam, small channels are formed in the myocardium to encourage new blood flow.
- **Atherectomy:** It is a surgical procedure in which the blocked area inside the artery is "shaved" away by a tiny device on the end of a catheter.
- **Coronary artery bypass grafting (CABG):** It is a surgical procedure in which a graft is surgically attached to the aorta and the other end of the graft is attached to a distal portion of a coronary vessel and bypasses obstructive lesions in the vessel and returns adequate blood flow to the heart muscle.

Nursing

- Encourage the patient to take a diet low in cholesterol and saturated fats to reduce the risk of atherosclerosis.
- Instruct the patient not to smoke.
- Motivate the patients to have their blood pressure and cholesterol checked regularly.
- Instruct the patient to maintain a healthy weight.
- Encourage the patient to do regular exercise.

Rehabilitation

There are four phases of cardiac rehabilitation in coronary artery disease as follows:

1. ***Inpatient phase***
   - It lasts between 5 days and 14 days.
   - Limiting physical and psychological consequences of the acute cardiac illness

- Educating patient and family members about measures to save life.
2. *Early-outpatient phase*
   - It lasts between 2-3 months after discharge.
   - Patients require close supervision and monitoring.
   - Providing referrals for self-help groups or community agencies.
3. *Late-outpatient phase*
   - It lasts after 6 months from discharge.
   - Patient and family members realize the importance of exercise, self- monitoring and lifestyle changes.
4. *Maintenance phase*
   - It lasts for lifelong.
   - Patients are more knowledgeable about their activity limits.

ENDOCARDITIS

Definition

Endocarditis is a microbial infection and inflammation of the endocardium and heart valves. The endocardium is the lining of the heart chambers containing small blood vessels and a few bundles of smooth muscle.

Etiology

- Bacterial infections
- Fungal infections
- Rheumatic heart disease
- Marfan's syndrome (a hereditary condition that affects the muscle skeletal system)
- Nosocomial bacteremia
- Catheters or needles
- Everyday oral activities
- Certain dental procedures.

Risk Factors

- Artificial heart valves
- Congenital heart defects
- History of endocarditis
- Damaged heart valves
- Intravenous illicit drug use.

Types

There are two types of endocarditis as follows:
1. **Subacute:** It has a long clinical course and insidious in onset and the causative organism is of low virulence.

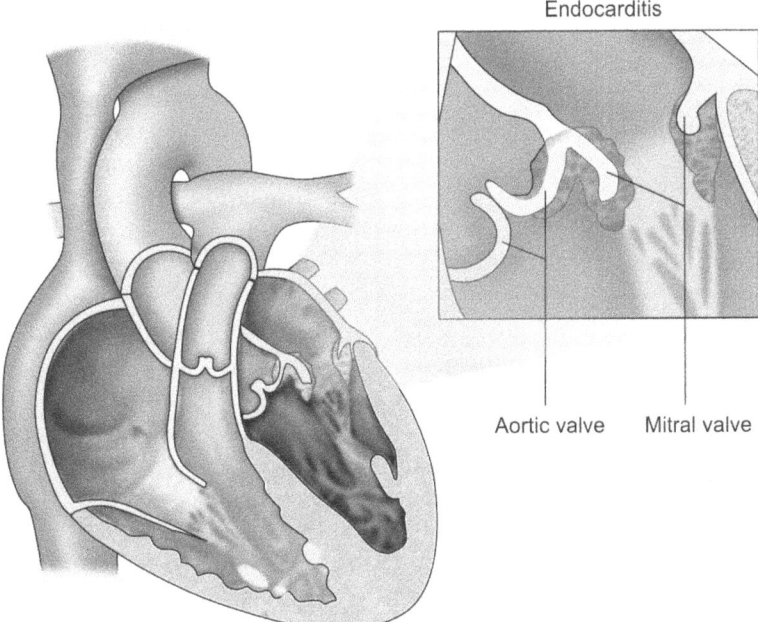

Fig. 7.9: Depicts inflamed endocardium and heart valves (Endocarditis).

2. ***Acute:*** It has a shorter clinical course and rapid in onset and the causative organism is more virulent.

Pathophysiology

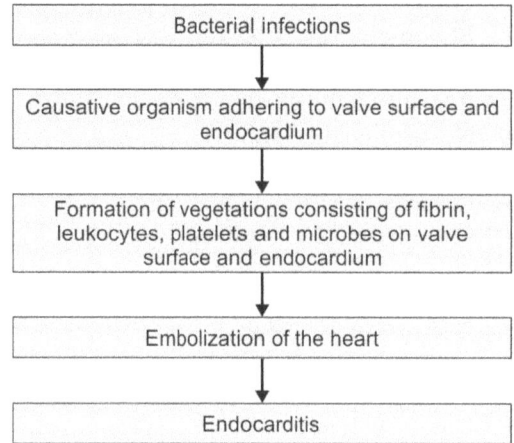

Clinical Features

- Fever and chills
- Weakness
- Night sweats
- Shortness of breath
- Malaise
- Fatigue
- Anorexia
- Aching joints and muscles
- Back pain
- Abdominal discomfort
- Weight loss
- Headache
- Clubbing of fingers
- Splinter hemorrhages (black longitudinal streaks)
- Petechiae in the conjunctiva, the lips, the buccal mucosa, the palate and over the ankles, the feet and the antecubital and popliteal areas.
- Osler's nodes (painful, tender, red or purple, pea-sized lesions) on the fingertips of toes.
- Janeway's lesions (flat, painless, small, red spots) may be found on the palms and soles.

Complications

- Heart failure
- Stroke
- Abscess of the spleen
- Aneurysm
- Infection in other parts of the body.

Diagnostic Tests

- History
- Physical examination
- Blood examination
- Chest X-ray
- Electrocardiogram
- Echocardiogram
- Cardiac catheterization
- Urine analysis.

Management

Medical

- **Antibiotics:** It inhibits the formation of peptidoglycan cross-inks in the bacterial cell wall and prevents any secondary infections. For example, penicillin G, ceftriaxone, amoxicillin, carbenicillin, cloxacillin, etc.
- **Antipyretics:** It causes the hypothalamus to override an interleukin-induced increase in fever and the body then works to lower the temperature, resulting in a reduction in fever. For example, acetaminophen, naproxen, ketoprofen, etc.
- **Antifungal agents:** It acts by binding to the ergosterol of the cell membrane of susceptible fungi and helps in preventing infection from fungal organisms. For example, amphotericin-B, amphocin, fungizone, etc.

Surgical

- **Valve replacement:** It is a procedure in which diseased valve is replaced with a new valve.
- **Valve repair:** It is a procedure in which mitral valves that become floppy and weak are surgically repaired.

Nursing
- Instruct the patient to pay attention to dental health.
- Instruct the patients to avoid procedures that may lead to skin infections such as body piercings or tattoos.
- Enforce prompt medical attention once they develop any type of skin infection or open cuts or sores that do not heal properly.

HYPERTENSION (SILENT KILLER)

Definition

Hypertension is sustained elevation of blood pressure (i.e., systolic blood pressure is equal to or greater than 140 mm Hg or diastolic blood pressure is equal to or greater than 90 mm Hg for extended periods of time) or it is a pressure generated in the peripheral channels (arteries) during contraction and relaxation of heart muscles.

Etiology

- Obstructive sleep apnea
- Kidney problems
- Adrenal gland tumors
- Thyroid problems
- Oral contraceptive pills
- Stress.

Risk Factors

- Age
- Alcohol
- Cigarette smoking
- Diabetes mellitus
- Fat-rich diet
- Excess dietary sodium
- Gender
- Family history
- Obesity
- Ethnicity
- Sedentary lifestyle or lack of exercise.

Classification

It was classified into two types as follows:
1. ***Primary (essential) hypertension:*** It has an elevated blood pressure without an identified cause and accounts for 90–95% of all cases.
2. ***Secondary (nonessential) hypertension:*** It has an elevated blood pressure with a specific identifiable cause and accounts for 5–10% of all cases.

Normal heart

Hypertensive heart

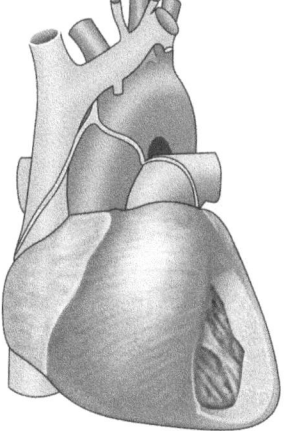
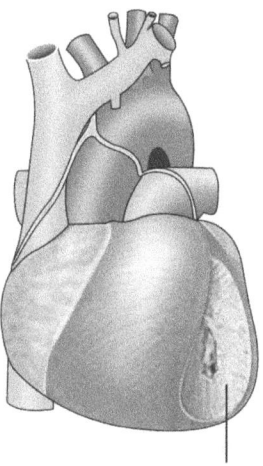

Thickening in walls of ventricles

Fig. 7.10: Shows the comparison of normal heart with that of thickened walls of the ventricles (Hypertensive heart).

Stages

It consists of three stages as follows:
- **Stage I**
  - Systolic BP → 140–159
  - Diastolic BP → 90–99.
- **Stage II**
  - Systolic BP → 140–159
  - Diastolic BP → 100–109.
- **Stage III**
  - Systolic BP → ≥180
  - Diastolic BP → ≥110.

Pathophysiology

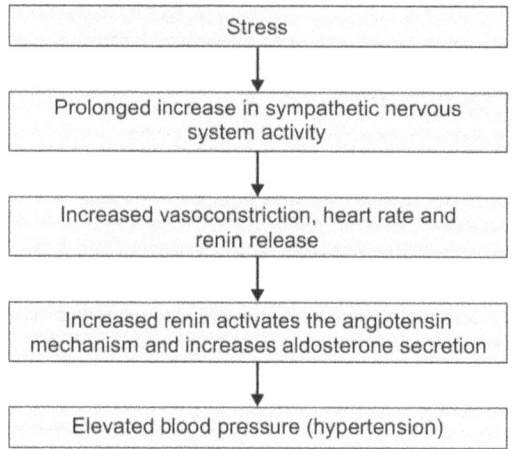

Clinical Features

- Fatigue
- Reduced activity tolerance
- Dizziness
- Palpitations
- Lightheadedness
- Tinnitus
- Visual disturbances
- Epistaxis
- Dyspnea.

Complications

- Coronary artery disease
- Left ventricular hypertrophy
- Heart failure
- Cerebrovascular disease
- Peripheral vascular disease
- Nephrosclerosis
- Retinal damage.

Diagnostic Tests

- History
- Physical examination
- Chest X-ray
- Serum electrolytes
- BUN and serum creatinine
- Serum lipid profile
- Complete blood count
- Electrocardiogram.

Management

Medical

- **Angiotensin-converting enzyme (ACE) inhibitors:** It prevents an enzyme in the body from producing angiotensin II, a substance in the body that narrows the blood vessels and releases hormones that raises the blood pressure. For example, captopril, enalapril, fosinopril, etc.
- **Beta blockers:** It helps blood vessels relax and open up to improve blood flow into the coronary artery. It works by blocking the effects of the hormone epinephrine, also known as adrenaline. As a result, the heart beats more slowly and with less force, thereby reducing blood pressure. For example, propranolol, metoprolol, atenolol, etc.
- **Angiotensin II receptor blockers (ARBs):** It lowers blood pressure and systemic vascular resistance. For example, losartan.
- **Calcium channel blockers:** It relaxes and widens blood vessels by affecting the muscle cells in the arterial walls and thus increases blood flow into the heart. For example, diltiazem, verapamil, nicardipine, etc.
- **Aldosterone antagonists:** It inhibits sodium resorption in the collecting duct of the nephron in the kidneys. This interferes

with sodium/potassium exchange, reducing urinary potassium excretion and increases water excretion (diuresis). For example, spironolactone, mexrenone, etc.
- **Thiazide diuretics:** It mobilizes edematous fluid, thereby reducing pulmonary venous pressure and in turn reduces preload. For example, metolazone, furosemide, etc.
- **Vasodilators:** It reduces the workload of the heart. For example, hydralazine, isosorbide dinitrate, etc.
- **Renin inhibitors:** It slows down the production of renin, an enzyme produced by the kidneys that starts a chain of chemical steps that increases blood pressure. For example, aliskiren, etc.
- **Alpha blockers:** It reduces nerve impulses to blood vessels, reducing the effects of natural chemicals that narrow blood vessels. For example, doxazosin, prazosin, etc.
- **Adrenergic inhibitors:** It prevents the brain from signaling the nervous system to increase the heart rate and narrow the blood vessels. For example, clonidine, guanfacine, methyldopa, etc.

Nursing

- Instruct the patient to eat a healthier diet with less salt.
- Instruct the patient not to smoke.
- Motivate the patients to have their blood pressure and cholesterol checked regularly.
- Instruct the patient to maintain a healthy weight.
- Encourage the patient to do regular exercise.

HYPOTENSION

Definition

Hypotension is defined as a systolic pressure of 90 mm Hg or below or as a 20% decrease from the patient's baseline measurement.

Etiology

- Fatigue
- Decreased preload secondary to hypovolemia
- Failure of the heart muscle to pump adequate blood
- Reduced peripheral vascular resistance
- Blood loss or inadequate fluid replacement
- Severe infection (septicemia)
- Severe allergic reaction (anaphylaxis)
- Lack of nutrients in the diet
- Ischemia
- Hypoxia
- Myocardial infarction
- Dysrhythmias
- Congestive heart failure
- Pregnancy
- Endocrine problems.

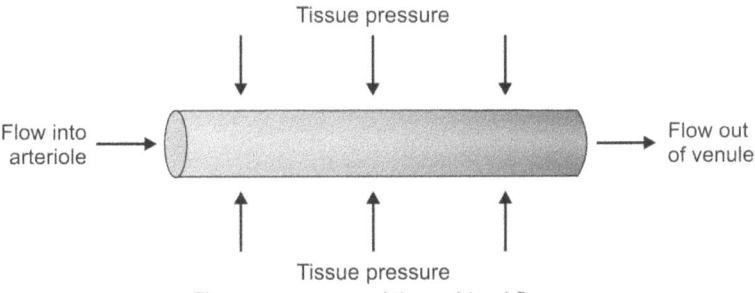

Fig. 7.11: Depicts hypotensive heart with a systolic pressure of 90 mm Hg or below.

Risk Factors

- Advancement in age
- Parkinson's disease
- Diabetes
- Certain medications (Alpha blockers).

Types

- ***Orthostatic or postural hypotension:*** This is a sudden drop in blood pressure when we stand up from a sitting position or if we stand up after lying down. It can occur for a variety of reasons, including dehydration, prolonged bedrest, pregnancy, diabetes, heart problems, burns, excessive heat, large varicose veins and certain neurological disorders.
- ***Postprandial hypotension:*** Postprandial hypotension is a sudden drop in blood pressure after eating. It affects mostly older adults. It is more likely to affect people with high blood pressure or autonomic nervous system disorders such as Parkinson's disease.
- ***Neurally mediated hypotension:*** This disorder causes blood pressure to drop after standing for long periods, leading to signs and symptoms such as dizziness, nausea and fainting. It mostly affects young people, and it seems to occur because of a miscommunication between the heart and the brain.
- ***Multiple system atrophy with orthostatic hypotension (also known as Shy-Drager syndrome):*** It causes progressive damage to the autonomic nervous system, which controls involuntary functions such as blood pressure, heart rate, breathing and digestion. It was associated with muscle tremors, slowed movement, problems with coordination and speech, and incontinence, its main characteristic is severe orthostatic hypotension in combination with very high blood pressure when lying down.

Pathophysiology

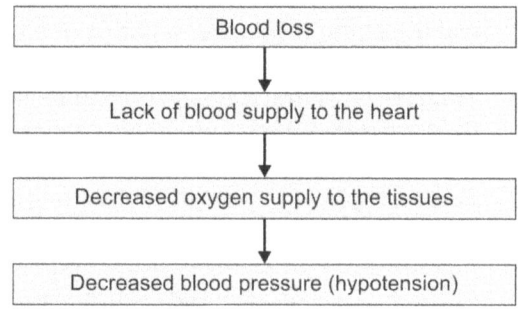

Clinical Features

- Increased heart rate
- Lack of concentration
- Blurred vision
- Nausea
- Cold, clammy, pale skin
- Rapid shallow breathing
- Fatigue
- Decreased urinary output
- Confusion
- Restlessness
- Thirst.

Complications

- Damages to heart and brain
- Risk of injury from falls
- Syncope (fainting)
- Dizziness or lightheadedness.

Diagnostic Tests

- History
- Physical examination
- Complete blood count
- Electrocardiogram
- Echocardiogram
- Stress test
- Tilt table test
- Valsalva maneuver test.

Management

Medical

- **Glucocorticoids:** It is an adrenal cortical steroid that has very high levels of

mineralocorticoid activity and moderate levels of glucocorticoid activity as it helps boosting blood volume, which raises blood pressure. For example, fludrocortisone, etc.
- **Antihypotensive/Vasopressor:** It raises standing blood pressure levels in people with chronic orthostatic hypotension by restricting the ability of our blood vessels to expand, which raises blood pressure. For example, midodrine hydrochloride, etc.

Nursing

- Instruct the patient to eat a healthier diet with adequate salt in it.
- Instruct the patient to drink more water.
- Ask the patient to go slowly while changing body positions.
- Educate the patient to eat small and low carbohydrate diet.
- Instruct the patient to maintain a healthy weight.

MYOCARDIAL INFARCTION

Definition

Myocardial infarction (also known as heart attack) is a devastating condition in which the myocardial cells in the heart are permanently destroyed and may lead to death of heart muscle.

Etiology

- Thrombosis (blood clot)
- Atheroma within the lining of the artery
- Coronary vasospasm
- Stab wound to the heart
- Blood clot forming elsewhere in the body (heart chamber)
- Cocaine intake
- Complications from heart surgery
- Elevated LDL ("bad") cholesterol
- Accumulation of homocysteine
- Inflammation.

Risk Factors

- Advancement in age
- Being men
- Diabetes
- Smoking
- High blood pressure
- Obesity
- High-fat diet
- Family history of heart attack
- Lack of exercise
- Stress.

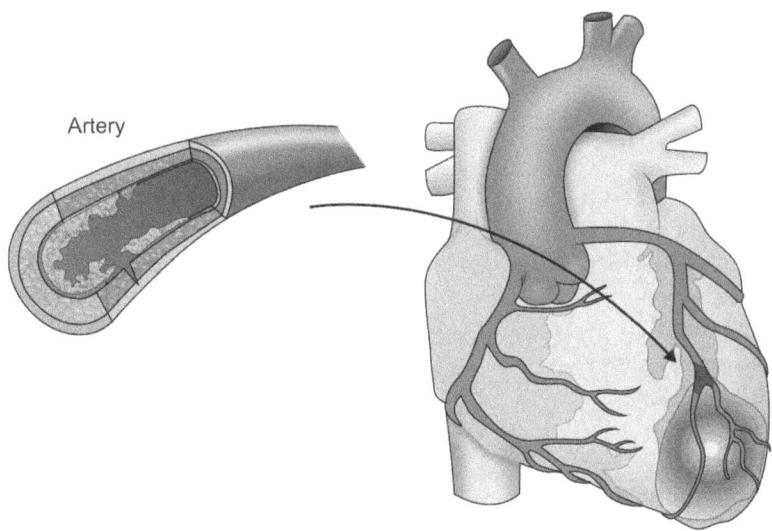

Fig. 7.12: Shows the destructed myocardial cells in the heart that leads to death of heart muscle (Myocardial infarction).

Pathophysiology

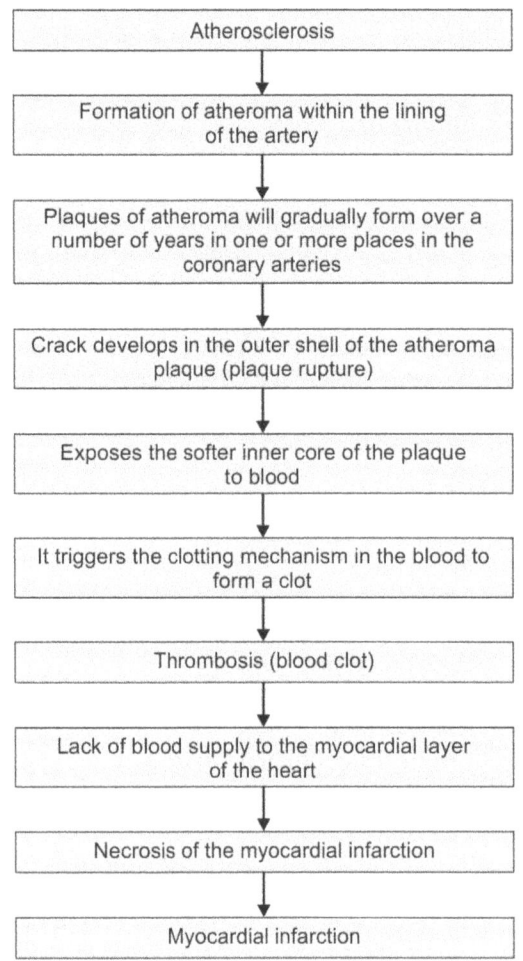

Clinical Features

- Squeezing pain, heaviness, tightness, pressure in center of chest
- Crushing chest pain which radiates to arm, shoulder, neck, jaw or back
- Shortness of breath
- Dizziness and weakness
- Nausea and vomiting
- Sweating
- Irregular heartbeat
- Feeling of impending doom
- Heartburn or pain in the abdomen
- Unusual fatigue
- Clammy skin.

Complications

- Dysrhythmias
- Heart failure
- Valvular insufficiency
- Cardiogenic shock.

Diagnostic Tests

- History
- Physical examination
- Complete blood count
- Electrocardiogram
- Echocardiogram
- Chest X-ray
- Stress test
- Coronary catheterization.

Management

Medical

- **Nitrates:** It relaxes and widens the blood vessels allowing more blood to flow into the heart muscle. For example, nitroglycerin, Nitrostat, Nitroquick, etc.
- **Aspirin:** It reduces the ability of the blood to clot, making it easier for blood to flow through narrowed heart arteries. For example, Astrix, Aspro, etc.
- **Beta blockers:** It helps blood vessels relax and open up to improve blood flow into the coronary artery. It works by blocking the effects of the hormone epinephrine, also known as adrenaline. As a result, the heart beats more slowly and with less force, thereby reducing blood pressure. For example, propranolol, metoprolol, atenolol, etc.
- **Bile acid sequestrants:** It binds bile acids in the intestine and increases the excretion of bile acids in the stool. This reduces the amount of bile acids returning to the liver and forces the liver to produce more bile acids to replace the bile acids lost in the stool. In order to produce more bile acids, the liver converts more cholesterol into bile acids, which lowers the level of cholesterol in the blood. For example, colestipol, cholestyramine, colesevelam, etc.

- **Fibrates (fibric acid derivatives):** It lowers blood triglyceride levels by reducing the liver's production of VLDL (the triglyceride-carrying particle that circulates in the blood) and by speeding up the removal of triglycerides from the blood. For example, gemfibrozil, fenofibrate, etc.
- **Glycoprotein receptor inhibitors:** It works by preventing platelet aggregation and thrombus formation in the blood vessels facilitating blood into the narrowed heart arteries. For example, abciximab, eptifibatide, tirofiban, etc.
- **Niacin:** It helps in lowering cholesterol and triglycerides. For example, Niaspan, Niacor, etc.
- **Ezetimibe:** It reduces blood cholesterol by inhibiting the absorption of cholesterol in the small intestine. For example, ezetrol, zetia, etc.
- **Statins or HMG-CoA reductase inhibitors:** These are drugs used to lower blood cholesterol by inhibiting the enzyme HMG-CoA reductase. It also helps the body to reabsorb cholesterol that has accumulated in plaques in the artery walls, helps in preventing further blockage in the blood vessels. For example, atorvastatin, lovastatin, simvastatin, etc.
- **Calcium channel blockers:** It relaxes and widens blood vessels by affecting the muscle cells in the arterial walls and thus increases blood flow into the heart. For example, diltiazem, verapamil, nicardipine, etc.
- **Angiotensin converting enzyme (ACE) inhibitors:** It prevents an enzyme in the body from producing angiotensin II, a substance in the body that narrows the blood vessels and releases hormones that raise the blood pressure. For example, captopril, enalapril, fosinopril, etc.
- **Blood-thinning agents:** It helps in preventing blood clots from forming by making the blood platelets less likely to stick together. For example, clopidogrel, warfarin, heparin, etc.
- **Analgesics:** It relieves pain, decreases anxiety, opens bronchioles and reduces preload and afterload and increases blood supply and oxygen to the myocardium. For example, morphine sulphate, etc.
- **Thrombolytics:** They dissolve blood clots by activating plasminogen, which forms a cleaved product called plasmin. Plasmin is a proteolytic enzyme that is capable of breaking cross-links between fibrin molecules, which provide the structural integrity of blood clots. For example, tissue plasminogen activator (t-PA), streptokinase, anistreplase, urokinase, etc.

Surgical

- **Percutaneous transluminous coronary angioplasty (PTCA):** It helps in compressing the plaque against the walls of the artery and dilutes the vessel.
- **Coronary artery bypass grafting (CABG):** It helps in improving blood flow to the myocardial tissue that is at risk for ischemia or infarction because of the occluded artery.

Nursing

- Encourage the patient to take a diet low in cholesterol and saturated fats to reduce the risk of atherosclerosis.
- Instruct the patient not to smoke.
- Motivate the patient to have their blood pressure and cholesterol checked regularly.
- Instruct the patient to maintain a healthy weight.
- Encourage the patient to do regular exercise.

MYOCARDITIS

Definition

It refers to an inflammatory process involving the myocardium, can cause heart dilation, thrombi on the heart wall (mural thrombi), infiltration of circulating blood cells around the coronary vessels and between the muscle fibers and degeneration of the muscle fibers themselves.

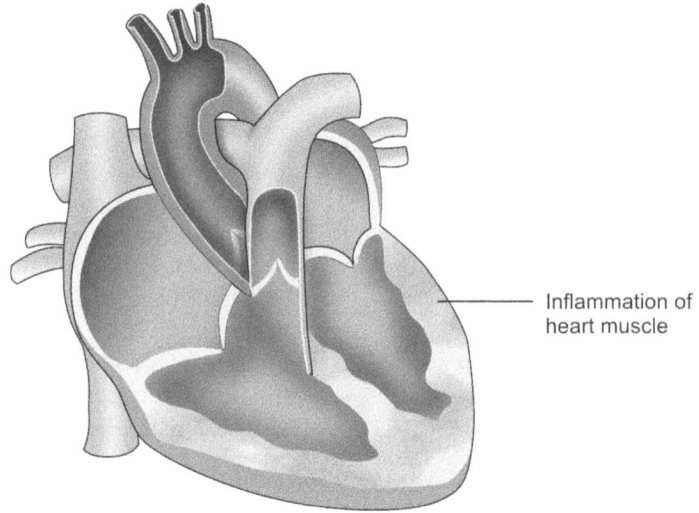

Fig. 7.13: Depicts inflamed myocardial cells in the heart (Myocarditis).

Etiology

- Viral infections (Coxsackie, Cytomegalovirus, Hepatitis C, Herpes, HIV, Parvovirus)
- Bacterial infections (*Chlamydia, Mycoplasma, Streptococcus, Treponema*)
- Fungal infections (*Aspergillus, Candida, Coccidioides, Cryptococcus, Histoplasma*)
- Allergic reactions to certain medicines or toxins (alcohol, cocaine, certain chemotherapy drugs, heavy metals and catecholamines)
- Being around certain chemicals
- Rheumatoid arthritis
- Sarcoidosis
- Debilitation
- Prolonged use of immunosuppressive agents
- After acute systemic infections such as rheumatic fever
- Increased invasive diagnostic procedures
- Prolonged IV antibiotic therapy
- Dental surgery
- Long-term use of steroids.

Risk Factors

- Patients with infective endocarditis
- Previous history of a heart attack
- An abnormal or damaged heart valve
- An artificial heart valve
- Congenital heart defects.

Pathophysiology

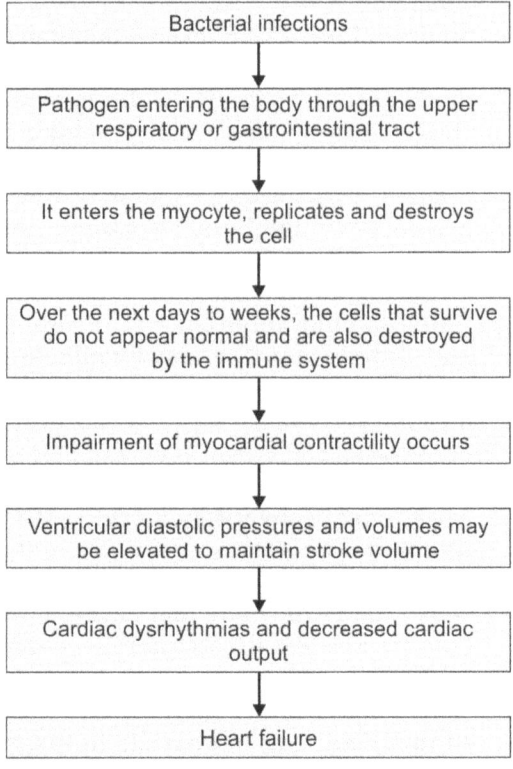

Clinical Features

- Abnormal heartbeat
- Chest pain that may resemble a heart attack
- Fatigue

- Fever
- Headache
- Muscle aches
- Sore throat
- Diarrhea or rashes
- Joint pain or swelling
- Leg swelling
- Shortness of breath
- Fainting
- Low urine output
- Fluid retention or swelling in the feet or legs.

Complications

- Cardiomyopathy
- Heart failure
- Pericarditis.

Diagnostic Tests

- History
- Physical examination
- Blood examination
- Blood culture
- Electrocardiogram
- Chest X-ray
- Echocardiogram
- Heart muscle biopsy (endomyocardial biopsy).

Management

Medical

- **Antibiotics:** It helps to prevent any secondary infection due to a bacterial agent. For example, benzyl penicillin, etc.
- **Angiotensin-converting enzyme (ACE) inhibitors:** It prevents an enzyme in the body from producing angiotensin II, a substance in the body that narrows the blood vessels and releases hormones that raise the blood pressure. For example, captopril, enalapril, fosinopril, etc.
- **Blood-thinning agents:** It helps in preventing blood clots from forming by making the blood platelets less likely to stick together. For example, clopidogrel, warfarin, heparin, etc.
- **Anti-inflammatory agents:** It helps to block the flow of pain signals from the central nervous system and thereby relieves pain and swelling. For example, Aspirin, ibuprofen, etc.
- **Corticosteroids:** It suppresses the immune system which mistakenly attacks its own tissues thereby reduces the severity of the disease. For example, dexamethasone, prednisone, etc.
- **Diuretics:** It mobilizes edematous fluid, thereby reducing pulmonary venous pressure and in turn reduces preload. For example, metolazone, furosemide, etc.

Surgical

Implantable cardioverter-defibrillator (ICD): It is a device that monitors the heart rhythm and delivers electric shocks when needed to control abnormal heart rhythms.

Nursing

- Instruct the patient to take complete bedrest as it reduces myocardial oxygen demand.
- Provide psychological support while the patient is confined to hospital or home with restrictive intravenous therapy.
- Instruct the patient and family about activity restrictions, medications, and signs and symptoms of infection.
- Instruct the patient to do proper oral hygiene.
- Provide postsurgical care and instruction if the patient received surgical treatment.

PERICARDITIS

Definition

It refers to an inflammation of the pericardium, the membranous sac enveloping the heart.

Etiology

- Viral infections
- Bacterial infections
- Fungal infections
- Tuberculosis
- Uremia (presence of nitrogenous wastes in blood)

Disorders of Cardiac System

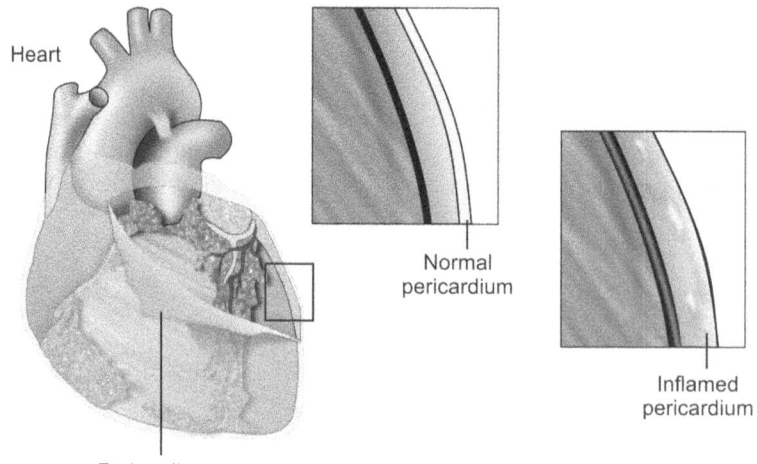

Fig. 7.14: Shows the normal pericardium with that of inflamed pericardium in the heart (Pericarditis).

- Acute myocardial infarction
- Neoplasm
- Trauma
- Dissecting aortic aneurysm
- Myxedema
- Rheumatic fever
- Rheumatic arthritis
- Ankylosing spondylitis (inflammatory condition affecting spine and the joints later)
- Post-myocardial infarction (Dressler syndrome)
- Renal failure.

Risk Factors

- Hypothyroidism
- Previous history of a heart attack
- Exposure to medications.

Types

Acute pericarditis: Inflammation can develop suddenly in acute pericarditis.

Chronic pericarditis: Inflammation develops gradually and is long-lasting in chronic pericarditis.

Constrictive pericarditis: In this type of pericarditis, the layers of the pericardium stiffen and develop scar tissue. The scar tissue thickens and sticks together. This makes it difficult for the heart to pump and work as it normally does.

Pathophysiology

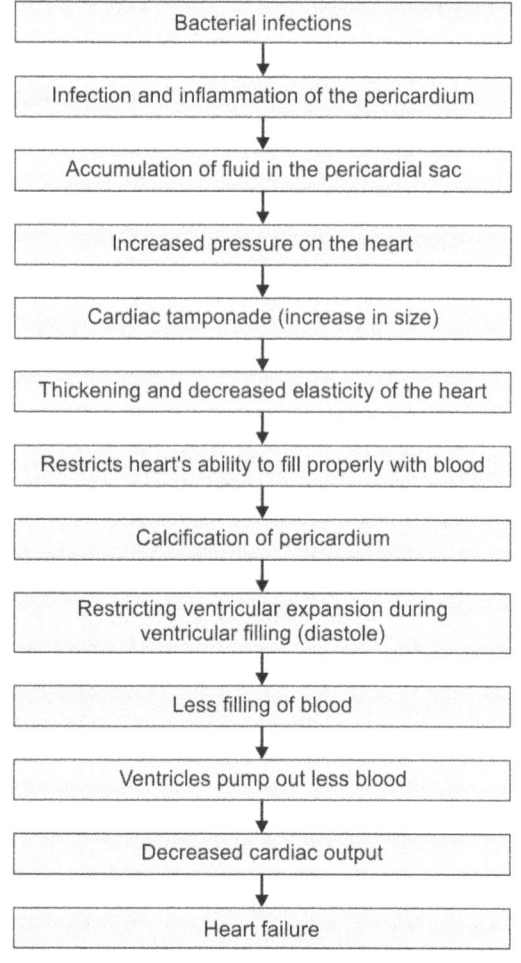

Clinical Features

- Pericardial pain in the anterior chest that radiates to the left side of the neck, shoulder or back.
- Pericardial friction rubs (high-pitched sound)
- Pain that is aggravated by breathing (particularly inspiration), coughing and swallowing.
- Pain is worse when in the supine position and may be relieved by learning forward.
- Dyspnea on exertion
- Low-grade fever
- Chills
- Malaise
- Fatigue
- Lower extremity edema
- Ascites
- Weight loss
- Elevated jugular venous pressure
- Heart palpitations.

Complications

- Pericardial effusion
- Cardiac tamponade
- Constrictive pericarditis.

Diagnostic Tests

- History
- Physical examination
- Blood examination
- Electrocardiogram
- Chest X-ray
- Echocardiogram
- Pericardial biopsy
- CT scan
- Cardiac magnetic resonance imaging (MRI) scan.

Management

Medical

- **Antibiotics:** It helps to prevent any secondary infection due to a bacterial agent. For example, benzyl penicillin, etc.
- **Analgesics:** It helps to block the flow of pain signals from the central nervous system and thereby relieves pain. For example, aspirin, ibuprofen, etc.
- **Antigout agents:** It responds to uric acid crystals, which reduces swelling and pain. For example, colchicine, etc.
- **Corticosteroids:** It suppresses the immune system which mistakenly attacks its own tissues thereby reduces the severity of the disease. For example, dexamethasone, prednisone, etc.
- **Diuretics:** It mobilizes edematous fluid, thereby reducing pulmonary venous pressure and in turn reduces preload. For example, metolazone, furosemide, etc.

Surgical

- **Pericardiocentesis:** It is a surgical procedure in which a sterile needle or a small tube (catheter) is inserted to remove and drain the excess fluid from the pericardial cavity.
- **Pericardiectomy:** It is a surgical procedure in which the entire pericardium that has become rigid and is making it hard for the heart to pump is removed.

Nursing

- Instruct the patient to take complete bed rest.
- Educate the patient to restrict the activity until pain subsides.
- Instruct the patient to take the medications properly.
- Instruct the patient not to smoke.
- Educate the patient to maintain a healthy weight.
- Instruct the patient to follow an exercise program.

RHEUMATIC FEVER

Definition

Rheumatic fever is an inflammatory disease of the heart potentially involving all layers

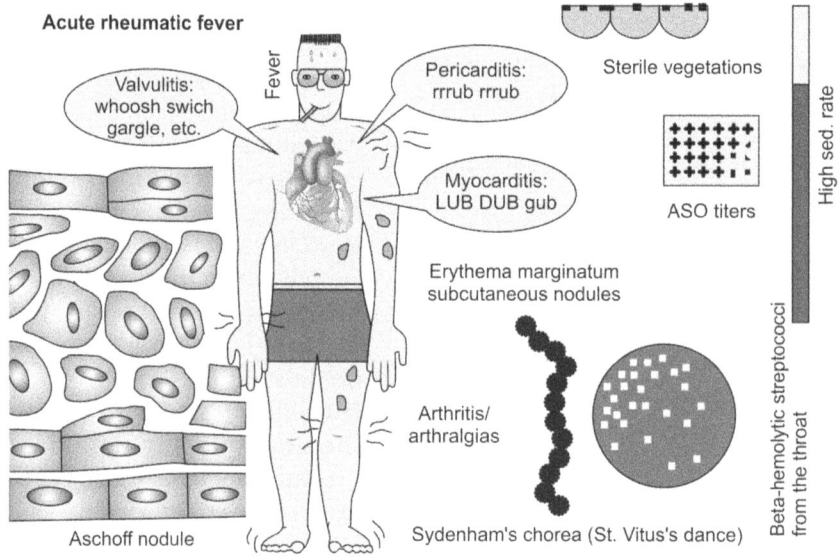

Fig. 7.15: Depicts the cardinal features of rheumatic fever.

(endocardium, myocardium and pericardium). The resulting damage to the heart from rheumatic fever is termed rheumatic heart disease, a chronic condition characterized by scarring and deformity of the heart valves.

Etiology
- Occurs 2–3 weeks after group A beta hemolytic streptococcal infection
- Pharyngeal infection
- Altered immune response.

Risk Factors
- Poverty
- Overcrowding
- Reduced access to medical care
- Children aged 5–15 years
- Underdeveloped or developing countries
- Family history
- Environmental factors
- Type of streptococcal bacteria.

Pathophysiology

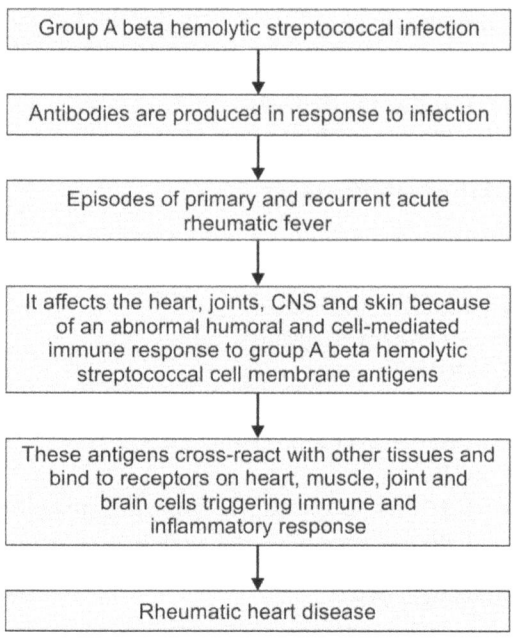

Clinical Features

As per Jones criteria.

Major Manifestations

- Carditis (heart inflammation)
- Polyarthritis (arthritis in several joints)
- Erythema marginatum (skin rash)
- Subcutaneous nodules or Aschoff bodies (nodules under the skin)
- Sydenham's chorea (rapid, jerky movements).

Minor Manifestations

- Fever
- Arthralgia
- Previous rheumatic heart disease
- Prolonged P-R interval on electrocardiogram
- Elevated ESR
- Abdominal pain
- Tachycardia
- Epistaxis.

Complications

- Chronic rheumatic carditis
- Rheumatic endocarditis
- Valve stenosis
- Valve regurgitation
- Damage to heart muscle
- Atrial fibrillation
- Heart failure.

Diagnostic Tests

- History
- Physical examination
- Blood examination
- Chest X-ray
- Echocardiogram
- Electrocardiogram
- Magnetic resonance imaging (MRI).

Management

Medical

- **Antibiotics:** It helps to prevent any secondary infection due to a bacterial agent. For example, penicillin, procaine penicillin, benzathine penicillin, etc.
- **Corticosteroids:** It suppresses the immune system which mistakenly attacks its own tissues thereby reduces the severity of the disease. For example, dexamethasone, prednisone, etc.
- **Nonsteroidal anti-inflammatory agents:** It helps to block the flow of pain signals from the central nervous system and thereby relieves pain. For example, aspirin, ibuprofen, naproxen, etc.
- **Anticonvulsants:** It helps in controlling the involuntary movements resulting from Sydenham's chorea. For example, valproic acid, carbamazepine, etc.

Nursing

- Provide patients with optimal bedrest to reduce cardiac overload.
- Position the patient comfortably in proper alignment.
- Provide psychological support to the patient.
- Encourage good nutrition and hygienic practices.

VALVULAR HEART DISEASE

Definition

Valvular heart disease is characterized by damage to or a defect in one of the four heart valves—the mitral, aortic, tricuspid or pulmonary.

Etiology

- Birth defects
- Infective endocarditis
- Rheumatic fever
- Age-related changes
- Heart attacks
- Coronary artery disease
- Cardiomyopathy
- Syphilis
- Hypertension
- Aortic aneurysms
- Atherosclerosis
- Myxomatous degeneration
- Lupus (a chronic autoimmune disorder).

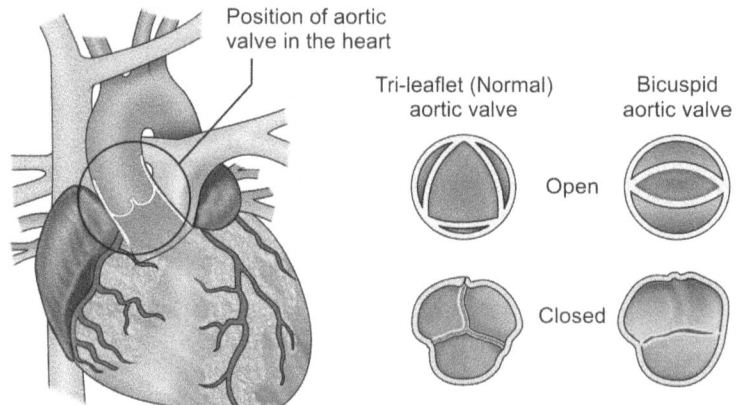

Fig. 7.16: Shows the comparison of normal heart valves with that of damaged or defective heart valves (Valvular heart disease).

Risk Factors

- Poverty
- Overcrowding
- Reduced access to medical care
- Children aged 5–15 years
- Underdeveloped or developing countries
- Family history
- Environmental factors
- Type of streptococcal bacteria.

Types

Aortic Regurgitation (AR)

Definition

It is incompetency of the aortic valve causing backflow from the aorta into the left ventricle during diastole.

Etiology

- Valvular degeneration and aortic root dilation (with or without a bicuspid valve)
- Rheumatic fever
- Endocarditis
- Myxomatous degeneration
- Aortic root dissection
- Connective tissue disorder (e.g., Marfan syndrome)
- Rheumatologic disorders.

Pathophysiology

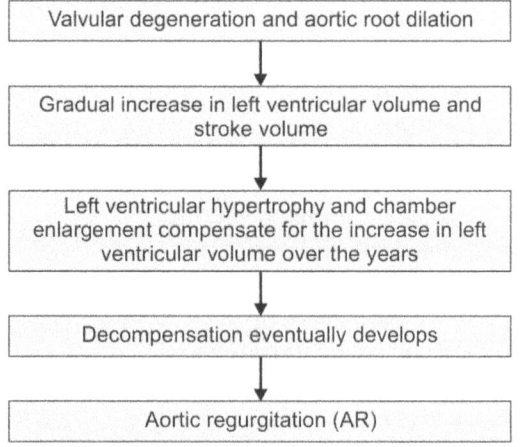

Clinical Features

- Exertional dyspnea
- Orthopnea
- Paroxysmal nocturnal dyspnea
- Palpitations
- Chest pain
- Widened pulse pressure
- Early diastolic murmur.

Diagnostic Tests

- History
- Physical examination
- Echocardiography.

Treatment
- Aortic valve replacement or repair
- Percutaneous valve replacement.

Aortic Stenosis (AS)

Definition

It is narrowing of the aortic valve, obstructing blood flow from the left ventricle to the ascending aorta during systole.

Etiology
- Congenital bicuspid valve
- Idiopathic degenerative sclerosis with calcification
- Rheumatic fever.

Pathophysiology

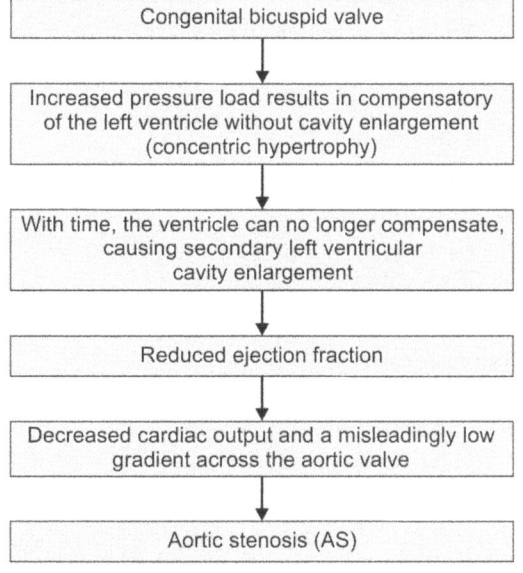

Clinical Features
- Syncope
- Angina
- Exertional dyspnea
- Heart failure
- Arrhythmias
- A crescendo-decrescendo ejection murmur.

Diagnostic Tests
- History
- Physical examination
- Echocardiography.

Treatment
- Surgical valve replacement (once symptoms develop)
- Balloon valvotomy (in severe cases).

Mitral Valve Prolapse (MVP)

Definition

It is a billowing of mitral valve leaflets into the left atrium during systole.

Etiology

Idiopathic myxomatous degeneration.

Pathophysiology

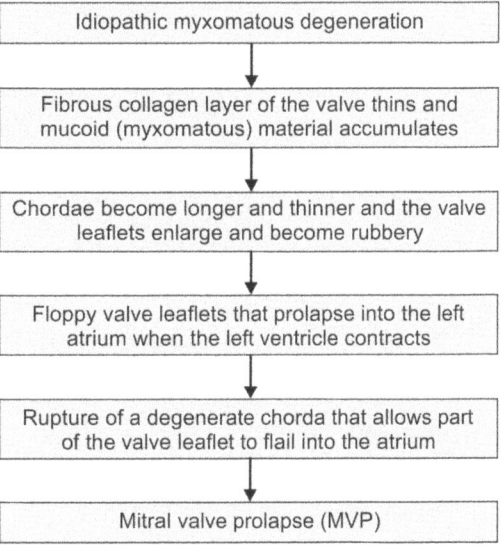

Clinical Features
- Chest pain
- Dyspnea
- Dizziness
- Palpitations
- Crisp midsystolic click followed by a late-systolic murmur.

Diagnostic Tests
- History
- Physical examination
- Echocardiography.

Treatment
- Valvuloplasty
- Valve replacement.

Mitral Regurgitation (MR)

Definition

It is incompetency of the mitral valve causing flow from the left ventricle (LV) into the left atrium during ventricular systole.

Etiology
- Mitral valve prolapse
- Rheumatic fever
- Left ventricular dilation or infarction.

Pathophysiology

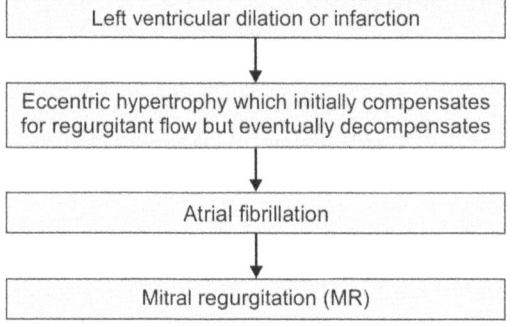

Clinical Features
- Dyspnea
- Palpitations
- Holosystolic murmur.

Diagnostic Tests
- History
- Physical examination
- Echocardiography.

Treatment

Mitral valve repair or replacement.

Mitral Stenosis (MS)

Definition

It is narrowing of the mitral orifice that impedes blood flow from the left atrium to the left ventricle.

Etiology

Rheumatic fever.

Pathophysiology

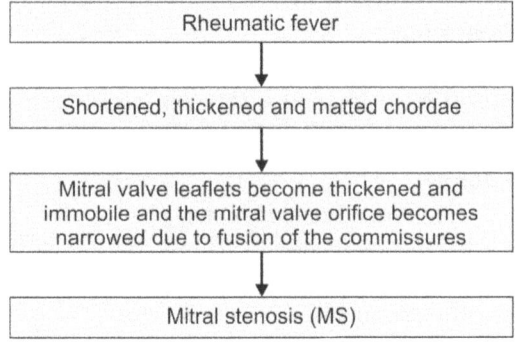

Clinical Features
- Pulmonary hypertension
- Atrial fibrillation
- Thromboembolism
- Heart failure
- Opening snap and a diastolic murmur.

Diagnostic Tests
- History
- Physical examination
- Echocardiography.

Treatment
- Balloon commissurotomy
- Surgical commissurotomy
- Valve replacement.

Pulmonic Regurgitation (PR)

Definition

It is incompetency of the pulmonic valve causing blood flow from the pulmonary artery into the right ventricle during diastole.

Etiology

Pulmonary hypertension.

Pathophysiology

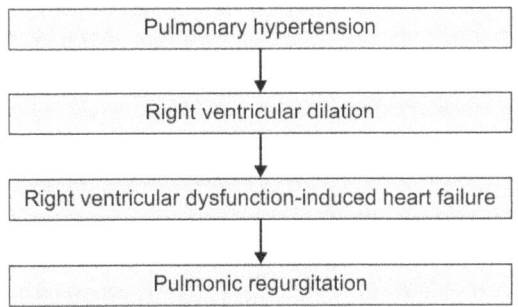

Clinical Features
Decrescendo diastolic murmur.

Diagnostic Tests
- History
- Physical examination
- Echocardiography.

Treatment
No specific treatment.

Pulmonic Stenosis (PS)

Definition
It is narrowing of the pulmonary outflow tract causing obstruction of blood flow from the right ventricle to the pulmonary artery during systole.

Etiology
Congenital.

Pathophysiology

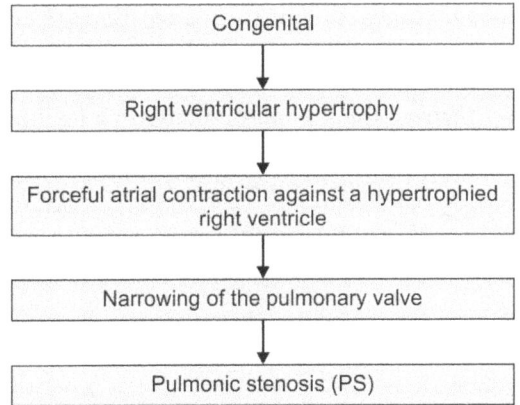

Clinical Features
Crescendo-decrescendo ejection murmur.

Diagnostic Tests
- History
- Physical examination
- Echocardiography.

Treatment
Balloon valvuloplasty.

Tricuspid Regurgitation (TR)

Definition
It is insufficiency of the tricuspid valve causing blood flow from the right ventricle to the right atrium during systole.

Etiology
Dilation of the right ventricle.

Pathophysiology

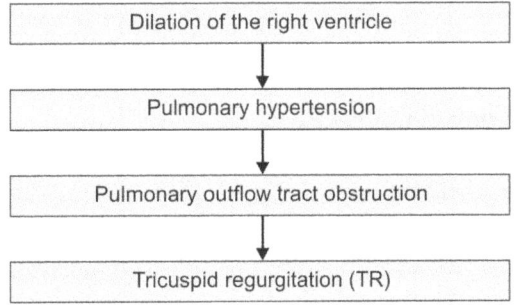

Clinical Features
- Neck pulsations
- Holosystolic murmur
- Right ventricular-induced heart failure
- Atrial fibrillation.

Diagnostic Tests
- History
- Physical examination
- Echocardiography.

Treatment
- Annuloplasty
- Valve repair or replacement.

Tricuspid Stenosis (TS)

Definition
It is narrowing of the tricuspid orifice that obstructs blood flow from the right atrium to the right ventricle.

Etiology
Rheumatic fever.

Pathophysiology

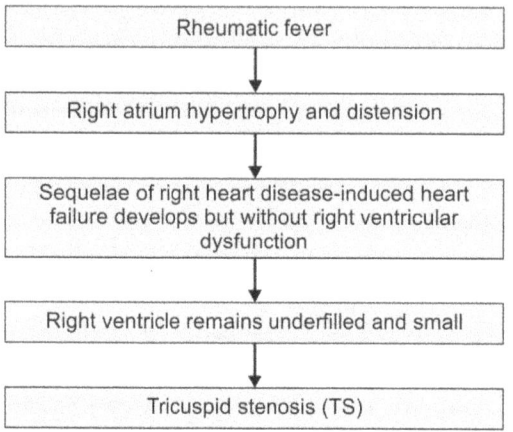

Clinical Features
- Fluttering discomfort in the neck
- Fatigue
- Cold skin
- Right upper quadrant abdominal discomfort
- Prominent jugular pulsations
- Presystolic murmur is often heard at the left sternal edge in the 4th intercostal space and is increased during inspiration.

Diagnostic Tests
- History
- Physical examination
- Echocardiography.

Treatment
No specific treatment.

Complications
- Heart failure
- Heart attack
- Stroke
- Aneurysm
- Peripheral artery disease
- Sudden cardiac arrest.

Management
In general, medical and surgical treatment for valvular heart disease includes:

Medical

If lifestyle changes alone are not enough, the doctor may prescribe medications to control the heart disease. The type of medication will depend on the type of heart disease.

Surgical

If medications are not enough, it is possible that the doctor will recommend specific procedures or surgery. The type of procedure will depend on the type of heart disease and the extent of the damage to the heart.

Nursing

- Instruct the patient not to smoke.
- Motivate the patients to have their blood pressure and cholesterol checked regularly.
- Instruct the patient to maintain a healthy weight.
- Encourage the patient to do regular exercise.

CHAPTER 8

Disorders of Vascular System

CHAPTER OUTLINE

- Acute blood loss
- Anemia
- Hemochromatosis
- Hemophilia
- Raynaud's phenomenon
- Thromboangiitis obliterans (Buerger's disease)
- Varicose veins
- Venous thrombosis
- Von Willebrand disease

ACUTE BLOOD LOSS

Definition

Acute blood loss is a state of vascular instability caused by external or internal hemorrhage and is a life-threatening condition that results when we lose more than 20% of our body's blood volume.

Etiology

- Accident
- Surgery
- Childbirth
- Stomach ulcers
- Blood vessel rupture
- Heavy menstrual bleeding for a long time.

Risk Factors

- Being women
- Certain conditions (e.g., Hemophilia, etc.)
- Certain medications (e.g., Warfarin, etc.)
- Older adults.

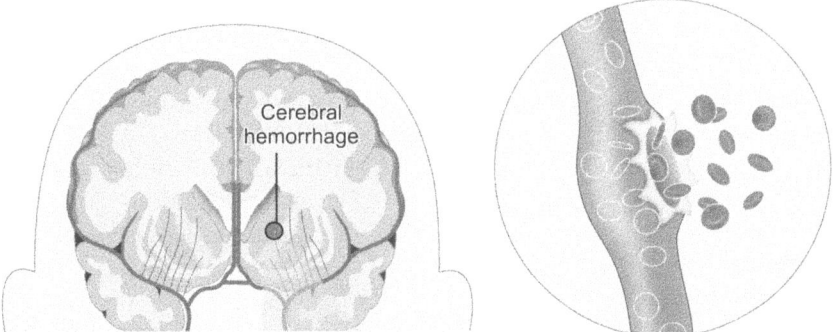

Fig. 8.1: Depicts blood loss by internal and external hemorrhage.

Pathophysiology

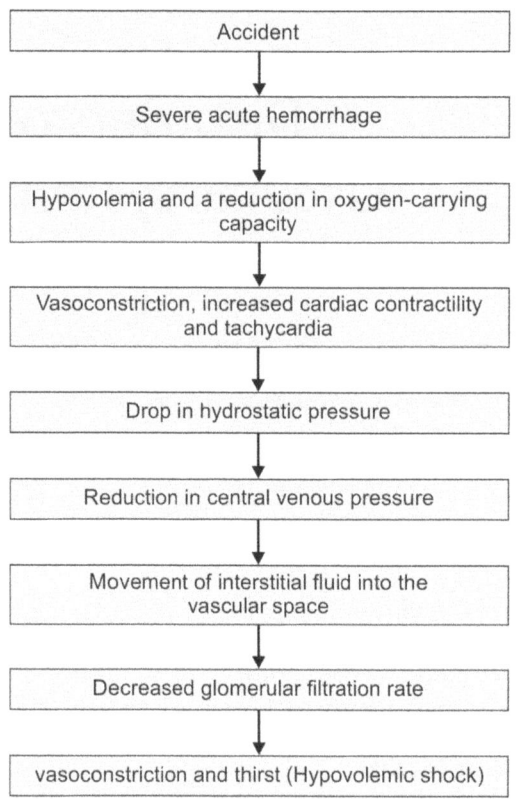

Clinical Features

- Bleeding coming from a break in the skin
- Pain at the injured site
- Bruising
- Cool, clammy skin
- Dizziness, weakness or confusion
- Headache
- Fatigue
- Fast, weak pulse
- Rapid heart rate
- Paleness
- Rapid, shallow breathing
- Nausea
- Blood vomiting
- Little or no urine output
- Profuse sweating
- Lightheadedness
- Extreme thirst
- Loss of consciousness.

Complications

- Hypovolemic shock
- Organ damage
- Heart attack
- Death.

Diagnostic Tests

- History
- Physical examination
- Blood examination
- Liver function test
- Kidney function test
- Echocardiogram
- Electrocardiogram
- Endoscopic examination
- Computed tomography (CT) scan
- Magnetic resonance imaging (MRI) scan.

Management

Medical

- **Sympathomimetic agents:** It is used to treat shock and low blood pressure caused by trauma. For example, dopamine, etc.
- **Inotropic agent:** Aminocaproic acid, Tranexamic acid, etc. It works by increasing the strength and force of the heartbeat, causing more blood to circulate throughout the body. For example, dobutamine, etc.
- **Sympathomimetic catecholamine:** It acts quickly to improve breathing, stimulate the heart and raise a dropping blood pressure. For example, epinephrine, adrenaline, etc.
- **Adrenergic agents:** It works by constricting the blood vessels and increasing the blood pressure. For example, norepinephrine, etc.
- **Antibiotics:** It helps in preventing the secondary infections. For example, ciprofloxacin, metronidazole, etc.

Surgical

- **Blood plasma transfusion:** It can be made from human blood (called plasma-derived products) or manufactured using genetically engineered cells that carry a

human factor gene (called recombinant products).
- **Platelet transfusion**: It is a life-saving procedure in preventing or treating serious complications from bleeding.
- **Intravenous crystalloids:** These are large molecular weight substances that largely remain in the intravascular compartment thereby generating oncotic pressure.

Nursing

- Check the conscious level of the patient using Glasgow coma scale.
- Monitor blood pressure for orthostatic changes.
- Make the patient to lie down.
- Do not give them anything to eat or drink.
- Offer reassurance to the patient.
- Administer intravenous fluids as ordered to help maintain adequate perfusion to vital organs and prevent shock.
- Administer all prescribed treatment as ordered by the physician.

ANEMIA

Definition

It is a condition in which the hemoglobin concentration is lower than normal, reflects the presence of fewer than normal RBCs within the circulation as a result the amount of oxygen delivered to body tissues is diminished.

Etiology

- Inadequate production of RBCs
- Premature or excessive destruction of red blood cells
- Blood loss
- Deficits in nutrients
- Hereditary factors
- Chronic diseases.

Risk Factors

- Being women
- Being children and adolescents
- Descendants from Africa, Caribbean islands, Mediterranean countries, India and Saudi Arabia
- Being vegetarian
- Have had part or all of the stomach removed
- Having autoimmune disorders
- Adults who have internal bleeding
- Family history of anemia and ancestry
- Older adults.

Types

- ***Iron-deficiency anemia:*** It is the most common type of anemia and it accounts for approximately 50% of the diagnosed cases of anemia. It can result from inadequate iron intake, decreased iron absorption, increased iron demand or increased iron loss. The infants and young children, women and adults who have internal bleeding are at the highest risk for iron-deficiency anemia. The symptoms of iron-deficiency anemia include the following: fatigue, shortness of breath, chest pain, dizziness, headache and pica (unusual cravings for substances with no nutritional value). It is treated with iron supplementation.
- ***Thalassemia***: It is a group of inherited blood disorders characterized by the body making an abnormal form of hemoglobin. It results in hemolysis or the destruction

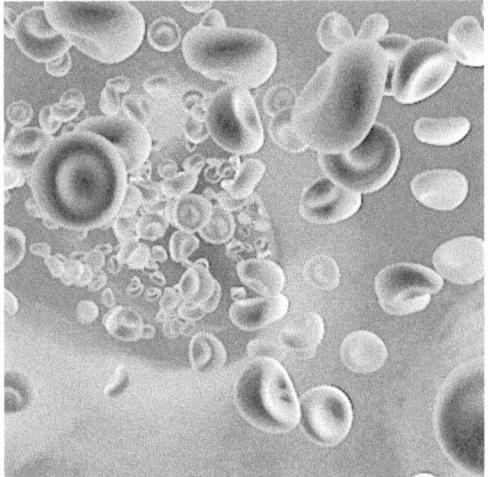

Fig. 8.2: Portrays low hemoglobin with fewer red blood cells (Anemia).

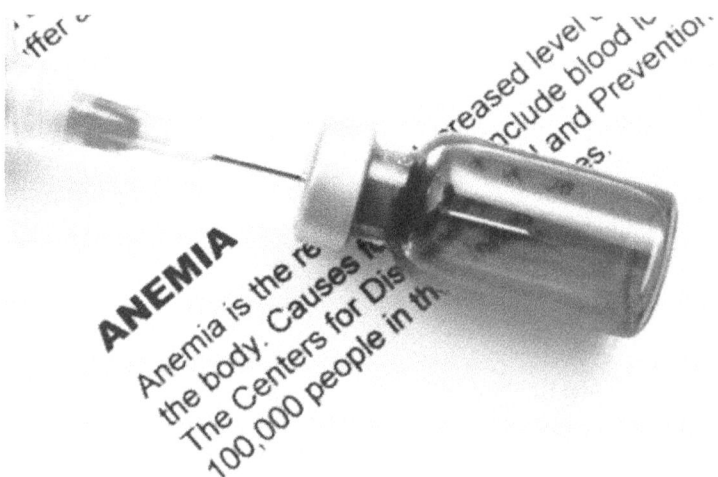

Fig. 8.3: Shows the iron supplementation in iron deficiency anemia.

of red blood cells. They are inherited disorders which pass on from parents to their children through genes. It is more common in individuals of Mediterranean, African, and Asian descent. The symptoms of thalassemia include the following: paleness, poor appetite, dark urine, slowed growth and delayed puberty, jaundice and enlarged liver, spleen and heart. The treatment for thalassemia depends on the type and severity of the disorder and it includes blood transfusion, iron chelation therapy and folic acid supplements.

- *Aplastic anemia:* It refers to a deficiency of all types of blood cells (red cells, white cells, and platelets) caused by bone marrow failure. It is a rare and serious condition that can develop at any age and can be fatal. It develops when a person's bone marrow is injured. It is more common in those exposed to toxins and taken certain medicines or had radiation or chemotherapy treatment. The symptoms of aplastic anemia include the following: fatigue, shortness of breath, dizziness, headache, coldness in the hands or feet, pale skin, gums and nail beds and chest pain. Treatment for aplastic anemia includes blood transfusions, blood and marrow stem cell transplants and medications.

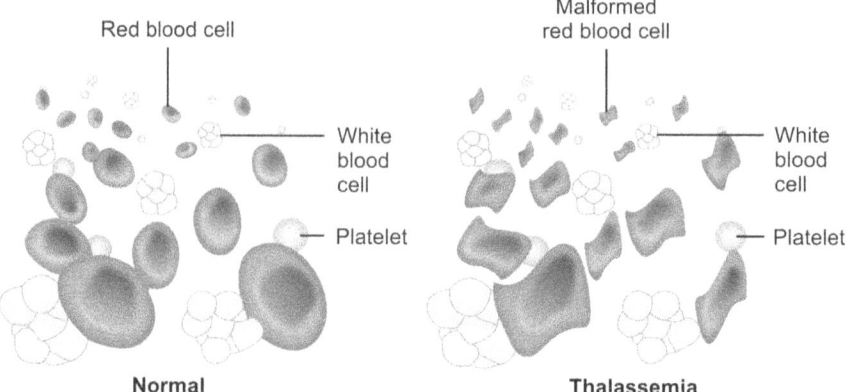

Fig. 8.4: Shows the normal red blood cells with that of malformed red blood cells (Thalassemia).

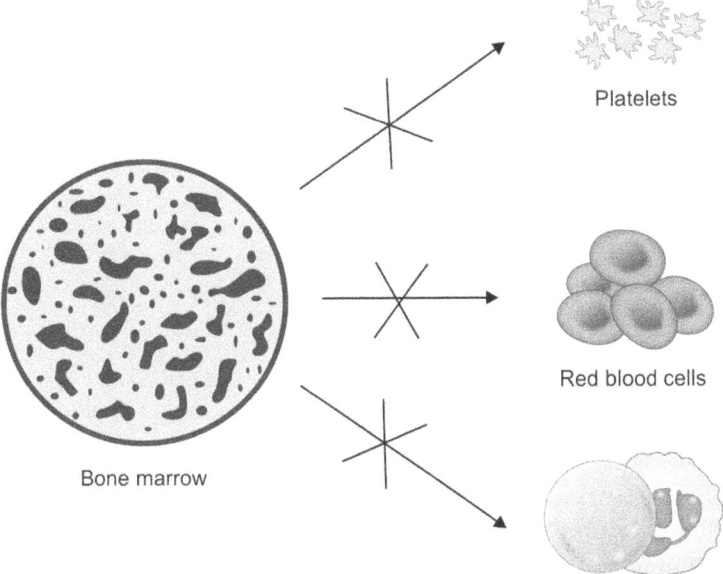

Fig. 8.5: Depicts deficiency of all types of blood cells (red cells, white cells and platelets) in aplastic anemia.

- **Hemolytic anemia:** It is a disease in which red blood cells are destroyed and removed from the bloodstream before their lifespan is over. The average lifespan of a red blood cell is 120 days. It can be inherited or acquired. Inherited means the disease is passed on due to genetic contributions from a person's parents. Acquired means the disease develops at some point in life after birth. It can affect people of all ages, races and sex. The symptoms of hemolytic anemia include the following: jaundice, pain in the upper abdomen, leg ulcers and pain and a severe reaction to a blood transfusion. Treatments for hemolytic anemia include blood transfusion, medicines, plasmapheresis, surgery, blood and marrow stem cell transplants and lifestyle changes.
- **Sickle cell anemia:** It is an inherited disorder of red blood cells. People with the disease have inherited two hemoglobin S

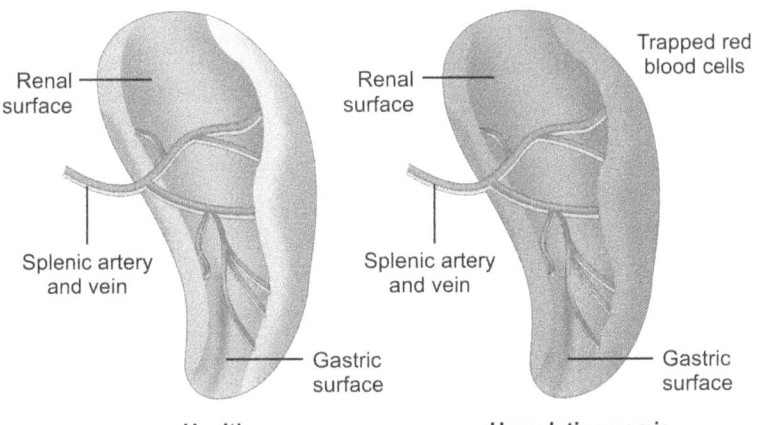

Fig. 8.6: Shows the comparison of healthy red blood cells with that of the trapped red blood cells (Hemolytic anemia).

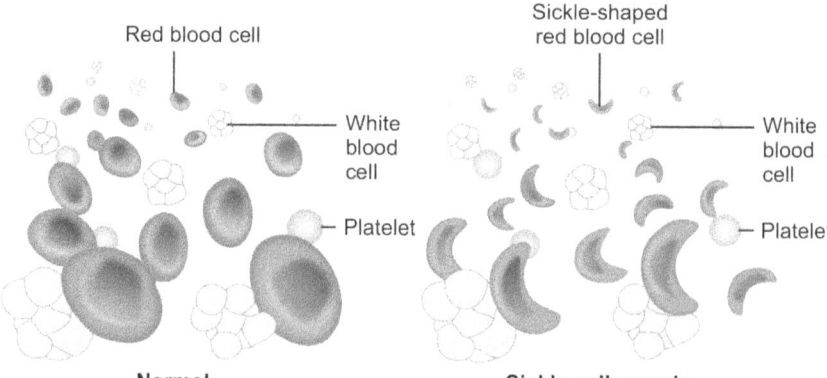

Fig. 8.7: Shows the comparison of normal red blood cell with that of the sickle-shaped red blood cell (Sickle cell anemia).

genes, one from each parent. The condition is termed hemoglobin SS and leads to sickle cell anemia. In this disease, red blood cells assume a crescent, or sickle shape. Under normal circumstances, red blood cells are disk-shaped. The sickle shaped red blood cells can slow or block the flow of blood to body tissues and organs. It is the most in people whose families descended from Africa, South or Central America, Caribbean islands, Mediterranean countries, India and Saudi Arabia. The common symptoms of sickle cell anemia include the following: fatigue, shortness of breath, dizziness, headache, coldness in the hands and feet, pale skin and chest pain. The only cure for sickle cell anemia is bone marrow transplantation.

- **Pernicious anemia:** It is a decrease in red blood cells that occurs when the intestines cannot properly absorb vitamin B_{12}. The body needs vitamin B_{12} to make red blood cells. The intestines cannot properly absorb vitamin B_{12} due to a deficiency of a special protein called intrinsic factor in the stomach. The disease is more common in individuals of Celtic (English, Irish or Scottish) or Scandinavian origin. The common symptoms of pernicious anemia include the following: nerve damage, confusion, dementia, depression, memory loss, nausea, vomiting, heartburn, abdominal bloating, constipation or diarrhea, loss of appetite, weight loss, enlarged liver and smooth beefy-red tongue. The treatment involves monthly injections, oral supplements or nasal administration of vitamin B_{12}.

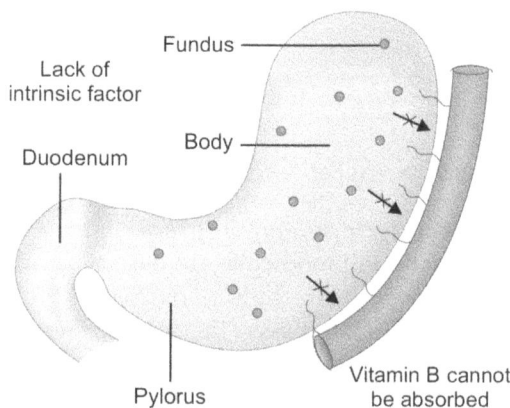

Fig. 8.8: Depicts decreased red blood cells due to the failure of vitamin B absorption (Pernicious anemia).

Pathophysiology

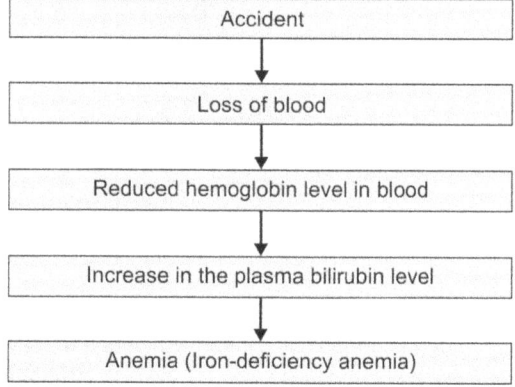

Clinical Features

- Headache
- Dizziness
- Body pain
- Shortness of breath
- Activity intolerance
- Coldness in the hands or feet
- Pale skin, gums and nail beds
- Tachycardia
- Fatigue
- Chest pain
- Poor appetite
- Dark urine
- Sore tongue
- Brittle nails.

Complications

- Confusion
- Paresthesia
- Enlarged spleen, liver and heart
- Restless legs syndrome
- Delayed growth and development.

Diagnostic Tests

- History
- Physical examination
- Blood examination
- Endoscopic examination
- Colonoscopic examination
- Fecal occult blood test
- Bone marrow examination
- Pelvic ultrasound.

Management

Medical

- **Oral iron supplements:** These are the best ways to restore iron levels for people who are iron-deficient, but they should be used only when dietary measures have failed. For example, ferrous fumarate, ferrous sulfate, ferrous gluconate, etc.
- **Intravenous or injected iron:** It is a way in which iron is administered through muscular injections or intravenously. For example, iron dextran, sodium ferric gluconate, etc.
- **Iron chelation therapy**: It removes the excess iron caused by blood transfusions. They take a drug that binds to the iron in the blood and the excess iron is then removed from the body by the kidneys.
- **Erythropoiesis-stimulating agents:** It is the hormone that acts in the bone marrow to increase the production of red blood cells. For example, epoetin alfa, darbepoetin alfa, Procrit, etc.
- **Vitamin replacements:** It prevents impaired absorption, or insufficient intake of folate. For example, folic acid supplements, etc.

Surgical

- **Blood transfusions:** It replaces blood loss due to injuries and during certain surgeries and they are commonly used to treat severe anemic patients.
- **Bone marrow transplantation (stem cell transplantation)**: It is a procedure in which unhealthy blood-forming cells are replaced with healthy ones to offer some patients the possibility of cure.
- **Plasmapheresis:** It is a procedure that removes antibodies from the blood. For this procedure, blood is taken from the body using a needle inserted into a vein. Then plasma, which contains the antibodies, is separated from the rest of the blood. The plasma, from a donor and the rest of the blood is put back into the body.
- **Surgery:** Some people who have hemolytic anemia may need surgery to remove their spleens. Removing the diseased spleen can stop or reduce high rates of red blood cell destruction.
- **Lifestyle changes**: Ask the people with anemia to avoid cold temperatures as this can help prevent the breakdown of red blood cells.

Nursing

- Encourage the patients to take foods rich in iron (red meat, liver and egg yolk).
- During times when the patient requires extra iron (such as pregnancy and breastfeeding) ask them to increase the amount of iron in the diet.

- Ask the patient to choose foods containing vitamin C to enhance iron absorption.
- Instruct the patient to avoid coffee, tea, egg yolk, milk, fiber and soy protein as they block the absorption of iron.
- Encourage the patient to take foods rich in vitamin B_{12}.

HEMOCHROMATOSIS

Definition

Hemochromatosis is an inherited blood disorder characterized by abnormally high absorption of iron by the intestinal tract, resulting in excess storage of iron particularly in the liver, skin, pancreas, heart, joints and testes.

Etiology

- Defects of the *HFE* gene
- Hemolytic anemia
- Regular consumption of iron-rich food or water
- Chronic liver disease
- Frequent blood transfusions
- Kidney dialysis
- Blood loss.

Risk Factors

- Age older than 50 years
- People of European descent
- Family history of hemochromatosis
- Being males
- Menopausal women
- Alcohol intake
- Vitamin C intake
- Consuming iron supplements or excessive amounts of iron fortified foods.

Pathophysiology

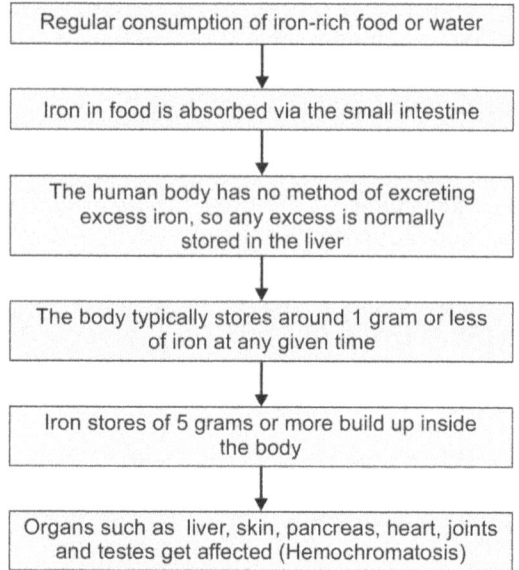

Clinical Features

- Chronic fatigue
- Weakness
- Lethargy
- Joint pain
- Abdominal pain
- Hepatomegaly
- Decrease in body hair
- Discoloration or bronzing of the skin
- Elevated liver enzymes
- Weight change
- Loss of libido (sex drive)
- Impaired memory

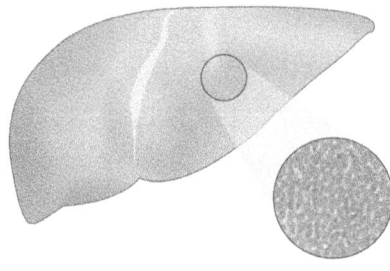
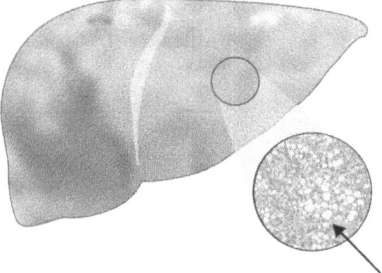

Healthy liver　　　　　　Hemochromatosis liver

Fig. 8.9: Shows the comparison of healthy liver with that of the liver with hemochromatosis.

- Mood swings
- Severe irritability
- Depression.

Complications
- Diabetes
- Hepatocellular carcinoma
- Hypogonadism
- Impotence
- Arthropathy
- Liver cirrhosis
- Congestive cardiac failure
- Premature death.

Diagnostic Tests
- History
- Physical examination
- Blood examination
- Genetic testing
- Liver function tests
- Magnetic resonance imaging (MRI)
- Computed tomography (CT) scan
- Liver biopsy
- Angiogram.

Management

Surgical

- **Phlebotomy**: It is the removal of blood by venesection and up to 500 mL of blood is removed at regular intervals until the iron levels in the blood return to within the normal range (The normal range is 20–300 micrograms per litre (µg/L) for men and 10–200 µg/L for women).

Nursing

- Instruct the patient to avoid iron supplements.
- Instruct the patient to avoid vitamin C supplements, as vitamin C increases iron absorption.
- Ask the patient to avoid the intake of alcohol.
- Ask the patient to refrain from iron-rich foods.

HEMOPHILIA (THE ROYAL DISEASE)

Definition

Hemophilia is a hereditary bleeding disorder caused by defective or deficient coagulation factors.

Etiology

- Inherited genetic condition (Majority of patients inherited X-linked recessive disorder)
- Mutations in the genes that encode clotting factors VIII, IX and XI (It is transmitted by an asymptomatic carrier female to an affected son).

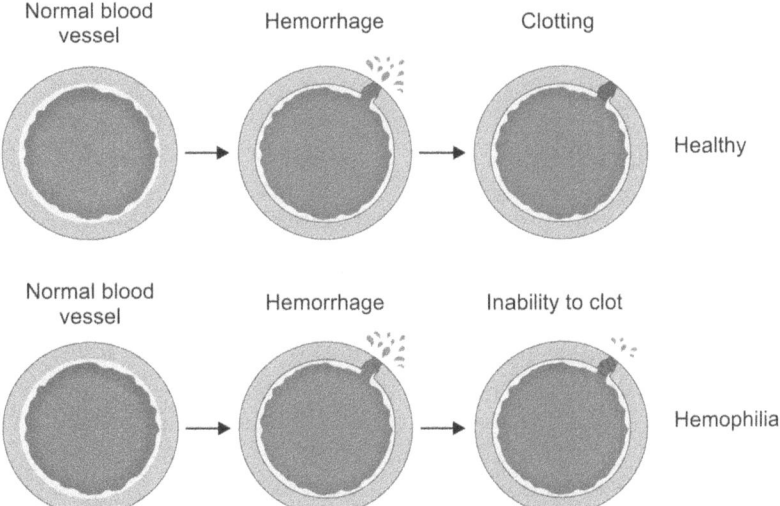

Fig. 8.10: Shows the comparison of healthy blood vessels which has the ability to clot with that of the blood vessels which has the inability to clot (Hemophilia).

Risk Factors

- Team sports
- People of Ashkenazi Jewish descent
- Being males
- Family history of hemophilia
- Royal families of Europe.

Types

- *Hemophilia A:* It is an X-linked recessive disease due to deficiency of clotting factor VIII. It is the most common type.
- *Hemophilia B:* It is X-linked recessive disease due to deficiency of clotting factor IX or Christmas factor.
- *Hemophilia C:* It is X-inked recessive disease due to deficiency of clotting factor XI. It is the least common type.
- *Acquired hemophilia:* It is a rare form of hemophilia and is not due to inheritance, but instead happens when the body launches an immune attack against clotting factor VIII.

Pathophysiology

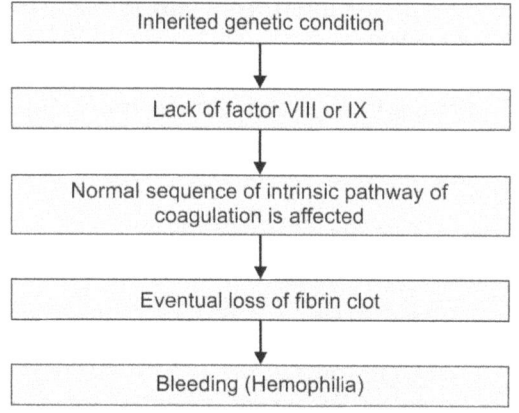

Clinical Features

- Slow, persistent, prolonged bleeding from minor trauma and small cuts delayed bleeding after minor injuries.
- Uncontrollable hemorrhage after dental extractions
- Epistaxis
- GI bleeding from ulcers and gastritis
- Hematuria
- Ecchymoses and subcutaneous hematomas
- Hemarthrosis (bleeding from joints)
- Neurologic signs such as pain, anesthesia and paralysis which may develop from nerve compression caused by hematoma formation
- Surface bruising
- Unusual bleeding after vaccination.

Complications

- Joint damages
- Deep internal bleeding
- Bleeding within the brain
- Blood-borne infections
- Death.

Diagnostic Tests

- History
- Physical examination
- Blood examination
- Genetic testing
- Activated partial thromboplastin time (APTT) test
- Prothrombin time (PT) test
- Fibrinogen test
- Clotting factor tests.

Management

Medical

- **Desmopressin:** It is a synthetic hormone that stimulates the release of factor VIII in an individual and facilitates clotting mechanism. For example, Stimate, etc.
- **Antifibrinolytics:** It helps in preventing clots from breaking down. Aminocaproic acid, tranexamic acid, etc.
- **Fibrin sealants:** It puts direct pressure to the wound sites to promote clotting and healing. Artiss, Tisseel, etc.
- **Analgesics:** It helps in reducing joint pain and swelling. For example, paracetamol, codeine, etc.
- **Corticosteroids:** It helps in reducing the severity of the disease. For example, prednisone, etc.

Surgical

- **Clotting factor concentrates**: It can be made from human blood (called plasma-derived products) or manufactured using genetically engineered cells that carry a human factor gene (called recombinant products).
- **Cryoprecipitate**: It is derived from blood and contains a moderately high concentration of clotting factor VIII (but not IX).
- **Fresh frozen plasma**: In this the red blood cells have been removed, leaving the blood proteins including clotting factors VIII and IX.

Nursing

- Instruct the patient to maintain a healthy weight because extra pounds can strain the body.
- Encourage the importance of exercise for a patient with hemophilia because it makes muscle stronger, which protects the joints and decreases bleeds.
- Instruct the patient not to take any product that contains ibuprofen, aspirin or naproxen sodium as these can keep blood from clotting.
- Ask the patient to wear a medic alert bracelet.
- Instruct the patient to carry a factor first wallet card in which the treatment information is detailed up to date.
- Teach every patient about their bleeding disorder, know what treatment they should receive in an emergency and carry the information with them.

RAYNAUD'S PHENOMENON

Definition

It is a condition that can cause discomfort as the blood supply to the fingers and toes becomes reduced in cold temperatures or emotionally stressful conditions, with a change in color of the affected areas.

Etiology

- Autoimmune disorders (rheumatoid arthritis, scleroderma, system lupus erythematosus)
- Emotional stress

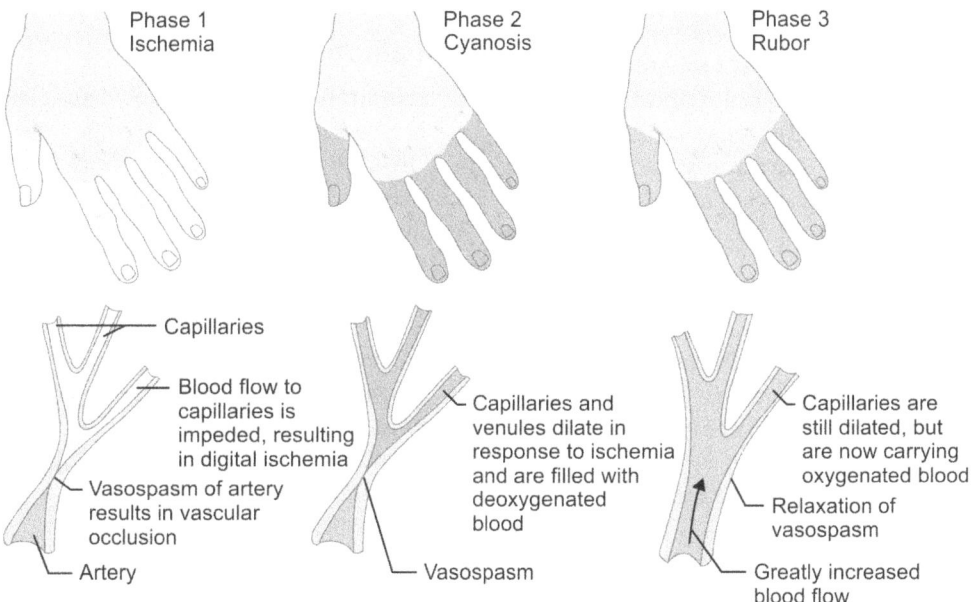

Fig. 8.11: Depicts the phases of Raynaud's phenomenon.

- Mechanical vibration (industrial white finger)
- Connective tissue disorders
- Buerger's disease
- Pulmonary hypertension
- Carpal tunnel syndrome
- Repetitive action or vibration (playing piano or doing similar movements)
- Atherosclerosis
- Injuries to the hands or feet
- Frostbite
- Certain medications (beta blockers, chemotherapy agents)
- Idiopathic.

Risk Factors

- Being women
- Age between 15 and 30
- People who live in colder climates
- Family history
- Exposure to cold.

Types

- *Primary Raynaud's phenomenon*: It is the most common form of Raynaud's phenomenon. It is called 'idiopathic' because there is no clear underlying cause. It is often so mild that the person never seeks medical attention.
- *Secondary Raynaud's phenomenon*: It is generally more complex and serious than primary type. The most common causes of secondary Raynaud's are underlying autoimmune disorders such as rheumatoid arthritis, scleroderma and systemic lupus erythematosus.

Stages

- *White stage:* It is the initial stage in which vasoconstriction occurs.
- *Blue stage*: It is the second stage in which cyanosis occurs.
- *Red stage*: It is the last stage in which rapid blood reflow occurs.

Pathophysiology

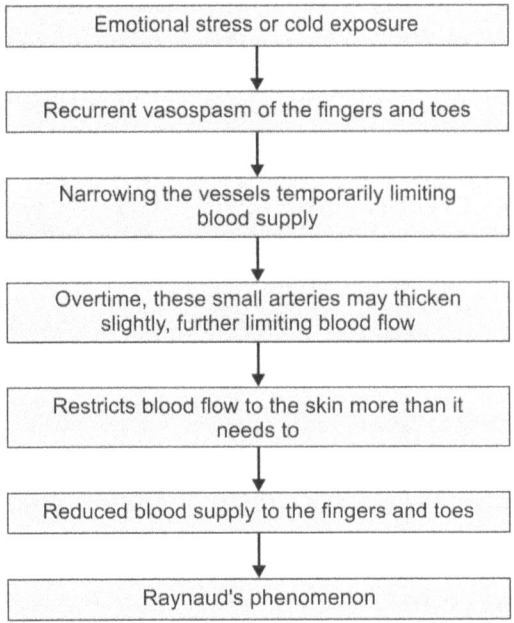

Clinical Features

- Cold fingers or toes
- Color changes in the skin in response to cold and stress
- Numb, prickly feeling or stinging pain upon warming or stress relief.

Complications

- Impaired healing of cuts and abrasions
- Increased susceptibility to infection
- Ulceration
- Tissue loss
- Scarring
- Gangrene.

Diagnostic Tests

- History
- Physical examination
- Blood examination
- Microscopic examination of fingernail tissues
- Cold stimulation test.

Management

Medical

- **Calcium channel blockers:** It relaxes and opens small blood vessels in the hands and feet decreasing the frequency and severity of attacks in most people. For example, nifedipine, amlodipine, felodipine, etc.
- **Alpha blockers:** It blocks the actions of norepinephrine, a hormone that constricts blood vessels. For example, prazosin, doxazosin, etc.
- **Vasodilators:** It relaxes and widens the blood vessels allowing more blood to flow into the hands and feet. For example, nitroglycerin, nitrostat, nitroquick, etc.
- **Beta blockers:** It helps blood vessels relax and open up to improve blood flow into the hands and feet. It works by blocking the effects of the hormone epinephrine, also known as adrenaline. For example, propranolol, metoprolol, atenolol, etc.

Surgical

- **Sympathectomy:** It is a surgical procedure in which a small incision is made on the affected hands or feet to strip away the tiny nerves around the blood vessels to control the opening and narrowing of blood vessels in the skin.
- **Chemical injection:** It is a procedure in which the sympathetic nerves in the affected hands or feet are blocked through injection chemicals such as local anesthetics or on a botulinum toxin type A (Botox) to control the opening and narrowing of blood vessels in the skin.

Nursing

- Instruct the patient to avoid known triggers, particularly exposure to cold temperatures.
- Educate the patient to avoid prolonged exposure to cold weather or sudden temperature changes, such as leaving a warm house on a cold day or air conditioned rooms in hot weather.
- Ensure patient to keep whole body warm, using several layers of clothing to trap body heat.
- Instruct the patient to keep their extremities warm with gloves and woollen socks.
- Educate the patients to moisturize their hands to prevent dryness and protect hands when in water with barrier creams.
- Instruct the patient not to smoke cigarettes or drink caffeinated beverages, since nicotine and caffeine constrict the arteries.
- Encourage the patient to do exercise regularly to maintain blood flow and skin condition.

THROMBOANGIITIS OBLITERANS (BUERGER'S DISEASE)

Definition

Thromboangiitis obliterans (Buerger's disease) is a non-atherosclerotic chronic disease characterized by segmental inflammation and thrombosis of the small- and medium-sized arteries, veins and nerves of both the peripheral upper and lower limbs.

Etiology

- Smoking
- Tobacco chewing
- Endarteritis
- Endophlebitis
- Autoimmune disorder.

Risk Factors

- Being male
- Genetic factors
- Infectious agents
- Mental stress
- Obesity.

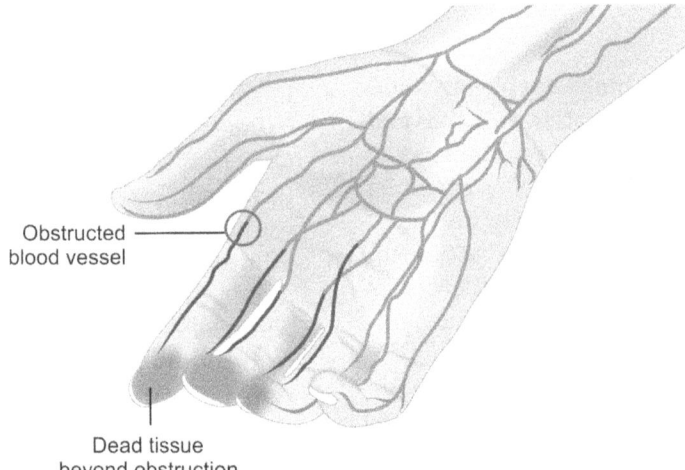

Fig. 8.12: Shows the segmental inflammation and thrombosis of the small and medium sized arteries, veins and nerves of both the peripheral upper and lower limbs (Thromboangiitis obliterans or Buerger's disease).

Pathophysiology

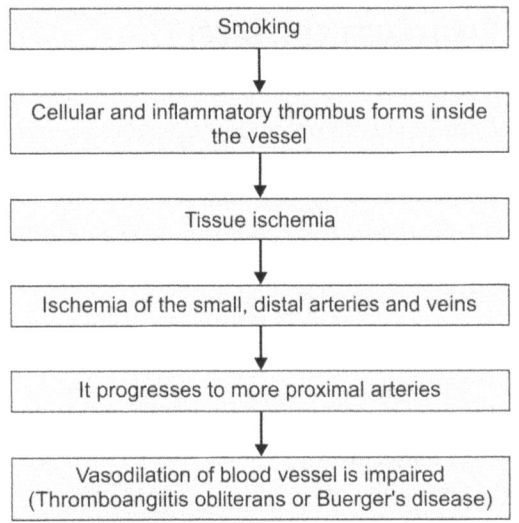

Clinical Features

- Intermittent claudication of feet, hands or arms
- Intermittent leg pains
- Color changes in the affected limb or limbs
- Paresthesia
- Superficial thrombophlebitis
- Cold sensitivity
- Leg pain worse with exertion
- Insomnia
- Sudden sweating
- Dyshidrosis (recurrent eczematous reaction).

Complications

- Ulceration
- Infection
- Amputation of fingers or toes
- Loss of blood flow in the limb of the affected fingers or toes
- Tissue death (Gangrene).

Diagnostic Tests

- History
- Physical examination
- Angiography
- Allen test
- Blood examination
- Doppler ultrasound scan
- Echocardiography
- Skin biopsy.

Management

Medical

- **Aspirin:** It reduces the ability of the blood to clot, making it easier for blood to flow through small and medium-sized arteries and veins of both the peripheral upper and lower limbs. For example, Astrix, Aspro, etc.
- **Endothelin receptor antagonist:** It is a potent vasoconstrictor that constricts

blood vessels and elevates blood pressure. For example, bosentan, macitentan, tezosentan, etc.

Surgical

- **Lumbar sympathectomy**: It is a surgical procedure that destroys nerves in the sympathetic nervous system. The procedure is performed to increase blood flow and decrease long-term pain in thromboangiitis obliterans disease that cause narrowed blood vessels. This surgical procedure cuts or destroys the sympathetic ganglia, which are collections of nerve cell bodies in clusters along the thoracic or lumbar spinal cord.
- **Periarterial sympathectomy**: It is a surgical removal of the sheath of an artery containing the sympathetic nerve fibers and it produces temporary vasodilation on small and medium-sized arteries and veins of both the peripheral upper and lower limbs.
- **Extended angioplasty**: It is a surgical procedure to open narrowed or blocked blood vessels that supply blood to the arteries and veins of both the peripheral upper and lower limbs.

- **Distal limb amputation**: It is a surgical procedure to remove a distal part of either of both the upper and lower limbs.

Nursing

- Instruct the patients to avoid conditions that reduce peripheral circulation like cold temperatures.
- Restrict the patient in sitting or standing in one position for long periods.
- Instruct the patient not to walk barefoot to avoid any injury.
- Instruct the patient to avoid tight or restrictive clothing.

VARICOSE VEINS

Definition

Varicose veins are veins that have become swollen with blood, leading to a tangled appearance and pain. The swelling in varicose veins arises from improper venous function, leading to inappropriate blood collection generally in the legs.

Etiology

- Chronic heart valve conditions
- Pregnancy
- Pressure on the midsection of the body

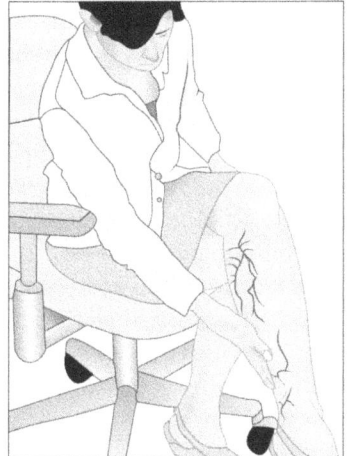 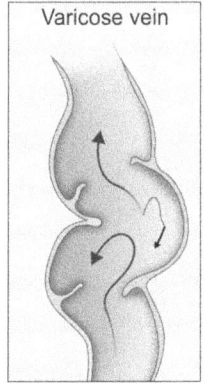 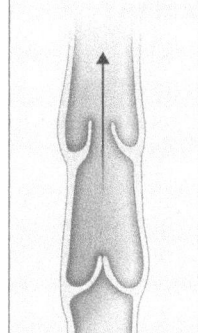

Fig. 8.13: Shows the comparison of normal veins with that of the veins with damaged valves allowing backflow of blood (Varicose veins).

- Trauma or injury to the skin
- Exposure to ultraviolet rays
- Use of birth control pills
- Postmenopausal hormonal replacement.

Risk Factors

- Age older than 50 years
- Excessive sun exposure
- Being women
- Family history
- Obesity
- Previous vein surgery
- History of blood clots
- Occupations that require prolonged standing.

Pathophysiology

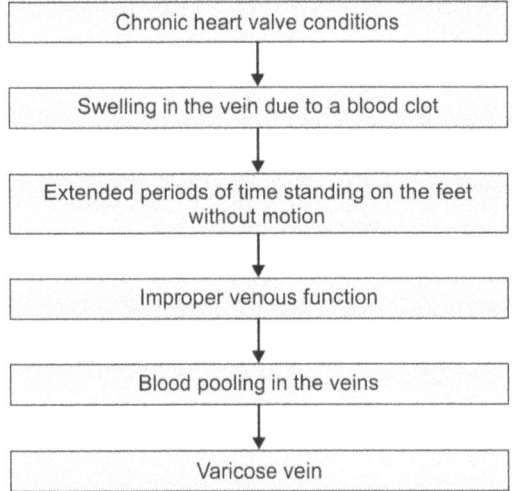

Clinical Features

- Enlarged veins
- Feeling of heaviness
- Hardened tissue under the skin
- Leg pain and swelling
- Rash
- Skin discoloration such as bruising
- Throbbing or cramping in the legs
- Visible veins.

Complications

- Ulcers of the leg
- Thrombosis
- Chronic leg swelling
- Cosmetic disfigurement
- Phlebitis
- Recurrence after treatment
- Venous rupturing and bleeding.

Diagnostic Tests

- History
- Physical examination
- Doppler ultrasound scan
- Duplex ultrasound scan
- Angiogram.

Management

Surgical

- **Sclerotherapy**: It is a non-surgical procedure in which a solution is injected into the problem varicose veins in order to cause its disappearance.
- **Endovenous laser treatment (EVLT)**: It is a procedure which works by heating the inside of the vein, which causes it to seal shut and disappear. This treatment requires that a very thin laser fiber be inserted into the damaged underlying vein.
- **Radiofrequency occlusion**: It is a method which treats the veins by heating them causing the vein to contract and then close.
- **Laser and pulsed light therapy**: It is a form of vein therapy that involves a light beam that is pulsed onto the veins in order to seal them off, causing them to dissolve.
- **Ambulatory phlebectomy**: It is a procedure in which tiny punctures or incisions are made through which the varicose veins are extracted. The incisions are so small no stitches are required.
- **Transilluminated powered phlebectomy (TIPP)**: It is a minimally invasive procedure for removing varicose veins.
- **Vein ligation**: It is a procedure in which incisions are made over the problem vein and the vein is tied off and this is done in

order to cut off the flow of blood to the varicose vein, which in turn causes it to become less visible.
- **Vein stripping:** It is a procedure that involves tying off the upper end of a problem vein and then removing the vein.

Nursing

- Instruct the patient to avoid standing for extended periods of time.
- Instruct the patient to avoid excessive sun exposure.
- Encourage the patient to eat a healthy, low-salt diet.
- Encourage the patient to refrain from crossing the legs for extended periods of time.
- Encourage the patient to do exercise to improve the leg strength.
- Facilitate the patients to sleep with their feet elevated.

VENOUS THROMBOSIS

Definition

Venous thrombosis is clotting of blood in a deep vein of an extremity (usually calf or thigh) or the pelvis.

Etiology

- Inheriting a blood clotting disorder
- Recent surgery (most commonly hip, knee, or female pelvic surgery)
- Cancer/chemotherapy
- Heart failure
- Inflammatory bowel disease
- Sitting for long periods of time, such as when driving
- Certain autoimmune disorders
- A broken hip or leg
- Prolonged bedrest, such as during a long hospital stay or paralysis
- A pacemaker catheter that has been passed through the vein in the groin.
- Having an indwelling (long-term) catheter in a blood vessel.

Risk Factors

- Any injury to the veins
- Polycythemia vera
- Pregnancy or recent birth
- Birth control pills or hormone replacement therapy
- Being overweight or obese
- Smoking
- Being overaged
- Alcohol consumption.

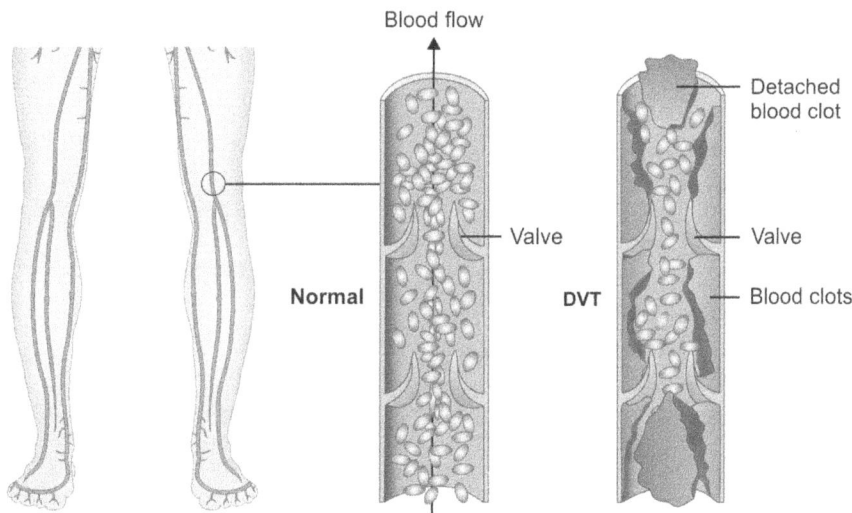

Fig. 8.14: Shows the normal veins with that of the veins with deep vein thrombosis (DVT).

Pathophysiology

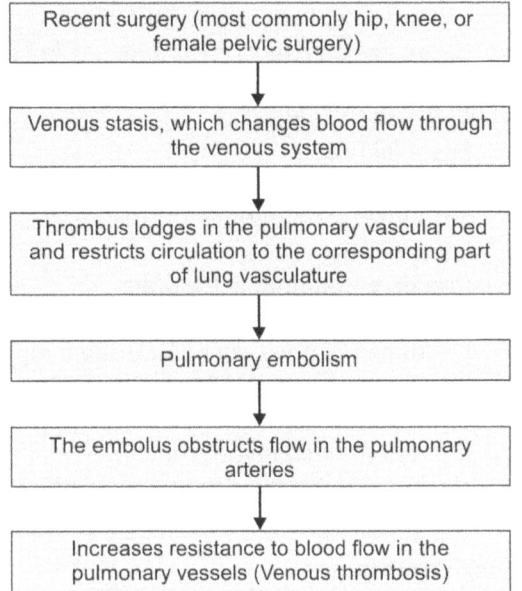

Clinical Features

- Pain or tenderness, often starting in the calf
- Swelling, including the ankle or foot
- Redness or noticeable discoloration
- Warmth
- Unexplained shortness of breath
- Rapid breathing
- Chest pain
- Rapid heart rate
- Lightheadedness or pass out.

Complications

- Chronic venous insufficiency
- Postphlebitic syndrome
- Pulmonary embolism
- Phlegmasia alba dolens (a rare complication during pregnancy in which the leg turns milky white)
- Phlegmasia cerulea dolens (massive iliofemoral venous thrombosis causing near-total venous occlusion)
- Lemierre syndrome.

Diagnostic Tests

- History
- Physical examination
- D-dimer blood test
- Doppler ultrasound examination
- Duplex ultrasound
- Venography.

Management

Medical

- **Blood-thinning agents:** It helps in preventing blood clots from forming by making the blood platelets less likely to stick together. For example, aspirin, warfarin, heparin, clopidogrel, etc.
- **Thrombolytics:** They dissolve blood clots by activating plasminogen, which forms a cleaved product called plasmin. Plasmin is a proteolytic enzyme that is capable of breaking cross-links between fibrin molecules, which provide the structural integrity of blood clots. For example, tissue plasminogen activator (t-PA), streptokinase, anistreplase, urokinase, etc.
- **Mechanical devices:** It helps in reducing the swelling and prevents blood from pooling into the veins of their legs. For example, compression stockings, etc.

Surgical

Venous thrombectomy: It is the surgical removal of the vein clot which does not respond to adequate non-surgical treatment.

Nursing

- Instruct the patient not to smoke.
- Moving the legs often during long plane trips, car trips, and other situations in which we are sitting or lying down for long periods.
- Instruct the patient to wear the pressure stockings as prescribed by the doctor.

VON WILLEBRAND DISEASE (VWD)

Definition

It is a genetic disorder caused by a missing or defective clotting protein in the blood called von Willebrand factor.

Etiology

- Inherited genetic disorder consisting of defective clotting protein (von Willebrand factor).

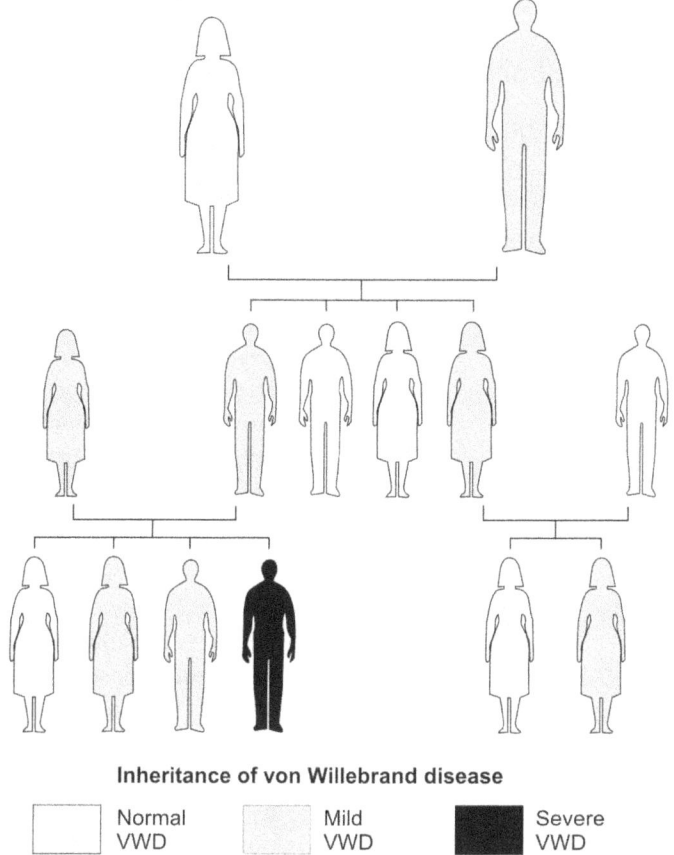

Fig. 8.15: Depicts the inheritance of von Willebrand disease (VWD).

Risk Factors

- Family history of von Willebrand disease
- Being girls after menarche
- Being children
- Factor VIII deficiency in blood
- Having an injury.

Types

- ***Type 1 VWD***: In this type, the body has low levels of von Willebrand factor and may also have low levels of factor VIII, which is another type of blood- clotting protein.
- ***Type 2 VWD***: In this type, the body makes normal amounts of von Willebrand factor, but it does not work the way it should.
- ***Type 3 VWD***: In this type, the body makes very little or no von Willebrand factor and has low levels of factor VIII.

Pathophysiology

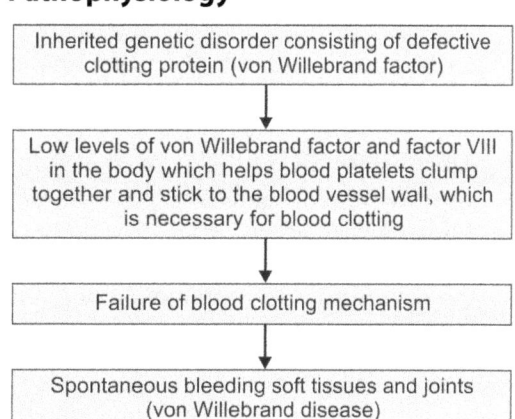

Clinical Features

- Frequent and prolonged nosebleeds
- Bleeding from the gums
- Easy bruising

- Excessive bleeding after surgery or dental procedures
- Spontaneous bleeding from soft tissue and joints
- Prolonged bleeding from cuts
- Heavy menstrual bleeding (in women)
- Blood in the stool or urine
- Bruises with lumps that form underneath the skin
- Skin rash.

Complications

- Deep internal bleeding
- Blood-borne infections
- Death.

Diagnostic Tests

- History
- Physical examination
- Genetic testing
- Blood examination
- von Willebrand factor antigen test
- von Willebrand factor activity test
- Factor VIII activity test
- Platelet aggregation test.

Management

Medical

- **Desmopressin:** It is a synthetic hormone that stimulates the release of von Willebrand antigen in an individual and facilitates clotting mechanism. For example, Stimate, etc.
- **Antifibrinolytics:** It helps in preventing clots from breaking down. Aminocaproic acid, tranexamic acid, etc.
- **Fibrin sealants:** It puts direct pressure to the wound sites to promote clotting and healing. Artiss, Tisseel, etc.
- **Corticosteroids:** It helps in reducing the severity of the disease. For example, prednisone, etc.

Surgical

- **Clotting factor concentrates:** It can be made from human blood (called plasma-derived products) or manufactured using genetically engineered cells that carry a human factor gene (called recombinant products).
- **Cryoprecipitate:** It is derived from blood and contains a moderately high concentration of von Willebrand factor antigen.
- **Fresh frozen plasma:** In this, the red blood cells have been removed, leaving the blood proteins which contain von Willebrand factor antigen and fresh frozen plasma if given.

Nursing

- Instruct the patient to avoid contact sports.
- Instruct the patient to maintain a healthy weight because extra pounds can strain the body.
- Encourage the importance of exercise for a patient with von Willebrand disease because it makes muscle stronger, and decreases bleeds.
- Instruct the patient not to take any product that contains ibuprofen, aspirin or naproxen sodium as these can keep blood from clotting.
- Ask the patient to wear a medic alert bracelet.
- Instruct the patient to carry a factor first wallet card in which the treatment information is detailed up to date.
- Teach every patient about their bleeding disorder, know what treatment they should receive in an emergency and carry the information with them.

9
CHAPTER

Disorders of Renal System

CHAPTER OUTLINE

- Acute kidney injury
- Chronic kidney disease
- Cystitis
- Glomerulonephritis
- Nephrosclerosis
- Nephrotic syndrome
- Polycystic kidney disease
- Pyelonephritis
- Renal calculi
- Uremic encephalopathy
- Urethral strictures
- Urethritis
- Urinary incontinence
- Urinary tract infection

ACUTE KIDNEY INJURY (ACUTE RENAL FAILURE)

Definition

Acute kidney injury (AKI) is a sudden and almost complete loss of kidney function (decreased glomerular filtration rate) over a period of hours to days.

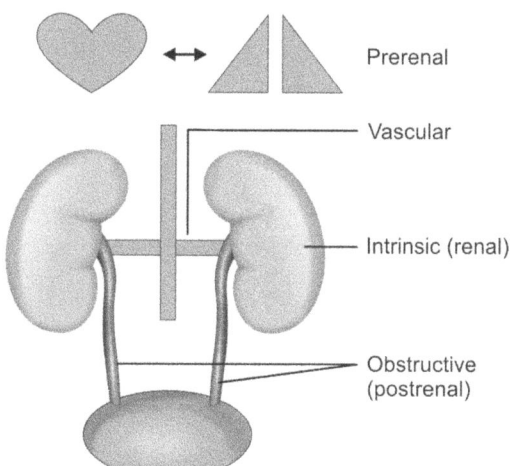

Fig. 9.1: Depicts various stages of acute kidney injury.

Etiology

- **Prerenal (hypoperfusion of kidney) cause:** It occurs as a result of impaired blood flow that leads to hypoperfusion of the kidney and a drop in the GFR.
  - Hemorrhage or GI losses
  - Cardiogenic shock or heart failure
  - Liver cirrhosis
  - Nephrotic syndrome
  - Sepsis or anaphylaxis
  - Renal hypoperfusion.
- **Intrarenal (parenchymal damage to the glomeruli) cause:** It occurs as a result of acute parenchymal damage to the glomeruli or kidney tubules.
  - Burns
  - Crush injuries
  - Infections
  - Nephrotoxic agents
  - Tubular injury
  - Eclampsia
  - Vasculitis.
- **Postrenal (obstruction somewhere distal to the kidney) cause:** It occurs as a result of any obstruction somewhere distal to the

kidney. Pressure rises in the kidney tubules and eventually the GFR decreases.

Urinary tract obstructions including:
- Calculi (stones)
- Tumors
- Benign prostatic hypertrophy (BPH)
- Urethral strictures
- Radiation fibrosis
- Retroperitoneal fibrosis
- Pelvic malignancy
- Papillary necrosis.

Risk Factors

- Being hospitalized, especially for a serious condition that requires intensive care
- Advanced age
- Diabetes mellitus
- Hypertension
- Peripheral artery disease
- Past history of acute kidney injury
- Nephrotoxic medication
- Intraperitoneal surgery
- Increased volume of contrast agent
- Proteinuria
- Use of iodinated contrast agents within the previous week
- Morbid obesity.

Phases of Acute Renal Failure

- ***Stage of initiation:*** This stage begins with the initial result and ends when oliguria develops.
- ***Stage of oliguria:*** In this stage, oliguria develops and there is a rise in the serum concentration of substances usually excreted by the kidneys (urea, creatinine, uric acid, organic acids and intracellular cations (potassium and magnesium). Uremic symptoms and hyperkalemia develop.
- ***Stage of diuresis:*** In this stage, there is gradual increase in the urine output and glomerular filtration starts to recover. Laboratory values stop rising and eventually decrease.
- ***Stage of recovery:*** In this stage, laboratory values return to normal and there is improvement of renal functions within 3–12 months.

Pathophysiology

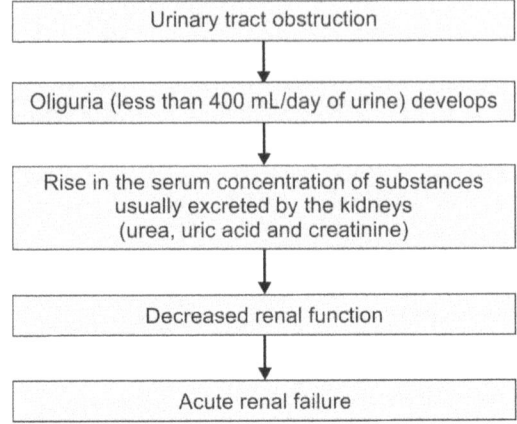

Clinical Features

- Drowsiness
- Headache
- Muscle twitching
- Seizures
- Lethargy
- Nausea
- Vomiting
- Diarrhea (or) dehydration
- Dry mucous membrane
- Oliguria
- Increased BUN and serum creatinine
- Breath may have the odor of urine (uremic fetor).

Complications

- Extracellular volume overload
- Hyponatremia
- Hyperkalemia
- Metabolic acidosis
- Hyperphosphatemia
- Hypocalcemia
- Hyperuricemia
- End-stage renal disease
- Death.

Diagnostic Tests

- History
- Physical examination

- Low specific gravity of urine (1.010 or less)
- Increased BUN and serum creatinine
- Increased potassium level (severe hyperkalemia)
- Increased serum phosphate and low serum calcium level
- Decreased hemoglobin level (anemia).

Management

Medical

- **Atrial natriuretic peptide (ANP):** It is a peptide hormone secreted by the cardiac atria that in pharmacological doses promotes salt and water excretion and lowers blood pressure and improves renal function. For example, glitazone, etc.
- **Diuretic agents:** It helps to manage fluid overload in acute kidney injury. For example, furosemide, bumetanide, ethacrynic acid, torsemide, etc.
- **Low-dose dopamine agents:** It helps to dilate the arteries and improves renal function. For example, Cardene, Corgard, Coumadin, Micardis, etc.
- **Free radical scavengers:** These are natural compounds that neutralize free radicals in the body. For example, astaxanthin, glutathione, etc.
- **Xathine oxidase inhibitors:** It is a substance that inhibits the activity of xanthine oxidase, an enzyme involved in purine metabolism. For example, Aloprim, Allopurinol, febuxostat, Uloric, Zyloprim, etc.
- **Calcium channel blockers:** It reduces the speed at which calcium moves into the heart muscle, blood vessels and cells in the heart that controls the heart rate and thereby reduces hypertension in acute renal injury. For example, diltiazem, nifedipine, verapamil, nisoldipine, etc.
- **Renal prostaglandins:** These are lipids made at sites of tissue damage or infection that are involved in dealing with injury and illness. For example, prostacyclin, thromboxane, etc.

Surgical

- **Hemodialysis (HD):** It is the artificial process of eliminating waste (diffusion) and unwanted water (ultrafiltration) from the blood by pumping the patient's blood against dialysate that may be generated by the dialysis machine or at a central location.
- **Continuous renal replacement therapy (CRRT):** It is a slow and continuous extracorporeal blood purification therapy and it mimics the function of the kidneys in regulating water, electrolytes and toxic products by the continuous slow removal of solutes and fluid that are provided 24 hour per day.
- **Sustained low-efficiency dialysis (SLED):** It is a procedure used as a renal replacement modality in critically ill patients with acute kidney injury and hemodynamic instability.
- **Peritoneal dialysis (PD):** It works using the body's peritoneal membrane as a filter which allows impurities to be drawn out of the blood.
- **Renal transplantation:** It is a procedure that involves a number of small incisions (1–3 cm) through which the faulty kidneys are removed and replaced with a healthy kidney from the donor.

Nursing

- Measure fluid input and output accurately.
- Weigh the patient every day, at the same time and on the same scale.
- Give them a variety of options in foods as well as fluids and get them involved in making their menu plan.
- Maintain good hygiene and ensure the patient also follows it.
- Provide emotional support and discuss the presence of continuous fatigue with patient.
- Limit the intake of protein to less than 1 g/day.
- Restrict the intake of potassium to 40–60 mEq/day.
- Restrict the intake of sodium to 2 mEq/day.

CHRONIC KIDNEY DISEASE (END-STAGE RENAL DISEASE)

Definition

Chronic kidney disease (or) end-stage renal disease (ESRD) is a progressive, irreversible deterioration in renal function in which the body's ability to maintain metabolic and fluid and electrolyte balance fails, resulting in uremia (or) azotemia (retention of urea and other nitrogenous wastes in the blood).

Etiology

- Chronic glomerulonephritis
- Polycystic kidney disease
- Urinary tract obstruction
- Urinary tract infection
- Nephrotoxic drugs
- Non-steroidal anti-inflammatory drugs.

Risk Factors

- Diabetes mellitus
- Hypertension
- Family history of kidney failure
- Smoking
- Obesity
- History of acute kidney injury
- Aboriginal or Torres Strait Islander origin
- Elders
- History of established cardiovascular disease.

Stages

- **Stage I: Nonazotemic stage**
  - In this stage, there is a reduced renal reserve.
  - It was characterized by 40–75% loss of nephron function.
  - The patient usually does not have symptoms because the remaining nephrons are unable to carry out the normal functions of the kidney.
- **Stage II: Renal insufficiency stage**
  - In this stage, there is renal insufficiency that prevails
  - 75–90% of nephron function is lost.
  - Serum creatinine and blood urea nitrogen rise, the kidney loses its ability to concentrate urine and anemia develops.
  - Patient may report polyuria and nocturia.
- **Stage III: Azotemic stage**
  - The final stage of chronic kidney disease occurs when there is less than 10% nephron function remaining.
  - Normal regulatory, excretory and hormonal functions of the kidney are severely impaired.
  - It is evidenced by elevated creatinine and blood urea nitrogen levels as well as electrolyte imbalances.

Pathophysiology

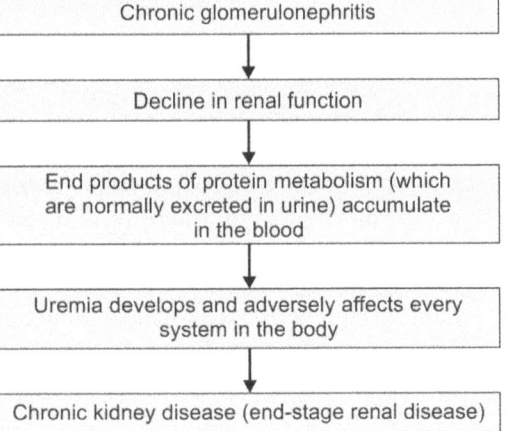

Chronic glomerulonephritis
↓
Decline in renal function
↓
End products of protein metabolism (which are normally excreted in urine) accumulate in the blood
↓
Uremia develops and adversely affects every system in the body
↓
Chronic kidney disease (end-stage renal disease)

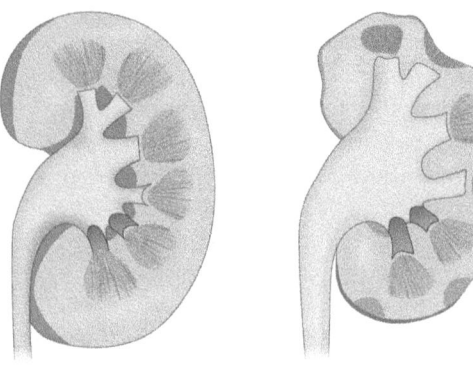

Normal kidney   Chronic renal failure affected kidney

Fig. 9.2: Shows the comparison of normal kidney with that of the kidney with chronic renal failure.

Clinical Features
- Hypertension
- Pruritus
- Nocturia
- Restless legs
- Hematuria
- Dyspnea
- Lethargy
- Frothy urine
- Loin pain
- Pallor
- Leukonychia
- Peripheral edema
- Pleural effusion
- Pulmonary edema
- Nausea
- Vomiting
- Malaise
- Anorexia
- Asterixis.

Complications
- Acidosis
- Albuminuria
- Anemia
- Depression
- Hyperkalemia
- Severe hypertension
- Mineral and bone disorder
- Sleep apnea
- Uremia.

Diagnostic Tests
- History
- Physical examination
- Blood examination
- Urine examination
- Urine microscopy and culture examination
- Kidney function test
- Ultrasonogram
- Computed tomography (CT) scan
- Magnetic resonance imaging (MRI) scan
- Cystoscopic examination
- Renal biopsy.

Management

Medical
- **Angiotensin-converting enzyme inhibitors:** It induces vasodilation which improves cardiac output and enhances the renal excretion of salt and water. For example, enalapril, captopril, ramipril, etc.
- **Calcium channel blockers:** They enhance glomerular filtration rate, renal blood flow and electrolyte excretion in the kidneys. For example, diltiazem, verapamil, etc.
- **Angiotensin receptor blockers:** It constricts the efferent arteriole more than the afferent arteriole within the kidney, which helps to maintain glomerular capillary pressure and filtration. For example, losartan, candesartan, etc.
- **Aldosterone antagonists:** It blocks the effects of aldosterone, therefore decreases sodium re-absorption and water retention by the kidneys and consequently leads to a decrease in blood pressure. For example, Aldactone, Inspra, etc.
- **Renin inhibitors:** It blocks the activity of renin and causes vasodilation. For example, Tekturna, etc.
- **Thiazide diuretics:** It decreases active re-absorption of sodium and chloride ions by inhibiting the sodium/chloride cotransporter in the distal convoluted tubule and also increases potassium ion loss. For example, Lozol, Thalitone, etc.
- **Antacids:** It binds dietary phosphorus in the GI tract. For example, cimetidine, etc.
- **Erythropoietin agents:** It binds to its receptor expressed on the surface of red blood progenitor cells and leads to increased production of RBCs. For example, recombinant human erythropoietin (Epogen), etc.
- **Antibiotics:** For example, doxycycline, clindamycin, metronidazole, etc. It helps to prevent any secondary infections.

Surgical
- **Hemodialysis (HD):** It is the artificial process of eliminating waste (diffusion) and unwanted water (ultrafiltration) from the blood by pumping the patient's blood against dialysate that may be generated by the dialysis machine or at a central location.
- **Continuous renal replacement therapy (CRRT):** It is a slow and continuous extra-

corporeal blood purification therapy and it mimics the function of the kidneys in regulating water, electrolytes and toxic products by the continuous slow removal of solutes and fluid that are provided 24 hour per day.
- **Peritoneal dialysis (PD):** It works using the body's peritoneal membrane as a filter which allows impurities to be drawn out of the blood.
- **Renal transplantation:** It is a procedure that involves a number of small incisions (1–3 cm) through which the faulty kidneys are removed and replaced with a healthy kidney from the donor.

Nursing

- Instruct the patient to stop smoking.
- Encourage the patient to participate in weight reduction program.
- Measure fluid input and output of the patient accurately.
- Monitor the weight of the patient at regular intervals.
- Encourage moderately intensive physical activity for at least 30 minutes in a day.
- Limit the intake of protein to less than 1g/day.
- Restrict the intake of potassium to 40–60 mEq/day.
- Restrict the intake of sodium to 2 mEq/day.
- Restrict dietary salt intake to 40–100 mmol/day.
- Provide emotional support to the patient.
- Allow proteins of high biologic value.
- Encourage fluid allowance of 500–600 mL more than the previous day's 24-hour urine output.
- Supplement the diet with vitamins that are necessary because of protein-restricted diet.
- Encourage supply of calories through carbohydrates and fat to prevent wasting.

CYSTITIS

Definition

It is a chronic infection and inflammation of the bladder wall that results in recurring discomfort or pain in the bladder and the surrounding pelvic region.

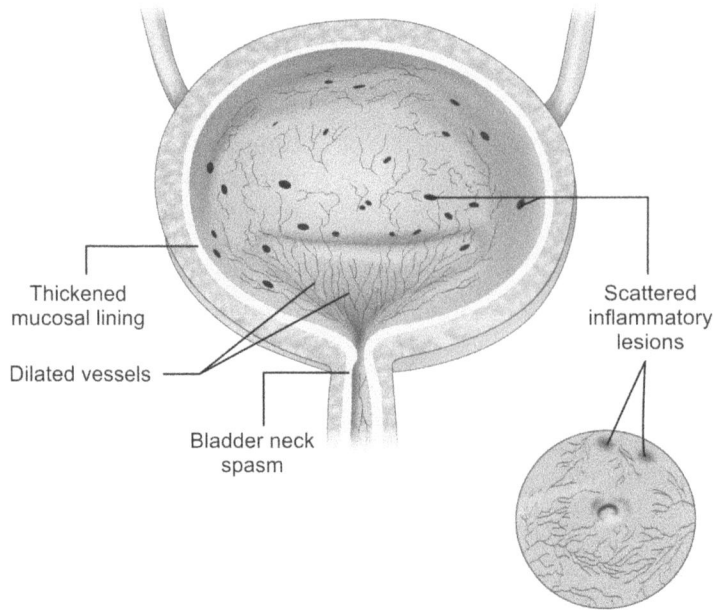

Fig. 9.3: Shows the inflamed bladder wall resulting in recurrent pain or discomfort (Cystitis).

Etiology

- Decrease in glycosaminoglycan (Urothelium)
- A defect in the bladder wall
- Chemicals released during an allergic reaction
- Autoimmune disorders
- Changes in the nerves that carry bladder sensations.

Risk Factors

- It is most common in women of all ages.
- Average age of onset is 40 years.
- Found in all ethnic groups.
- Being pregnant
- Being sexually active
- Using spermicide with contraception
- Having had the menopause
- Diabetes
- Having a catheter in the bladder.

Pathophysiology

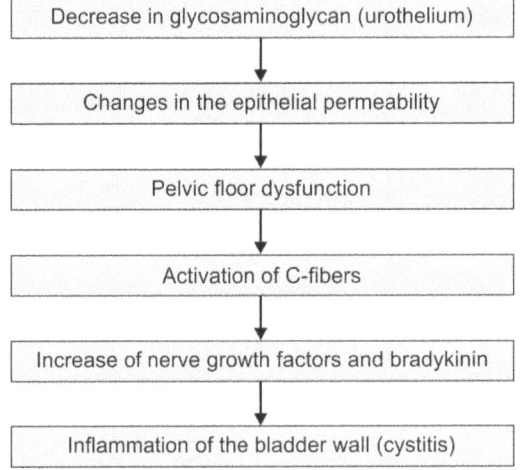

Clinical Features

- Frequent pain
- Burning micturition
- Frequency of urination
- An urge to pass urine most often
- Nocturia
- Pass only small amount of urine
- Feel that the bladder is still full after passing urine, dark or bloody urine
- Smelly, cloudy
- Pain low down in the abdomen
- Feeling unwell with nausea, fever and headache
- Pain during sexual intercourse.

Complications

- Reduced bladder capacity
- Urinary tract infections
- Pyelonephritis
- Sepsis.

Diagnostic Tests

- History
- Physical examination
- Pelvic examination
- Blood examination
- Urine examination
- Potassium sensitivity test
- Biopsy examination
- Cystoscopy
- Ultrasonography
- Computed tomography (CT) scan.

Management

Medical

- **Antibiotics:** It helps to prevent secondary infections. For example, norfloxacin, trimethoprim, nitrofurantoin, etc.
- **Urinary analgesics:** It helps to reduce mild bladder pain. For example, phenazopyridine, paracetamol, codeine, etc.
- **Bladder protectants:** It helps to ease symptoms by restoring the inner surface of the bladder and protecting the bladder wall from irritating substances. For example, pentosan polysulfate sodium, etc.
- **Antispasmodic agents:** It causes direct smooth muscle relaxation of the urinary bladder and increases the bladder outlet resistance at the level of the bladder neck. For example, oxybutynin, etc.
- **Antidepressants:** It helps to increase bladder capacity and blocks pain. For example, amitriptyline, etc.
- **Antihistamines:** These are drugs that inhibit the action of histamine in the body

by blocking the receptors of histamine. For example, hydramine, diphenhydramine, Diphen, etc.

Nursing

- Educate the patient to completely empty the bladder each time when they urinate.
- Place a warm pack, such as a hot water bottle wrapped in a towel on the abdomen to help in relieving pain.
- Encourage the patient to take plenty of rest.
- Ask the patient to drink plenty of water.
- Encourage the patient to take cranberry juice daily to prevent infections.
- Educate the patient to wipe from front to back (urethra to anus) after going to the toilet to prevent infections.
- Educate the patient to pass urine often and not to "hold on".

GLOMERULONEPHRITIS

Definition

The infection and inflammation of the glomerular capillaries is known as glomerulonephritis.

Etiology

- Group A beta hemolytic streptococcal infection of the throat precedes the onset of glomerulonephritis by 2–3 weeks.
- Systemic lupus erythematosus
- Goodpasture's syndrome
- Wegener's granulomatosis
- Amyloidosis
- Polyarteritis nodosa
- Cryoglobulinemia
- Impetigo (infection of the skin)
- Mumps
- Heredity nephritis
- Certain medications (e.g., Quinine, Gemcitabine, Mitomycin C, etc.).

Risk Factors

- Exposure to hydrocarbon solvents
- Immunocompromised individuals
- Family history of cancer
- Smoking
- Diabetes.

Types

- ***Acute glomerulonephritis:*** It is sudden in onset and occurs most often as a

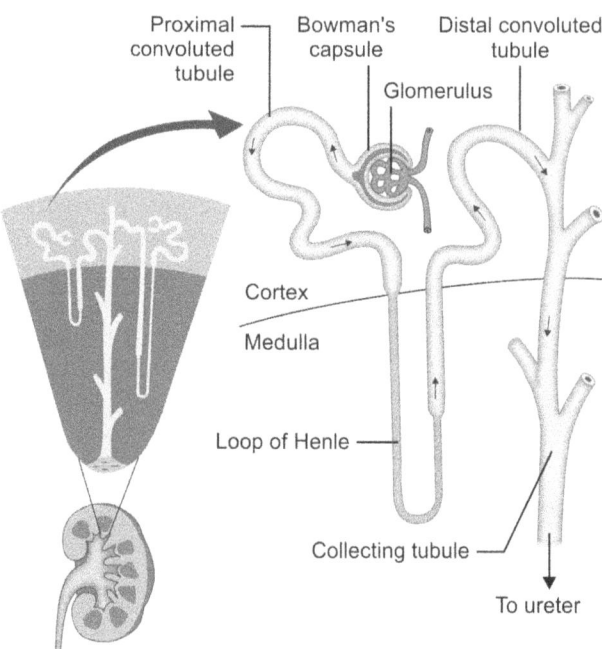

Fig. 9.4: Depicts inflamed glomerular capillaries.

complication of a throat or skin infection with Streptococcus, a type of bacteria. It typically develops in children between the ages of 2–10 after recovery from the infection.
- **Chronic glomerulonephritis:** It is gradual in onset and is caused by hereditary nephritis, an inherited genetic disorder.

Pathophysiology

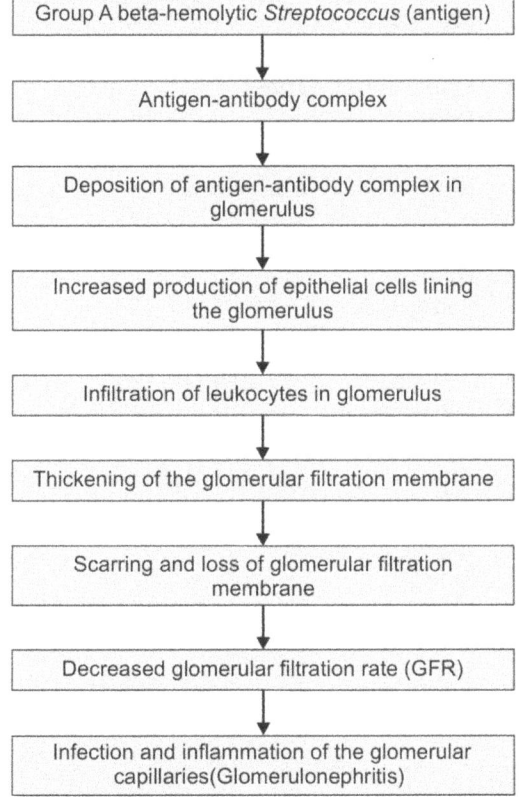

Clinical Features
- Hematuria (blood in the urine)
- Cola-colored urine (due to RBCs)
- Oliguria
- Proteinuria
- Increased serum creatinine
- Increased blood urea nitrogen (BUN)
- Edema
- Hypertension
- Headache
- Malaise
- Flank pain

- Tenderness over CVA (Costovertebral angle)
- Confusion
- Increased irritability
- Sudden severe nosebleed (or) seizure
- Nocturia
- Anemia.

Complications
- Nephrotic syndrome
- End-stage renal disease
- Hypertensive encephalopathy
- Heart failure
- Pulmonary edema
- Optic neuropathy.

Diagnostic Tests
- History
- Physical examination
- Blood examination
- Urine examination
- Immunology testing
- Kidney biopsy
- Kidney ultrasonogram
- Chest X-ray examination
- Intravenous pyelogram
- Computed tomography (CT) scan.

Management

Medical
- **Angiotensin-converting enzyme inhibitors:** It induces vasodilation which improves cardiac output and enhances the renal excretion of salt and water. For example, enalapril, captopril, ramipril, etc.
- **Angiotensin receptor blockers:** It constricts the efferent arteriole more than the afferent arteriole within the kidney, which helps to maintain glomerular capillary pressure and filtration. For example, losartan, candesartan, etc.
- **Aldosterone antagonists:** It blocks the effects of aldosterone, therefore, decreases sodium re-absorption and water retention by the kidneys and consequently lead to a decrease in blood pressure. For example, Aldactone, eplerenone, etc.

- **Thiazide diuretics:** It decreases active re-absorption of sodium and chloride ions by inhibiting the sodium/chloride cotransporter in the distal convoluted tubule and also increases potassium ion loss. For example, Lozol (indapamide), Thalitone (chlorthalidone), etc.
- **Antibiotics:** It helps to prevent any secondary infections. For example, penicillin, doxycycline, clindamycin, metronidazole, etc.
- **Corticosteroids:** It helps in reducing the severity of the disease. For example, prednisone, etc.
- **Immunosuppressant agents:** It lowers the body's ability to reject a transplanted organ from the donor. For example, cyclophosphamide, etc.

Surgical

- **Hemodialysis (HD):** It is the artificial process of eliminating waste (diffusion) and unwanted water (ultrafiltration) from the blood by pumping the patient's blood against dialysate that may be generated by the dialysis machine or at a central location.
- **Renal transplantation:** It is a procedure that involves a number of small incisions (1–3 cm) through which the faulty kidneys are removed and replaced with a healthy kidney from the donor.

Nursing

- Encourage the patient to restrict salt in the diet.
- Encourage the patient to restrict protein in the diet.
- Maintain intake output chart.
- Provide adequate calories to the patient to promote nutritional status.
- Encourage the patient to maintain a healthy body weight.
- Instruct the patient to avoid smoking.

NEPHROSCLEROSIS

Definition

Nephrosclerosis is a condition characterized by a thickening and hardening of the blood vessels in the kidneys.

Etiology

- Chronic high blood pressure
- Certain medications (e.g., Cocaine, amphetamines, etc)
- Pre-eclampsia
- Autoimmune disorders
- Spinal cord injuries
- Renal stenosis
- Aortic dissection
- Intake of birth control pills.

Risk Factors

- Diabetes
- Being males
- Older age
- Preexisting renal disease
- Smoking
- Alcohol consumption.

Types

- **Benign nephrosclerosis:** It is most present in people over 60 years old.

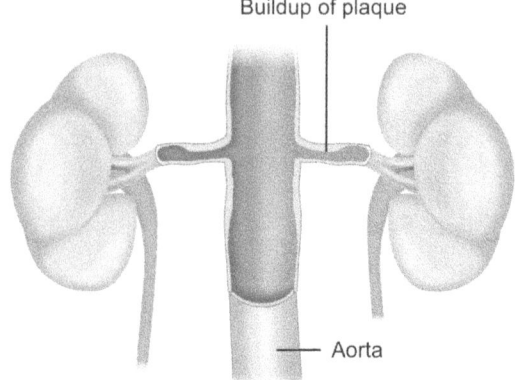

Fig. 9.5: Shows the narrowed renal artery due to built-up of plaque in the artery (Nephrosclerosis).

- **Chronic glomerulonephritis:** It occurs only in a case of hypertension with diastolic blood pressure exceeding 130 mm Hg.

Pathophysiology

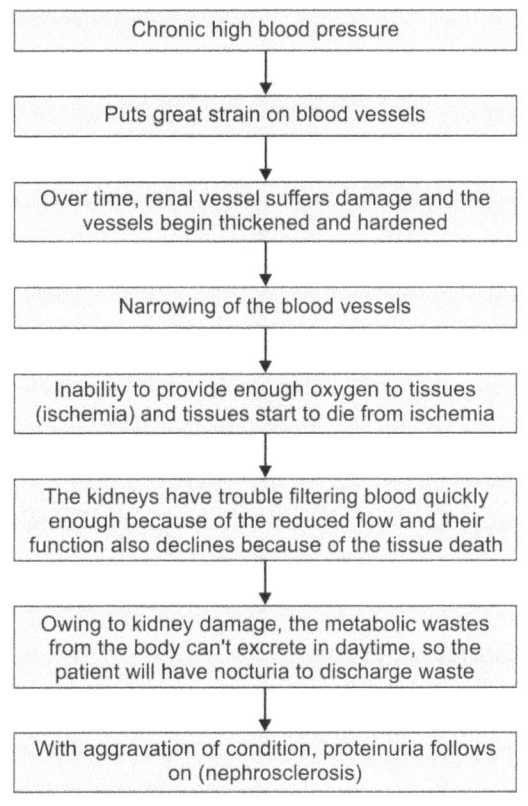

Clinical Features

- Frequent urination at night (nocturia)
- Proteinuria
- Hematuria
- Color change of urine
- Foamy urine
- Tiredness
- Headache
- Nausea
- Vomiting
- Protein in urine
- Reduced urine output.

Complications

- Organ damage
- End-stage renal disease

- Loss of vision
- Heart failure
- Stroke.

Diagnostic Tests

- History
- Physical examination
- Blood examination
- Urine examination
- Kidney biopsy
- Kidney function test
- Kidney ultrasonogram
- Echocardiogram
- Computed tomography (CT) scan.

Management

Medical

- **Angiotensin-converting enzyme inhibitors:** It induces vasodilation which improves cardiac output and enhances the renal excretion of salt and water. For example, enalapril, captopril, ramipril, etc.
- **Angiotensin receptor blockers:** It constricts the efferent arteriole more than the afferent arteriole within the kidney, which helps to maintain glomerular capillary pressure and filtration. For example, losartan, candesartan, etc.
- **Aldosterone antagonists:** It blocks the effects of aldosterone, therefore decreases sodium re-absorption and water retention by the kidneys and consequently leads to a decrease in blood pressure. For example, Aldactone, Inspra, etc.

Surgical

- **Hemodialysis (HD):** It is the artificial process of eliminating waste (diffusion) and unwanted water (ultrafiltration) from the blood by pumping the patient's blood against dialysate that may be generated by the dialysis machine or at a central location.

Nursing

- Encourage the patient to restrict salt in the diet.

- Encourage the patient to restrict protein in the diet.
- Instruct the patient to avoid intake of alcohol.
- Encourage the patient to maintain a healthy body weight.
- Encourage the patient to perform regular exercise for a minimum of 30 minutes per day.
- Instruct the patient to avoid smoking.
- Teach stress management techniques to the patient.

NEPHROTIC SYNDROME

Definition

Nephrotic syndrome is a primary glomerular disease characterized by proteinuria (marked increase in protein in the urine), hypoalbuminemia (decrease in albumin in the blood), hyperlipidemia (high serum cholesterol and low-density lipoprotein) and edema.

Etiology

- Membranous nephropathy
- Focal segmental glomerulosclerosis
- Glomerulopathy
- IgA nephropathy
- Fibrillar glomerulopathy
- Congenital podocyte anomaly
- Membranoproliferative glomerulonephritis.

Risk Factors

- Being children
- Hispanic and black race people
- Diabetes
- Long-term use of NSAIDs
- Immunocompromised individuals
- Systemic lupus erythematosus
- Multiple myeloma
- Hepatitis
- Amyloidosis.

Pathophysiology

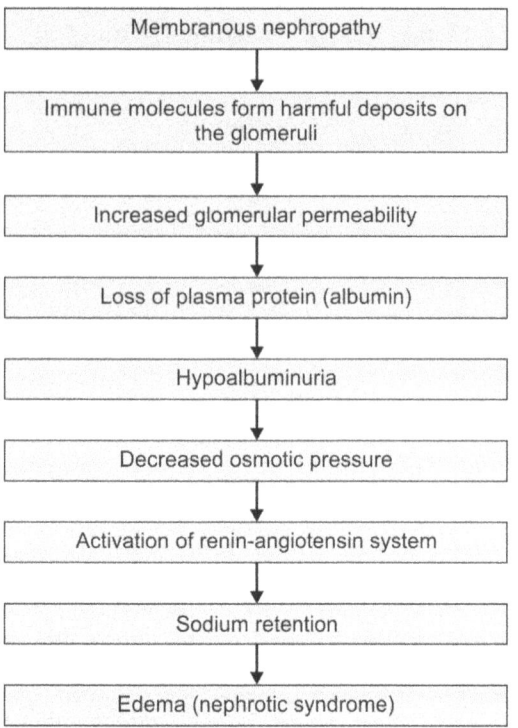

Clinical Features

- Hypoalbuminemia
- Hyperlipidemia
- Proteinuria
- Soft and pitting edema in dependent (sacrum, ankles and hands and in the abdomen) and periorbital areas
- Headache
- Malaise
- Irritability
- Fatigue
- Weight gain
- Foamy urine
- Loss of appetite.

Complications

- Infection
- Hypovolemia
- Thrombosis

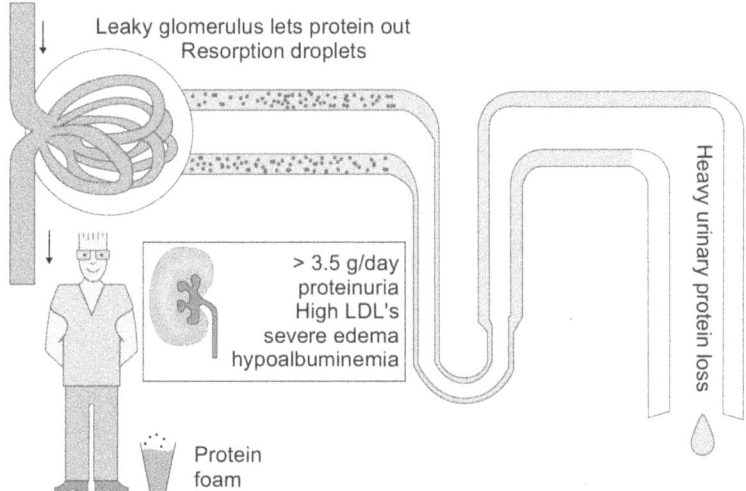

Fig. 9.6: Depicts primary glomerular disease characterized by proteinuria, hypoalbuminemia, hyperlipidemia and edema (Nephrotic syndrome).

- Acute kidney injury
- Hypertension.

Diagnostic Tests

- History
- Physical examination
- Blood examination
- Urine examination
- Kidney function test
- Coagulation tests
- Renal duplex echography
- Lipid profile tests
- Kidney biopsy.

Management

Medical

- **Diuretic agents:** It aids the kidneys in removing fluid from the blood and thereby reduces edema. For example, furosemide, bumetanide, ethacrynic acid, torsemide, etc.
- **Angiotensin-converting enzyme inhibitors:** It induces vasodilation which improves cardiac output and enhances the renal excretion of salt and water. For example, enalapril, captopril, ramipril, etc.
- **Angiotensin receptor blockers:** It slows down the progression of kidney disease by reducing the pressure inside the glomeruli and thereby reducing proteinuria. For example, losartan, candesartan, etc.
- **Calcium channel blockers:** They enhance glomerular filtration rate, renal blood flow and electrolyte excretion in the kidneys. For example, diltiazem, verapamil, etc.
- **Beta blockers:** They slow down the heart beat, decrease the force of contraction of the heart muscles and reduce blood vessel contraction in various parts of the body. For example, atenolol, labetalol, carvedilol, etc.
- **Statins:** It helps to lower the level of low-density lipoprotein (LDL) cholesterol in the blood. For example, atorvastatin, lovastatin, fluvastatin, etc.
- **Antibiotics:** It helps to prevent any secondary infections. For example, doxycycline, clindamycin, metronidazole, etc.
- **Corticosteroids:** It helps in reducing the severity of the disease. For example, prednisone, etc.

Nursing

- Encourage the patient to take high protein and low sodium diet.
- Encourage the patient to take liberal potassium diet to enhance sodium elimination thereby reducing edema.
- Instruct the patient to take low saturated fat diet.

- Explain the patient about the administration of the medicine and its continuation.
- Explain the patient about the follow-up and the risk of relapse.
- Demonstrate urine testing for albumin to patient.

POLYCYSTIC KIDNEY DISEASE

Definition

Polycystic kidney disease (PKD) is a genetic disorder characterized by the growth of numerous cysts in the kidneys.

Etiology

Genetic defects (Mutations in the genes PKD1 and PKD2).

Risk Factors

- Being babies and children
- Being males
- Tuberous sclerosis
- Von Hippel-Lindau syndrome
- Women with hypertension.

Types

- ***Autosomal dominant polycystic kidney disease:*** It is the most common inherited form and it constitutes about 90% of all PKD diseases. Its symptoms usually develop between the ages of 30 and 40 years, but they also can begin earlier in childhood.
- ***Autosomal recessive polycystic kidney disease:*** It is a rare inherited form and its symptoms begin in the earliest months of life, even in the womb.

Pathophysiology

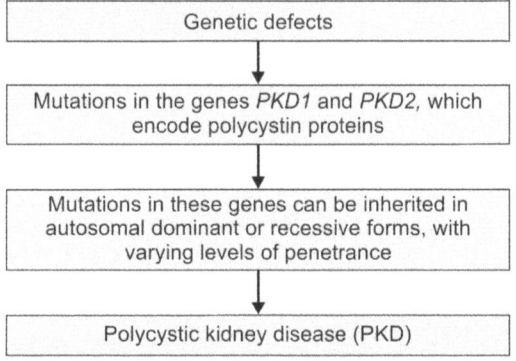

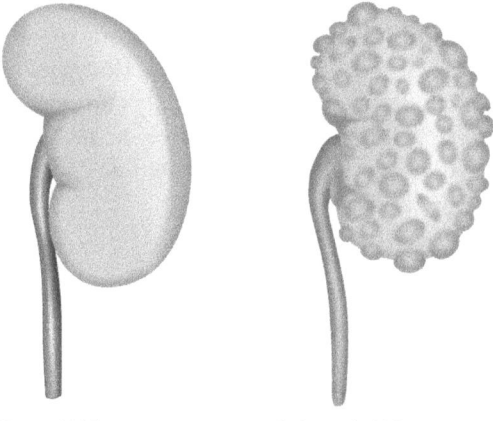

Fig. 9.7: Shows the comparison of normal kidney with that of the polycystic kidney.

Clinical Features

- Pain in the back and the lower sides
- A lump in the tummy on one or both sides
- Feeling of fullness or indigestion
- Headaches
- Frequent urinary tract infections
- Blood in the urine
- Protein in the urine
- Cysts in the kidneys and other organs
- Fluttering or pounding in the chest
- High blood pressure
- Kidney failure requiring dialysis.

Complications

- Abnormal heart valves
- Hernias
- Kidney stones
- Diverticulosis (small pouches bulge outward through the colon)
- Aneurysms.

Diagnostic Tests

- History
- Physical examination
- Blood examination
- Urinalysis
- Kidney imaging studies

- Kidney function test
- Ultrasound
- Computed tomography (CT) scan
- Magnetic resonance imaging (MRI) scan.

Management

Medical

- **Angiotensin-converting enzyme inhibitors:** It induces vasodilation which improves cardiac output and enhances the renal excretion of salt and water. For example, enalapril, captopril, ramipril, etc.
- **Angiotensin receptor blockers:** It constricts the efferent arteriole more than the afferent arteriole within the kidney, which helps to maintain glomerular capillary pressure and filtration. For example, losartan, candesartan, etc.
- **Aldosterone antagonists:** It blocks the effects of aldosterone, therefore decreases sodium re-absorption and water retention by the kidneys and consequently leads to a decrease in blood pressure. For example, Aldactone, Inspra, etc.
- **Urinary analgesics:** It helps to reduce the pain to a certain extent. For example, paracetamol, ibuprofen, etc.
- **Antibiotics:** It helps to prevent any secondary infections. For example, ciprofloxacin, gentamicin, cephalosporins, etc.
- **Statins:** It helps to lower the level of low-density lipoprotein (LDL) cholesterol in the blood. For example, atorvastatin, lovastatin, fluvastatin, etc.

Surgical

- **Hemodialysis (HD):** It is the artificial process of eliminating waste (diffusion) and unwanted water (ultrafiltration) from the blood by pumping the patient's blood against dialysate that may be generated by the dialysis machine or at a central location.
- **Renal transplantation:** It is a procedure that involves a number of small incisions (1–3 cm) through which the faulty kidneys are removed and replaced with a healthy kidney from the donor.

Nursing

- Encourage the patient to maintain a healthy weight.
- Encourage the patient to eat well-balanced diet.
- Instruct the patient to reduce the intake of salt in the diet.
- Instruct the patient to do regular exercise.
- Explain the patient about the administration of the medicine and its continuation.
- Instruct the patient to stop smoking.
- Encourage the patient to drink lots of plain water throughout the day.
- Instruct the patient to avoid caffeinated drinks.

PYELONEPHRITIS

Definition

Pyelonephritis is a bacterial infection of the renal pelvis, tubules and interstitial tissue of one or both kidneys.

Etiology

- Bacterial infection (*Escherichia coli*)
- Ureterovesical reflux (backup of urine into ureters)
- Urinary tract obstruction (tumor, stones, etc).

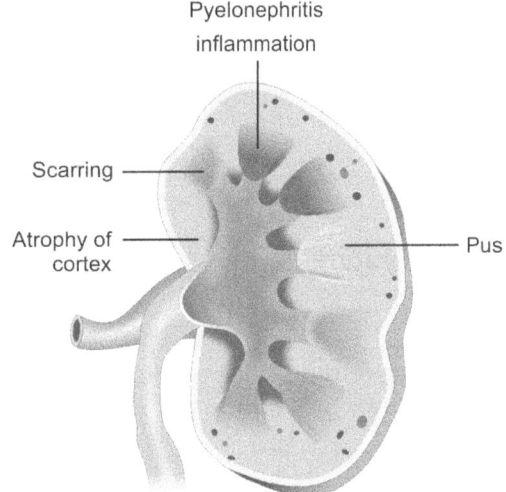

Fig. 9.8: Depicts inflamed renal pelvis, tubules and interstitial tissue of a kidney.

Risk Factors

- Being females
- Being children
- Previous history of urinary tract infection
- Siblings who have a history of urinary tract infection
- An indwelling urinary catheter
- An intact prepuce in boys
- Structural abnormalities of the kidneys and lower urinary tract
- Neuropathic bladder
- People with a weakened immune system
- Diabetes
- Pregnancy
- Prostate enlargement
- Primary biliary cirrhosis.

Types

- *Acute pyelonephritis:* It is sudden in onset and it occurs within the renal pelvis, usually accompanied by infection within the renal parenchyma and is caused by the bacteria.
- *Chronic pyelonephritis:* It is a repeated bouts of acute attack and is due to chronic obstruction or chronic reflux.

Pathophysiology

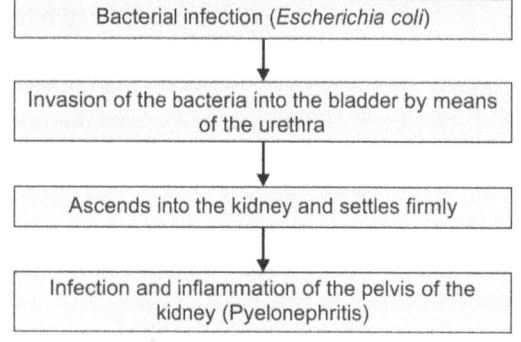

Clinical Features

- Fever
- Chills
- Leukocytosis
- Bacteriuria
- Pyuria
- Flank pain
- CVA tenderness
- Dysuria
- Frequency of urination
- Urine that smells bad
- Blood or pus in the urine
- Nausea
- Vomiting.

Complications

- Bacteremia
- Recurrence
- Renal scarring
- Hypertension
- Formation of kidney stones.

Diagnostic Tests

- History
- Physical examination
- Blood examination
- Urinalysis
- Urine culture
- Kidney function test
- Ultrasound
- Computed tomography (CT) scan
- Intravenous pyelogram
- Dimercaptosuccinic acid (DMSA) scintigraphy
- Voiding cystourethrogram (VCUG)
- Digital rectal examination (DRE).

Management

Medical

- **Fluid replacement therapy:** It is the administration of fluids to a patient as a treatment or preventive measure usually 3–4 liters per day to dilute the urine and to expel the bacteria from the urinary tract.
- **Antibiotics:** It helps to prevent any secondary infections. For example, ciprofloxacins, gentamicin, cephalosporin, etc.
- **Corticosteroids:** It helps in reducing the severity of the disease. For example, prednisone, etc.
- **Urinary analgesics:** It helps to reduce the pain to a certain extent. For example, phenazopyridine, paracetamol, codeine, etc.

Disorders of Renal System

Nursing

- Encourage the patient to drink 8–12 glasses of fluid every day.
- Instruct the patient to avoid holding urine in the bladder for a long time.
- Instruct the patient to keep the genital area clean.
- Explain the patient about the administration of the medicine and its continuation.
- Encourage the patient to drink cranberry juice daily.
- Instruct the patient to urinate as soon as they feel the need.

RENAL CALCULI (KIDNEY STONES)

Definition

A kidney stone is a solid piece of material that forms in a kidney when substances that are normally found in the urine (calcium, oxalate and phosphorus) become highly concentrated.

Etiology

- Caffeinated and sugary drinks
- People who do not drink enough fluids
- Low urine volume
- Vitamin C supplements.

Risk Factors

- Being males
- Non-Hispanic white people
- Obesity
- Hypercalciuria
- Cystic kidney diseases
- Hyperparathyroidism
- Renal tubular acidosis
- Cystinuria
- Hyperoxaluria
- Hyperuricosuria
- Gout
- Blockage of the urinary tract
- Bowel disease
- Excess dietary meat
- Prolonged immobilization
- Insulin resistance.

Types

- ***Calcium stones:*** These are the most common type of kidney stones and occur in two major forms: calcium oxalate and calcium phosphate.
- ***Uric acid stones:*** They form when the urine is persistently acidic.
- ***Struvite stones:*** These result from kidney infections.

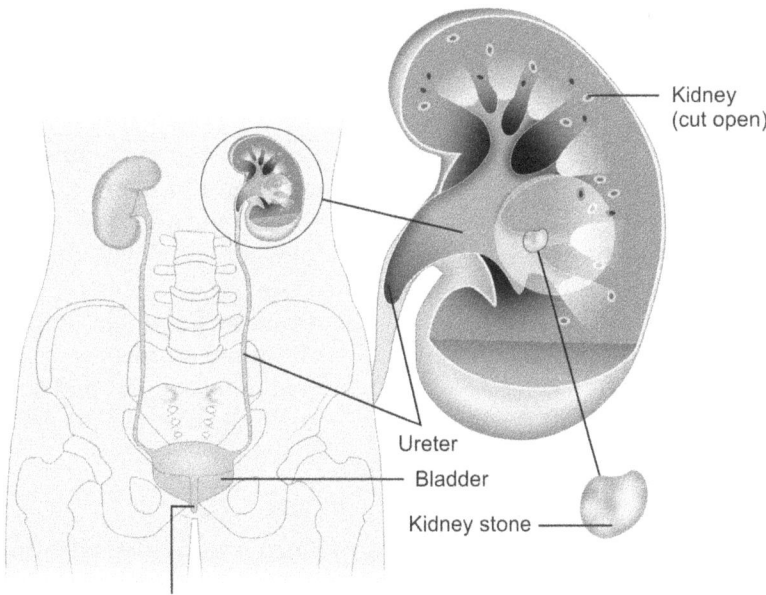

Fig. 9.9: Show kidney with stones in it.

- **Cystine stones:** These result from a genetic disorder that causes cystine to leak the kidneys and into the urine, forming crystals that tend to accumulate into stones.

Pathophysiology

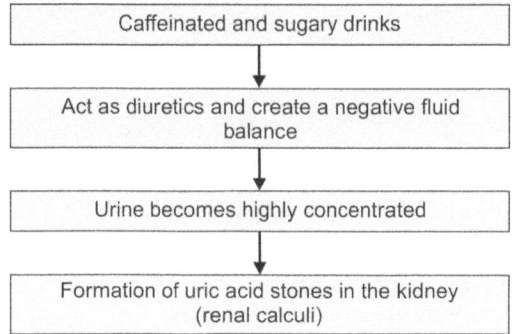

Clinical Features

- Severe loin pain that comes and goes (colicky pain)
- Difficulty in passing urine
- Nausea
- Vomiting
- Abnormal urine color
- Blood in the urine
- Cloudy or foul-smelling urine
- Fever
- Chills
- Diaphoresis.

Complications

- Sepsis
- Urinary tract infections
- Pyelonephritis
- Permanent kidney damage.

Diagnostic Tests

- History
- Physical examination
- Blood examination
- Urinalysis
- Kidney function test
- Ultrasound
- Computed tomography (CT) scan
- Intravenous pyelogram.

Management

Medical

- **Fluid replacement therapy:** It is the administration of fluids to a patient as a treatment or preventive measure usually 2–3 liters per day to dilute the urine.
- **Antibiotics:** It helps to prevent any secondary infections. For example, ciprofloxacin, cephalosporins, etc.
- **Urinary analgesics:** It helps to reduce the colicky pain prevailing in renal calculi. For example, ibuprofen, hydrocodone, etc.
- **Adrenergic receptor antagonists:** It relaxes the ureters, making it easier for the stone to pass. For example, tamsulosin, etc.

Surgical

- **Extracorporeal shock wave lithotripsy (ESWL):** It is a procedure in which ultrasound waves are used to break the kidney stone into smaller pieces, which can pass out with the urine. It is used for stones less than 2 cm in size.
- **Percutaneous nephrostolithotomy (PCNL):** It is a procedure in which a small cut is made at the back and then a special instrument is used to remove the kidney stone.
- **Ureteroscopy with lithotripsy:** It is a procedure in which an instrument is inserted into the urethra, passed into the bladder and then to where the stone is located and it allows the surgeon to remove the stone or break it up so it can pass more easily.
- **Open surgery:** It is a procedure in which the renal stones are removed through traditional surgery and it requires a cut at the back to access the kidney and ureters to remove the stone.

Nursing

- Encourage the patient to drink 8–12 glasses of fluid everyday.

- Instruct the patient to avoid holding urine in the bladder for a long time.
- Instruct the patient to reduce the intake of salt in the diet.
- Explain the patient about the administration of the medicine and its continuation.
- Instruct the patient to avoid excess intake of caffeinated drinks.
- Encourage the patient to eat plenty of fruits and vegetables.

UREMIC ENCEPHALOPATHY

Definition

Uremic encephalopathy is an acute organic brain syndrome that regularly occurs in patients with acute renal failure when glomerular filtration rate declines.

Etiology

- Acute kidney injury (AKI)
- Infection (Bacteria, viruses or prions)
- Lack of oxygen to the brain
- Increased intracranial pressure
- Renal artery stenosis
- Polycystic kidney disease.

Risk Factors

- Being males
- Person older than 65 years
- Alcohol/drug overdose
- Poor nutrition
- Metabolic diseases
- Long-term use of aspirin
- Prolonged exposure to toxic chemicals.

Pathophysiology

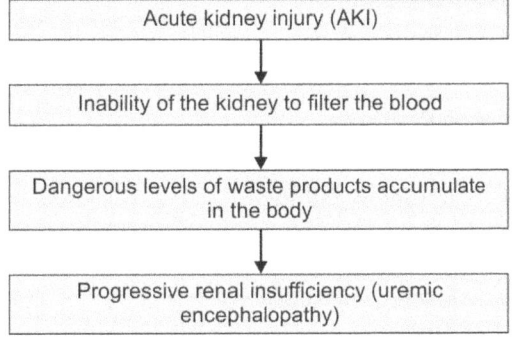

Clinical Features

- Altered mental state
- Anorexia

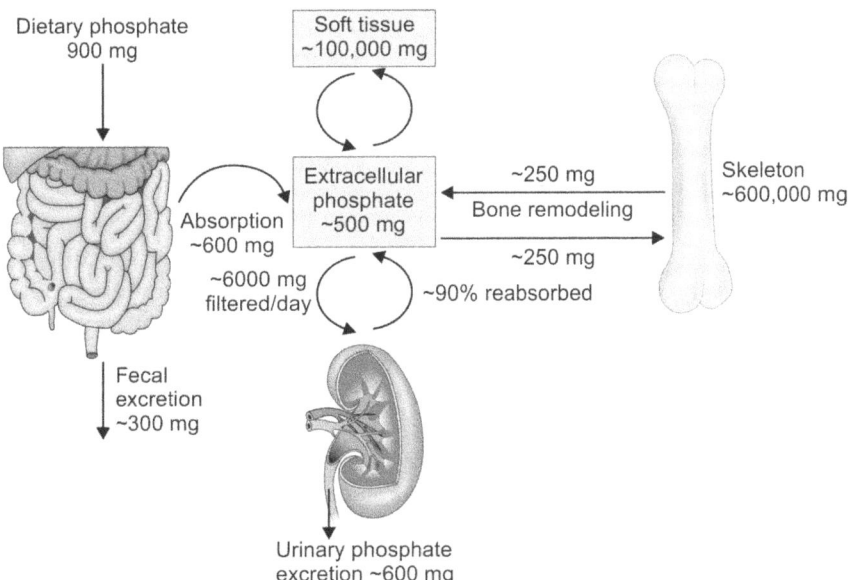

Fig. 9.10: Shows the declined rate of glomerular filtration (Uremic encephalopathy).

- Nausea
- Restlessness
- Gradual but progressive drowsiness
- Diminished ability to concentrate
- Vomiting
- Emotional volatility
- Disorientation
- Confusion
- Myoclonus
- Asterixis
- Prolonged hypotension
- Hyponatremia
- Hypocalcemia
- Metabolic alkalosis.

Complications

- Sepsis
- Circulatory failure
- Stupor
- Hallucinations
- Muscle twitching
- Coma
- Death.

Diagnostic Tests

- History
- Physical examination
- Blood examination
- Urinalysis
- Kidney function test
- Ultrasound
- Computed tomography (CT) scan
- Intravenous pyelogram.

Management

Medical

- **Angiotensin-converting enzyme inhibitors:** It induces vasodilation which improves cardiac output and enhances the renal excretion of salt and water. For example, enalapril, captopril, ramipril, etc.
- **Calcium channel blockers:** They enhance glomerular filtration rate, renal blood flow and electrolyte excretion in the kidneys. For example, diltiazem, verapamil, etc.
- **Angiotensin receptor blockers:** It constricts the efferent arteriole more than the afferent arteriole within the kidney, which helps to maintain glomerular capillary pressure and filtration. For example, losartan, candesartan, etc.
- **Aldosterone antagonists:** It blocks the effects of aldosterone, therefore decreases sodium re-absorption and water retention by the kidneys and consequently leads to a decrease in blood pressure. For example, Aldactone, Inspra, etc.
- **Renin inhibitors:** It blocks the activity of renin and causes vasodilation. For example, Tekturna, etc.
- **Thiazide diuretics:** It decreases active re-absorption of sodium and chloride ions by inhibiting the sodium/chloride cotransporter in the distal convoluted tubule and also increases potassium ion loss. For example, lozol, thalitone, etc.
- **Antibiotics:** It helps to prevent any secondary infections. For example, doxycycline, clindamycin, metronidazole, etc.

Surgical

- **Hemodialysis (HD):** It is the artificial process of eliminating waste (diffusion) and unwanted water (ultrafiltration) from the blood by pumping the patient's blood against dialysate that may be generated by the dialysis machine or at a central location.
- **Continuous renal replacement therapy (CRRT):** It is a slow and continuous extracorporeal blood purification therapy and it mimics the function of the kidneys in regulating water, electrolytes and toxic products by the continuous slow removal of solutes and fluid that are provided 24 hours per day.
- **Sustained low-efficiency dialysis (SLED):** It is a procedure used as a renal replacement modality in critically ill patients with acute kidney injury and hemodynamic instability.
- **Peritoneal dialysis (PD):** It works using the body's peritoneal membrane as a filter which allows impurities to be drawn out of the blood.

- **Renal transplantation:** It is a procedure that involves a number of small incisions (1–3 cm) through which the faulty kidneys are removed and replaced with a healthy kidney from the donor.

Nursing

- Measure fluid input and output accurately.
- Weigh the patient every day, at the same time and on the same scale.
- Limit the intake of protein to less than 1 g/day.
- Restrict the intake of potassium to 40–60 mEq/day.
- Restrict the intake of sodium to 2 mEq/day.

URETHRAL STRICTURES

Definition

Urethral stricture is a narrowing of the urethra due to scar tissue, which leads to obstructive voiding dysfunction with potentially serious consequences for the entire urinary tract.

Etiology

- A straddle injury
- Hypospadias surgery
- Pelvic bone fractures
- Balanitis xerotica obliterans (BXO)
- Men who have penile implants
- A tumor located in close proximity to the urethra.

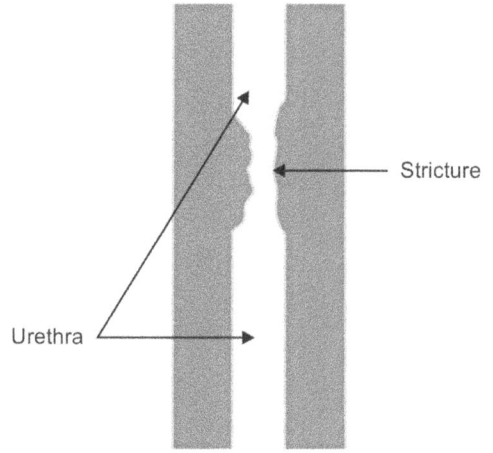

Fig. 9.11: Depicts narrowing of the urethra due to scar tissue (Urethral stricture).

Risk Factors

- Being males
- History of sexually transmitted diseases
- Surgeries performed on the prostate
- History of urethritis
- Untreated or repetitive urinary infections
- Radiation
- Urethral catheterization.

Pathophysiology

Straddle trauma injury to the urethra caused by falling from a bicycle, being kicked, hit by a ball or any other impact to the scrotal area

↓

Tear of the membranous portion of the posterior urethra

↓

Stricture in the bulbar urethra (a portion of the urethra)

↓

Inability to pass urine (urethral strictures)

Clinical Features

- Reduced urine flow
- Pain on passing urine
- Blood in the urine
- Spraying or dribbling of the urine stream
- Slow urine stream
- Urinary tract infections
- Abdominal pain
- Urethral discharge
- Urinary incontinence.

Complications

- Abscess formation
- Stricture recurrence
- Incomplete emptying of the bladder
- Cancer of the urethra (rare).

Diagnostic Tests

- History
- Physical examination
- Blood examination
- Urinalysis
- Urine culture
- Urethral culture

- Ultrasound of the urethra
- Retrograde urethrogram
- Anterograde cystourethrogram
- Cystourethroscopy.

Management

Medical

- **Antibiotics:** It helps to prevent any secondary infections. For example, trimethoprim, nitrofurantoin, metronidazole, etc.
- **Urinary analgesics:** It helps to relieve pain and burning caused by the urethral stricture. For example, phenazopyridine, etc.

Surgical

- **Urethral dilation:** It is a surgical procedure in which thin rods of increasing diameters are gently inserted into the urethra in order to open the urethral narrowing without causing further injury.
- **Urethrostomy:** It is an endoscopic procedure in which a thin tube with a camera (endoscope) is inserted into the urethra to visualize the stricture and then a tiny knife is passed through the endoscope to cut the stricture lengthwise and open the flow of urine.
- **Urethral stent placement:** It is an endoscopic procedure where a closed tube (stent) is passed through an endoscope to the area of the stricture and once it reaches the proper location, the stent can be opened to form a tube to enable urine to flow.
- **Open urethral reconstruction:** It is a surgical procedure in which the area of scarring is cut out and the remaining urethra is reconstructed through a graft.

Nursing

- Assist the patient in making healthy lifestyle choices.
- Explain the patient about the administration of the medicine and its continuation.
- Instruct the patient to maintain a good personal hygiene.
- Ask the patient to limit the number of sexual partners by practicing monogamy.
- Place a warm pack, such as a hot water bottle wrapped in a towel on the abdomen to help in relieving pain.
- Encourage the patient to take cranberry juice daily to prevent infections.

URETHRITIS

Definition

Urethritis is an inflammation (irritation) of the urethra, the tube that drains the bladder.

Etiology

- Bacterial infection (*Neisseria gonorrhoeae, Mycoplasma genitalium, Chlamydia trachomatis*, etc.)

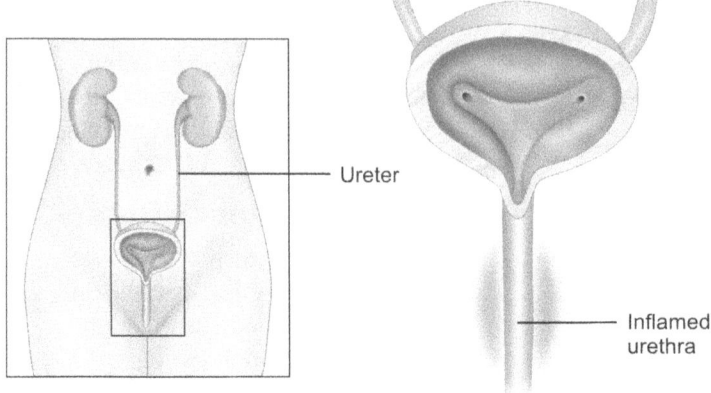

Fig. 9.12: Shows the inflamed urethra, the tube that drains the bladder (Urethritis).

- Viral infection (Herpes simplex virus, adenovirus, etc.)
- Parasitic infection (*Trichomonas vaginalis*)
- Injury to the urethra
- Sensitivity to the chemicals in spermicides or contraceptives
- Autoimmune diseases.

Risk Factors

- Being young men aged 20–35 years
- Having multiple sexual partners
- Women who are in their reproductive ages
- Unprotected sex (without using contraceptives)
- History of sexually transmitted diseases
- High-risk sexual behavior (anal sex)
- Urethral catheterization.

Pathophysiology

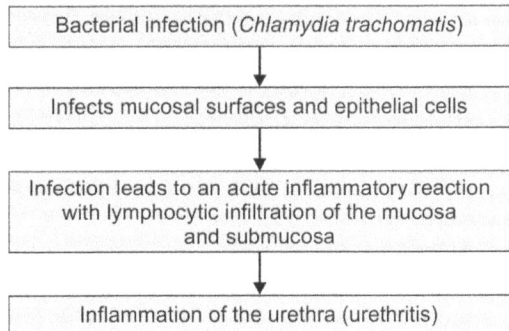

Clinical Features

In Women
- Burning pain while passing urine (Dysuria)
- Pain in the lower abdomen and pelvis
- Frequent or urgent urination
- Pus-filled urethral discharge
- Blood in the urine
- Unusual vaginal discharge
- Urine that appears cloudy
- Fever
- Chills
- Pain during sex.

In Men
- Blood in the urine or semen
- Burning pain while passing urine (Dysuria)
- Pus or whitish mucus discharge from the penis
- Frequent or urgent urination
- Itching, pain or discomfort in the penis or groin area
- Pain during intercourse or ejaculation
- Fever (rare).

Complications

- Urethral stricture
- Infertility
- Renal impairment
- Cystitis
- Orchitis
- Prostatitis
- Cervicitis.

Diagnostic Tests

- History
- Physical examination
- Blood examination
- Urinalysis
- Urine culture
- Urethral swab
- Nucleic acid amplification test
- Cystoscopy
- Pelvic ultrasound.

Management

Medical

- **Fluid replacement therapy:** It is the administration of fluids to a patient as a treatment or preventive measure usually 2–3 liters per day to dilute the urine.
- **Antibiotics:** For example, metronidazole, trimethoprim, nitrofurantoin, azithromycin, erythromycin, etc. It helps to prevent any secondary infections.
- **Urinary analgesics:** For example, phenazopyridine, etc. It helps to relieve pain and burning caused by the infection.

Nursing

- Instruct the patient to avoid irritants (lotion, detergents, spermicides or contraceptives) causing the condition.
- Instruct the patient to maintain a good personal hygiene.
- Ask the patient to limit the number of sexual partners by practicing monogamy.

- Encourage the patient to drink plenty of fluids.
- Assist the patient in making healthy lifestyle choices.
- Teach the patient to practice pelvic floor exercises.

URINARY INCONTINENCE

Definition
Urinary incontinence is unintentional loss of urine that is sufficient enough in frequency and amount to cause physical or emotional distress in the person experiencing it.

Etiology
- Nerve damage
- Infection of the urinary tract and bladder
- Caffeine and alcohol
- Chronic constipation
- Excess weight
- Certain medications (e.g., Furosemide)
- Pregnancy
- Childbirth
- Menopause
- Urinary tract infection.

Risk Factors
- Being females
- Brain injury
- Birth defects
- Stroke
- Diabetes
- Multiple sclerosis
- Physical changes associated with aging.

Types
- ***Stress incontinence:*** In this, the leakage happens with coughing, sneezing, exercising, laughing, lifting heavy things and other movements that put pressure on the bladder. This is the most common type of incontinence in women.
- ***Urge incontinence:*** In this the leakage usually happens after a strong, sudden urge to urinate. This may occur when we do not expect it, such as during sleep, after drinking water, or when touch running water.
- ***Functional incontinence:*** People with this type of incontinence may have problems thinking, moving, or speaking that keep them from reaching to a toilet. For example, a person with Alzheimer's disease may not plan a trip to the bathroom in time to urinate and a person in a wheelchair may be unable to get to a toilet in time.
- ***Overflow incontinence:*** In this, the urine leakage happens because the bladder does not empty completely. It is less common in women.
- ***Mixed incontinence:*** This is due to the combination of two or more types of incontinence together (usually stress and urge incontinence).
- ***Transient incontinence:*** In this, the urine leakage happens for a short time due to an illness (bladder infection). The leaking stops when the illness is treated.

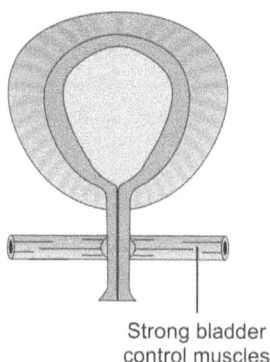 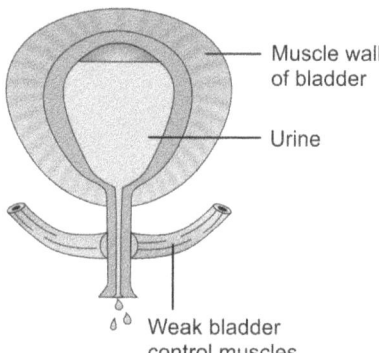

Fig. 9.13: Shows the comparison of strong bladder with control muscles with that of the weak bladder with control muscles.

Pathophysiology

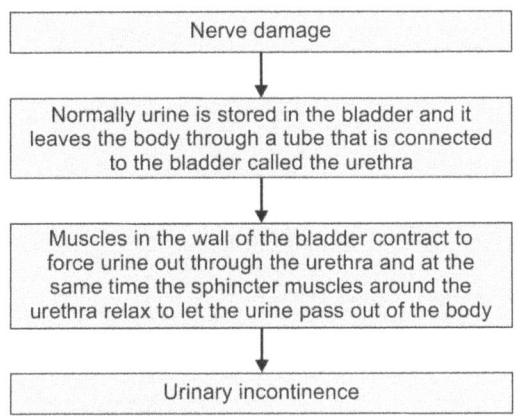

Clinical Features

- Strong urge to urinate
- Frequent micturition
- Nocturia
- Dysuria
- Nocturnal enuresis
- Inability to get to the toilet in time
- Passing small amount of urine many times a day
- A burning or stinging sensation when passing urine.

Complications

- Urinary tract infection
- Skin problems
- Bladder stones
- Renal impairment.

Diagnostic Tests

- History
- Physical examination
- Blood examination
- Urinalysis
- Bladder stress test
- Ultrasound
- Urodynamic testing
- Cystoscopy.

Management

Medical

- **Anti-spasm agents:** It helps to control muscle spasms or unwanted bladder contractions and helps in preventing leakage from urgency urinary incontinence. For example, methenamine, flavoxate, etc.
- **Beta-3 adrenergic receptor:** It relaxes the bladder muscle and allows the bladder to store more urine. For example, Mirabegron, etc.
- **Neurotoxin agents:** It helps to stop unwanted bladder muscle contractions. For example, onabotulinumtoxinA, etc.

Surgical

- **Colposuspension:** In this procedure, stitches are placed on either side of the bladder neck and attached to nearby supporting structures to lift up the urethra and hold it in place.
- **Bladder slings:** It is a narrow strap made of synthetic mesh that is placed under the urethra to provide support to it.
- **Sacral neuromodulation:** This is a technique in which a thin wire is placed under the skin of the low back and close to the nerve that controls the bladder. The wire is attached to a battery device placed under the skin nearby. The device sends a mild electrical signal along the wire to improve bladder function.
- **Percutaneous tibial nerve stimulation (PTNS):** It is a procedure in which a slender needle is inserted near a nerve in the ankle and connected to a special machine. A signal is sent through the needle to the nerve, which sends the signal to the pelvic floor.

Nursing

- Instruct the patient to maintain a healthy weight.
- Teach the patient to practice pelvic floor exercises.
- Instruct the patient to avoid caffeine and alcohol.
- Encourage the patient to take more roughages in the diet to prevent constipation.
- Ask the patient to be physically active.

- Enforce the patient to practice good toilet habits.
- Assist the patient in making healthy lifestyle choices.

URINARY TRACT INFECTION

Definition
Urinary tract infection is the microbial invasion of any tissue of the urinary tract, extending from the urethral meatus to the renal cortex.

Etiology
- Bacterial infection (*Escherichia coli*)
- Waiting to urinate
- Making too little urine
- Constipation.

Risk Factors
- Young women who are sexually active.
- Elderly men with prostate problems
- Young boys
- History of renal calculi
- Diabetes that is poorly controlled
- Patients treated with antibiotics
- Neurogenic bladder retention
- Structural abnormality of urinary tract
- People with spinal cord injury
- Women using diaphragm for birth control.

Pathophysiology

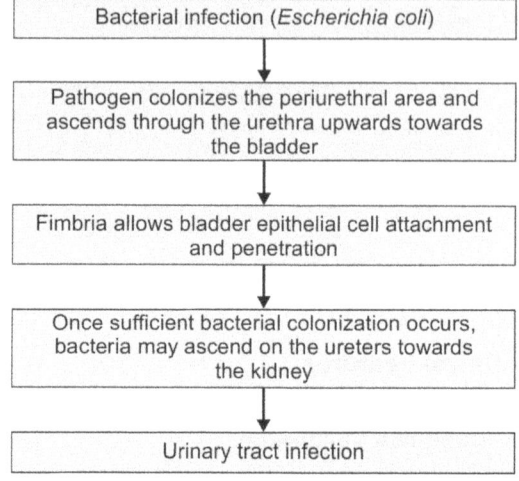

Clinical Features
- Dysuria
- Hematuria
- Cloudy urine
- Frequent and intense urge to urinate
- Nausea
- Vomiting
- Tiredness
- Fever
- Chills
- Pain in the back or side below the ribs
- Delirium
- Functional decline.

Complications
- Recurrent infections
- Sepsis
- Pyelonephritis.

Diagnostic Tests
- History
- Physical examination
- Blood examination
- Urinalysis
- Ultrasound
- Urodynamic testing

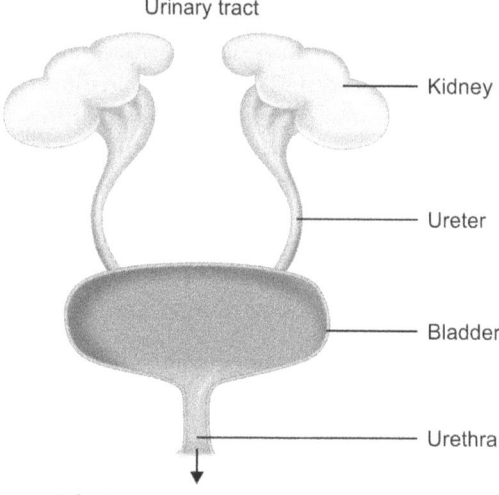

Fig. 9.14: Depicts microbial invasion of the urinary tract (Urinary tract infection).

- Cystourethrogram
- Computed tomography (CT) scan
- Magnetic resonance imaging (MRI) scan
- Radionuclide scan
- Cystoscopy.

Management

Medical

- **Fluid replacement therapy:** It is the administration of fluids to a patient as a treatment or preventive measure usually 2–3 liters per day to dilute the urine.
- **Antibiotics:** It helps to prevent any secondary infections. For example, trimethoprim sulfamethoxazole, penicillin, cephalosporins, fluoroquinolones, tetracycline, aminoglycosides, nitrofurantoin, etc.
- **Urinary analgesics:** It helps to relieve pain and burning caused by the infection. For example, phenazopyridine, etc.
- **Anti-spasm agents:** It helps to reduce the bladder spasm. For example, methenamine, flavoxate, etc.

Nursing

- Encourage the patient to drink 8–12 glasses of fluid everyday.
- Instruct the patient to avoid holding urine in the bladder for a long time.
- Explain the patient about the administration of the medicine and its continuation.
- Ask the patient to urinate often and when the urge arises.
- Encourage the patient wear loose-fitted clothes.

10

CHAPTER

Disorders of Reproductive System

CHAPTER OUTLINE

MALE REPRODUCTIVE SYSTEM
- Benign prostatic hyperplasia (BPH)
- Cryptorchidism
- Epididymitis
- Erectile dysfunction
- Male infertility
- Prostatitis
- Varicocele

FEMALE REPRODUCTIVE SYSTEM
- Abortion
- Bartholin's abscess
- Dysmenorrhea
- Ectopic pregnancy
- Endometritis
- Female infertility
- Fibroid uterus
- Pelvic inflammatory disease
- Premenstrual syndrome
- Polycystic ovary disease
- Toxic shock syndrome
- Uterine prolapse

MALE REPRODUCTIVE SYSTEM

BENIGN PROSTATIC HYPERPLASIA

Definition

Benign prostatic hyperplasia (BPH) is a nonmalignant (noncancerous) enlargement of the prostate gland, a common occurrence in older men. It is also known as BPH.

Etiology

- Drop in blood testosterone level and subsequent rise in the estrogen level.
- High levels of dihydrotestosterone (DHT) in the prostate gland
- Neoplasm
- Arteriosclerosis
- Metabolic or nutritional disturbances.

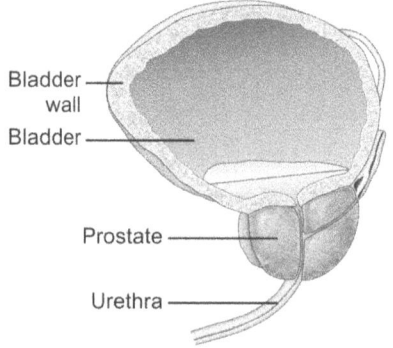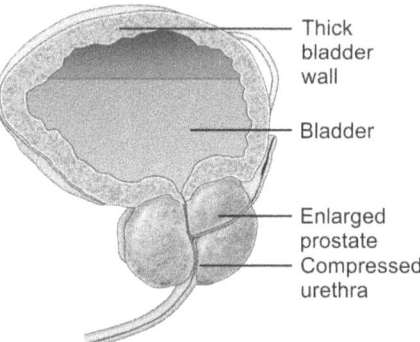

Fig. 10.1: Shows the comparison of normal prostate with enlarged prostate (Benign prostatic hyperplasia).

Risk Factors

- Males aged 40 years and older
- Type 2 diabetes mellitus
- Lack of physical exercise
- Family history of BPH
- Ethnic background
- Erectile dysfunction
- Obesity.

Pathophysiology

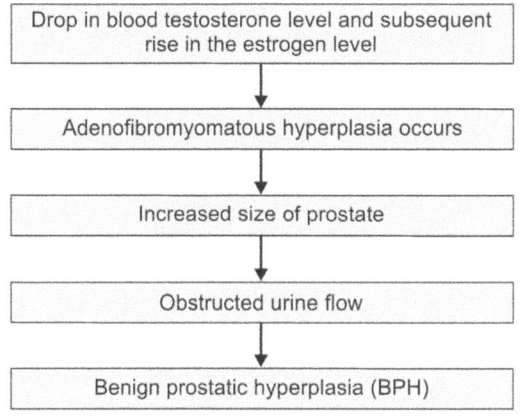

Clinical Features

- Weak urine stream
- Difficulty in starting urination
- Dribbling of urine
- Frequency and urgency of urination
- Nocturia (a need to pass urine more than twice at night)
- Perineal pain (pain in between the scrotum and penis)
- Not being able to completely empty the bladder
- Paradoxical incontinence (urine overflows from a full bladder uncontrollably even though normal urination cannot be started)
- Impaired kidney function

Complications

- Acute urinary retention
- Bladder diverticula
- Cystolithiasis
- Hydronephrosis
- Hematuria.

Diagnostic Tests

- History
- Physical examination
- Neurological examination
- Digital rectal exam (DRE)
- Urine examination
- Prostate-specific antigen (PSA) blood test
- Urinary flow test
- Post-void residual volume test
- Transrectal ultrasound
- Prostate biopsy
- Cystoscopy
- Intravenous pyelogram or CT urogram.

Management

Medical

- **Alpha blockers:** It relaxes the smooth muscles of the prostate and the bladder neck, which helps to relieve urinary obstruction caused by an enlarged prostate in BPH. For example, tamsulosin, alfuzosin, etc.
- **5 Alpha reductase inhibitors:** It shrinks the prostate by preventing hormonal changes that causes prostate growth. For example, finasteride, dutasteride, etc.
- **Phosphodiesterase 5 inhibitors:** It reduces lower urinary tract symptoms relaxing smooth muscles in the lower urinary tract. For example, tadalafil, etc.

Surgical

- **Transurethral resection of prostate (TURP):** It is the surgical procedure in which a surgeon places a special lighted scope (resectoscope) into the urethra and uses small cutting tools to remove all but the outer part of the prostate (prostate resection) to facilitate urine flow.
- **Transurethral incision of prostate (TUIP or TIP):** It is the surgical procedure in which the surgeon makes one or two small cuts in the prostate gland to open up a channel in the urethra with the help of special instruments to facilitate urine flow.
- **Open prostatectomy:** It is the surgical procedure in which the surgeon makes an

incision in the lower abdomen to reach the prostate and to facilitate urination.
- **Minimal invasive surgical treatments:** These are treatments which are less likely to cause blood loss during surgery and also do not require a hospital stay. They are as follows:
  - *Laser surgery*: In this, they use high energy lasers to destroy or remove overgrown prostate tissue.
  - *Ablative procedure including vaporization*: In this procedure, prostate tissue is removed by pressing on the urethra by burning it away and facilitating urine flow.
  - *Enucleative procedure*: In this procedure, the prostate tissue is removed and facilitates urine flow and also prevents regrowth of tissue.
- **Transurethral microwave therapy (TUMT):** In this procedure, the surgeon inserts a special electrode through the urethra into the prostate area. Microwave energy from the electrode generates heat and destroys the inner portion of the enlarged prostate gland causing it to shrink and ease urine flow.
- **Transurethral needle ablation (TUNA):** It is the surgical procedure in which a lighted scope (cystoscope) is passed into the urethra and a needle is placed in the prostate gland with the help of it. When the needles are in place radiowaves pass through them, heating and destroying excess prostate tissue that's blocking urine flow.
- **Prostatic stents:** A prostatic stent is a tiny metal or plastic device that's inserted into the urethra to keep it open. Tissue grows over the metallic stent to hold it in place and also facilitates urination.

Nursing

- Educate the patient to limit beverages in the evening.
- Instruct to limit decongestants or antihistamines as it worsens the situation.
- Encourage them to be in warm environment as it enhances the urge to void.
- Instruct them to have mild exercise as it avoids urine retention.
- Encourage the patient to take 2–4 liters of fluids daily as tolerated.
- Encourage the patient to use hot sitz bath.
- Ask the patient to take adequate rest.

CRYPTORCHIDISM (UNDESCENDED TESTES)

Definition

When one or both testicles fail to move into the scrotum before birth, the condition is referred to as cryptorchidism or undescended testes.

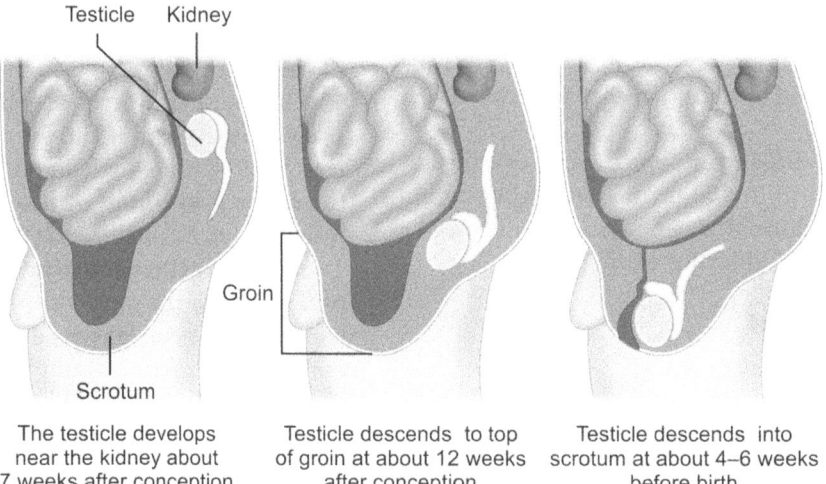

The testicle develops near the kidney about 7 weeks after conception

Testicle descends to top of groin at about 12 weeks after conception

Testicle descends into scrotum at about 4–6 weeks before birth

Fig. 10.2: Depicts how testicle descends into the scrotum before birth.

Etiology

- Premature infants with hormonal imbalance
- Low levels of androgens
- Developmental delay
- Aarskog syndrome (genetic disorder affecting person's stature and genitalia)
- Idiopathic
- Congenital
- Down's syndrome.

Risk Factors

- Being male infants
- Klinefelter's syndrome
- Spina bifida
- Maternal obesity
- Low birth weight
- Exposure to pesticides during pregnancy.

Pathophysiology

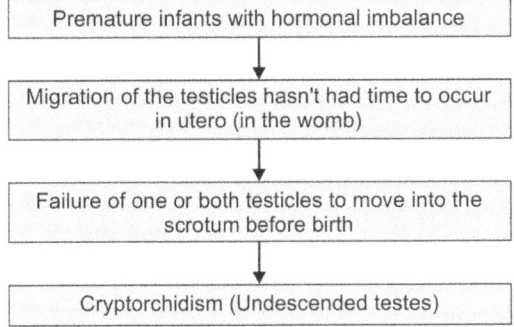

Clinical Features

- Empty scrotum
- Incomplete descent or ectopic testicle (s)
- Infertility
- Severe groin pain (rare)
- Hydrocele testis
- Inguinal hernia
- Depressed mood
- Insomnia
- Fatigue
- Anxiety.

Complications

- Testicular injury
- Testicular cancer
- Spermatic cord torsion
- Poor self-image.

Diagnostic Tests

- History
- Physical examination
- Blood examination
- Testicular self-examination
- Ultrasonogram
- HCG stimulation test.

Management

Medical

Human chorionic gonadotropin (hCG) or gonadotropin-releasing analogs: It increases the level of the male sex hormone testosterone which increases the likelihood of moving the undescended testicles into the scrotum. For example, B-hCG, testosterone, etc.

Surgical

- **Orchidopexy:** It is the surgical procedure which secures the proper position of a testicle into the scrotum.
- **Two-stage orchidopexy:** It is an alternative procedure in which the surgeon brings the testicle down into the scrotal sac and stitches it to the thigh; then 2–3 months later, it is embedded into the scrotal sac.

Nursing

- Instruct the mother to avoid tobacco consumption during fetal development.
- Restrict themselves from exposure to environmental toxins and pesticides.
- Ask the mother to stay away from second-hand smoke during fetal development.
- Instruct the mother to take plenty of rest and to spend time to relax during fetal development.

EPIDIDYMITIS

Definition

Epididymitis is an inflammation of the epididymis, the tubular structure that connects the testicle with the vas deferens.

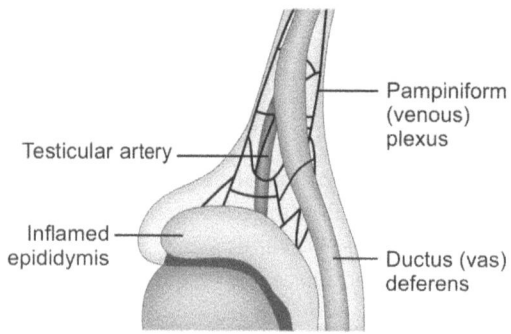

Fig. 10.3: Shows inflamed epididymis, the tubular structure connecting the testicle with the vas deferens.

Etiology

- Urinary tract infections
- Sexually transmitted infections (*Chlamydia* and *Gonorrhea*)
- Tuberculosis
- Long-term use of anti-arrhythmic medications
- Use of chronic indwelling urethral catheter
- Groin injury.

Risk Factors

- Sexually active men who are not monogamous and do not use condoms.
- Men who underwent surgery on the genitourinary tract recently.
- Uncircumcised men
- Personal history of sexually transmitted diseases
- Previous history of prostate enlargement
- Vasectomy.

Pathophysiology

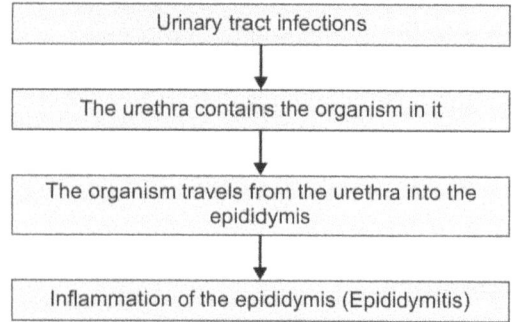

Clinical Features

- Enlarged testes
- Painful scrotum
- Testicular lump
- Tender and swollen testicle on the affected side
- Testicle pain which aggravates by bowel movement
- Fever
- Chills
- Burning pain during micturition
- Pain on ejaculation
- Discharge from the urethra
- Blood in the semen
- Groin pain.

Complications

- Testicular infarction
- Scrotal abscess
- Cutaneous scrotal fistula
- Infertility
- Acute scrotal pain.

Diagnostic Tests

- History
- Physical examination
- Rectal examination
- Urine analysis
- Urine culture
- Blood examination
- Doppler ultrasound
- Testicular scan.

Management

Medical

- **Antibiotics:** It helps in fighting the inflammation. For example, doxycycline, ciprofloxacin, levofloxacin, etc.
- **Analgesics:** It helps in alleviating pain caused by epididymitis. For example, paracetamol, ibuprofen, etc.

Nursing

- Encourage the patient to take complete bedrest for 3–4 days till the fever and pain subside.
- Instruct the patient to avoid lifting heavy objects.
- Instruct the patient to avoid sex until the infection is cleared.
- Apply cold packs to the scrotal area as tolerated.

- Encourage the patient to drink plenty of fluids to keep well hydrated which facilitates speedy recovery.
- Provide scrotal support by placing a pillow under the scrotum to elevate the scrotum while lying down.

ERECTILE DYSFUNCTION (IMPOTENCE)

Definition

The inability to get or maintain an erection that is firm enough for a man to have sexual intercourse is known as erectile dysfunction or impotence.

Etiology

- High cholesterol
- Spinal cord injury
- Multiple sclerosis
- Diabetic neuropathy
- Pelvic surgery
- Parkinson's disease
- Alzheimer's disease
- Peyronie's disease
- Pelvic trauma
- Thyroid disease
- Cortisone excess
- Hypogonadism
- Hypertension
- Heart or thyroid problems
- Poor blood circulation
- Low testosterone level in blood.

Risk Factors

- Medications such as beta blockers, digoxin, antidepressants, pantocid, sleeping pills, etc.
- Nicotine, alcohol and cocaine
- Poor communication with the partner
- Stress, fear, anxiety or anger
- Unrealistic sexual expectations
- Vicious cycle of doubt, failure or negative communication
- Hypertension
- Obesity
- Sleep apnea
- Lack of exercise or physical activity.

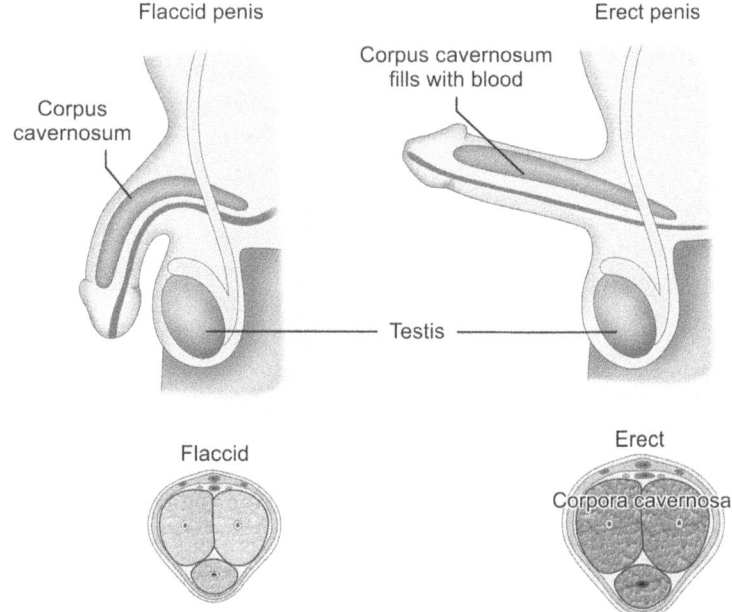

Fig. 10.4: Shows the comparison of erect penis with that of the flaccid penis (Erectile dysfunction).

Pathophysiology

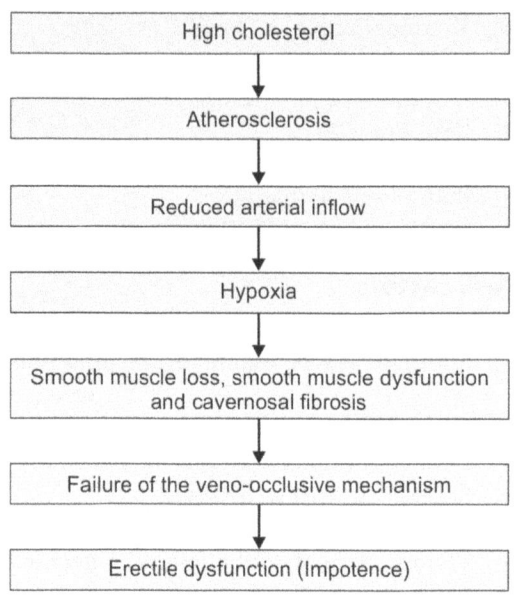

Clinical Features

- Inability to get and maintain an erection for satisfactory intercourse
- Premature ejaculation (may or may not be)
- Low levels of testosterone
- Depression
- Anxiety
- Low self-esteem
- Changes in libido.

Complications

- Stress
- Embarrassment
- Relationship problems
- Dissatisfaction in sexual life.

Diagnostic Tests

- History
- Physical examination
- Neurological testing
- Psychometric testing
- Blood examination
- Urine analysis
- Penile ultrasound
- Nocturnal penile tumescence (NPT)
- Rigidity testing (Rigiscan).

Management

Medical

- **Hormone replacement therapy:** Testosterone replacement therapy is performed when the testosterone level is too low in the blood.
- **Phosphodiesterase type 5 (PDE-5) inhibitors:** They work to relax muscles in the penis for better blood flow and to produce a rigid erection. For example, sildenafil citrate (Viagra), Vardenafil HCl (Levitra), tadalafil (Cialis), etc.
- **Self-injecting prostaglandin medication:** It is injected into the base of the penis before sexual activity. The medication goes directly into the corpus cavernosum, where it relaxes smooth muscle and produces an erection. For example, alprostadil, etc.
- **Intraurethral therapy:** This treatment is a variation on self-injection therapy. Instead of injecting the penis, a man inserts a tiny medicated pellet of alprostadil into the urethra.

Surgical

- **Vacuum erection devices:** It is a procedure in which a pump is connected to the cylinder that draws out air. This creates a negative pressure that draws blood into the penis, causing an erection to form. Once an erection occurs, an elastic ring is slipped around the base of the penis. The ring helps hold the blood in the penis. The ring can be left in place safely for up to 30 minutes. Wearing the ring for longer than 30 minutes could result in tissue damage.
- **Penile implants:** In this procedure, a man bends his penis upward into an erect position. With an inflatable implant, a pair of inflatable cylinders is attached to a fluid reservoir and a pump hidden inside the body. To have an erection, a man presses on the pump and this transfers fluid into the cylinders, making the penis rigid.

Nursing

- Educate the patient to cut down smoking, alcohol and illegal drugs.
- Instruct the patient to take plenty of rest and to take time to relax.
- Encourage the patient to eat a healthy balanced diet.
- Instruct the patient to avoid smoking.
- Ask the patient to get involved with adequate exercise.
- Encourage the patient to participate in stress reduction program.
- Ask the patient to communicate freely with the partner about the sexual issues.

MALE INFERTILITY

Definition

Infertility is the inability of the couple to become pregnant after 12 months of unprotected sex.

Etiology

- Varicocele
- Genetic and chromosomal defects
- Immunologic factor
- Ejaculatory disorders
- Undescended testes
- Infections
- Torsion (twisting of the testes in scrotum)
- Certain medicines and chemicals
- Radiation damage
- Spinal cord injury
- Prostate surgery
- Idiopathic.

Risk Factors

- Advanced age
- Smoking
- Obesity
- Occupational exposure
- Lack of exercise

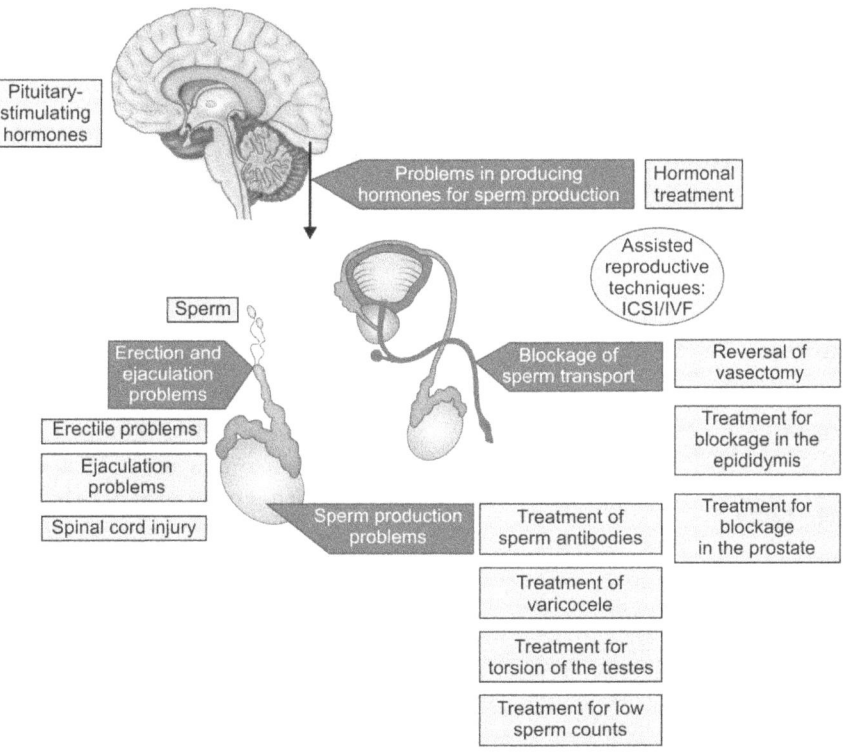

Fig. 10.5: Depicts erection and ejaculation problems with management.

- Consumption of alcohol and caffeinated beverages
- Long-time exposure to electronic devices (laptop)
- Stress.

Pathophysiology

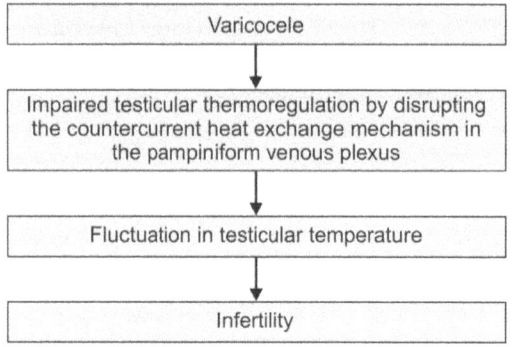

Clinical Features

Most infertile men will not show any clinical features. However, the problem is caused by a particular health condition, it may cause symptoms. These could include:
- Pain and swelling in the testicles (when infection prevails)
- Blood in the semen
- Pain after ejaculation
- Not being able to get or keep an erection
- Not being able to ejaculate when they have sex
- Difficulty in emptying the bladder.

Complications

- Marital disharmony
- Depression
- Anxiety.

Diagnostic Tests

- History
- Physical examination
- Blood examination
- Urine examination
- Ultrasound
- Venogram
- Testicular self-examination.

Management

Medical

- **Hormone replacement therapy:** Testosterone replacement therapy is performed when the testosterone level is too low in the blood.
- **Phosphodiesterase type 5 (PDE-5) inhibitors:** They work to relax muscles in the penis for better blood flow and to produce a rigid erection. For example, sildenafil citrate (Viagra), vardenafil HCl (Levitra), tadalafil (Cialis), etc.
- **Self-injecting prostaglandin medication:** It is injected into the base of the penis before sexual activity. The medication goes directly into the corpus cavernosum, where it relaxes smooth muscle and produces an erection. For example, alprostadil, etc.
- **Intraurethral therapy:** This treatment is a variation on self-injection therapy. Instead of injecting the penis, a man inserts a tiny medicated pellet of alprostadil into the urethra.

Surgical

- **Varicocelectomy:** It is a surgical procedure in which a surgeon will go through the abdomen and clamp the abnormal veins and blood can then flow around the abnormal veins to the normal ones.
- **Varicocele embolization:** It is a surgical procedure in which a small catheter is inserted into a groin or neck vein. A coil is then placed into the catheter and into the varicocele and this blocks from getting into the abnormal veins.
- **Laparoscopic varicocele ligation:** It is a surgical procedure in which a camera and small instruments are introduced to the abdomen where the veins feeding the varicocele are clipped.
- **Subinguinal varicocele ligation:** In this surgical procedure, an incision is made in the lower groin area and the spermatic cord is isolated. All of the veins feeding the

varicocele are identified and divided, while important structures for testicular function are preserved.
- **Vacuum erection devices:** It is a procedure in which a pump is connected to the cylinder that draws out air. This creates a negative pressure that draws blood into the penis, causing an erection to form. Once an erection occurs, an elastic ring is slipped around the base of the penis. The ring helps hold the blood in the penis. The ring can be left in place safely for up to 30 minutes. Wearing the ring for longer than 30 minutes could result in tissue damage.
- **Penile implants:** In this procedure, a man bends his penis upward into an erect position. With an inflatable implant, a pair of inflatable cylinders is attached to a fluid reservoir and a pump hidden inside the body. To have an erection, a man presses on the pump and this transfers fluid into the cylinders, making the penis rigid.

Nursing

- Instruct the patient to avoid smoking.
- Ask the patient to get involved with adequate exercise.
- Educate the patient to cut down smoking, alcohol and illegal drugs.
- Instruct the patient to take plenty of rest and to take time to relax.
- Encourage the patient to eat a healthy balanced diet.
- Encourage the patient to participate in stress reduction program.
- Ask the patient to communicate freely with the partner about the sexual issues.

PROSTATITIS

Definition

Prostatitis is the inflammation of the prostate gland, which means the prostate can feel sore and irritated.

Etiology

- Bacterial infection (*Escherichia coli*)
- Urethritis
- Phimosis
- Injury to the peritoneum
- Bladder outlet obstruction
- Having a catheter to drain urine.

Risk Factors

- Being males
- Black men
- Frequent urinary infections
- Family history of prostatitis

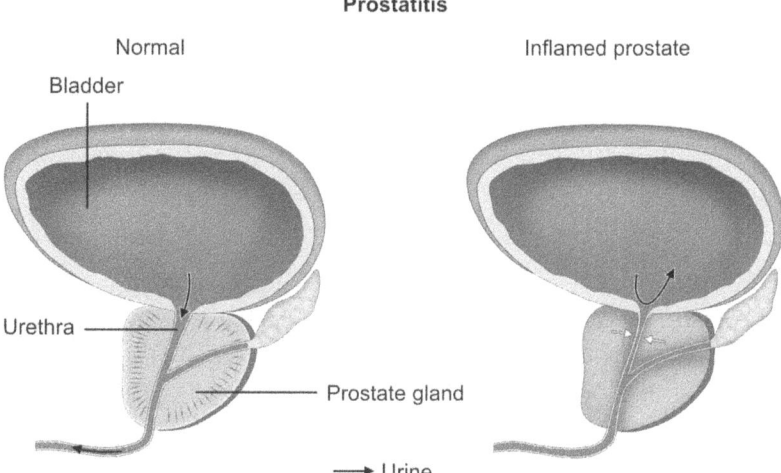

Fig. 10.6: Shows the comparison of normal and inflamed prostate (Prostatitis).

- Following a bout of acute bacterial prostatitis
- Obesity
- Having a catheter to drain urine
- Orchitis
- Being under psychological stress
- Having more than one sexual partners
- Those who don't drink enough fluids.

Types

- **Bacterial prostatitis:** It is caused by bacteria and is the easiest form of prostatitis to diagnose and treat, although serious complications may develop if it is not treated quickly.
- **Non-bacterial prostatitis:** It is an inflammed prostate without bacteria and is the form of prostatitis that is not well understood.

Pathophysiology

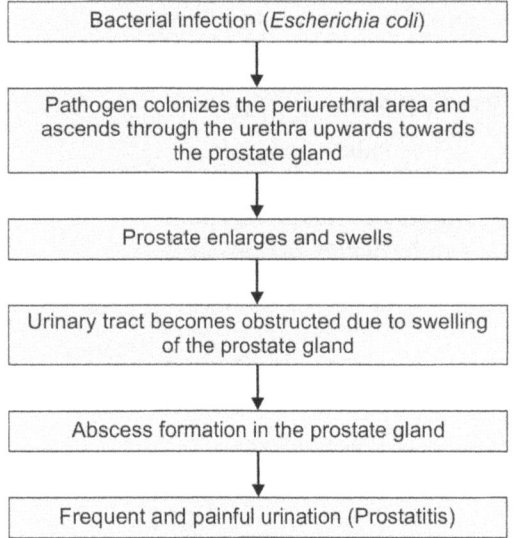

Clinical Features

- Dysuria (painful urination)
- Urgency of passing urine
- Frequent and painful urination
- Painful ejaculation
- Lower back pain
- Perineal pain (pain at the base of the scrotum and penis)
- Chills
- Fever
- Muscle pain
- Fatigue.

Complications

- Bacteremia
- Epididymitis
- Prostatic abscess
- Infertility
- Acute urinary retention.

Diagnostic Tests

- History
- Physical examination
- Digital rectal examination
- Urine analysis
- Prostate-specific antigen (PSA) test
- Urine PCR (Polymerase chain reaction) test.

Management

Medical

- **Antibiotics:** It helps in preventing the infections. For example, norfloxacin, doxycycline, ciprofloxacin, etc.
- **Alpha blockers:** It is used to relax the muscles in the upper part of the urethra which helps with pain. For example, tamsulosin, alfuzosin, etc.
- **Nonsteroidal anti-inflammatory drugs (NSAIDs):** It helps in relieving the symptoms of prostatitis. For example, ibuprofen, naproxen, etc.
- **Mild laxatives:** It helps to pass any hard stools and stop them from pressing the prostate. For example, dulcolax, etc.

Surgical

Transurethral resection of prostate (TURP): It is a surgical procedure in which prostate is removed in small pieces through the penis by introducing an endoscope into the urethra to the prostate and bladder.

Nursing

- Instruct the patient to include more roughages in the diet to prevent constipation

which can press on the sore prostate and can be quite painful.
- Instruct the patient to drink plenty of fluids.
- Encourage the patient to have a warm bath which helps in minimizing the pain in the lower back.
- Instruct the patient to eat a well balanced diet.
- Instruct the patient to avoid caffeine, alcohol and spicy foods.
- Encourage the patient to perform exercise to a moderate level.
- Ask the patient to wash the hands thoroughly after the bowel movement to help bacteria stop travelling up the urethra inside the penis and so reaching the prostate.

VARICOCELE

Definition

A varicocele is a bundle of enlarged veins in a man's scrotum, which is the sac that holds the two testicles.

Etiology

- Defective valves in the veins within the scrotum
- Kidney tumor
- Increased reflux from compression of the renal vein (nutcracker syndrome)
- High-cholesterol diet.

Risk Factors

- Being males between the ages of 15 and 35 years
- Infertile males
- Smoking
- Being overweight
- Prior surgery or trauma
- Leg crossing
- Abdominal straining.

Types

- ***Primary varicocele:*** It is an abnormal tortuosity and dilatation of the testicular veins and pampiniform plexus.
- ***Secondary varicocele:*** It results from increased pressure on the spermatic vein produced by disease processes such as hydronephrosis, cirrhosis or abdominal neoplasm.

Pathophysiology

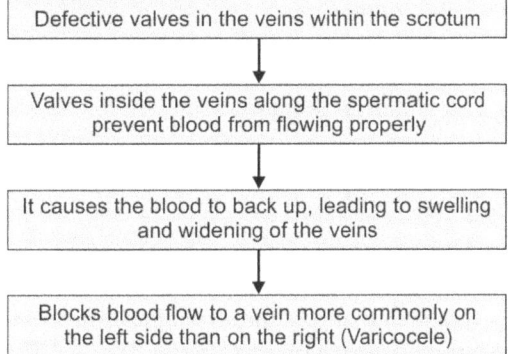

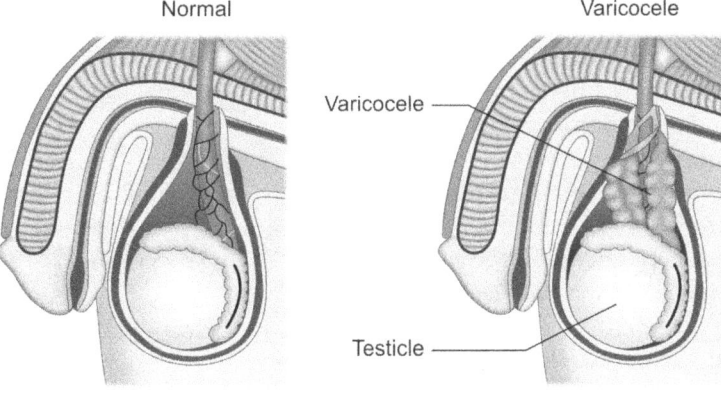

Fig. 10.7: Shows the comparison of normal and enlarged veins in scrotum (Varicocele).

Clinical Features

- Enlarged, twisted veins in the scrotum
- Painless testicle lump
- Scrotal swelling or bulge in the scrotum
- A dull ache in the testicle (s)
- Feeling of heaviness in the scrotum
- Discomfort in the testicle
- Testicle is smaller on the side where the dilated veins are.

Complications

- Infertility
- Testicular atrophy
- Blood clot formation
- Infection.

Diagnostic Tests

- History
- Physical examination
- Blood examination
- Urine examination
- Ultrasound
- Venogram
- Testicular self-examination
- hCG stimulation test.

Management

Surgical

- **Varicocelectomy:** It is a surgical procedure in which a surgeon will go through the abdomen and clamp the abnormal veins and blood can then flow around the abnormal veins to the normal ones.
- **Varicocele embolization:** It is a surgical procedure in which a small catheter is inserted into a groin or neck vein. A coil is then placed into the catheter and into the varicocele and this block from getting into the abnormal veins.
- **Laparoscopic varicocele ligation:** It is a surgical procedure in which a camera and small instruments are introduced to the abdomen where the veins feeding the varicocele are clipped.
- **Subinguinal varicocele ligation:** In this surgical procedure, an incision is made in the lower groin area and the spermatic cord is isolated. All of the veins feeding the varicocele are identified and divided, while important structures for testicular function are preserved.

Nursing

- Encourage the patient to eat a whole foods as they act as catalysts for antioxidants.
- Educate the patient to avoid exposure to environmental toxins.
- Encourage the patient to include cod liver oil in the diet as it facilitates proper maturation of sperm.
- Ask the patient wear a comfortable underwear or jockstrap as it eases the discomfort.

FEMALE REPRODUCTIVE SYSTEM

ABORTION

Definition

Abortion is the expulsion or extraction of an embryo/fetus from the womb weighing 500 g or less when it is not capable of independent survival.

Etiology

- Induced to preserve the health of the pregnant female
- Fetal factors with chromosomal abnormalities
- Maternal infections
- Maternal systemic diseases
- Cervicouterine factors
- Autoimmune factors
- Rh –ve pregnancy

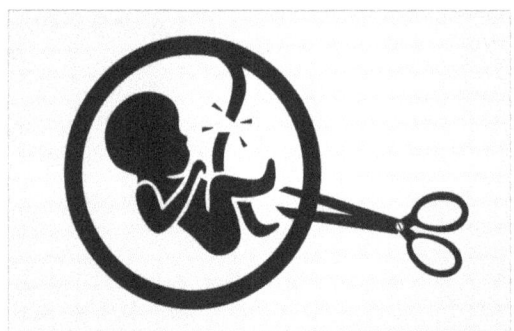

Fig. 10.8: Depicts termination of pregnancy either spontaneous or induced.

- ABO incompatibility
- Surgical trauma due to any operation
- Premature rupture of the membrane
- Accidental trauma or intentional trauma.

Risk Factors
- Frequent travelling during first trimester
- Previous history of spontaneous abortions
- Low progesterone level
- Advancing maternal age
- Cigarette smoking
- Alcohol consumption
- Any complications during pregnancy
- Any exposure to radiations
- Antineoplastic drugs
- Anesthetic agents.

Types
The following are the different types of abortion:
1. **Spontaneous abortion (miscarriage):** These are abortions that occur without any medical or surgical interventions. It constitutes nearly 25% of abortions. It is further subdivided as follows:
   - *Threatened abortion:* These are abortions occurring before the 20th week of gestation, the patient usually experiences vaginal bleeding with or without some cramps, and the cervix is closed.
   - *Inevitable abortion:* These are abortions in which the process of expulsion of fetus is in progress with rupture of the membrane dilating the cervical canal.
   - *Complete abortion:* These are abortions in which the embryonic and placental components have been expelled completely from the uterus.
   - *Incomplete abortion:* These are abortions in which part of the products of conception is expelled and some part of the gestational tissue is retained within the uterus.
   - *Habitual abortion (recurrent):* These are abortions which have occurred more than 3 times consecutively and spontaneously.
   - *Missed abortion:* These are abortions in which there is no uterine growth over a prolonged period of time, typically 6 weeks after its (fetus) death.
   - *Septic abortion:* This is a type of abortion in which there is sepsis or infection of the uterus and its contents.
2. **Induced abortion:** These are abortions in which drugs or instruments used to stop the normal course of pregnancy. The procedure is performed under the supervision of a licensed physician. It is grouped as follows:
   - *Therapeutic abortion:* These are abortions induced for the welfare of the pregnant female.
   - *Elective abortion:* These are abortions induced for any other reasons.

Pathophysiology

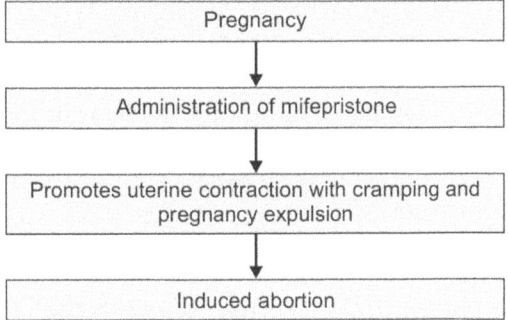

Clinical Features
- Prolonged or heavy menstrual period
- Several days of severe bleeding
- Tachycardia
- High fever with chills
- Severe lower abdominal pain
- Abdominal cramping
- Backache
- Hypotension
- Oliguria
- Respiratory distress.

Complications
- Excessive blood loss
- Uterine perforation
- Infection
- Death.

Diagnostic Tests

- History
- Physical examination
- Pelvic examination
- Blood examination
- Vaginal or abdominal ultrasound
- Pregnancy tests.

Management

Medical

- **Abortion-inducing agents:** It works by blocking the hormone progesterone, which is necessary to sustain pregnancy. Without this hormone, the lining of the uterus breaks down, the cervix softens and bleeding begins. For example, mifepristone, etc.
- **Antimetabolite agents:** It stops the ongoing implantation process that occurs during the first several weeks after conception. For example, methotrexate, etc.
- **Synthetic prostaglandin E_1 analog:** Within a few days after taking either mifepristone or methotrexate, misoprostol is taken and it causes the uterus to contract and empty and this ends the pregnancy. For example, misoprostol, etc.

Surgical

- **Menstrual extraction (endometrial or vacuum aspiration):** It is a method in which suctioning is done on the lining of the uterus (endometrium) through a thin opening of the undilated cervix. This is mostly performed in the first trimester and mostly done on women who just missed a period till eight weeks of pregnancy.
- **Dilation and evacuation (vacuum suction or suction curettage):** In this method suction is used to remove the fetus and placenta. The cervix is first dilated under local anesthesia using a suction tube that is firm and a stronger suction is used than in menstrual extraction.
- **Dilation and curettage (D&C):** In this method, curette is used to remove the fetus and placenta. The cervix is first dilated under local anesthesia using a curette that is firm and a stronger.
- **Prostaglandin or saline administration:** In this method injection prostaglandins or saline solution is injected through the uterine wall and into the amniotic sac holding the fetus to induce labor and delivery of a nonviable fetus.
- **Hysterectomy:** In this method the uterus is opened through a small abdominal incision and the fetus is removed and it is performed under general anesthesia.

Nursing

- Provide complete bedrest to the patient till bleeding stops.
- Provide reassurance to the patient and her partner.
- Recommend iron supplements to replace iron lost from bleeding.
- Educate the woman who chooses to terminate pregnancy regarding the endangers it may have on her health.
- Instruct the woman regarding improved methods of contraception available to prevent unplanned pregnancies.
- Measure the maternal blood loss by saving and weighing the used pads.
- Measure intake and output to establish renal function.

BARTHOLIN'S ABSCESS

Definition

Bartholin's abscess is the inflammation of Bartholin's glands containing pus that formed as a result of infection.

Etiology

- Any blockage in the small opening of the gland
- Bacterial infection (*Escherichia coli*)
- Poor personal hygiene
- Use of restrictive pants and garments
- Gonorrheal infection
- Chlamydial infection
- Endometritis

Disorders of Reproductive System

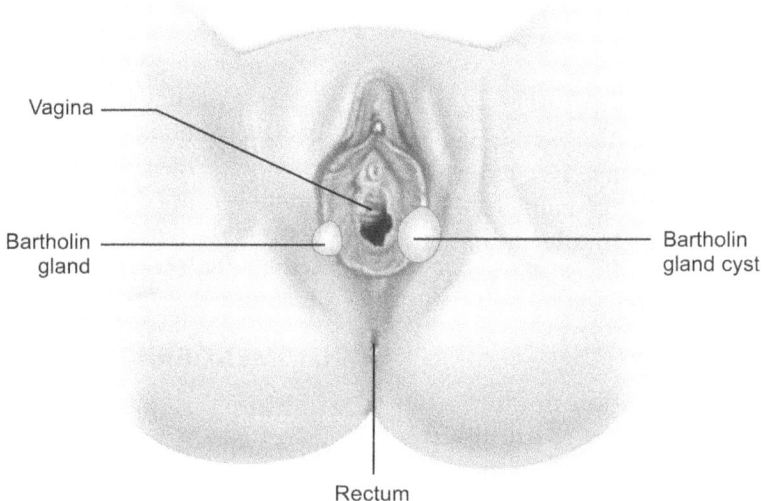

Fig. 10.9: Depicts inflamed Bartholin's glands containing pus as a result of infection (Bartholin's abscess).

- Candidiasis
- Contraceptive creams and jellies
- Drugs
- Radiation therapy.

Risk Factors

- Being women of reproductive age group especially between the ages of 20–30 years.
- Previous history of Bartholin's abscess
- Being sexually active
- Direct trauma or surgery.

Pathophysiology

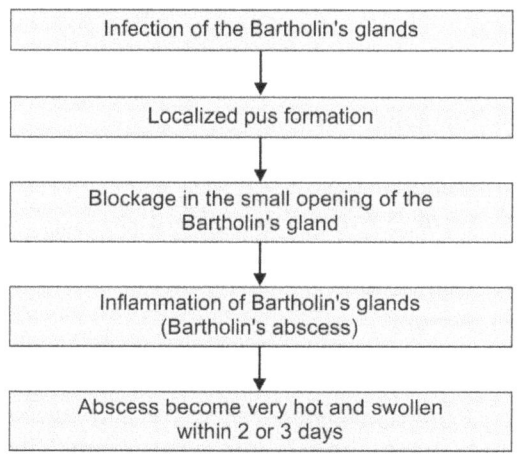

Clinical Features

- Fever
- Chills
- A tender lump on either side of the vaginal opening
- Discomfort while walking or sitting
- Pain with sexual intercourse
- Foul smelling pus oozing from the abscess
- Discomfort when passing urine (stinging sensation)
- Drainage from the cyst
- Swollen groin lymph nodes.

Complications

- Tumor formation
- Abscess
- Chronic Bartholin's duct cyst formation.

Diagnostic Tests

- History
- Physical examination
- Pelvic examination
- Blood examination
- Urine examination
- Electrocardiogram
- Chest X-ray

- Culture and sensitivity of the fluid
- Biopsy of the gland.

Management

Medical

- **Antibiotics:** It helps to prevent against secondary infections. For example, penicillin, amoxicillin, gentamicin, etc.
- **Analgesics:** It helps in alleviating pain caused by Bartholin's abscess. For example, paracetamol, ibuprofen, etc.

Surgical

- **Sitz bath:** It is a procedure in which a tub filled with a few inches of warm water several times a day for three or four days helps the infected cyst to rupture and drain on its own.
- **Surgical drainage:** It is a procedure in which an infected cyst requires drainage by a surgeon. It is done under local anesthesia. In order to facilitate drainage, a small incision in the cyst is made to allow it to drain. Then a small rubber tube (catheter) is placed in position and it is retained for up to 6 weeks to keep the opening from closing and to allow complete drainage. After that the catheter is removed and the incision heals completely.
- **Marsupialization:** It is a procedure in which a small permanent opening less than 5 mm is surgically created to drain the gland on each side of the gland. The catheter is inserted to promote draining for few days to prevent recurrence.
- **Gland excision:** It is the surgical removal of the Bartholin's glands.

Nursing

- Instruct to maintain good hygienic activities to prevent infection of a cyst and formation of an abscess.
- Use a warm compress (clothes or cotton wool warmed with hot water) held against the area.
- Instruct the patient to avoid using tight-fitted clothings around the genital area as this causes friction which decreases circulation and invites infection.
- Encourage the patient to go for yearly pelvic examinations and Pap smears.
- Educate the patient to practice safe sex by using a condom.
- Encourage the patient to shower or bathe carefully every day with a mild soap.
- Instruct the patient to abstain from sexual activity for 3 weeks during the process of healing.

DYSMENORRHEA

Definition

Dysmenorrhea is defined as difficult menstrual flow or painful menstruation.

Etiology

- Endometriosis
- Inflammation of the fallopian tube
- Fibroid uterus
- Adenomyosis
- Pelvic inflammatory disease (PID)
- Adhesions
- Endometrial polyps
- Structural abnormalities of the genital tract
- Pelvic congestion syndrome
- Cervical stenosis
- Intrauterine device.

Risk Factors

- Being females
- Long menstrual periods
- Young age
- Never having been pregnant
- Menarche attainment before 12 years of age
- Smoking
- Obesity
- Underweight
- Family history of dysmenorrhea
- High levels of stress
- Depression
- Anxiety.

Types

- ***Primary dysmenorrhea:*** It is pain during menstruation where there is no underlying

Disorders of Reproductive System

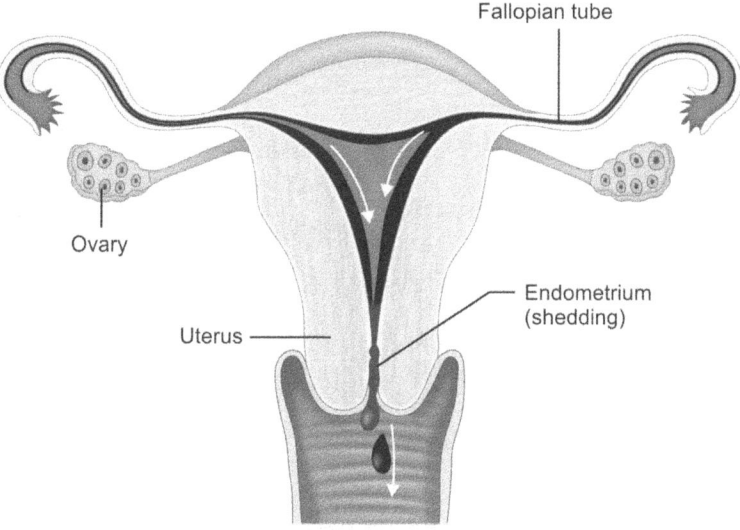

Fig. 10.10: Depicts painful menstruation (Dysmenorrhea).

disease or disorder of the uterus (womb) or in the pelvis.
- **Secondary dysmenorrhea:** It is painful menstruation that occurs in the presence of an underlying disorder or pelvic pathology.

Pathophysiology

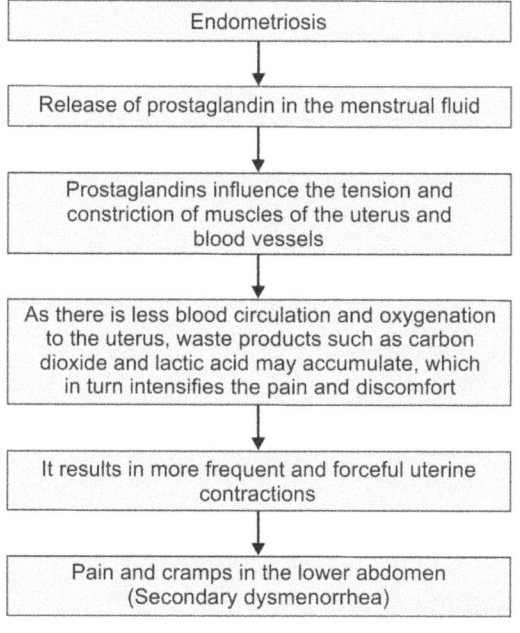

Clinical Features
- Pain and cramps in the lower abdomen
- Sever pain and discomfort for a day or two
- Headache
- Nausea
- Vomiting
- Bloating
- Loose stools
- Fatigue
- Dizziness.

Complications
- Fainting
- Back pain
- Infection
- Severe bleeding.

Diagnostic Tests
- History
- Physical examination
- Pelvic examination
- Laparoscopy
- Hysteroscopy
- Ultrasound examination.

Management

Medical

- **Antibiotics:** It helps in preventing the infections. For example, norfloxacin, doxycycline, ciprofloxacin, etc.
- **Non-steroidal anti-inflammatory drugs:** It helps to relieve pain and cramps due to excessively heavy bleeding. For example, ibuprofen, naprosyn, etc.
- **Iron supplements:** It helps to prevent anemia due to heavy periods. For example, Bifera, Femiron, Fergon, etc.
- **Oral contraceptives (birth control pills):** It helps to control heavy bleeding. For example, mifepristone, Mirena, etc.

Nursing

- Instruct the patients to lie on their back, supporting the knees with a pillow.
- Ask them to hold a hot water bottle over the abdomen or lower back.
- Instruct them to take a warm bath.
- Encourage them to take plenty of rest and avoid stressful situations as the period approaches.
- Recommend iron supplements to replace iron lost from bleeding.

ECTOPIC PREGNANCY

Definition

An ectopic pregnancy is one that occurs anywhere outside the uterus.

Etiology

- Sexually transmitted infections (*Chlamydia* and *Gonorrhea*)
- Endometriosis
- Conceiving after having a tubal ligation or while an intrauterine device is in place.
- Previous pelvic or abdominal surgery
- Pelvic inflammatory disease.

Risk Factors

- Being females
- Maternal age of 35–44 years
- Previous ectopic pregnancy
- Several induced abortions
- Smoking
- Exposure to the drug diethylstilbesterol (DES)
- Increased age
- Those who become pregnant by IVF.

Pathophysiology

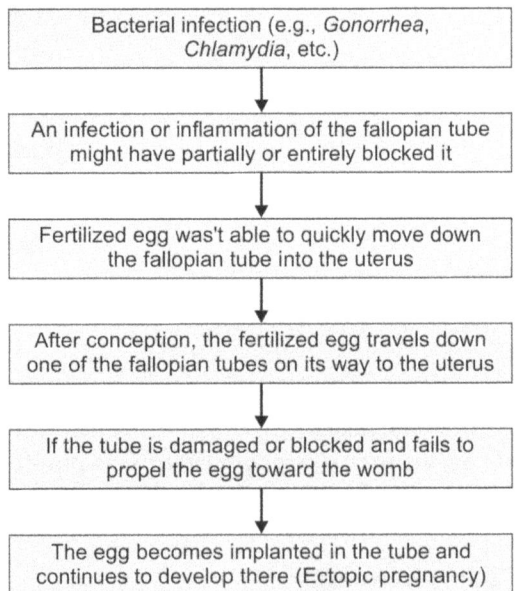

Clinical Features

- Mild to severe sharp pain in the pelvis or abdomen
- Abnormal vaginal bleeding
- Breast tenderness
- Urinary symptoms
- Shoulder tip pain
- Vaginal spotting
- Dizziness
- Weakness
- Low back pain
- Hypotension
- Fainting
- Paleness
- Diarrhea
- Rectal pain or pressure on defecation.

Complications

- Tubal rupture
- Massive hemorrhage

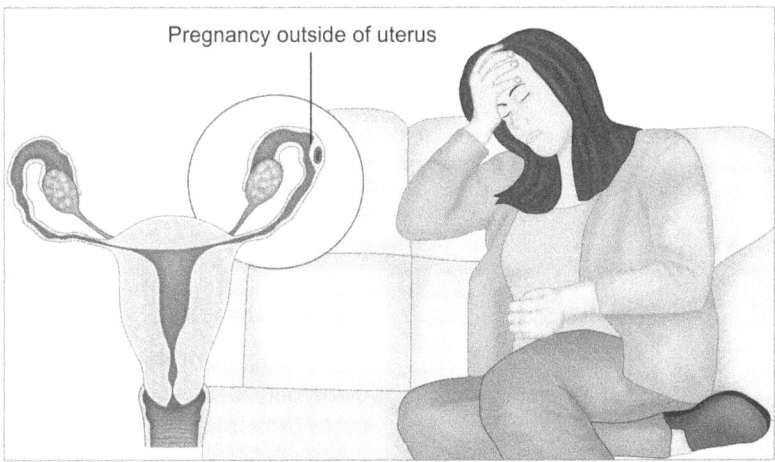

Fig. 10.11: Depicts pregnancy outside of uterus (Ectopic pregnancy).

- Disseminated intravascular coagulopathy
- Septic shock
- Death.

Diagnostic Tests

- History
- Physical examination
- Pelvic examination
- Blood examination
- Human chorionic gonadotropin (hCG) test
- Laparoscopy
- Transvaginal ultrasound
- Computed tomography (CT) scan.

Management

Medical

- **Abortion-inducing agents:** It works by blocking the hormone progesterone, which is necessary to sustain pregnancy. For example, mifepristone, etc.
- **Antimetabolite agents:** It stops the ongoing implantation process that occurs during the first several weeks after conception. For example, methotrexate, etc.

Surgical

- **Dilation and evacuation (vacuum suction or suction curettage):** In this method suction is used to remove the fetus and placenta. The cervix is first dilated under local anesthesia using a suction tube that is firm and a stronger suction is used than in menstrual extraction.
- **Dilation and curettage (D&C):** In this method, curette is used to remove the fetus and placenta. The cervix is first dilated under local anesthesia using a curette that is firm and a stronger.
- **Prostaglandin or saline administration:** In this method injection prostaglandins or saline solution is injected through the uterine wall and into the amniotic sac holding the fetus to induce labor and delivery of a nonviable fetus.

Nursing

- Provide complete bedrest to the patient till bleeding stops.
- Provide reassurance to the patient and her partner.
- Recommend iron supplements to replace iron lost from bleeding.
- Measure the maternal blood loss by saving and weighing the used pads.
- Measure intake and output to establish renal function.

ENDOMETRITIS

Definition

The inflammation or irritation of the lining of the uterus (endometrium) is known as endometritis.

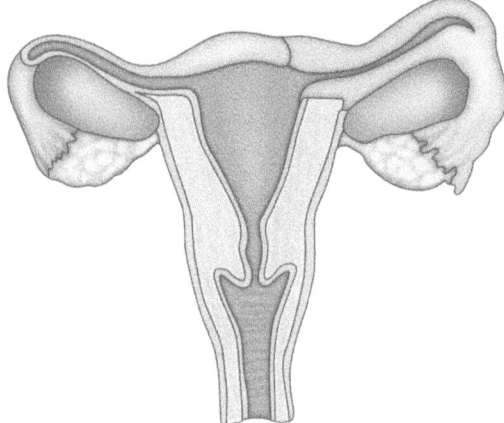

Fig. 10.12: Shows the inflamed or irritated lining of the uterus (Endometrium).

Etiology

- Sexually transmitted infections (*Chlamydia* and *Gonorrhea*)
- Salpingitis
- Tuberculosis
- Childbirth
- Surgery or other gynecological procedures that require insertion of medical instruments.

Risk Factors

- History of acute salpingitis
- Acute cervicitis
- Pelvic infections
- Hysteroscopy
- Intrauterine device insertion
- Abortion (therapeutic, elective or spontaneous).

Pathophysiology

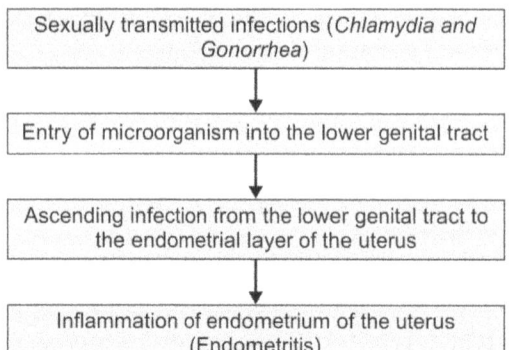

Clinical Features

- Abnormal vaginal bleeding or discharge
- Lower abdominal or pelvic pain
- Abdominal distention
- Discomfort when having a bowel movement
- Constipation
- Fever
- Malaise.

Complications

- Pelvic peritonitis
- Pelvic or uterine abscess formation
- Septicemia
- Septic shock
- Infertility.

Diagnostic Tests

- History
- Physical examination
- Pelvic examination
- Blood examination
- Endocervical culture
- Endometrial biopsy
- Laparoscopy
- Hysteroscopy
- Computed tomography (CT) scan
- Vaginal ultrasonogram.

Management

Medical

- **Antibiotics:** It helps in fighting the inflammation. For example, gentamicin, clindamycin, cephalosporin, metronidazole, etc.
- **Analgesics:** It helps in alleviating pain caused by endometritis. For example, paracetamol, ibuprofen, etc.

Nursing

- Enforce early diagnosis and complete treatment for sexually transmitted infections.
- Educate the patient to practice safe sex by following appropriate contraceptive method.
- Ensure adequate rest and hydration to the patient.
- Ensure proper follow-up by the patient to the hospital.

FEMALE INFERTILITY

Definition
Infertility is the inability of the couple to become pregnant after 12 months of unprotected sex.

Etiology
- Environmental pollutants
- Scarring from sexually transmitted diseases
- Use of drugs such as cimetidine, spironolactone and nitrofurantoin
- Pelvic infections
- Hormonal imbalance
- Ovarian cysts
- Intrauterine devices
- Problems with ovulation
- Poor nutrition
- Tumor
- Abnormal egg transport from the cervix through the fallopian tubes.

Risk Factors
- Women's age of more than 35 years
- Anovulatory menstrual cycles
- Autoimmune disorders such as antiphospholipid syndrome (APS)
- Clotting disorders
- Defects of the uterus (Myomas) or blockage of the cervix
- Eating disorders
- Endometriosis
- Long-term use of drugs such as diethylstilbestrol (DES)
- Chronic diseases such as diabetes mellitus
- Pelvic inflammatory diseases (PID).

Types
- ***Primary infertility:*** It is the term used to describe a couple who has never been able to achieve a pregnancy after 1 year of unprotected sex.
- ***Secondary infertility:*** It is the term used to describe a couple who has been pregnant at least once, but has not been able to achieve a pregnancy again.

Pathophysiology

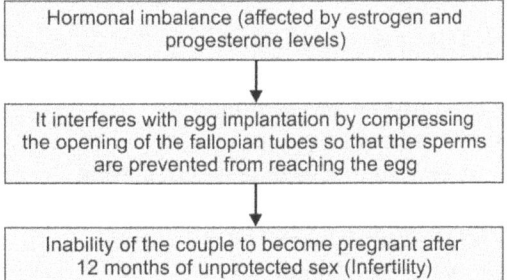

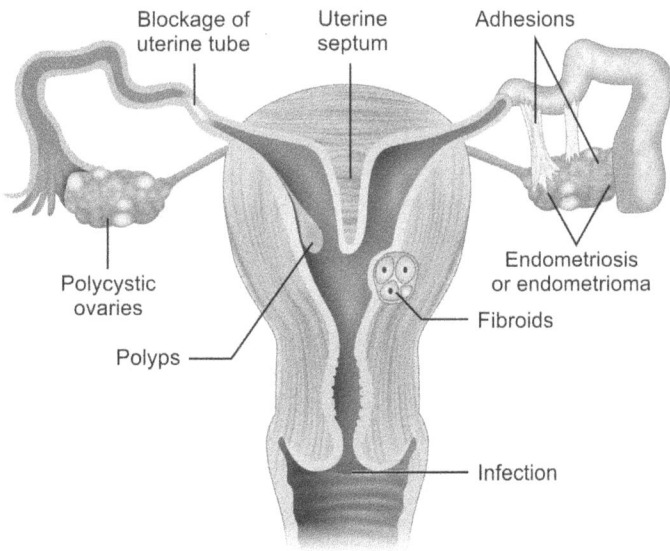

Fig. 10.13: Denotes possible causes of infertility in a women (Female infertility).

Clinical Features

- Emotional disturbance
- Inability to become pregnant
- Loss of hair
- Weight gain
- Noticed dark hair growing in new places of the body
- Sudden onset of severe acne
- Painful menstruation
- Amenorrhea or irregular menses
- Anhedonia (loss of interest).

Complications

- Marital disharmony
- Depression
- Anxiety.

Diagnostic Tests

- History
- Physical examination
- Endometrial biopsy
- Laparoscopic examination
- Blood examination
- Cervical mucus to detect ovulation
- Hysterosalpingography
- Luteinizing hormone urine test
- Pelvic examination.

Management

Medical

- **Fertility promoting agents:** It stimulates the ovary to release one or more eggs and it works by adjusting levels of the natural hormones. Also it works only if the infertility is caused by failure of the ovary to release eggs. For example, clomiphene, etc.
- **Gonadotropin-releasing hormone (GnRH) agonists:** It prepares the body for a precisely timed cycle of ovulation. For example, Zoladex, Synarel, lupron, etc.
- **Hormone replacement therapy:** It stimulates the follicle growth in the ovaries and promotes ovulation. For example, follicle-stimulating hormone, bromocriptine, etc.
- **Antibiotics:** It helps in treating genital tract infections, either in the male or in the female. For example, doxycycline, tetracycline, etc.

Surgical

Assisted conception technique

- **Intrauterine insemination (IUI):** It is a procedure in which sperm are directly inserted into the uterus using a special catheter or a syringe.
- **In vitro fertilization (IVF):** It is a procedure in which the eggs that the ovary has been stimulated to release are collected surgically. The eggs and sperms are combined in the laboratory to produce embryos. One or more embryos are then inserted into the uterus.
- **Intracytoplasmic sperm injection (ICSI):** It involves the injection of a single sperm into the cytoplasm of an egg with a fine glass needle in case of poor sperm quality and azoospermia.
- **Gamete intrafallopian transfer (GIFT):** It is a technique in which male and female gametes are injected through a laparoscope into the fimbriated ends of the fallopian tubes.
- **Zygote intrafallopian transfer (ZIFT):** It is a retrieval of oocytes from the ovary followed by their fertilization and culture in the laboratory and placement of the resulting zygotes in the fallopian tubes by the laparoscopy 24 hrs after the oocytes retrieval.
- **Myomectomy:** It is a surgical procedure in which the fibroids are removed and also the fertility of the women is preserved by leaving the uterus in place.

Nursing

- Facilitate marital counseling to the patient and the spouse.
- Facilitate sex education to the patient and the spouse.
- Instruct the patients to avoid drugs and alcohol.
- Instruct the patient to maintain a healthy weight.

- Instruct the patient to avoid exposure to certain environmental toxins.
- Instruct the patient to eat a well-balanced diet.
- Encourage the patient to perform exercise to a moderate level.
- Promote the idea of getting pregnant when the couples are in young age.

FIBROID UTERUS

Definition

Fibroid uterus is a noncancerous tumor that develops within the walls of the uterus, which is a female reproductive organ and attaches to it.

Etiology

- Hormonal imbalance (affected by estrogen and progesterone levels)
- Genetic predisposition (runs in families)
- Nulliparity
- Long-term use of synthetic estrogen (Tamoxifen) for the treatment of cancer breast.

Risk Factors

- Being women over 35 years
- African American women
- Family history of fibroid uterus
- Overweight
- Eating a lot of red meat (beef)
- Exposure to exogenous hormones
- Early menarche
- Late menopause.

Types

- ***Submucosal:*** These fibroids grow into the uterine cavity.
- ***Intramural:*** These fibroids grow within the wall of the uterus.
- ***Subserosal:*** These fibroids grow on the outside of the uterus.

Pathophysiology

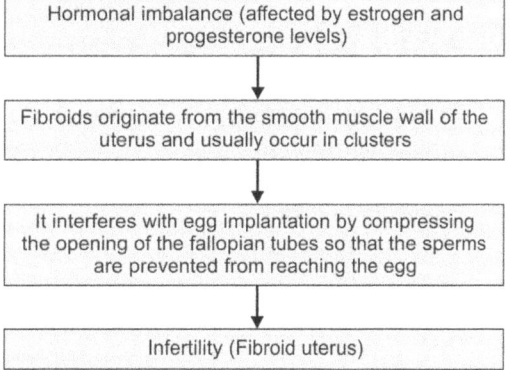

Clinical Features

- Sensation of fullness or pressure over the lower abdomen
- Heavy menstrual bleeding (menorrhagia), sometimes with passage of blood clots

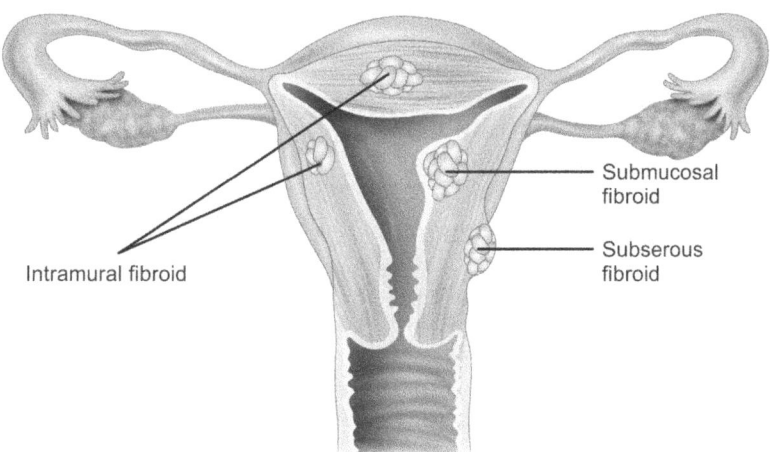

Fig. 10.14: Shows the noncancerous tumor that develops within the walls of the uterus (Fibroid uterus).

- Pelvic cramping or pain with periods
- Increase in urine frequency
- Fullness of abdomen (gas)
- Bleeding between periods or very prolonged bleeding with periods
- Pain during sex
- Miscarriages
- Anemia.

Complications

- Infertility
- Premature delivery
- Severe pain with excessively heavy bleeding
- Cancerous changes will occur.

Diagnostic Tests

- History
- Physical examination
- Pelvic examination
- Transvaginal or pelvic ultrasound
- Pelvic laparoscopy
- Endometrial biopsy
- Hysteroscopy
- Sonohysterography
- Hysterosalpingography.

Management

Medical

- **Nonsteroidal anti-inflammatory drugs:** It helps to relieve pain and cramps due to excessively heavy bleeding. For example, ibuprofen, naprosyn, etc.
- **Iron supplements:** It helps to prevent anemia due to heavy periods. For example, Bifera, Femiron, Fergon, etc.
- **Oral contraceptives (birth control pills):** It helps to control heavy bleeding. For example, mifepristone, Mirena, etc.
- **Hormonal therapy:** It reduces the production of the hormones estrogen and progesterone and finally shrinks the fibroids. For example, depot leuprolide, etc.

Surgical

- **Hysteroscopic resection of fibroids:** In this procedure a small camera and instruments are inserted through the cervix into the uterus to remove the fibroid tumors.
- **Uterine artery embolization:** It is a procedure in which the blood supply to the fibroid is stopped causing the fibroid to shrink and die.
- **Myomectomy:** It is a surgical procedure in which the fibroids are removed and also the fertility of the women is preserved by leaving the uterus in place.
- **Hysterectomy:** It is a surgical procedure in which the uterus is surgically removed to control pain or excessive bleeding due to fibroid uterus.

Nursing

- Encourage the patient to include more vegetables in the diet.
- Encourage the patient to eat organic foods.
- Instruct the patient to avoid exposure to pesticides and synthetic fertilizers.
- Instruct the patient to avoid food preservatives and dyes.
- Encourage the patient to include good sources of fiber (broccoli, dark leafy greens, beans, etc.) in the diet.
- Encourage the patient to maintain a healthy weight.

PELVIC INFLAMMATORY DISEASE

Definition

Pelvic inflammation disease (PID) is an infection of the female reproductive organs.

Etiology

- Sexually transmitted infections (e.g: *Chlamydia, Gonorrhea*, etc.)
- A recent miscarriage or abortion
- A recent operation or procedure on the womb (uterus)
- A contraceptive coil inserted recently.

Risk Factors

- Being females
- Women who are sexually active

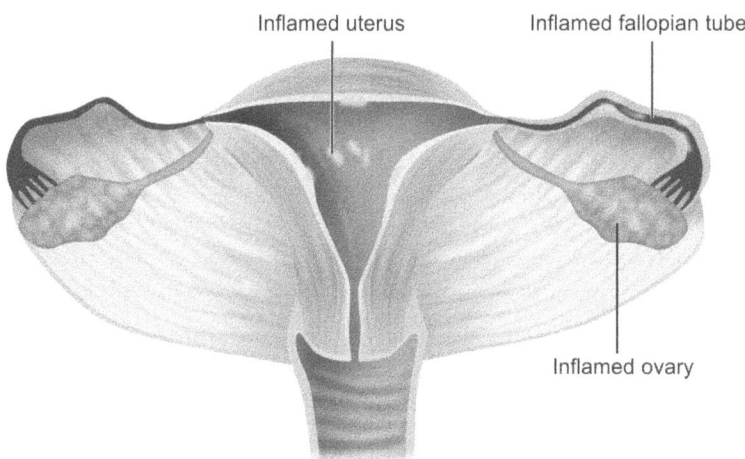

Fig. 10.15: Shows the inflamed uterus, fallopian tube and ovary (Pelvic inflammatory disease).

- Past pelvic inflammatory disease
- Multiple sex partners
- Those women using douche
- Those women have an STD and do not get treated.

Pathophysiology

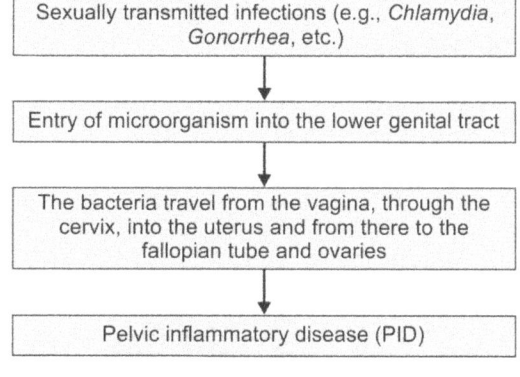

Clinical Features

- Abnormal vaginal discharge
- Pain in the lower abdomen
- Pain in the upper right abdomen
- Abnormal menstrual bleeding
- Painful urination
- Chills
- Fever
- Painful sexual intercourse
- Nausea
- Vomiting.

Complications

- Infertility
- Scarring of the fallopian tube
- Ectopic pregnancy
- Chronic pelvic pain
- Pelvic abscess
- Fitz-Hugh-Curtis syndrome.

Diagnostic Tests

- History
- Physical examination
- Pelvic examination
- Blood examination
- Swab test
- Ultrasonography
- Endometrial biopsy
- Laparoscopy
- Computed tomography (CT) scan
- Magnetic resonance imaging (MRI) scan.

Management

Medical

Antibiotics: It helps in preventing the infections. For example, ceftriaxone, azithromycin, doxycycline, cefixime, etc.

Nursing

- Instruct the patient to avoid sexual contact until the patients and their partner(s) have completed screening and treatment.

- Instruct the patient to limit the number of sexual partners.
- Ask the patient to seek medical care if symptoms have not resolved by 3–7 days after starting treatment.
- Instruct the patient to drink plenty of fluids.
- Encourage the patient to go for yearly pelvic examinations and Pap smears.
- Educate the patient to practice safe sex by using a condom.
- Encourage the patient to shower or bathe carefully every day with a mild soap.
- Instruct the patient to be monogamous.
- Ensure the patient understands the importance of compliance with medication.

POLYCYSTIC OVARY DISEASE (STEIN-LEVENTHAL SYNDROME)

Definition

The presence of tiny small cysts in the ovaries which can affect a woman's ability to get pregnant is known as polycystic ovary disease.

Etiology

- Low levels of follicular stimulating hormone
- Production of androgens (male hormones) higher than normal in the ovary
- Insulin resistance
- Genetic predisposition.

Risk Factors

- Being women of reproductive age
- Family history of polycystic ovary disease
- Being overweight
- Those women with high blood pressure
- Those women with heart attack.

Pathophysiology

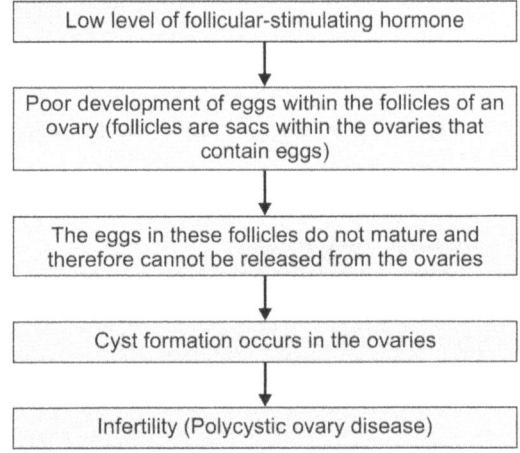

Clinical Features

- Abnormal, irregular or very light or infrequent menstrual periods

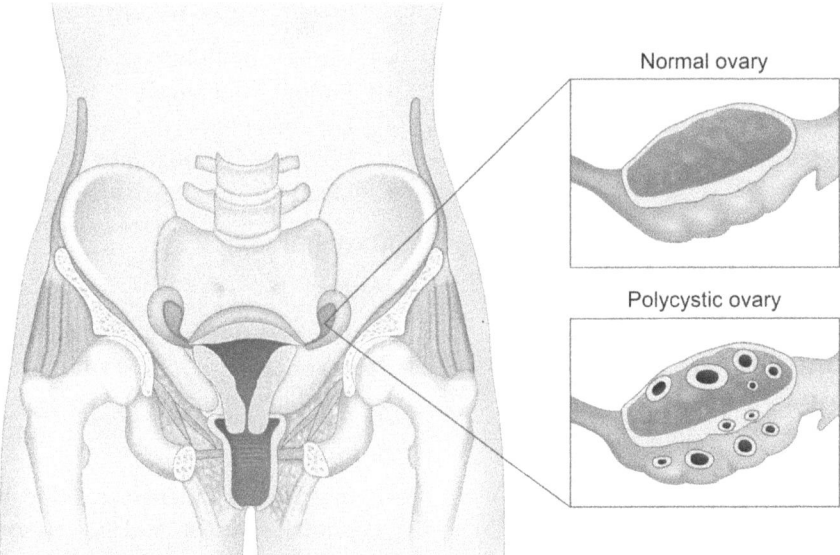

Fig. 10.16: Depicts normal ovary with that of polycystic ovary (Polycystic ovary disease).

- Secondary amenorrhea
- Acne that gets worsened
- Decreased breast size
- Deeper voice
- Virilization (development of male sex characteristics like increased body hair, facial hair, change in the voice and enlargement of the clitoris)
- Increased glucose level in blood
- Thinning hair on the scalp
- Poor response to the hormone insulin in the blood
- Weight gain around the waist.

Complications

- Uterine cancer
- Breast cancer
- High blood pressure
- Sleep apnea
- Infertility.

Diagnostic Tests

- History
- Physical examination
- Pelvic examination
- Blood examination
- Abdominal ultrasound
- Abdominal MRI scan
- Tissue biopsy of the ovary
- Laparoscopic examination
- Vaginal ultrasound
- Thyroid function tests.

Management

Medical

- **Fertility agents:** It causes the pituitary gland to produce more follicular-stimulating hormone and stimulates ovulation. For example, clomiphene citrate, letrozole, etc.
- **Oral hypoglycemic agents:** It improves the cells response to insulin and helps move glucose into the cell, which allows the body to make less insulin and also lowers testosterone levels. For example, metformin, etc.
- **Birth control pills:** It regulates or controls menstrual cycles and also helps with ovulation and future conception. For example, desogestrel, levonorgestrel, norethindrone, etc.
- **Nonsteroidal anti-androgen agents:** It works in the body to prevent the actions of androgens. For example, flutamide, drogenil, etc.
- **Potassium-sparing diuretics:** It slows down the action of androgens and treats female-pattern hair loss and hirsutism. For example, spironolactone, etc.

Surgical

- **Ovarian drilling:** It is a surgical procedure in which a small cut above or below the navel is made and a telescope is introduced into the abdomen, also known as laparoscopy. The ovary is punctured with a small needle carrying an electric current to destroy a small portion of the ovary. It lowers male hormone levels and helps with ovulation.
- **Oophorectomy:** It is a surgical procedure where one or both ovaries are removed.
- **Hysterectomy:** It is a surgical procedure in which a woman's uterus and cervix is removed.
- **Cyst aspiration:** It is a surgical procedure intended to relieve discomfort and improve fertility in women with polycystic ovary syndrome (PCOS).

Nursing

- Instruct the patient to limit processed foods and foods with added sugar.
- Instruct the patient to maintain a healthy weight.
- Instruct the patient to eat a well-balanced diet.
- Instruct the patient to avoid tobacco chewing.
- Encourage the patient to perform exercise to a moderate level.

PREMENSTRUAL SYNDROME

Definition

Premenstrual syndrome (PMS) is defined as a recurrent, cyclical set of varying physical and behavioral symptoms that appear 7–14 days before menses and usually subside with onset.

Etiology

- Changing hormone levels during the menstrual cycle
- Hypoglycemia
- Allergies
- Catecholamine alterations
- Endorphin withdrawal
- Fluid retention
- Increased adrenal activity
- Increased aldosterone activity
- Increased renin-angiotensin activity
- Nutritional deficiencies
- Prostaglandin impact
- Psychological or psychogenic effects.

Risk Factors

- Stress
- Emotional problems
- Being a menstruating women
- Those who have at least one child
- Those who have a family history of depression
- Those who have a past medical history of either postpartum depression or a mood disorder.
- Those who are between their late 20s and early 40s.

Pathophysiology

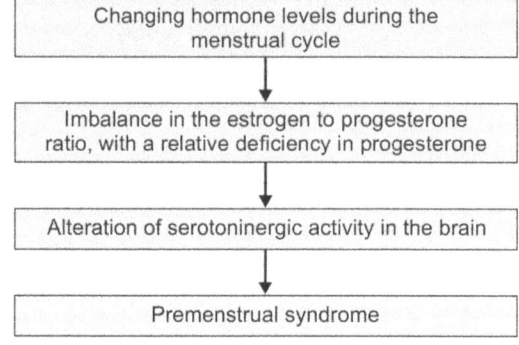

Clinical Features

Physical Symptoms

- Breast tenderness
- Thirst and appetite changes (food cravings)
- Bloating and weight gain
- Headache
- Swelling of the hands or feet
- Aches and pains
- Fatigue
- Gastrointestinal symptoms

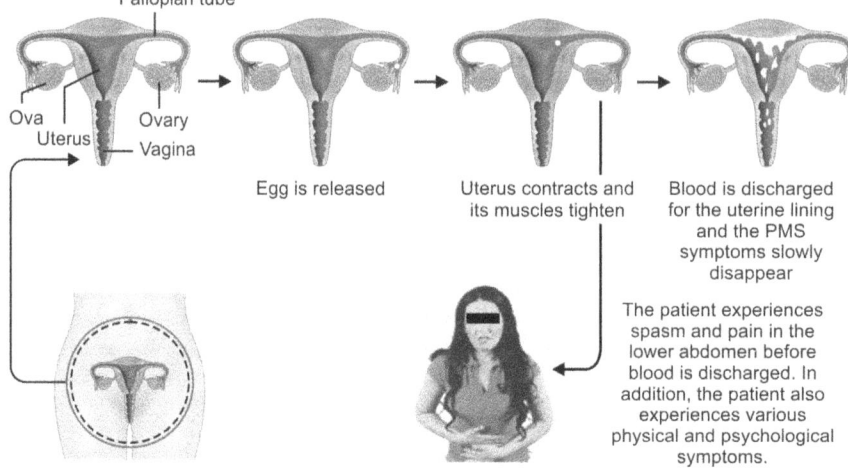

Fig. 10.17: Depicts the process of pre-menstrual syndrome (PMS).

- Skin problems
- Abdominal pain.

Emotional Symptoms
- Angry outbursts
- Irritability
- Crying spells
- Confusion
- Social withdrawal
- Poor concentration
- Insomnia
- Increased nap-taking
- Changes in sexual desire.

Complications
- Premenstrual dysphoric disorder (PMDD)
- Anxiety
- Depression
- Substance abuse disorder.

Diagnostic Tests
- History
- Physical examination
- Prospective charting information for a 2-month period
- Blood examination.

Management

Medical
- **Selective serotonin reuptake inhibitors (SSRIs):** It changes serotonin levels in the brain and is beneficial for women with premenstrual syndrome. For example, sertraline, fluoxetine, paroxetine, etc.
- **Birth control pills:** It helps to reduce dysmenorrhea, intensity and duration of menstrual flow. For example, desogestrel, levonorgestrel, norethindrone, etc.
- **Nonsteroidal anti-inflammatory drugs (NSAIDs):** It helps to ease cramps, headaches, backaches and breast tenderness. For example, ibuprofen, aspirin, naproxen, etc.

Nursing
- Encourage the patient to eat a diet rich in complex carbohydrates as it may reduce mood symptoms and food cravings.
- Encourage the patient to take 1200 mg of calcium per day which reduces the physical and emotional symptoms associated with premenstrual syndrome.
- Ask the patient to reduce the intake of fat, salt and sugar.
- Instruct the patient to avoid caffeine intake.
- Encourage the patient to eat six small meals a day rather than three large ones.
- Ask the patient to get enough sleep (8 hours of sleep each night).
- Encourage the patient to perform regular exercise.
- Ask the patient to include vegetables, fruits and food grains in the diet.

TOXIC SHOCK SYNDROME

Definition
Toxic shock syndrome (TSS) is an acute, noncontagious systemic illness characterized by high fever, hypotension, rash, multiorgan dysfunction and cutaneous desquamation during early convalescent period.

Etiology
- Bacterial infection (*Staphylococcus aureus, Streptococcus pyogenes, Clostridium sordellii*, etc.)
- Sinusitis
- Tracheitis
- Allergic contact dermatitis
- Burns
- Boils
- Recreational intravenous drug use.

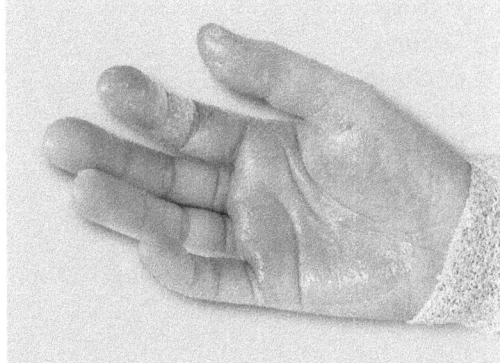

Fig. 10.18: Depicts toxic shock syndrome (TSS).

Risk Factors

- Being young people
- Use of barrier contraceptives such as diaphragm or vaginal sponge
- Menstruating women using tampons or other inserted devices
- Foreign bodies or packings which are used to stop nosebleeds
- Puerperal sepsis
- A local infection in the skin or deep tissue
- Surgical wounds
- Persons with weakened immune system.

Pathophysiology

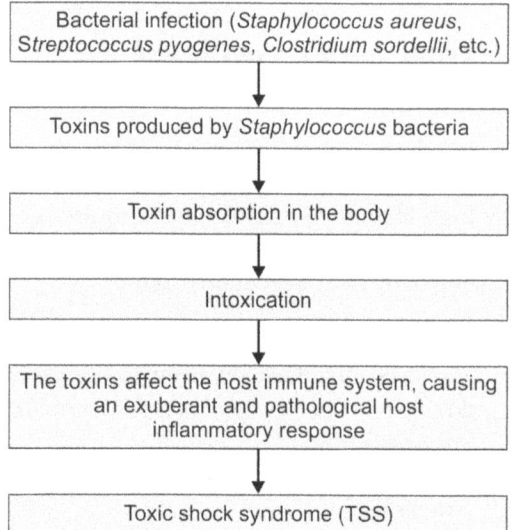

Clinical Features

- High fever sometimes accompanied by chills
- Malaise
- Seizures
- Confusion
- Headache
- Redness of eyes, mouth and throat
- Nausea
- Vomiting
- Profuse watery diarrhea
- Widespread red rash resembling sunburn
- Muscle ache
- Tenderness
- Rashes followed by peeling of the skin after 1 or 2 weeks particularly on the palms of the hand and bottom of the feet
- Confusion
- Sensitivity to light
- Sore throat.

Complications

- Hypotension
- Severe organ dysfunction (kidney, heart or liver failure)
- Shock
- Death.

Diagnostic Tests

- History
- Physical examination
- Blood examination
- Blood culture
- Urine examination
- Kidney function tests
- Throat swab
- Chest X-ray
- Lumbar puncture.

Management

Medical

- **Oxygen therapy:** It increases the concentration of oxygen being inhaled which increases the partial pressure of oxygen in the blood and corrects hypoxia.
- **Identification and decontamination of the site of toxin production:** Drain or debride the lesion, remove foreign material and irrigate copiously. Recent surgical wounds should be explored and irrigated even when signs of inflammation are absent.
- **Aggressive fluid resuscitation:** Loss of fluid into the extravascular compartment can be very substantial to increase blood pressure and treat dehydration. Maintenance of

cardiac filling pressures is critical in order to prevent end-organ damage. Adult patients with toxic shock syndrome require up to 10 L of fluid in the first 24 hours.

- **Antibiotics:** It helps to control the infection. For example, penicillin, clindamycin, etc.
- **Administration of pooled human immunoglobin:** A single infusion of 400 mg/kg intravenously will generate a protective titer in a nonimmune patient.
- **Beta blockers:** They slow down the heartbeat, decrease the force of contraction of the heart muscles and reduce blood vessel contraction in various parts of the body. For example, atenolol, labetalol, carvedilol, etc.

Surgical

- **Hemodialysis (PV):** It is the artificial process of eliminating waste (diffusion) and unwanted water (ultrafiltration) from the blood by pumping the patient's blood against dialysate that may be generated by the dialysis machine or at a central location mostly done in patients who are at risk of acute kidney injury.

Nursing

- Instruct the patient not to use highly absorbent vaginal tampons.
- Educate the patient not to leave the diaphragms and contraceptive sponges for more than 12 hours.
- Ask the patient to keep all skin wounds clean to prevent infection.
- Wash the hands with soap and water before inserting or removing a tampon, diaphragm or contraceptive sponge.
- Ask the patient to follow the directions on package inserts when using tampons, diaphragm and contraceptive sponges.
- Instruct the women who are menstruating and develop a high fever with vomiting and diarrhea must discontinue any vaginal tampon use immediately.

UTERINE PROLAPSE

Definition

The falling or sliding of uterus from its normal position in the pelvic cavity into the vaginal canal is known as uterine prolapse.

Etiology

- Tissue trauma sustained during childbirth (Post-hysterectomy)
- Decreased estrogen level
- Pelvic tumor
- Chronic bronchitis
- Asthma.

Risk Factors

- Being overweight
- Caucasian women
- Menopausal women
- Chronic coughing or straining
- Chronic constipation
- Mother who had one or more vaginal births
- Tobacco consumption.

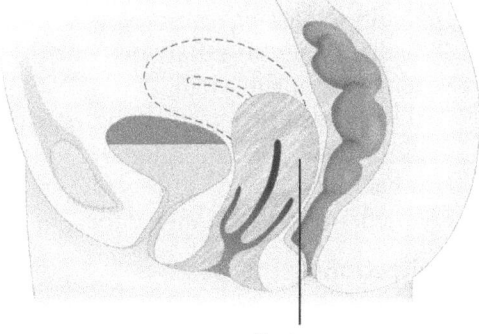

Fig. 10.19: Shows the fallen or slided uterus from its normal position in the pelvic cavity into the vaginal canal (Uterine prolapse).

Degree of Prolapse

- *Stage I:* The uterus is in the upper half of the vagina.
- *Stage II:* The uterus has descended nearly to the opening of the vagina.
- *Stage III:* The uterus protrudes out of the vagina.
- *Stage IV:* The uterus is completely out of the vagina.

Pathophysiology

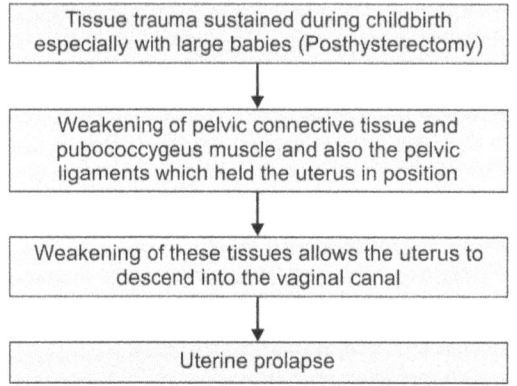

Clinical Features

- Sensation of heaviness or pulling in the pelvis
- Greater than normal amount of vaginal discharge
- Protrusion from the vaginal opening
- Difficulty in passing urine
- Difficult or painful sexual intercourse
- Feeling of sitting in a ball
- Leakage of urine when coughing, laughing or lifting heavy objects
- Low backache
- Frequent urinary tract infections.

Complications

- Urinary tract infection
- Ulceration and infection of the cervix
- Constipation
- Hemorrhoids.

Diagnostic Tests

- History
- Physical examination
- Pelvic examination
- Ultrasound scan
- Computed tomography (CT) scan
- Magnetic resonance imaging (MRI) scan.

Management

Medical

Estrogen replacement therapy: It replaces the hormone estrogen among post-menopausal women. For example, estrogen hormone, etc.

Surgical

- **Vaginal pessary:** It is a procedure in which an object is inserted into the vagina to hold the uterus in place as a temporary or permanent form of treatment.
- **Sacral colpopexy:** It is a surgical procedure which involves the use of surgical mesh for supporting the uterus without removing the uterus.
- **Vaginal hysterectomy:** It is a surgical procedure in which the vaginal walls, urethra, bladder or rectum are sagged and corrected at the same time.

Nursing

- Instruct the patient to avoid heavy lifting of objects.
- Ask the patient to avoid high-impact exercises.
- Instruct the patient to avoid tobacco chewing.
- Encourage the patient to take more roughages in the diet to prevent constipation.
- Encourage the patient to perform pelvic floor exercises to strengthen the pelvic floor muscles.

11 CHAPTER

Disorders of Skin

CHAPTER OUTLINE

- Acne vulgaris
- Athlete's foot (Tinea pedis)
- Burns
- Candidiasis
- Cellulitis
- Dermatitis (Eczema)
- Impetigo
- Onychomycosis
- Psoriasis
- Tinea corporis
- Scabies
- Shingles

ACNE VULGARIS

Definition

Acne vulgaris is a skin condition that occurs when our hair follicles become plugged with oil and dead skin cells. It usually appears on our face, neck, chest, back and shoulders.

Etiology

Bacterial infection (*Propionibacterium acnes*).

Risk Factors

- Stress
- Pregnancy
- High humidity and heavy sweating

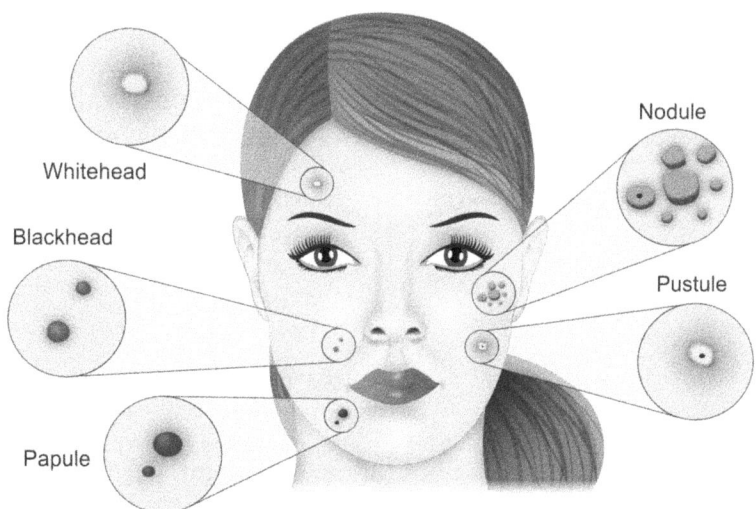

Fig. 11.1: Shows the cardinal features of acne vulgaris.

- Diets high refined sugars or dairy products
- Hormonal imbalance in teenage years
- Hormone changes during pregnancy
- Starting or stopping birth control pills
- Heredity
- Greasy makeup
- Certain medications (Corticosteroids, androgens, lithium, etc).

Pathophysiology

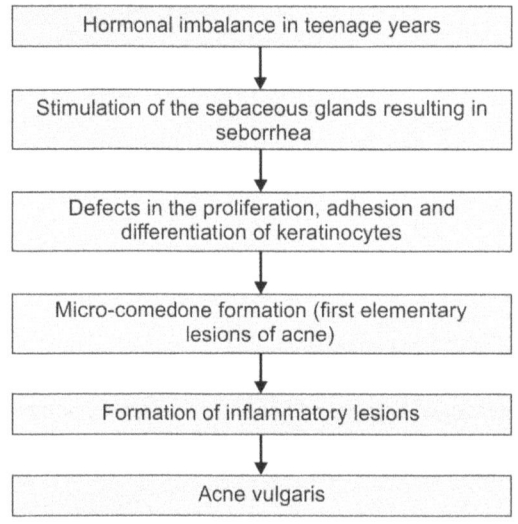

Clinical Features

Acne usually occurs on the face and shoulders, but may also occur on the arms, legs and back. The symptoms of acne, in increasing order of severity as follows:
- Blackheads (open comedone)
- Whiteheads (closed comedone)
- Papules (small red bumps)
- Pustules
- Cysts
- Scarring of the skin
- Crusting of skin bumps
- Redness around the skin eruptions.

Complications

- Cutaneous abscess
- Acne fulminans (pimples break open and ulcerate)
- Scarring
- Lowers self-esteem.

Diagnostic Tests

- History
- Physical examination
- Blood examination
- Hormonal examination
- Liver function test
- Lipid profile test.

Management

Medical

- **Retinoids (topical):** It acts by normalizing follicular epithelial cell turnover and preventing comedone formation. For example, tretinoin, Retin-A, Atralin, Renova, etc.
- **Oral antibiotics:** It helps to reduce bacteria and fights inflammation. For example, tetracycline, doxycycline, minocycline, erythromycin, trimethoprim, amoxicillin, etc.
- **Topical antibiotics:** It works by killing excess skin bacteria and reducing redness. For example, clindamycin, erythromycin, dapsone, etc.
- **Anti-androgen agents:** It works by blocking the effect of androgen hormones on the sebaceous glands. For example, spironolactone, etc.
- **Benzoyl peroxide:** It reduces the number of comedones and acts by sterilizing the follicle via its antibacterial effects on *Propionibacterium acnes*.
- **Photodynamic therapy:** It is a procedure that utilizes a photosensitizing molecule (frequently a drug that becomes activated by light exposure) and a light source to activate the applied drug and targets the bacteria that cause acne inflammation.

Surgical

- **Laser resurfacing:** It is a skin resurfacing procedure that uses a laser to improve the appearance of your skin.
- **Soft tissue fillers:** It is a procedure in which soft tissue fillers, such as collagen or fat, are injected under the skin and into indented

scars to fill out or stretch the skin. This makes the scars less noticeable.
- **Chemical peel:** It is a procedure in which high-potency acid is applied to the skin to remove the top layer and minimize deeper scars.
- **Punch excision:** It is a procedure in which the surgeon cuts out individual acne scars and repairs the hole at the scar site with stitches or a skin graft.
- **Extraction of whiteheads and blackheads:** It is a procedure that gently removes whiteheads and blackheads (comedones) that haven't cleared up with topical medications and also cause scarring.

Nursing

- Ask the patient not to squeeze, scratch, pick or rub the pimples.
- Instruct to avoid greasy cosmetics or creams.
- Ask not to leave make-up on overnight.
- Instruct them to avoid touching their face with hands or fingers.
- Instruct them to avoid wearing tight headbands and other hats.
- Ask them to avoid scrubbing or repeated skin washing.
- Encourage small amount of sun exposure as it improves the condition slightly better.

ATHLETE'S FOOT (TINEA PEDIS)

Definition

It is a contagious fungal infection that affects the skin on the feet and can spread to the toenails and sometimes the hands.

Etiology

Fungal infection (Trichophyton rubrum).

Risk Factors

- Being male
- Heavy sweating

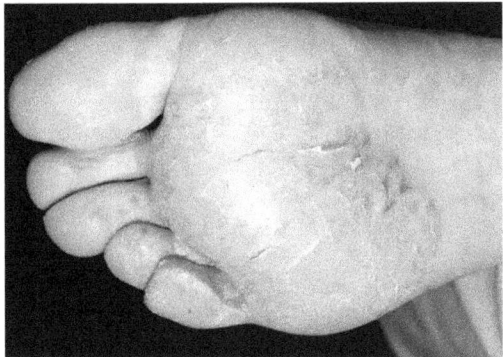

Fig. 11.2: Depicts contagious fungal infection that affects the skin on the feet (Athlete's foot).

- Keeping the feet wet for long periods
- Develop a minor skin or nail injury
- Wearing plastic-lined closed shoes
- Walking barefoot in public areas
- Having a weakened immune system.

Types

There are three types of athlete's foot as follows:
1. *Moccasin:* It doesn't cause itching or inflammation. The entire sole and heel becomes dry and flaky with loose, white scales that appear in a moccasin-like pattern. Sometimes the toenails can also become infected, which makes it more difficult to treat.
2. *Vesicular or blistered:* People with this type suffer from sore, fluid-filled blisters that occur between the toes and on the arch and sides of the foot. These blisters form in response to an allergic reaction to the fungi causing the athlete's foot.
3. *Interdigital or ulcerative:* It is the most common type and presents as maceration (softened tissue caused by soaking) and scales in the web spaces between the toes. Ulceration develops when a secondary bacterial infection occurs. Its symptoms include painful ulcers between the toes, which often take a long time to heal.

Pathophysiology

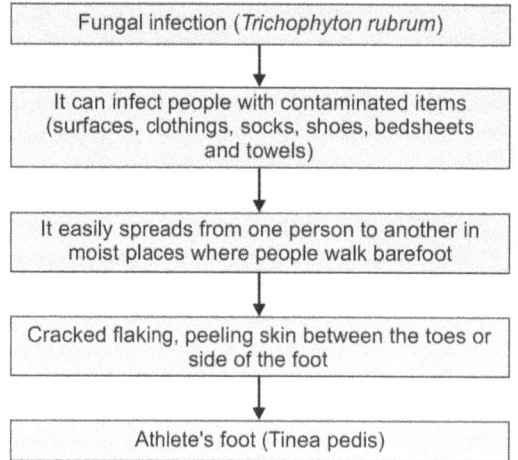

Clinical Features

- Cracked flaking, peeling skin between the toes or side of the foot
- Red and itchy skin
- Burning or stinging pain
- Blisters that ooze or get crusty
- Discolored, thick and crumbly toenails
- Toenails that pull away from the nail bed.

Complications

- Allergic reaction
- Lymphangitis (infection of the lymph vessels)
- Lymphadenitis (infection of the lymph nodes).

Diagnostic Tests

- History
- Physical examination
- Skin scraping
- Wood's lamp (black light) examination.

Management

Medical

Topical antifungal agents: It works by killing the fungus causing the infection. For example, miconazole, clotrimazole, terbinafine, tolnaftate, etc.

Nursing

- Instruct the patient to keep the feet clean and dry.
- Ask them to wear shoes that are well-ventilated and made of natural materials such as leather.
- Instruct them to change the shoes and socks often to keep the feet dry.
- Instruct the patient to wash the feet with soap and water every day and dry them thoroughly.
- Ask them not to share shoes, socks and towel with others.

BURNS

Definition

Any injury to the tissues of the body which leads to cell destruction of the layers of the skin and the resultant of fluid and electrolytes is known as burns.

Etiology

- Hot objects (or) flames (thermal burns)
- Electricity (electrical burns)
- Chemical (chemical burns)
- Radiations (radiation burns)
- Gases
- Overexposure to the sun.

Risk Factors

- Adults with greater than 15% of burn injury
- Children's greater than 10% of burn injury
- Use of alcohol or drugs
- Delay in resuscitation
- Being elders
- Smoke inhalation injury
- Associated injuries.

Types

1. **Classification based on depth of burns:** Burns are often categorized as first-degree, second-degree, or third-degree, depending

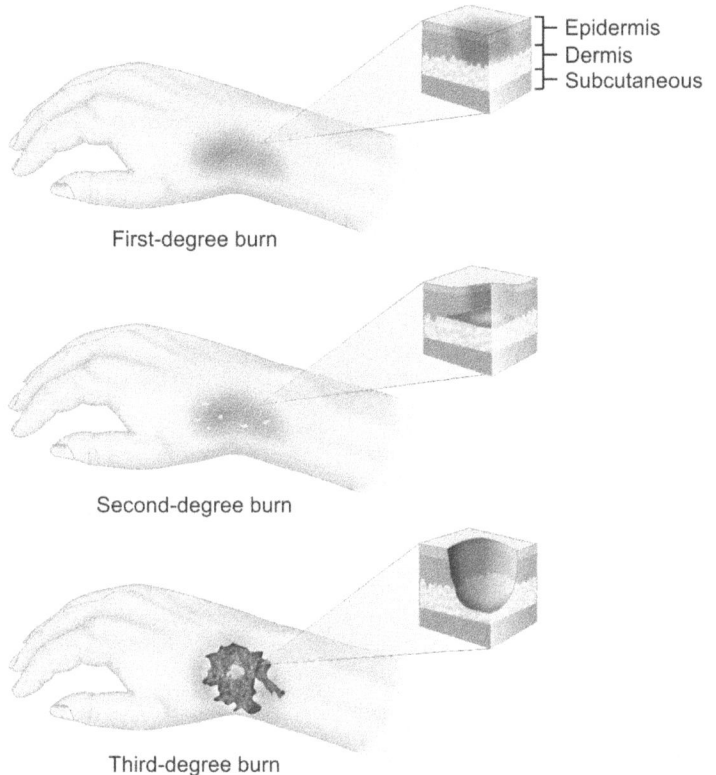

Fig. 11.3: Depicts classification of burns based on depth of the injury.

on how badly the skin is damaged as follows:
- **First-degree burns:** It is the mildest of the three and is limited to the top layer of the skin. These burns produce redness, pain and minor swelling. The skin is dry without blisters. Healing time is about 3–6 days and the superficial skin layer may peel off in 1 or 2 days.
- **Second-degree burns:** These are more serious and involve the skin layers beneath the top layer. These burns produce blisters, severe pain, and redness. The blisters sometimes break open and the area is wet looking with a bright pink to cherry red color. Healing time varies depending on the severity of the burn and it can take upto 3 weeks or more.
- **Third-degree burns (full-thickness burns):** These are the most serious type of burn and involve all the layers of the skin and the underlying tissue. The surface appears dry, and can look waxy white, leathery, brown or charred. There may be little or no pain or the area may feel numb at first because of nerve damage. Healing time depends on the severity of the burn. It (also known as full-thickness burns) will likely need to be treated with skin grafts, in which healthy skin is taken from another part of the body and surgically placed over the burn wound to help the area heal.

2. **Classification based on extent of burns:** Burns are often categorized as first-degree, second-degree, or third-degree, depending on how badly the skin is damaged as follows:
   - *Minor burns:* These are partial-thickness burns; are no greater than 15% of the total surface area in an adult and full-thickness burn of less than 2% of the total body surface area in an adult. These do not involve the eyes, ears, hands, face, feet or perineum. There are no electrical burns or inhalation injuries. The patient is an adult younger than 60 years of age. The patient has no preexisting medical conditions at the time of burn injury and no other injury occurred with the burn.
   - *Moderate burns:* These are partial-thickness burns that are deep and are 15%–25% of the total body surface areas in the adult and full-thickness burns of 2%–10% of the total body surface area in the adult. They do not involve the eyes, ears, hands, face, feet or perineum. There are no electrical burns or inhalation injuries. The client is an adult younger than 60 years of age. The patient has no chronic cardiac, pulmonary or endocrine disorder at the time of burn injury and no other complicated injury occurred with the burn.
   - *Major burns:* These are partial-thickness burns of more than 25% of the total body surface area in the adult and full-thickness burns of more than 10% of the total body surface area. The burn areas involve the eyes, ears, hands, face, feet or perineum. The burn injury was an electrical injury or inhalation injury. The patient is older than 60 years of age. The patient has a chronic cardiac, pulmonary or metabolic disorder at the time of the burn injury and is accompanied by other injuries.

Pathophysiology

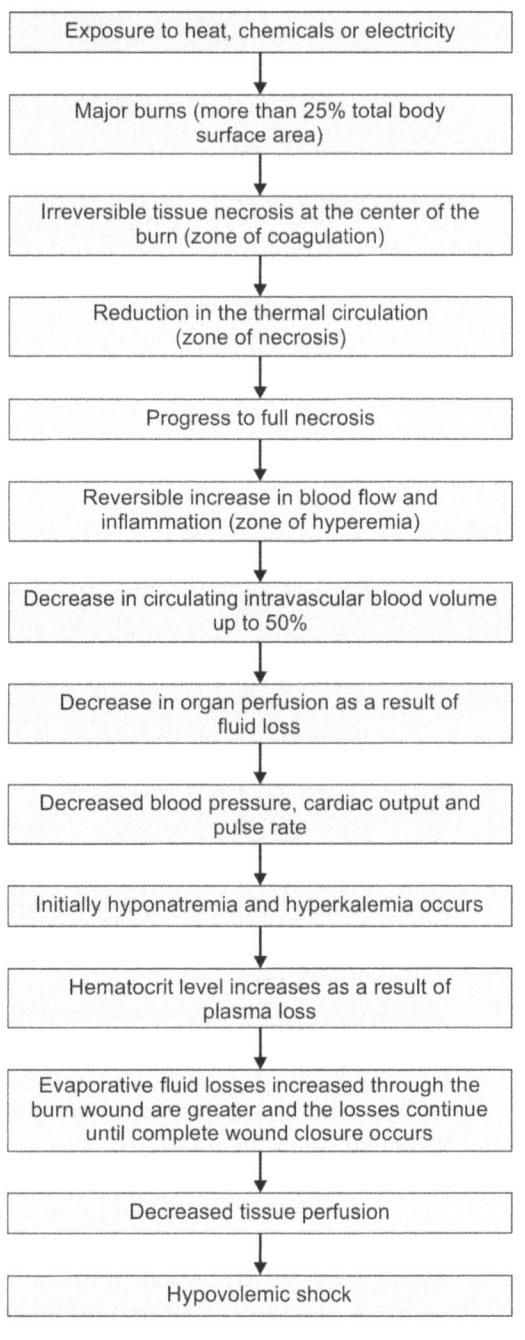

Clinical Features

- Loss of skin barrier
- Impaired immune response

Disorders of Skin

- Hemolysis
- Hyperkalemia
- Hyponatremia
- Increased capillary permeability
- Hemoglobin (or) myoglobin in urine
- Increased concentration of RBCs
- Increased blood viscosity
- Decreased circulating blood volume
- Decreased blood pressure
- Hypoxemia
- Hyperglycemia
- Decreased cardiac output
- Decreased GI blood flow
- Decreased tissue perfusion
- Metabolic acidosis.

Complications

- Hypovolemia
- Infection
- Metabolic abnormalities
- Hypothermia
- Ileus
- Eschar
- Scarring and contractures.

Diagnostic Tests

- History
- Physical examination
- Rule of nine
- Blood examination
- Electrolyte levels
- X-rays.

Management

Medical

- **Topical antibiotics:** It reduces the risk of infection in smaller burns and may facilitate the development of multi-resistant bacteria. For example, silver sulfadiazine, silver nitrate, mafenide acetate, etc.
- **Opioid agonists:** They are potent and provide some dose-dependent degree of sedation that can be advantageous to burns patients. For example, nalbuphine, butorphanol, etc.
- **Anesthetics:** It provides safe and effective analgesia without loss of consciousness for moderately painful procedures for the treatment of burn pain. For example, nitrous oxide, prilocaine, lidocaine, etc.

Surgical

- **Escharotomy:** It is a surgical procedure in which an incision is made lengthwise through the eschar of the burned area to facilitate circulation.
- **Fasciotomy:** It is a surgical procedure in which an incision is made, extending through the subcutaneous tissue and fascia.
- **Hydrotherapy:** Showers given to clean the wounds and to prevent infection and sepsis. Tap water is used and the temperature of the water is maintained at 37.8°C (100°F). The temperature of the room is maintained at 80°F–85°F and performed for about 20–30 minutes.
- **Wound closure:** It is a permanent wound covering which is made and grafting is performed. Amnion, skin of donated cadaver (allograft) and porcine skin (heterograft) are used for grafting.

Nursing

- Instruct them to keep electrical appliances away from water.
- Instruct them to unplug iron box and similar devices when not in use.
- Instruct them to keep hot liquids out of the reach of children.
- Ask them not to cook while wearing loose-fitted clothes.
- Ask them not to leave items cooking on the stove unattended.
- Educate them to keep a fire extinguisher on every floor of the house.
- Ask them to keep chemicals, lighters and matches out of the reach of children.
- Ask them to set their water heater's thermostat below 120°F to prevent scalding.
- Encourage them to change the batteries regularly.

CANDIDIASIS

Definition
It is a localized mucocutaneous infection caused by a yeast-like fungus *Candida albicans*.

Etiology
Fungal infection (*Candida albicans*).

Risk Factors
- Warm weather
- Tight clothing
- Poor hygiene
- Infrequent undergarment changes
- Certain drugs (Antibiotics, corticosteroids, etc.)
- Weakened immune system
- Birth control pills
- Diabetes mellitus
- Pregnancy
- Being overweight
- Altered flora resulting from antibiotic therapy
- Incomplete drying of damp or wet skin
- Inflammatory diseases (Psoriasis).
- Stress.

Types
- ***Oropharyngeal/Esophageal candidiasis (Thrush):*** The candidiasis that develops in the mouth or throat is called "thrush" or oropharyngeal candidiasis. The most common symptom of oral thrush is white patches or plaques on the tongue and other oral mucous membranes. This infection is uncommon among healthy adults.
- ***Genital/Vulvovaginal candidiasis (Yeast infection):*** It occurs when there is overgrowth of the normal yeast in the vagina. This infection is relatively common and nearly 75% of all adult women have had at least one "yeast infection" in their lifetime.
- ***Invasive candidiasis:*** It is a serious infection that can affect the blood, heart, brain, eyes, bones, and other parts of the body.

Pathophysiology

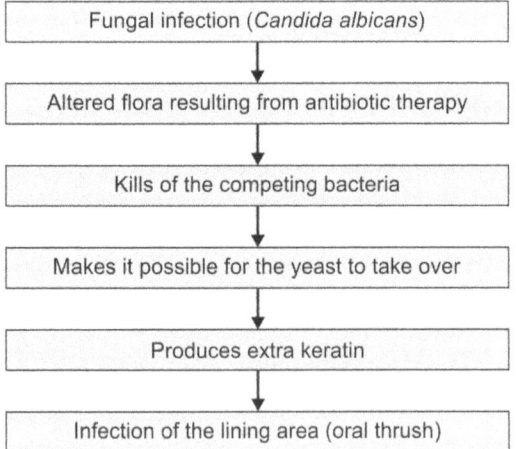

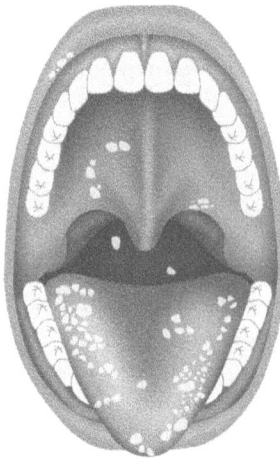

Fig. 11.4: Shows the appearance of oral thrush in candidiasis.

Clinical Features
- Creamy white patches in the mouth or throat (oral thrush)
- Painful cracks at the corners of the mouth (oral thrush)
- Skin rashes, patches and blisters found most commonly in the groin, between fingers and toes and under the breasts.
- Vaginal itching and irritation with a white discharge resembling cheese (vaginal yeast infection).
- Slight bleeding if the lesions are rubbed or scraped.

- A cottony feeling in the mouth.
- Loss of taste.

Complications
- Onychomycosis
- Tinea corporis
- Tinea pedis
- Vaginitis
- Thrush.

Diagnostic Tests
- History
- Physical examination
- Blood examination
- Skin scraping or biopsy.

Management

Medical
Antifungal agents: It helps in reducing the severity of candidiasis infection and its associated symptoms. For example, miconazole, ticonazole, clotrimazole, Renova, etc.

Nursing
- Ask the patient to practice good hygiene.
- Instruct them to wear the right clothes.
- Instruct them to avoid the use of cosmetics.
- Encourage them to have proper diet, sleep and exercise.
- Ask them to change the underwear often to prevent dampness.

CELLULITIS

Definition
Cellulitis is an infection of the deep subcutaneous tissue of the skin which is caused by normal skin flora or by exogenous bacteria.

Etiology
Bacterial infection (*Staphylococcus* and *Streptococcus* organisms).

Risk Factors
- Insect bites
- Blisters
- Animal bites
- Tattoos
- Athlete's foot
- Eczema
- Burns and boils
- Intravenous catheter insertion
- Cracks or peeling skin between the toes

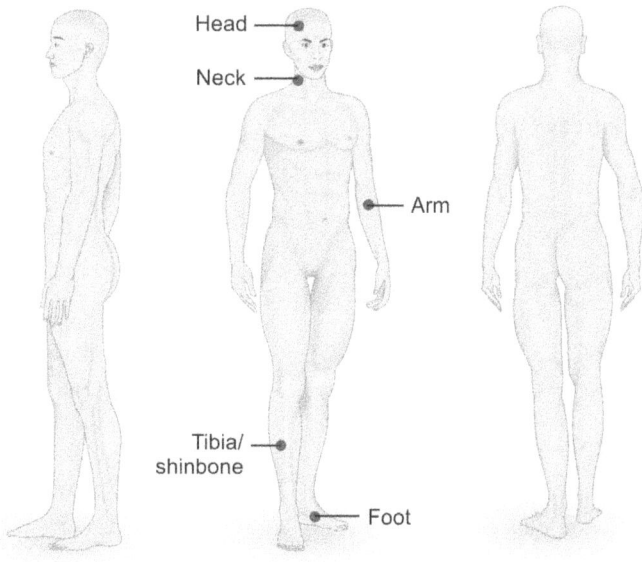

Fig. 11.5: Shows the most common sites for cellulitis.

- History of peripheral vascular disease
- Injury or trauma with a break in the skin
- Ulcers from certain diseases (diabetes and vascular disease)
- Use of corticosteroids
- Wound from a recent surgery
- Elderly people
- Diabetics
- Chickenpox
- Shingles
- Varicose veins.

Types

There are five common forms of cellulitis as follows:

1. **Hand cellulitis:** It is a medical condition that occurs on arms which is mainly caused by bacteria entering a break on the surface of the skin.
2. **Leg cellulitis:** It is an infection of the legs occurs from bacteria permeating the skin surface.
3. **Facial cellulitis:** People with compromised lymphatic systems, upper respiratory infections or tooth infections are at risk for this type.
4. **Periorbital cellulitis:** It affects the tissues around the eye and is most common in children.
5. **Orbital cellulitis:** It is less common than the periorbital infection and is more dangerous of it spreads to the brain.

Pathophysiology

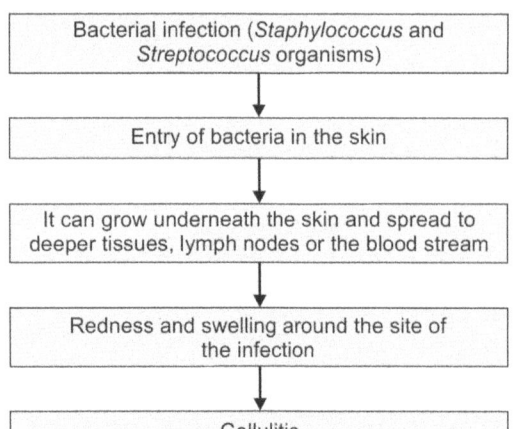

Clinical Features

- It occurs on exposed areas of the body such as the arms, legs, feet and face.
- Fever
- Chills
- Headache
- Nausea
- Vomiting
- Itching
- Redness on the affected area that gets bigger as the infection spreads
- Skin sore or rash that starts suddenly, and grows quickly in the first 24 hours.
- Tight, glossy, stretched appearance of the skin
- Warm skin in the area of redness
- Hair loss at the site of infection
- Joint stiffness caused by swelling of the tissue over the joint
- Pain or tenderness in the affected area.

Complications

- Necrotizing fasciitis
- Chronic swelling of the affected limb
- Erysipelas
- Gangrene.

Diagnostic Tests

- History
- Physical examination
- Blood culture
- Ultrasound of leg
- X-ray examination.

Management

Medical

- **Antibiotics:** It prevents the bacterial infection from spreading rapidly and reaching the blood and internal organs. For example, dicloxacillin, cephalexin, etc.
- **Analgesics:** It helps to decrease pain and keep fever down. For example, ibuprofen, acetaminophen, etc.

Nursing

- Instruct them to keep the skin moist with lotions or ointments to prevent cracking.

- Ask them to wear shoes that fit well and provide enough room for the feet.
- Educate them how to trim their nails to avoid harming the skin around them.
- Ask them to wear appropriate protective equipment when participating in work or sports.
- Ask them to clean the break in the skin carefully with soap and water.

DERMATITIS (ECZEMA)

Definition

It is a long-term (chronic) skin disorder that involves scaly and itchy rashes.

Etiology

- Emotional stress
- Cold and dry air in the winter
- Allergies to pollen, mold, dust mites or animals.

Risk Factors

- Colds or the flu
- Contact with irritants or chemicals
- Contact with rough materials, such as wool
- Dry skin
- Drying out of the skin from taking too much baths or showers and swimming too often
- Getting too hot or too cold, as well as sudden changes of temperature
- Perfumes.

Types

There are eight common forms of dermatitis as follows:

1. **Atopic dermatitis:** It refers to personal and family tendency to develop eczema. They are hereditary and are not always passed directly from parent to child and may skip a generation.
2. **Contact dermatitis:** It occurs as a result of contact with irritants or allergens in the environment.
3. **Adult seborrheic dermatitis:** The rash appears in those areas of the skin with large numbers of grease (sebaceous) glands, such as the scalp and side of the nose.
4. **Infantile seborrheic dermatitis:** It is a common skin condition seen in infants under the age of one year. It usually appears quite suddenly between two weeks and six months after birth.
5. **Discoid dermatitis:** It is usually seen in adults with dry skin although it can affect teenagers and young children, but this is rare.
6. **Pompholyx dermatitis:** It is a form of dermatitis in which blistering that is restricted

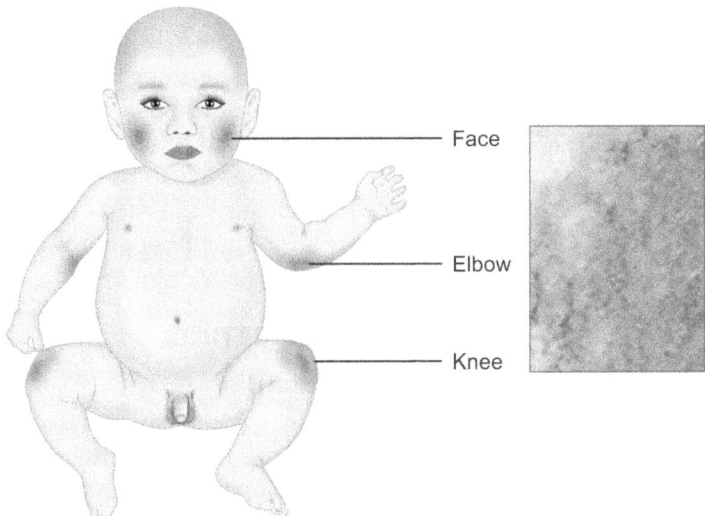

Fig. 11.6: Portrays scaly and itchy rashes at different sites of the body.

to the hands and feet.
7. *Asteatotic dermatitis:* It almost always affects people over the age of 60.
8. *Varicose dermatitis:* It common in later life, particularly in women but can occur from the teenage years onwards.

Pathophysiology

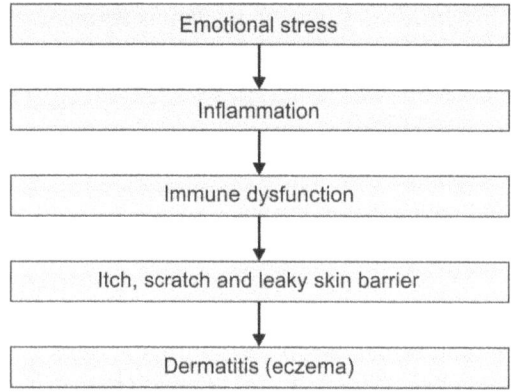

Emotional stress → Inflammation → Immune dysfunction → Itch, scratch and leaky skin barrier → Dermatitis (eczema)

Clinical Features

- Blisters with oozing and crusting
- Dry skin all over the body or areas of bumpy skin on the back of the arms and front of the thighs
- Ear discharge or bleeding
- Raw areas of the skin from scratching
- Skin coloring changes, such as more or less color than the normal skin tone
- Skin redness or inflammation around the blisters
- Thickened or leather-like areas (lichenification), which can occur after long-term irritation and scratching.

Complications

- Infection of the skin
- Permanent scars.

Diagnostic Tests

- History
- Physical examination
- Blood culture
- Allergy skin testing
- Skin biopsy.

Management

Medical

- **Antihistamines**: It helps in reducing itch. For example, chlorpheniramine, cyclizine, etc.
- **Topical corticosteroids**: It helps in reducing pain and speeding healing of the rash, especially when the rash covers large areas of the body. For example, hydrocortisone, prednisone, etc.
- **Calcineurin inhibitors (topical immunosuppressants)**: It inhibits production of inflammatory cytokines in the skin. For example, tacrolimus, pimecrolimus, etc.
- **Oral antibiotics**: It helps to prevent any secondary infections. For example, tetracycline, doxycycline, minocycline, erythromycin, trimethoprim, amoxicillin, etc.
- **Immunosuppressants**: It inhibits or prevents activity of the immune system. For example, cyclosporine, methotrexate, mycophenolate mofetil, etc.
- **Phototherapy**: It is a medical treatment in which the skin is carefully exposed to ultraviolet light.

Nursing

- Ask them to avoid scratching the rash or skin.
- Instruct them to keep the skin moist with lotions or ointments to prevent cracking.
- Educate them how to trim their nails to avoid harming the skin around them.
- Expose the skin to water for as short a time as possible.
- Encourage to use gentle body washes and cleansers instead of regular soaps.
- Instruct them not to scrub or dry the skin too hard or for too long.

IMPETIGO

Definition

It is a highly contagious bacterial skin infection causing blisters and sores most common among preschool children.

Disorders of Skin

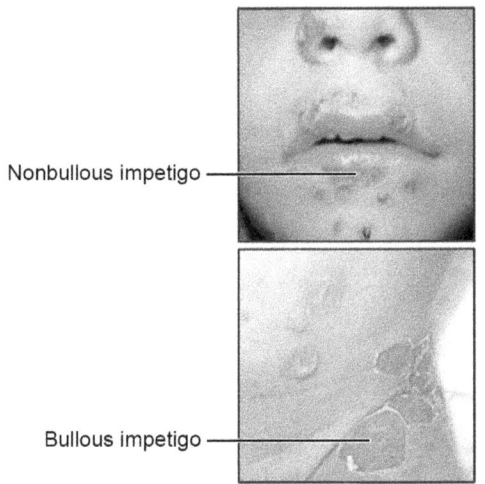

Fig. 11.7: Depicts nonbullous and bullous impetigo.

blisters that appear clear, then cloudy. These blisters are more likely to stay longer on the skin without bursting.

Pathophysiology

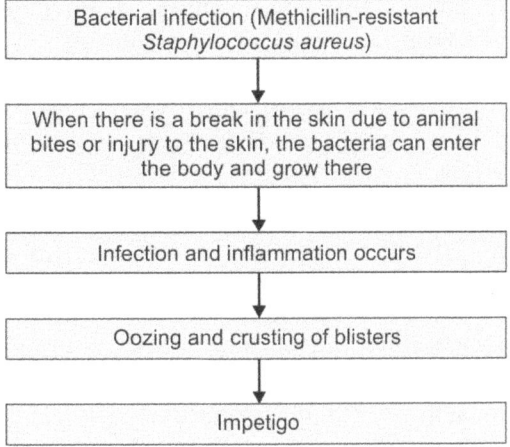

Etiology

Bacterial infection (Methicillin-resistant *Staphylococcus aureus*).

Risk Factors

- Being children
- Residing in crowded area
- Warm, humid weather
- Participating in sports involving skin-to-skin contact
- Broken skin.

Types

There are two types of impetigo as follows:
1. ***Nonbullous (crusted) impetigo:*** It is the most common type. It is usually caused by *Staphylococcus aureus* but also can be due to infection with *Staphylococcus pyogenes*. It begins as tiny blisters that eventually burst and leave small wet patches of red skin that may weep fluid. Gradually, a yellowish-brown or tan crust covers the affected area, making it look like it has been coated with honey or brown sugar.
2. ***Bullous (large blisters) impetigo:*** It is nearly always caused by *Staphylococcus aureus*, which releases toxins that trigger the formation of larger fluid-containing

Clinical Features

- One or many blisters filled with pus that are easy to pop
- Blisters filled with yellow or honey-colored fluid
- Oozing and crusting over of blisters
- Rash that may begin as a single spot, but spreads to other areas with scratching
- Skin sores on the face, lips, arms or legs that spread to other areas.
- Swollen lymph nodes near the infection.

Complications

- Post-streptococcal glomerulonephritis
- Cellulitis
- Scarlet fever
- Guttate psoriasis
- Septicemia.

Diagnostic Tests

- History
- Physical examination
- Swab examination
- Blood examination
- Skin biopsy
- Culture and sensitivity test.

Management

Medical

- **Oral antibiotics:** It helps to reduce bacteria and fights inflammation. For example, tetracycline, doxycycline, minocycline, erythromycin, trimethoprim, amoxicillin, etc.
- **Topical antibiotics:** It works by killing excess skin bacteria and reducing blisters. For example, clindamycin, erythromycin, etc.

Nursing

- Encourage them to use a clean washcloth and towel each time.
- Ask them not to share towels, clothing, razors and other personal care products with other family members.
- Instruct them to avoid touching blisters that are oozing.
- Educate them to wash hands thoroughly after touching infected skin.
- Instruct them to keep the skin clean to prevent getting the infection.
- Ask them to avoid scratching the rash or skin.
- Encourage to use gentle body washes and cleansers instead of regular soaps.
- Isolate the patient until sure they are not contagious.

ONYCHOMYCOSIS (FUNGAL NAIL INFECTION)

Definition

These are common infections of the fingernails or toenails that can cause the nail to become discolored, thick and more likely to crack and break.

Etiology

Fungal infection (*Trichophyton rubrum*).

Risk Factors

- Have minor skin or nail injuries
- Get manicures or pedicures with tools that have been used on other people

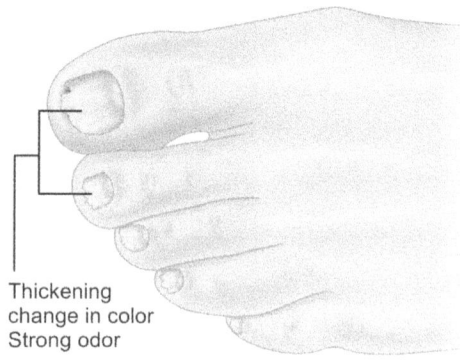

Fig. 11.8: Depicts infection of the toenails that causes the nails to become discolored, thick and break (Onychomycosis).

- Have deformed nail or nail disease
- Have moist skin for a long time
- Have weakened immune system
- Wearing closed-in footwear
- Being older
- Perspiring heavily
- Being male
- Walking barefoot in damp community areas
- Having athlete's foot.

Types

There are five types of onychomycosis as follows:

1. ***Distal/lateral subungual onychomycosis:*** The most common variant of onychomycosis is distal/lateral subungual onychomycosis, a condition usually caused by *Trichophyton rubrum*. The nail is abnormally colored (white or brown) along the lateral edges of the upper distal areas and may be eroded.
2. ***Superficial white onychomycosis:*** This uncommon toenail fungus is usually caused by *Tinea mentagrophytes*. It initially affects the upper nail surface, extending to the nail bed and area beneath the nail.
3. ***Proximal subungual onychomycosis:*** This toenail fungus involves the proximal area beneath the nail bed; it is most common in immunosuppressed patients and is usually caused by *Trichophyton rubrum*.

4. **Candidal onychomycosis:** This may be seen in patients whose feet are constantly wet. With continued water exposure, the cuticle loosens from the nail plate, and microorganisms enter the exposed area.
5. **Total dystrophic onychomycosis:** In this condition, the nail plate is virtually eradicated.

Pathophysiology

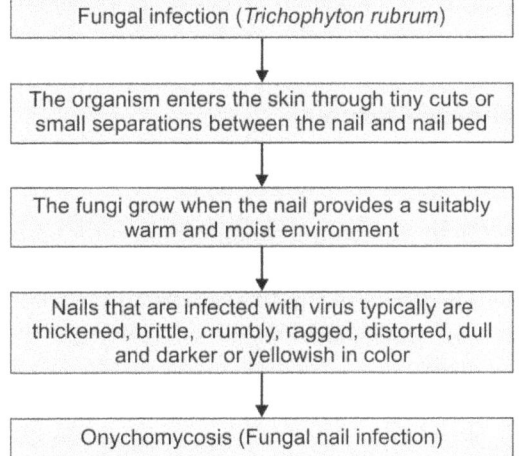

Clinical Features

- Brittleness of nails
- Change in nail shape
- Crumbling of the outside edges of the nail
- Debris trapped under the nail
- Loosening or lifting up of the nail
- Loss of luster and shine
- Thickening of the nail
- White or yellow streaks on the side of the nail.

Complications

- Post-streptococcal glomerulonephritis
- Cellulitis
- Scarlet fever
- Guttate psoriasis
- Septicemia.

Diagnostic Tests

- History
- Physical examination
- Skin scraping
- Skin biopsy
- Fungal culture.

Management

Medical

Topical antifungal agents: It helps in controlling *Trichophyton rubrum* and its related symptoms. For example, terbinafine, fluconazole, griseofulvin, itraconazole, etc.

Nursing

- Ask them not to share tools used for manicures and pedicures.
- Encourage them to keep the skin clean and dry.
- Ask them to take care of their nails properly.
- Encourage them to use a clean wash cloth and towel each time.
- Educate them to wash hands thoroughly after touching the infected skin.
- Ask them not to share nail clippers with other people.

PSORIASIS

Definition

Psoriasis is a chronic autoimmune condition that causes the rapid buildup of skin cells. This buildup of cells causes scaling on the skin's surface.

Etiology

Fungal infection (*Trichophyton rubrum*).

Risk Factors

- Bacterial or viral infections (Streptococcal tonsillitis and other infections)
- Change in weather that dries the skin
- Certain medications (antimalarials, lithium, beta-blockers, etc).
- Stressful event
- Sun exposure
- Obesity
- Excessive alcohol
- Smoking

Disorders of Skin

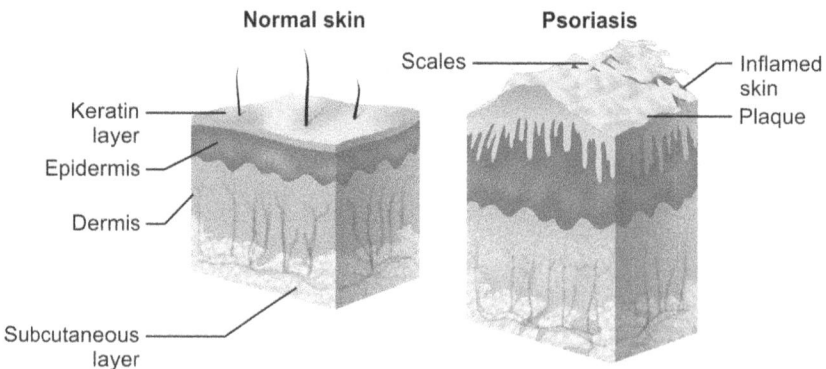

Fig. 11.9: Shows the comparison of normal skin with that of the inflamed skin (Psoriasis).

- Having a weakened immune system
- Stopping oral steroids.

Types
There are five types of psoriasis as follows:
1. **Erythrodermic:** In this, the skin redness is very intense and covers a large area.
2. **Guttate:** Small, pink-red spots appear on the skin.
3. **Inverse:** In this, skin redness and irritation occurs in the armpits, groin, and in between overlapping skin.
4. **Plaque:** Thick, red patches of skin are covered by flaky, silver-white scales. This is the most common type of psoriasis.
5. **Pustular:** White blisters are surrounded by red, irritated skin.

Pathophysiology

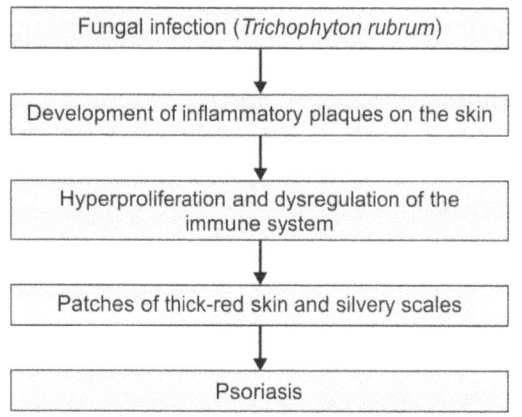

Clinical Features
- Patches of thick-red skin and silvery scales
- Itchy and painful plaques that sometimes crack and bleed
- Disorders of the fingernails and toenails including discoloration and pitting of the nails
- Nails begin to crumble or detach from the nail bed
- Scaly plaques on the scalp
- Small areas of bleeding where the involved skin is scratched
- Swollen and stiff joints.

Complications
- Psoriatic arthritis
- Obesity
- Type-2 diabetes
- Hypertension
- Metabolic syndrome
- Parkinson's disease.

Diagnostic Tests
- History
- Physical examination
- Blood examination
- Skin biopsy
- X-ray examination.

Management

Medical

- **Topical steroids:** It decreases inflammation, relieves itching and blocks the production of cells that are overproduced in psoriasis. For example, hydrocortisone, prednisone, etc.
- **Calcipotriene:** It is effective for treating psoriasis and works by slowing down the growth of skin cells. For example, Dovonex, Sorilux, etc.
- **Retinoids (topical):** It helps in improving the condition by reducing the severity of the disease. For example, tretinoin, Retin-A, Atralin, Renova, etc.
- **Topical acetylsalicylic acid:** It helps to clear and prevent pimples and skin blemishes that involve scaling and overgrowth of skin cells. For example, aspirin, etc.

Nursing

- Instruct them not to scrub too hard.
- Ask them to keep the skin in a moist condition.
- Encourage to maintain proper hygiene as it promotes cell turnover and reduces the likelihood of plaque development.
- Instruct them not to smoke.
- Strictly prohibit alcohol consumption in them.

TINEA CORPORIS (RINGWORM OF THE BODY)

Definition

It is a dermatophytosis that causes pink-to-red annular (O-shaped) patches and plaques with raised scaly borders that expand peripherally and tend to clear centrally.

Etiology

- Fungal infection (*Trichophyton rubrum*).
- Household pets
- Going barefoot

Risk Factors

- Being children
- Have wet skin for a long time (as in sweating)
- Those who have minor skin and nail injuries.

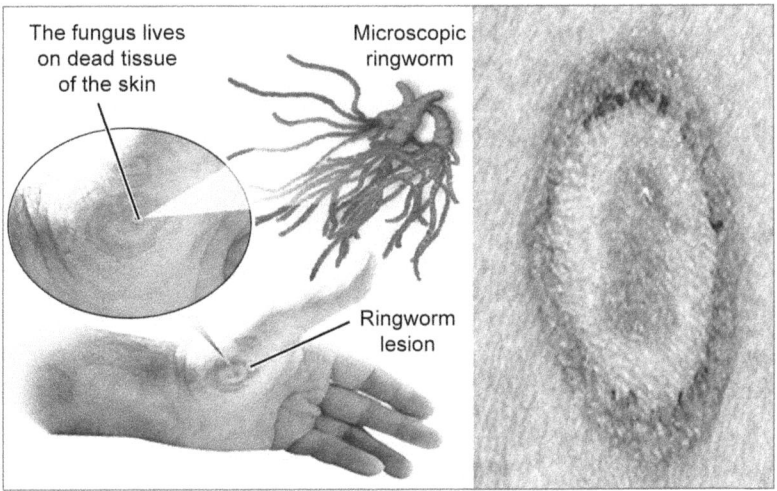

Fig. 11.10: Depicts pink-to-red annular patches and plaques with raised scaly borders due to fungal infection (Tinea corporis or ring worm).

- Come in close contact with other people.
- Wear tight or restricted clothing.
- Live in damp, humid or crowded conditions.
- Have a weakened immune system.
- Participating in sports featuring skin-to-skin contact (wrestling).
- Lack of hygiene.

Pathophysiology

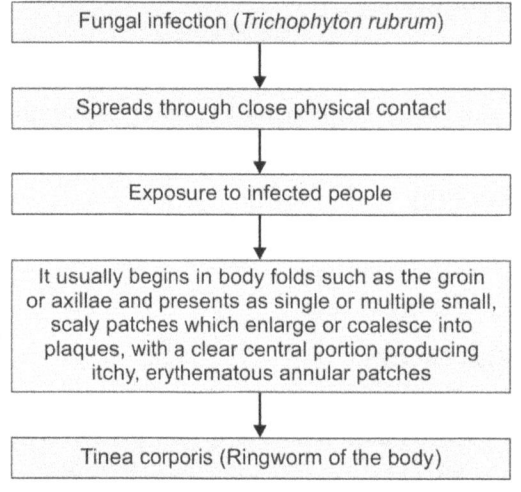

Clinical Features

- Small area of red, raised spots and pimples and it slowly becomes ring-shaped, with a red colored, raised border and a clearer center.
- Border looks scaly.
- Rash occurs on the arms, legs, face or other exposed body areas
- Itching.

Complications

- Skin infection from scratching too much
- Pyoderma or dermatophytid
- Majocchi's granuloma.

Diagnostic Tests

- History
- Physical examination
- Skin scraping
- Skin biopsy
- Fungal culture.

Management

Medical

Topical antifungal agents: It helps in controlling tinea corporis and its related symptoms. For example, miconazole, clotrimazole, ketoconazole, terbinafine, oxiconazole, etc.

Nursing

- Instruct the patient to avoid touching or scratching the rash.
- Instruct them to wash towels in warm, soapy water and then dry them.
- Ask them to clean sinks, bathtubs and bathroom floors well after using.
- Ask them to wear loose-fitted clothing.
- Encourage them to wear clean clothes every day and also instruct them not to share clothes.
- Instruct them to avoid infected pets.

SCABIES

Definition

It is a skin infestation caused by a very tiny mite known as the *Sarcoptes scabiei*.

Etiology

Mites (*Sarcoptes scabiei*).

Risk Factors

- Shared clothes or bedding
- Being in nursing homes or prison
- Weakened immune system
- Elderly and children
- People who underwent organ transplant
- Crowded areas.

Disorders of Skin

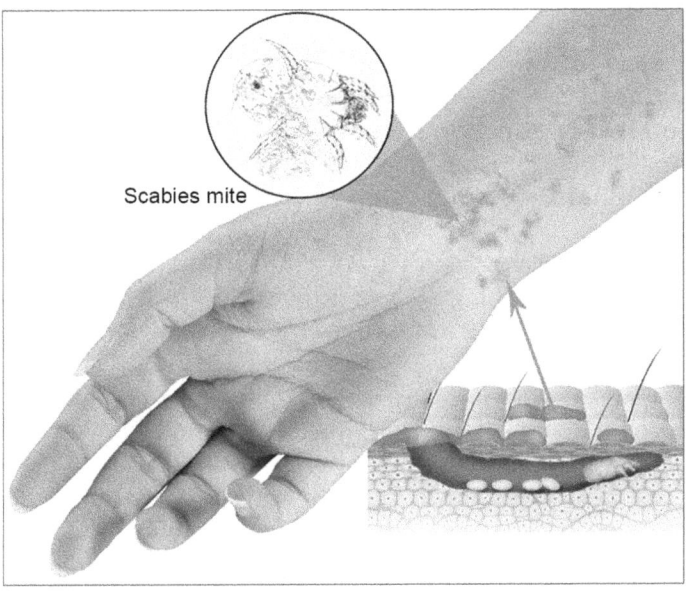

Fig. 11.11: Depicts the scabies mite burrow under the skin and lay eggs (Scabies).

Pathophysiology

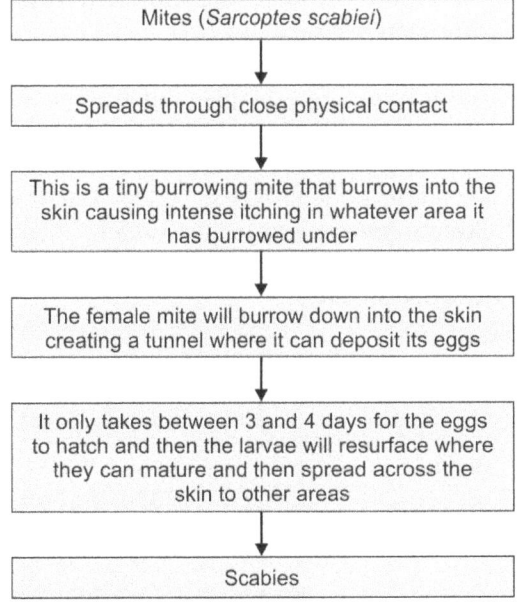

Clinical Features

- Itching, most commonly at night
- Rashes, mostly between the fingers
- Sores (abrasions) on the skin from scratching and digging
- Thin, pencil-mark lines on the skin
- Small blisters over the palms and soles.

Complications

- Impetigo
- Crusted scabies.

Diagnostic Tests

- History
- Physical examination
- Skin scraping
- Skin biopsy.

Management

Medical

- **Topical scabicidal agents:** It helps to get rid of the mites, eliminate symptoms such as itch and to treat the infection. For example, crotamiton, malathion, sulfur-based, benzyl benzoate, lindane, etc.
- **Antihistamines:** It helps in reducing itch and promotes sleep. For example, chlorpheniramine, cyclizine, etc.
- **Oral corticosteroids:** It helps to ease the redness, swelling and itch. For example, prednisolone, prednisone, etc.

Nursing

- Instruct the patient to avoid touching or scratching the rash.
- Instruct them to wash underwear and towels in hot water.
- Ask them to vacuum the carpets and upholstered furniture.
- Encourage them to use calamine lotion and soak in a cool bath to ease itching.
- Encourage the whole family to get involved in the treatment.
- Restrict the patient from having salty or citrus foods.

SHINGLES

Definition

It is an infection of a nerve area caused by the varicella-zoster virus characterized by a painful skin rash with blisters involving a limited area.

Etiology

Viral infection (Varicella zoster).

Risk Factors

- Being elders
- Being under stress
- Undergoing cancer treatment
- Those with infections that threaten the eye
- Weakened immune system by medicines or disease
- Occurrence of chicken pox before age 1
- Pregnancy
- Premature babies.

Types

There are three types of stages as follows:

1. **Prodromal stage:** It occurs before the rash appears. This is characterized by burning, itching, or tingling numbness. This can last several days or weeks before the rash appears. It is accompanied by fever, chills and flu-like symptoms and swelling of lymph nodes.
2. **Active stage:** In this stage the rash and blisters appear. Clear fluid-filled clustered blisters appear. The clear fluid may become cloudy after 3 to 4 days. Crops of rash appear for initial 3–5 days. These break-open and ooze finally forming dried crusts. The rash heals in 2–4 weeks.
3. **Postherpetic neuralgia:** It is a long-term condition after shingles much after the rash has disappeared. There may be burning, stabbing or dull pain over the area sometimes persisting for years. The area shows extreme sensitivity to touch.

Pathophysiology

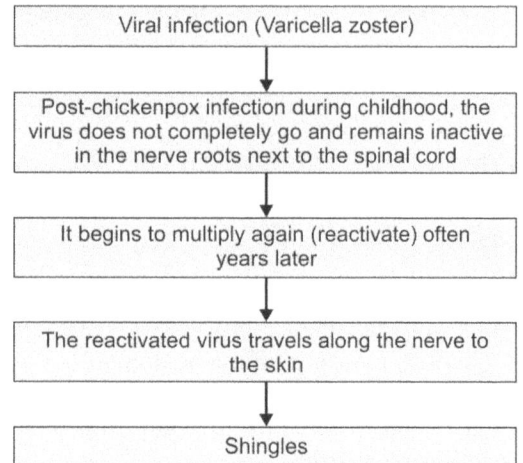

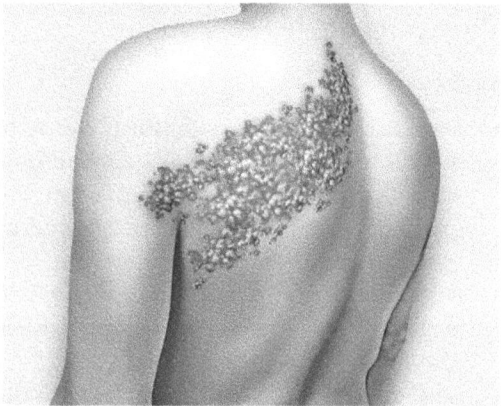

Fig. 11.12: Shows the skin rash with blisters involving a limited area of the body (Shingles).

Clinical Features

- Pain, tingling, or burning that occurs one side of the body
- Red patches on the skin followed by small blisters in it
- Fever
- Chills
- Malaise
- Headache
- Joint pain
- Swollen lymph nodes
- Difficulty moving some of the muscles in the face
- Drooping eyelid (Ptosis)
- Hearing loss
- Loss of eye motion.

Complications

- Postherpetic neuralgia (PHN)
- Ramsay Hunt syndrome (involvement of the geniculate ganglion of the facial nerve)
- Pneumonia
- Hearing problems
- Blindness
- Encephalitis
- Death.

Diagnostic Tests

- History
- Physical examination
- Blood examination
- Skin scraping
- Electromyography (EMG)
- CSF examination
- Magnetic resonance imaging (MRI) scan
- Nerve conduction velocity (NCV).

Management

Medical

- **Analgesics:** It helps in relieving pain in an acute shingles attack. For example, ibuprofen, aspirin, paracetamol, tramadol, etc.
- **Antiviral agents:** It blocks viral reproduction and reduces the severity of the disease. For example, acyclovir, famciclovir, valacyclovir, brivudine, etc.
- **Tricyclic antidepressants:** It eases neuralgia (nerve pain) separate to the action for depression. For example, amitriptyline, nortriptyline, imipramine, etc.
- **Anticonvulsants:** It eases neuralgic pain separate to the action to control convulsions. For example, gabapentin, etc.
- **Antihistamines:** It helps in reducing itch. For example, chlorpheniramine, cyclizine, etc.
- **Oral corticosteroids:** It helps in reducing pain and speeding healing of the rash. For example, prednisolone, prednisone, etc.

Nursing

- Instruct the patient to avoid touching or scratching the rash.
- Ask them to keep the rash covered to avoid spreading to others.
- Encourage them to wash their hands frequently.
- Encourage the patient to use cool wet compresses or give baths in cool or lukewarm water every 3-4 hours for the first few days.
- Restrict the patient from having salty or citrus foods.

12

CHAPTER

Disorders of Musculoskeletal System

CHAPTER OUTLINE

- Acute low back pain
- Ankylosing spondylitis
- Carpal tunnel syndrome
- Fracture
- Gout
- Herniated lumbar disk
- Muscular dystrophy
- Myositis ossificans
- Osteoarthritis
- Osteomalacia
- Osteomyelitis
- Osteoporosis
- Paget's disease
- Rheumatoid arthritis
- Sprain
- Strain
- Systemic lupus erythematosus

ACUTE LOW BACK PAIN

Definition

Acute low back pain is defined as low back pain present for up to six weeks. It may be experienced as aching, burning, stabbing, sharp or dull, well-defined or vague.

Etiology

- Carrying too much weight
- Lumbar herniated disk
- Back muscle strain
- Degenerative disk disease
- Isthmic spondylolisthesis
- Sacroiliac joint disease
- Facet joint osteoarthritis
- Lumbar spinal stenosis
- Spinal compression fracture
- Piriformis syndrome
- Spinal tumor
- Fibromyalgia
- Ankylosing spondylitis
- Coccydynia.

Risk Factors

- More common in individuals over age 50
- Those with a history of cancer
- Those with severe pain at rest with associated fever
- Diabetes
- Heavy alcohol or drug use
- Long-term use of corticosteroids
- Osteoporosis
- Lack of exercise
- Improper lifting
- Smoking
- Pregnancy
- Overweight.

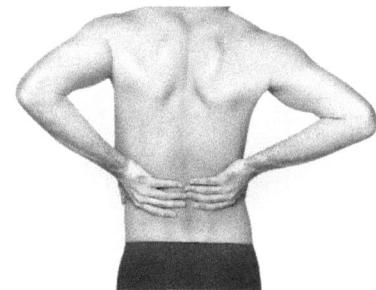

Fig. 12.1: Portrays aching, burning, stabbing, sharp or dull low back pain.

Pathophysiology

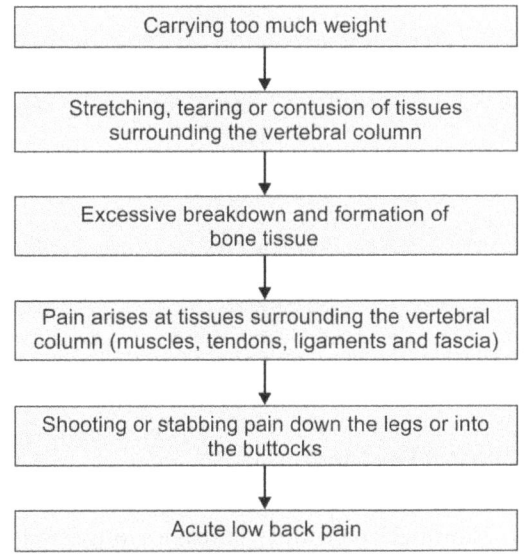

Clinical Features

- Muscle ache
- Shooting or stabbing pain down the legs or into the buttocks
- Limited flexibility or range of motion of the back
- Tingling or burning sensation around the groin
- Change in the bowel or bladder function
- Weakness in the legs
- Muscle stiffness.

Complications

- Disability
- Nerve root impingement
- Depression
- Weight gain.

Diagnostic Tests

- History
- Physical examination
- Blood examination
- X-ray examination
- Bone scan
- Computed tomography (CT) scan
- Magnetic resonance imaging (MRI) scan
- Myelogram.

Management

Medical

- **Analgesics:** It helps to provide effective reduction of acute low back pain and thereby promotes recovery. For example, paracetamol, ibuprofen, etc.
- **Muscle relaxants:** They calm or sedate the central nervous system and facilitate sleep and secondarily reduce contributing emotional or muscular tension in the setting of severe pain. For example, carisoprodol, baclofen, chlorzoxazone, dantrolene, etc.
- **Narcotics (Also known as opioids):** It reduces the symptoms of acute low back pain and minimizes the pain caused by acute low back pain in the tissues surrounding the vertebral column. For example, codeine, fentanyl, methadose, etc.

Surgical

- **Laminectomy:** It is a surgical procedure designed to remove a small portion of the bone over the nerve root or disk material from under the nerve root to give the nerve root more space and a better healing environment.
- **Microdiscectomy:** It is a surgical procedure designed to remove a small portion of the bone over the nerve root or disk material from under the nerve root is removed to relieve neural impingement and provide more room for the nerve to heal.

Nursing

- Instruct the patient to perform low impact aerobic exercise.
- Encourage the patient to take adequate rest as it allows injured tissue and even nerve roots to begin to heal which, in turn, will help to relieve lower back pain.
- Reduce the activity of the patient to the level of pain-free functioning.
- Apply ice packs to reduce pain and swelling caused by low back pain.

- Ask the patient to maintain a neutral pelvic position.
- Instruct the patient to maintain a healthy weight.
- Instruct the patient to avoid heavy lifting.
- Ask the patient to use a firm mattress.
- Ask the patient to wear a special back support device.

ANKYLOSING SPONDYLITIS

Definition

Ankylosing spondylitis (AS) is a chronic progressive painful inflammatory rheumatic disease that involves the back (i.e. the spine and sacroiliac joints).

Etiology

- Crohn's disease
- Bacterial infection (*Shigella, Salmonella, Yersinia, Campylobacter*, etc.)
- Genetic predisposition
- Idiopathic.

Risk Factors

- Being males
- Those with a family history of ankylosing spondylitis
- Young people between ages 15 and 35 years
- Smoking
- Those who have *HLA-B27* gene
- Frequent gastrointestinal infections.

Pathophysiology

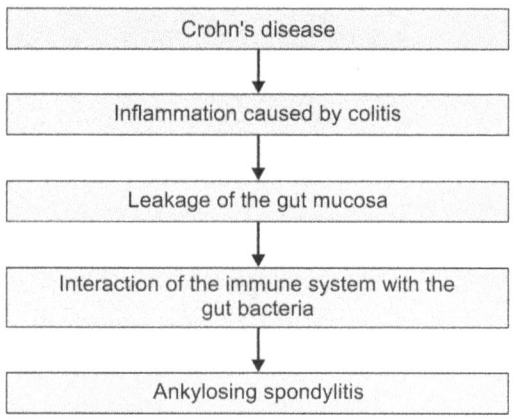

Clinical Features

- Sacroiliitis
- Low back pain and stiffness for longer than 3 months which improve with exercise but are not relieved by rest.
- Restriction of motion of the lumbar spine in both the sagittal and lumbar planes
- Restriction of chest expansion relative to normal values correlated for age and sex
- Morning stiffness of greater than 30 minutes
- Awakening because of back pain during the second half of the night only
- Alternating buttock pain
- Inflammation of tendons and ligaments.

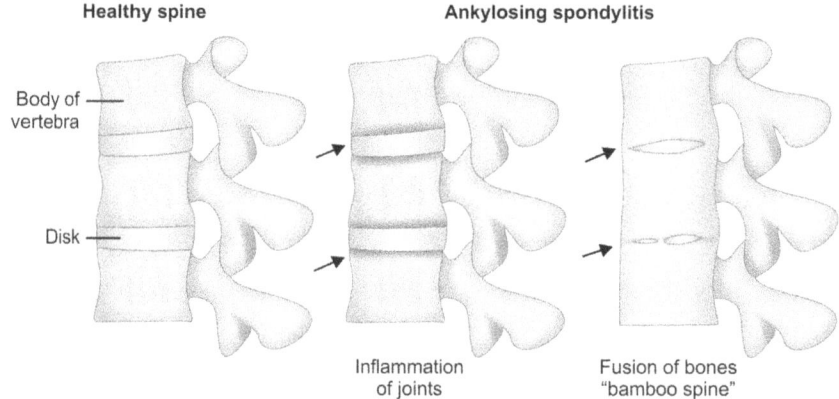

Fig. 12.2: Shows the comparison of healthy spine with that of ankylosing spondylitis.

Complications

- Uveitis
- Compression fractures
- Dyspnea
- Heart damage
- Enthesitis
- Cauda equina syndrome
- Amyloidosis.

Diagnostic Tests

- History
- Physical examination
- Blood examination
- X-ray examination
- Bone scan
- Computed tomography (CT) scan
- Magnetic resonance imaging (MRI) scan.

Management

Medical

- **Analgesics:** It helps to lessen pain and stiffness by reducing inflammation. For example, paracetamol, ibuprofen, etc.
- **Disease-modifying antirheumatic drugs (DMARDs):** They block proteins involved with inflammation in the body and reduce inflammation in ankylosing spondylitis. For example, adalimumab, etanercept, infliximab, etc.

Nursing

- Instruct the patient to maintain a good posture when standing and sitting.
- Instruct the patient to keep themselves physically active.
- Ask the patient to plan and pace daily activities, varying tasks and allowing time to rest and relax.
- Instruct the patient to stop smoking.
- Instruct the patient to sleep in a position that is most comfortable.
- Encourage the patient to eat a balanced diet.
- Reduce the activity of the patient to the level of pain-free functioning.
- Instruct the patient to maintain a healthy weight.
- Instruct the patient to avoid heavy lifting.

CARPAL TUNNEL SYNDROME

Definition

Carpal tunnel syndrome (CTS) or median neuropathy at the wrist is a medical condition in which the median nerve is squeezed where it passes through the wrist.

Etiology

- Congenital predisposition
- Trauma or injury to the wrist
- Sprain or fracture
- Obesity
- Overactivity of the pituitary gland
- Rheumatoid arthritis
- Hypothyroidism
- Repetitive hand movements or any mechanical problems in the wrist joint
- Fluid retention during pregnancy or menopause
- Work stress
- Double crush syndrome (It is during compression or irritation of nerve branches contributing to the median nerve in the neck or anywhere above the wrist, this then increases the sensitivity of the nerve to compression in the wrist)
- Development of cyst or tumor in the canal
- Multiple myeloma
- Writer's cramp (lack of fine motor skill coordination)
- Mucopolysaccharidoses
- Idiopathic.

Risk Factors

- Being females
- Metabolic disorders
- Those performing assembly line work
- Data entry personnel
- Those who pack meat, poultry or fish.

Disorders of Musculoskeletal System

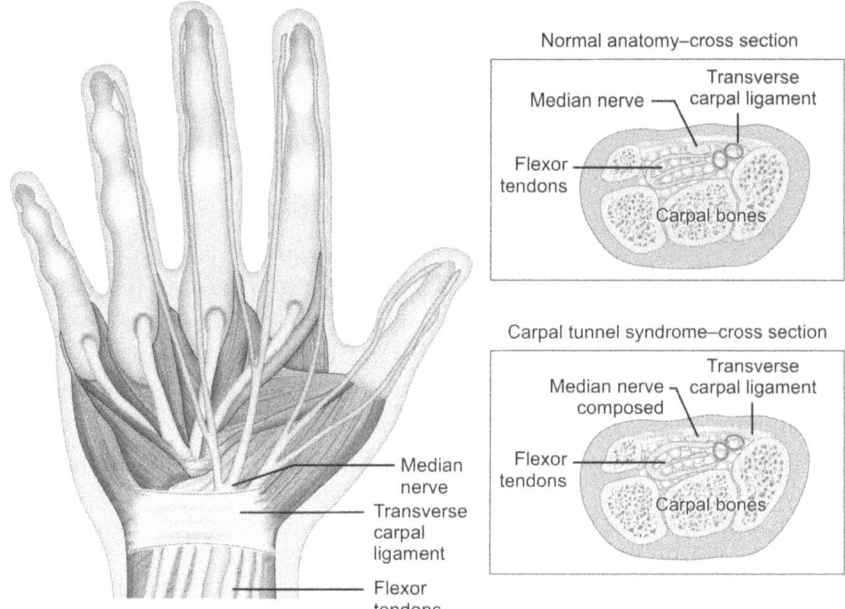

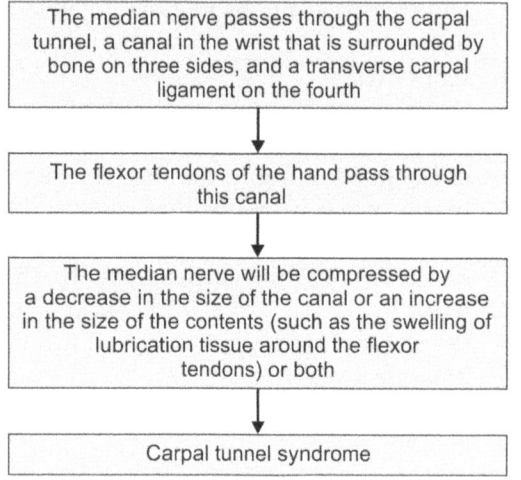

Fig. 12.3: Shows the cross section view of normal wrist with that of the carpal tunnel syndrome.

Pathophysiology

The median nerve passes through the carpal tunnel, a canal in the wrist that is surrounded by bone on three sides, and a transverse carpal ligament on the fourth

↓

The flexor tendons of the hand pass through this canal

↓

The median nerve will be compressed by a decrease in the size of the canal or an increase in the size of the contents (such as the swelling of lubrication tissue around the flexor tendons) or both

↓

Carpal tunnel syndrome

Clinical Features

- Numbness and paresthesia (a burning and tingling sensation) in the thumb, index and middle fingers
- Frequently accompanied by sharp pains, radiating through the arm or shoulder
- Increased pain with increased use of the hand, such as while driving or reading the newspaper
- Muscle weakness
- It appears in one or both hands during night as people tend to bend their wrists when they sleep, which further compresses the carpal tunnel
- Increased pain at night
- Fingers feel useless and swollen
- Wasting of the thenar muscles (the body of muscles which are connected to the thumb)
- Fine motor deficits
- Sensitivity to cold.

Complications

- Nerve injury
- Persistent painful tingling
- Weak grip tendency to drop objects held in the hand
- Muscles at the base of the thumb waste away.

Diagnostic Tests

- History
- Physical examination
- Phalen's test: It is a test which is performed by flexing the wrist gently as far as possible, then holding this position and awaiting for symptoms. A positive test is one that results in numbness in the median nerve distribution when holding the wrist in acute flexion position within 60 seconds. The quicker the numbness starts, the more advanced the condition is.
- Tinel's test: It is a test which is performed by lightly tapping the area over the nerve to elicit a sensation of tingling or "pins and needles" in the nerve distribution.
- Durkan test (carpal compression test): It is a test in which firm pressure is applied on the palm over the nerve for up to 30 seconds to elicit symptoms.
- Nerve conduction studies
- Electromyography
- Ultrasonography
- Magnetic resonance imaging.

Management

Medical

- **Nonsteroidal anti-inflammatory drugs:** It helps to relieve pain caused by strenuous activity. For example, aspirin, ibuprofen, etc.
- **Diuretics:** It helps to reduce swelling. For example, furosemide, etc.
- **Corticosteroids:** It helps to relieve pressure on median nerve and provides immediate, temporary relief to persons with mild or intermittent symptoms. For example, prednisone, etc.
- **Vitamin B-6 supplements:** It helps to ease the symptoms of carpal tunnel syndrome. For example, methylcobalamine, pyridoxine, etc.

Surgical

- **Carpal tunnel release:** It is a simple procedure involving releasing the ligament that forms the top of the tunnel on the palm side of the hand, therefore easing the pressure on the nerve.
- **Open release surgery:** It is a traditional surgical procedure in which an incision is made up to 2 inches in the wrist and then cutting the carpal ligament to enlarge the carpal tunnel.
- **Endoscopic surgery:** It is an endoscopic procedure in which two incisions are made in the wrist and palm, a camera attached to the tube observes the tissue on the screen and cuts the carpal ligament (the tissue that holds joints together).
- **Immobilizing braces:** A wrist splint helps to limit numbness by limiting wrist flexion.

Nursing

- Instruct to elevate the arm with pillows while lying down.
- Instruct to avoid activities that overuse the hand.
- Encourage to use the other hand.
- Instruct to avoid bending the wrists.
- Encourage to take regular breaks from the repetitive motion.
- Instruct to avoid resting the wrists on hard or ridged surfaces for prolonged periods.

FRACTURE

Definition

A bone fracture is a medical condition in which a bone is cracked or broken and it occurs in any age and in any bone. It is a break in the continuity of the bone.

Etiology

- Trauma from either a fall or accident
- Osteosarcoma

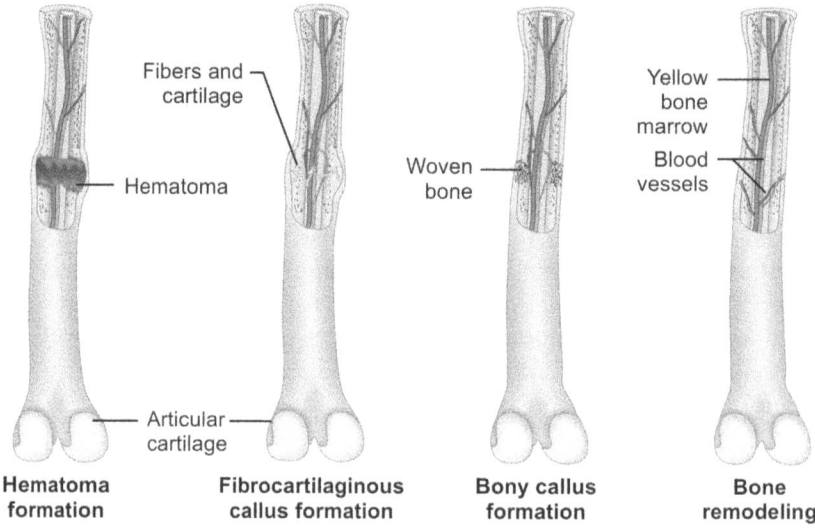

Fig. 12.4: Depicts the stages of bone healing.

- Paget's disease
- Ewing's sarcoma
- Multiple myeloma
- Sports injuries
- Osteoporosis
- Osteomalacia
- Osteogenesis imperfecta (Brittle bone disease).

Risk Factors

- Elders above 65 years
- Family history of osteoporosis
- Smoking
- Excessive alcohol use
- Lack of exercise
- Low body weight
- Poor nutrition
- People with small, thin builds
- Physical frailty
- Arthritis
- Poor eyesight
- Unsteady balance
- Regular drinking of soda pop (phosphoric acid added to pop may interfere with calcium absorption)
- Certain drugs which are used to treat HIV and endometriosis
- High stress.

Stages of Bone Healing

- ***Hematoma formation:*** Blood vessels in the broken bone tear and hemorrhage resulting in the formation of clotted blood (hematoma) occurs at the site of the break. The severed blood vessels at the broken ends of the bone are sealed by the clotting process. Bone cells deprived of nutrients begin to die.
- ***Bone generation:*** Within days of the fracture, capillaries grow into the hematoma, while phagocytic cells begin to clear away the dead cells. Though fragments of the blood clot may remain, fibroblasts and osteoblasts enter the area and begin to reform bone. Fibroblasts produce collagen fibers that connect the broken bone ends, the fibrocartilaginous callus, is composed of both hyaline and fibrocartilage.
- ***Bone callus formation:*** The fibrocartilaginous callus is converted into a bony callus of spongy bone. It takes about two months for the broken bone ends to be firmly joined together after the fracture.
- ***Bone remodeling:*** The bony callus is then remodeled by osteoclasts and osteoblasts,

with excess material on the exterior of the bone and within the medullary cavity being removed. Compact bone is added to create bone tissue that is similar to the original, unbroken bone. This remodeling can take many months; the bone may remain uneven for years.

Types

- **Complete fracture:** A fracture in which bone fragments separate completely.
- **Incomplete (Greenstick) fracture:** A fracture in which the bone fragments are still partially joined.
- **Longitudinal fracture:** A fracture that is parallel to the bone's long axis.
- **Transverse fracture:** A fracture that is at a right angle to the bone's long axis.
- **Oblique fracture:** A fracture that is diagonal to a bone's long axis.
- **Compression fracture:** A fracture that usually occurs in the vertebrae.
- **Spiral fracture:** A fracture where at least one part of the bone has been twisted.
- **Comminuted fracture:** A fracture which results in several fragments.
- **Impacted fracture:** A fracture caused when bone fragments are driven into each other.
- **Open fracture:** A fracture when the bone is in contact with air either by piercing the skin or by severe tissue injury.
- **Closed fracture:** A fracture which does not disrupt the skin.
- **Pathological fracture:** A fracture in which bone is weakened either by pressure from a tumor within the bone.
- **Stress fracture:** A fracture resulting in a bone across one cortex.
- **Displaced fracture:** A fracture in which bone pieces are out of normal alignment.
- **Avulsion fracture:** A fracture in which a piece of bone is torn away from the main bone but still attached to a ligament or tendon.

Pathophysiology

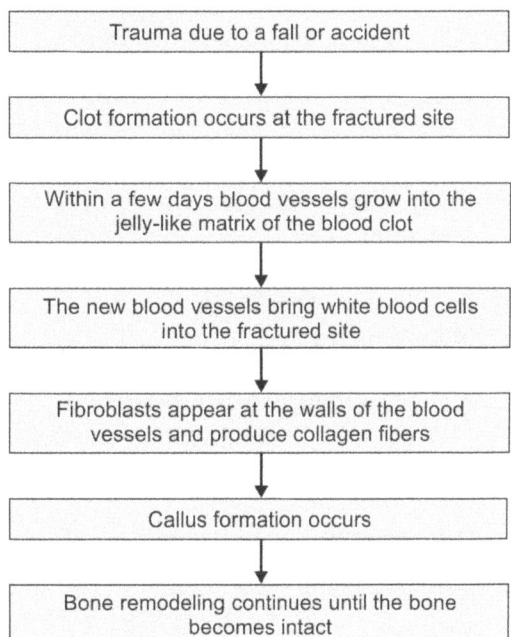

Clinical Features

- Intense pain
- Tenderness over the site of the injury
- A visibly out-of-place or misshapen limb or joint
- Decreased range of motion
- Ecchymosis (bruising)
- Swelling
- Fever
- Numbness
- Tingling
- Broken skin with bone protruding.

Complications

Early

- Impaired neurovascular status
- Hemorrhage
- Hemarthrosis
- Compartment syndrome (Volkmann's ischemia)
- Infection
- Deep vein thrombosis or pulmonary embolus

- Fat embolism
- Hypovolemic shock
- Acute respiratory distress syndrome
- Crush syndrome
- Pneumonia.

Late

- Delayed and nonunion
- Malunion
- Shortening of limbs
- Avascular necrosis
- Stiffness of joints
- Contractures
- Algodystrophy (Sudeck's dystrophy)
- Myositis ossificans (Post-traumatic ossification)
- Osteomyelitis
- Osteoarthritis.

Diagnostic Tests

- History
- Physical examination
- X-ray examination
- Blood examination
- Bone scintigraphy
- Computed tomography
- Magnetic resonance imaging
- Ultrasonogram.

Management

Medical

- **Antibiotics:** It helps to prevent any secondary infections. For example, cephalexin, cephalosporins, etc.
- **Analgesics:** It helps to relieve against bone pain. For example, voveran, tramadol etc.
- **Muscle relaxants:** It helps to relieve pain associated with muscle spasm. For example, Carisoprodol, cyclobenzaprine, methocarbamol, etc.

Surgical

- **Reduction followed by immobilization:** It is a surgical procedure in which the fractured bones are anatomically realigned by feeling it through the soft tissues and then the fractured bone is kept immobilized to prevent movement that might interfere with the union.
- **Immobilization:** It is a procedure in which the fractured bone is immobilized where it is without any significant displacement and to prevent movement that might interfere with the union with the help of strapping, sling, cast, braces and traction.
- **Open reduction and internal fixation (ORIF):** It is a surgical procedure in which the fragments are reduced under direct vision and also fixed internally with the help of devices such as screws, nails, pins, plates, etc.
- **Open reduction and external fixation:** It is a procedure in which the fracture is held in a frame outside the limb with the help of external fixator devices such as steel pins, clamps, etc. An external fixator is a metallic device composed of metal pins that are inserted into the bone and attached to external rods to stabilize the fracture while it heals.
- **Casts:** It is a temporary circumferential immobilization device which allows the client to perform the normal activities of daily living and also provides sufficient immobilization to ensure stability. It is of 4 types like sugar-tong splint (wrist injuries), posterior splint (forearm and phalangeal injuries), short-arm cast (wrist or metacarpal fractures) and long-arm cast (elbow fractures).
- **Traction:** It is a device which applies pulling force on the fractured extremity to attain realignment while counteraction pulls in the opposite direction. There are two types of traction as follows: *(a) Skin traction* [Short term of 48–72 hours] and *(b) Skeletal traction* [Long-term and weight ranges from 5–45 pounds].

Nursing

- Reduce the activity of the patient to the level of pain-free functioning.

- Increase the activity of the patient in graduated fashion after several weeks of rest and improved symptoms.
- Check the person's airway and breathing and if necessary begin rescue.
- Examine the person closely for other injuries.
- Keep the person still and calm.
- Apply ice packs on injured area to reduce pain and swelling.
- Check the person's blood circulation and press firmly over the skin beyond the fracture site.
- Place a dry, clean cloth over the wound to dress it.
- Do not move the person unless the broken bone is stable.
- Do not attempt to straighten a bone or change its position unless blood circulation appears hampered.
- Instruct the patient to prevent falls by not standing on unstable objects.

GOUT

Definition

Gout is an inflammatory arthritis caused by a buildup of uric acid crystals in the joints.

Etiology

- Chronic kidney disease
- Certain medications (Aspirin, cyclosporine, levodopa, etc.)
- Genetic predisposition
- Surgery or sudden, severe illness
- Joint injury
- Chemotherapy
- Long-term exposure to lead.

Risk Factors

- Family history of gout
- Being males
- Overweight
- Drinking too much alcohol
- Those who take excessive purine rich foods.
- Those who are exposed to lead in the environment.
- Those who have had an organ transplant.
- Those who take the vitamin niacin.
- Those who have an enzyme defect that makes it hard for the body to break down purines.
- Excessive weight gain
- High blood pressure
- High cholesterol
- Diabetes.

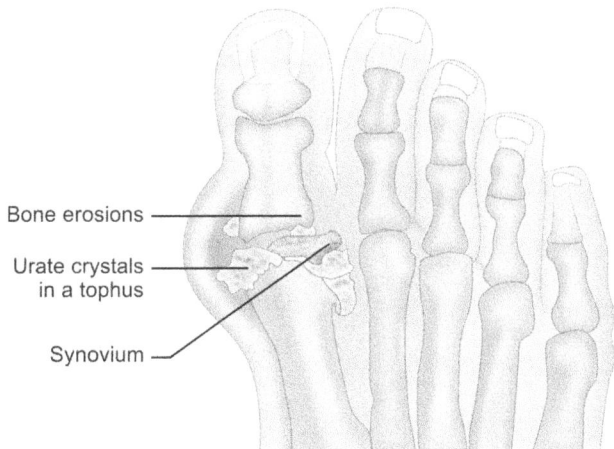

Fig. 12.5: Shows the cardinal features of gout.

Pathophysiology

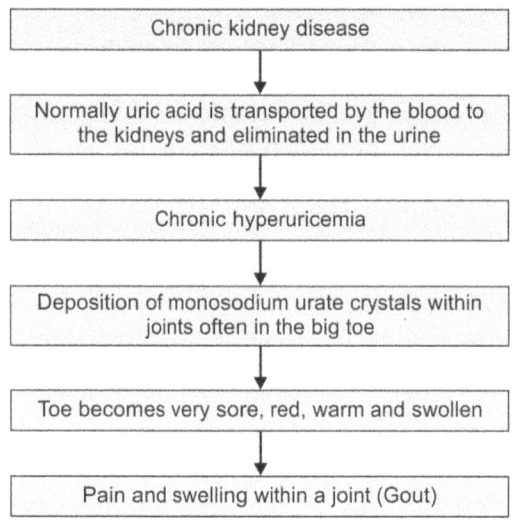

Clinical Features

- Pain and swelling within a joint
- Shiny red or purple skin around the affected joint
- Extreme tenderness around the joint
- Warmth over a joint
- Mild fever
- Chills
- Loss of appetite
- Nausea.

Complications

- Chronic gouty arthritis (recurrent gout)
- Tophi (chalky lumps under the skin)
- Kidney stones
- Insomnia
- Disability.

Diagnostic Tests

- History
- Physical examination
- Blood examination
- Urine examination
- X-ray examination
- Ultrasound
- Computed tomography (CT) scan
- Magnetic resonance imaging (MRI) scan.

Management

Medical

- **Nonsteroidal anti-inflammatory drugs (NSAIDs):** It helps to quickly relieve the pain and swelling of an acute gout episode and can shorten the attack, especially if taken in the first 24 hours. For example, ibuprofen, naproxen, etc.
- **Corticosteroids:** It helps to relieve the pain and swelling of an acute gout attack. For example, prednisone, etc.
- **Anti-gout agents:** It helps to relieve the pain and swelling of acute attacks. For example, colchicine, allopurinol, febuxostat, probenecid, pegloticase, etc.

Nursing

- Instruct the patient to maintain a healthy weight.
- Encourage the patient to develop a lifelong eating strategy that focuses on following a heart-healthy diet.
- Encourage the patient to take vitamin C supplements (500–1000 mg daily).
- Instruct the patient to avoid the intake of alcohol.
- Instruct the patient to perform low-impact aerobic exercise.
- Encourage the patient to include more vegetables and fruits in the diet.
- Ask the patient to adopt a healthy lifestyle habits.
- Instruct the patient to drink plenty of fluids.

HERNIATED LUMBAR DISK

Definition

Disk herniation is a rupture of fibrocartilaginous material (annulus fibrosis) that surrounds the intervertebral disk.

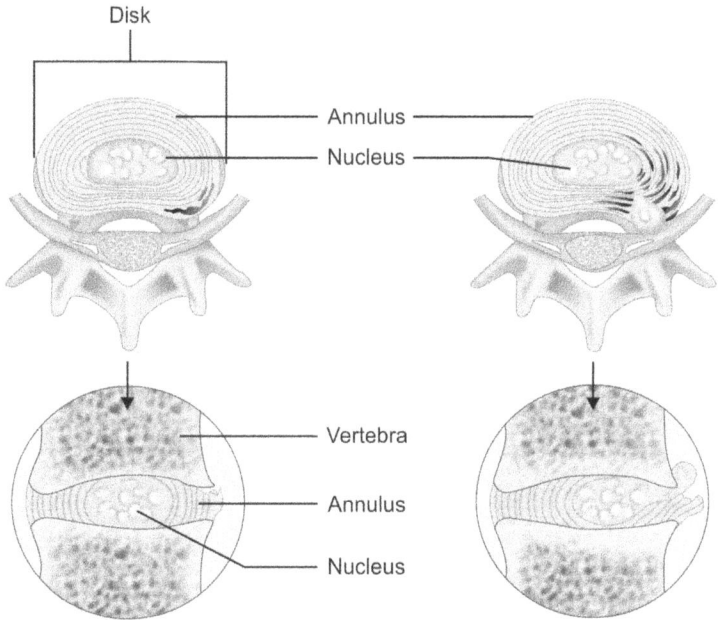

Fig. 12.6: Lumbar disk herniation.

Etiology

- Aging and degeneration
- A sudden strain from improper lifting or from twisting violently
- Excessive weight
- Osteoarthritis.

Risk Factors

- More common in people between 35 and 55 years
- Being males
- People with physically demanding jobs
- Excessive back and neck strain
- Being taller
- Poor posture
- An unhealthy diet
- Inactivity
- Smoking
- Dehydration.

Pathophysiology

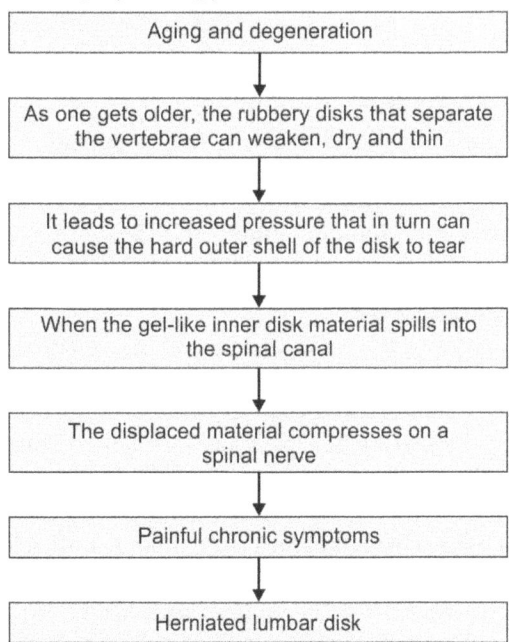

Clinical Features

- Intermittent or continuous back pain
- Spasm of the back muscles
- Pain that starts near the back or buttock and radiates down the leg to the calf or into the foot
- Muscle weakness in the legs
- Numbness in the leg or foot
- Decreased reflexes at the knee or ankle
- Muscle atrophy
- Difficulty in walking
- Difficulty with fine-motor skills such as buttoning, handwriting, or picking up small objects.

Complications

- Cauda equina syndrome
- Bladder of bowel incontinence
- Chronic back or leg pain
- Numbness in the legs.

Diagnostic Tests

- History
- Physical examination
- Blood examination
- Myelogram
- Electromyography
- Nerve conduction tests
- X-ray examination
- Computed tomography (CT) scan
- Magnetic resonance imaging (MRI) scan.

Management

Medical

- **Nonsteroidal anti-inflammatory drugs (NSAIDs):** It helps to quickly relieve inflammation and reduce pain. For example, ibuprofen, naproxen, aspirin, etc.
- **Muscle relaxants:** It helps to control muscle spasms. For example, methocarbamol, Carisoprodol, cyclobenzaprine, etc.
- **Corticosteroids:** It helps to reduce the swelling and inflammation of the nerves. For example, prednisone, etc.
- **Analgesics:** It helps to quickly relieve inflammation and reduce pain. For example, acetaminophen, paracetamol, etc.

Surgical

- **Microdiscectomy:** It is a surgical procedure in which the spinal muscles are dissected and moved aside to expose the vertebra and a portion of the bone is removed to expose the nerve root and disk.
- **Laminectomy:** It is a surgical procedure designed to remove a small portion of the bone over the nerve root or disk material from under the nerve root to give the nerve root more space and a better healing environment.

Nursing

- Instruct the patient to maintain a healthy weight and lean body mass.
- Instruct the patient to practice proper lifting techniques.
- Instruct the patient to avoid smoking.
- Encourage a positive attitude and stress management among patients.
- Instruct the patient to perform appropriate exercise program to strengthen weak abdominal muscles and prevent re-injury.
- Encourage the patient to maintain good posture during sitting, standing, moving and sleeping.

MUSCULAR DYSTROPHY

Definition

Muscular dystrophies are genetic disorders characterized by progressive muscle wasting and weakness that begin with microscopic changes in the muscle. As muscles degenerate over time, the person's muscle strength declines.

Etiology

Genetic predisposition (inherited genetic abnormality).

Risk Factors

- Family history of muscular dystrophy
- Being males
- Most common in children with 2–6 years of age
- Having a partner with a family history of the disease.

Disorders of Musculoskeletal System

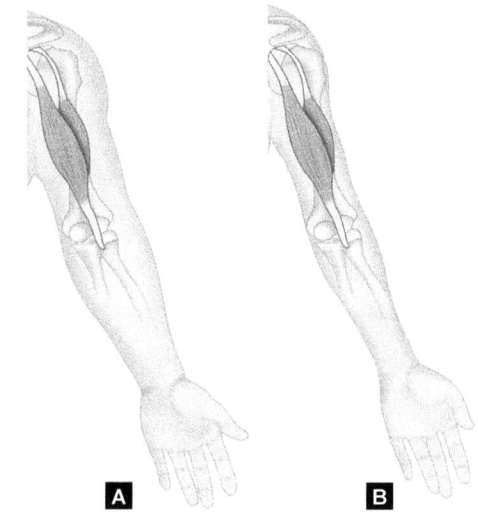

Figs. 12.7A and B: (A) Normal biceps; (B) Muscular dystrophy.

Pathophysiology

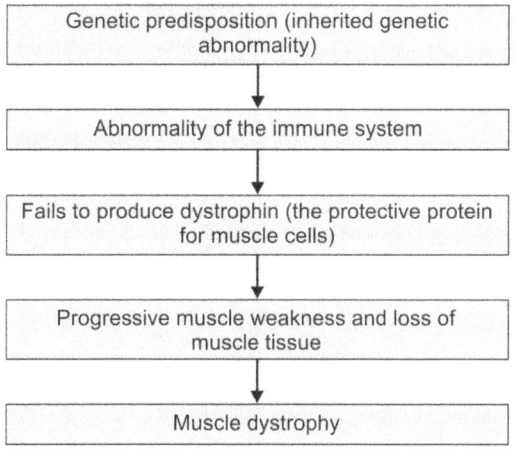

Clinical Features

- Muscle pain and stiffness
- Joint stiffness
- Walking on the toes
- Learning disabilities
- Waddling gait
- Large calf muscles
- Trouble running and jumping
- Difficulty in getting up from a lying or sitting position
- Difficulty in walking
- Loss of ability to walk
- Lack of motor skills development
- Fatigue
- Rapidly worsening weakness in the legs, pelvis, arms and neck
- Drooling
- Drooping eyelids (Ptosis)
- Hypotonia.

Complications

- Pseudohypertrophy
- Contractures
- Scoliosis
- Lung failure
- Cardiomyopathy.

Diagnostic Tests

- History
- Physical examination
- Blood examination
- Genetic testing
- Muscle biopsy
- Electromyogram
- Nerve conduction studies
- Bone scan
- Pulmonary function test.

Management

Medical

- **Physical therapy:** It helps in slowing the development of contractures or reduced flexibility in the muscles and joints.
- **Corticosteroids:** It slows down the early course of illness. For example, Prednisone, etc.
- **Analgesics:** It helps to reduce the pain caused by muscular dystrophy. For example, acetaminophen, paracetamol, etc.
- **Assistive devices:** It includes devices such as canes, walkers, wheelchairs, strollers and power wheelchairs that help to maintain the child's mobility and independence.

Surgical

- **Surgical release of contractures:** It is a surgical procedure in which the surgeon lengthens the tendon to relieve the muscle

tension. The tendon then heals at the longer length and helps the child to continue walk.
- **Spinal fusion for scoliosis:** It lessens back pain and improves sitting balance as these factors improve the child's quality of life.

Nursing

- Encourage the patient to use orthopedic appliances to help in achieving mobility.
- Encourage the patient to take low-calorie, high-protein and high-fiber diet.
- Encourage the patient to drink a lot of fluid.
- Motivate the patient to perform exercise as tolerated.
- Encourage the patient to perform activities of daily living without muscle fatigue or intolerance.
- Encourage coughing and deep breathing exercises among patients.
- Encourage the patient and his family to verbalize their concerns and feelings and allow time for the patient and their family to process the information.
- Encourage the patient and family participation in care activities to promote feelings of self-esteem and control over the situation.
- Allow for frequent rest periods among patients and cluster care activities to prevent overtiring the patient.

MYOSITIS OSSIFICANS (HETEROTOPIC OSSIFICATION)

Definition

Myositis ossificans refers to the deposition of extraskeletal bone with soft tissue and results due to a bad muscle strain or contusion is neglected.

Etiology

- Trauma
- Failing to apply cold therapy and compression immediately after the injury
- Applying heat too soon
- Having intensive physiotherapy or massage too soon after the injury
- Returning too soon to training after exercise.

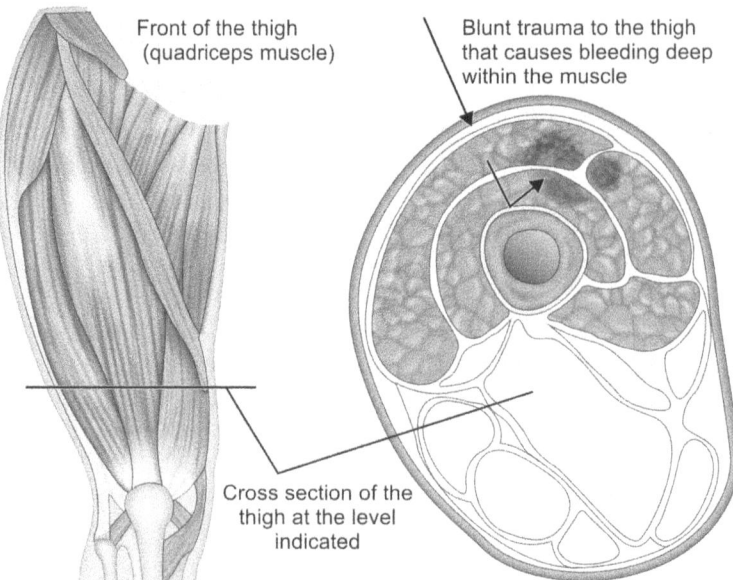

Fig. 12.8: Shows the deposition of extraskeletal bone with soft tissue resulting from a bad muscle strain (Myositis ossificans).

Risk Factors

- Contusions that are severe.
- Contusions that are inappropriately managed.
- Re-injury to the contusion.
- Contusion resulting in a large loss of movement.
- Those who do not rest sufficiently following a contusion.
- Those who continue to play through an injury.
- Those who perform stretching hard follwing an injury.

Pathophysiology

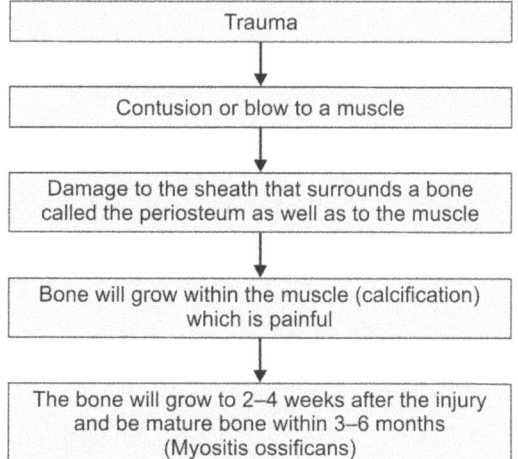

Clinical Features

- Pain in the muscle during exercise
- Restricted range of movement
- Hard lump felt deep in the muscle
- Bone growth
- Swelling
- Tenderness
- Bruising
- Inability to sleep
- Escalating pain especially in morning.

Complications

- Ectopic calcification
- Raised alkaline phosphatase bone isoenzyme levels
- Myalgia
- Alopecia
- Heterotopic ossification.

Diagnostic Tests

- History
- Physical examination
- Blood examination
- X-ray examination
- Computed tomography (CT) scan
- Magnetic resonance imaging (MRI) scan
- Bone scan.

Management

Medical

- **Apply ice packs:** It helps to relieve against swelling of the joint muscles and it should be done immediately after the injury.
- **Physiotherapy:** It helps to provide maximal stability and strength to the injured joint and should not be taken immediately following an injury.
- **Analgesics:** It helps to relieve pain. For example, ibuprofen, acetaminophen, naproxen, etc.

Surgical

- **Immobilization:** It is practiced in any contusion of the muscles following an injury and the part is immobilized for 4-6 weeks.
- **Splints/Braces:** It helps in immobilizing the affected part either temporarily or during transportation.

Nursing

- Encourage the patient to take adequate rest.
- Instruct the patient to immobilize the part which gets affected (usually the thigh).
- Instruct the patient not to opt for any massage immediately after the injury.
- Ask the patient to avoid applying heat too soon after the injury.
- Encourage the patient to perform activities of daily living without muscle fatigue or intolerance.
- Instruct the patient not to return for training immediately.

OSTEOARTHRITIS

Definition

Osteoarthritis (OA) is a progressive degenerative disorder of joints caused by gradual loss of cartilage and resulting in the development of bony spurs and cysts at the margins of the joints.

Etiology

- Rheumatoid arthritis
- Metabolic disorders (Hemochromatosis)
- Acromegaly
- Being overweight
- Heavy lifting
- Genes.

Risk Factors

- Most common in people older than 65 years of age
- Obesity
- Previous joint injury
- Overuse of the joint
- Weak thigh muscles
- Smoking
- Alcohol and drug use
- Sedentary lifestyle
- Mechanical stress.

Pathophysiology

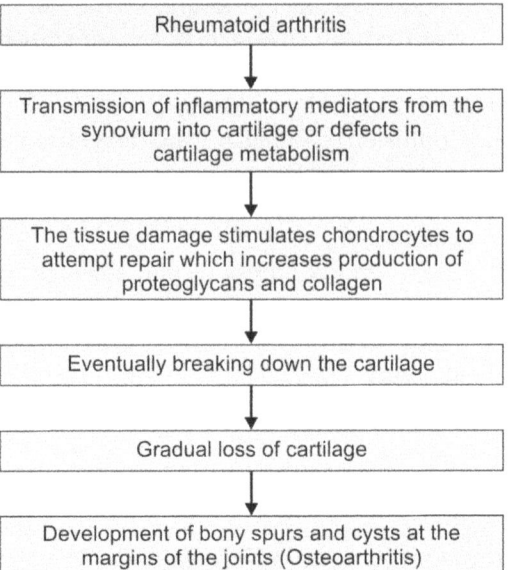

Clinical Features

- Pain and stiffness in the morning or after the rest
- Swollen joints, especially after extended activity
- Sore or stiff joints
- Limited range of motion or stiffness that go away after movement
- Clicking or cracking sound when a joint bends
- Mild swelling around a joint
- Pain that is worse after activity or toward the end of the day
- Pain is felt in the groin area or buttocks
- A grating or scraping sensation occurs when moving the knee
- Bony growths (spurs) at the edge of joints
- Swelling in ankles or toes.

Complications

- Gout
- Chondrocalcinosis
- Osteonecrosis
- Stress fracture
- Bleeding inside the joint.

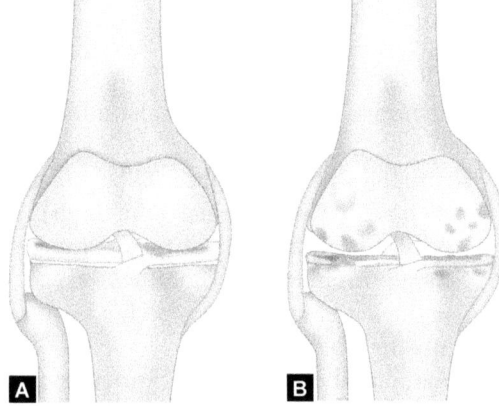

Figs. 12.9A and B: (A) Healthy knee joint; (B) Osteoarthritis.

Diagnostic Tests

- History
- Physical examination
- Blood examination
- Genetic testing
- Joint aspiration
- X-ray examination
- Magnetic resonance imaging (MRI) scan
- Bone scan.

Management

Medical

- **Simple analgesics:** It helps to quickly relieve inflammation and reduces pain. For example, paracetamol, acetaminophen, etc.
- **Nonsteroidal anti-inflammatory drugs (NSAIDs):** It helps to quickly relieve inflammation and reduce pain. For example, ibuprofen, naproxen, aspirin, etc.
- **Selective COX-2 inhibitors:** It prevents the synthesis of a chemical called prostaglandin by inhibiting an enzyme called cyclo-oxygenase 2 (COX-2). Prostaglandins are important mediators of pain and inflammation in the body. For example, celecoxib, etoricoxib, etc.
- **Weak opioids:** It is used to treat moderate to severe pain. For example, codeine, tramadol, etc.

Surgical

- **Arthroscopy:** It is a surgical procedure in which the surgeon makes a small incision in the knee thereby irrigating and removing loose pieces of cartilage.
- **Partial knee replacement:** It is a surgical procedure in which the surgeon replaces only the part of the knee that is worn out.
- **Total knee replacement:** It involves resecting the ends of the bones of the knee and replacing them with a combination of metal and plastic.
- **Osteotomy:** It involves cutting the bone and reorienting the alignment of the knee.
- **Cartilage procedure:** It involves harvesting cartilage cells and transplanting them into the area of disease in the knee.

Nursing

- Encourage the patient to take low-calorie, high-protein and high-fiber diet.
- Instruct them to avoid any falls or accidents in their routine day-to-day life.
- Encourage use of braces to prevent pathological fractures.
- Motivate the patient to perform exercise as tolerated.
- Instruct the patient to participate in weight reduction program.
- Encourage the patient and his family to verbalize their concerns and feelings and allow time for the patient and their family to process the information.
- Encourage the patient and family participation in care activities to promote feelings of self-esteem and control over the situation.

OSTEOMALACIA

Definition

Osteomalacia is a vitamin D deficiency in adults that results in a shortage or loss of calcium salts, causing bones to become increasingly soft, flexible, brittle and deformed. It is characterized by defective bone mineralization, bone pain, increased bone fragility and fractures.

Etiology

- Vitamin D deficiency
- Calcium deficiency
- Hypophosphatemia
- Fanconi syndrome
- Hypophosphatasia
- Malabsorption syndrome
- Wilson disease
- Cystinosis
- Chronic renal failure
- Phenytoin
- Glucocorticoids
- Heavy metals
- Cancer drugs.

Risk Factors

- Breastfed infants
- Having very little exposure to sunlight

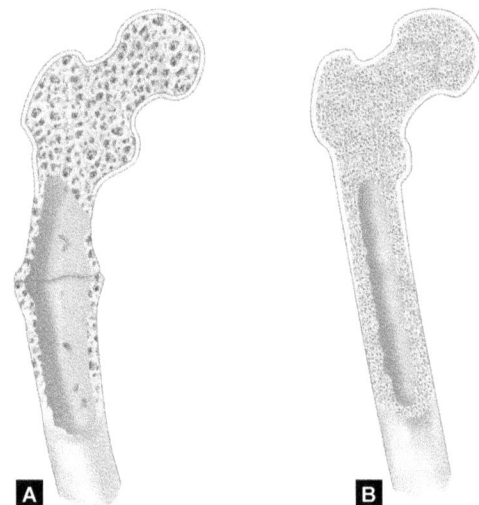

Figs. 12.10A and B: (A) Osteomalacia; (B) Normal bone.

- Shorter days of sunlight
- Smog
- Using very strong sunscreen
- Elderly people who do not drink milk.

Pathophysiology

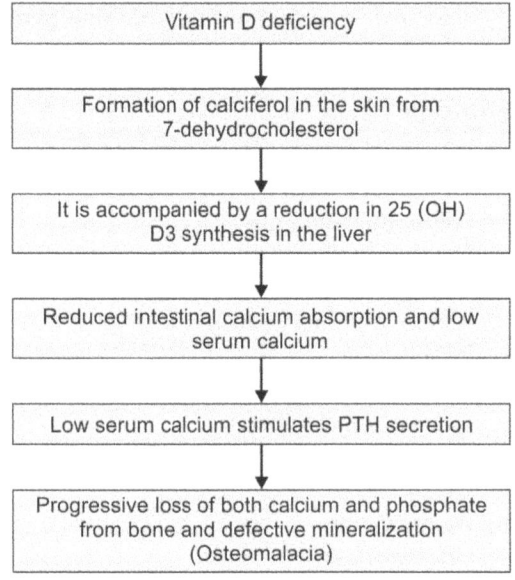

Clinical Features

- Restlessness/Irritability
- Head sweating
- Head somewhat square
- Fontanels opened
- Frontal bossing
- Osseous borders soft (Craniotabes)
- Teething delayed
- Enlargement of costochondral junctions
- Muscles flabby
- Upper respiratory tract infections
- Anemia
- Carpal pedal spasms
- Seizure.

Complications

- Stress fractures
- Hypocalcemia
- Hypophosphatemia
- Chronic pain
- Spontaneous fractures.

Diagnostic Tests

- History
- Physical examination
- Blood examination
- Urine examination
- X-ray examination
- Bone biopsy
- Bone density test.

Management

Medical

Vitamin D supplements: It improves the signs and symptoms of osteomalacia. For example, calcifediol, calcitriol, etc.

Nursing

- Encourage the patient to eat foods rich in calcium and vitamin D.
- Encourage to take daily supplements containing 10 micrograms of vitamin D which helps to prevent osteomalacia.

- Instruct the patient to expose to sun for at least 15 minutes in a day as most of vitamin D comes from it.
- Encourage the patient and his family to verbalize their concerns and feelings and allow time for the patient and their family to process the information.

OSTEOMYELITIS

Definition
Osteomyelitis is an infection and inflammation of the bone or bone marrow which is caused by pyogenic bacteria or mycobacteria. It may be either acute (lasting less than 4 weeks) or chronic (lasting more than 4 weeks).

Etiology
- Bacterial infections (*Pseudomonas aeruginosa, Staphylococcus aureus* and *Proteus, Haemophilus influenzae, Escherichia coli*, Group-A and B *Streptococcus* species, *Enterobacter* species)
- Penetrating trauma
- Slow healing foot ulcer
- Peripheral vascular disease

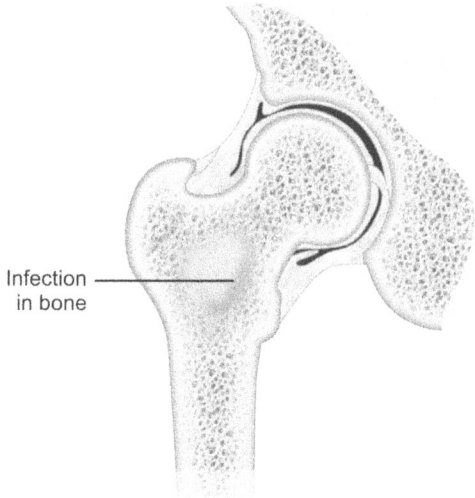

Fig. 12.11: Depicts infected or inflamed bone or bone marrow leading to necrosis (Osteomyelitis).

- Long-term intravenous catheters
- Pulmonary tuberculosis.

Risk Factors
- Weakened immune system
- Poor circulation
- Diabetes
- Orthopedic surgery
- Smoking
- Sickle cell disease
- Peripheral arterial disease
- Hemodialysis.

Pathophysiology

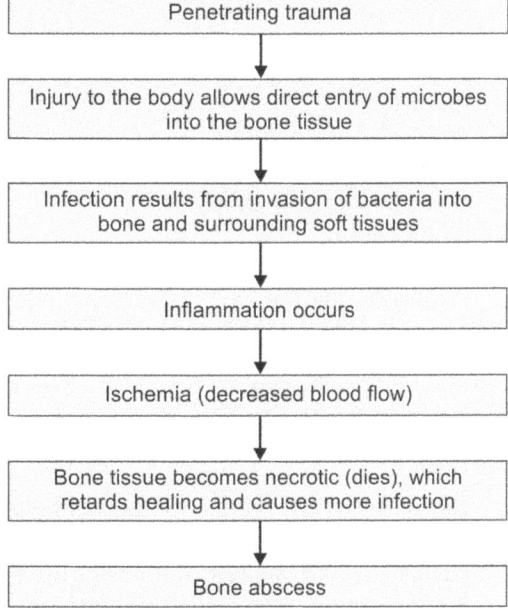

Clinical Features
- Pain over the area of infection which is unrelieved by rest and worsens with activity
- Night sweats
- Chills
- Malaise
- Nausea
- Warmth at the infection site
- Restricted movement of the affected part
- Redness
- Tenderness

- Heat
- Swelling
- Fever.

Complications

- Septicemia
- Pyemia
- Acute pyogenic arthritis
- Pathological fracture
- Growth abnormalities
- Acute exacerbation
- Joint stiffness
- Sinus tract malignancy
- Amyloidosis
- Squamous cell carcinoma
- Septic arthritis.

Diagnostic Tests

- History
- Physical examination
- Blood examination
- Bone or soft tissue biopsy
- Blood culture
- Magnetic resonance imaging
- X-ray examination
- Radionuclide bone scans
- Bone aspiration.

Management

Medical

- **Oxygen therapy:** Hyperbaric oxygen helps to promote antibiotic activity and stimulate circulation and healing in the infected tissue.
- **Antibiotics:** It helps to prevent secondary infections. For example, cefotaxime, amikacin, penicillin, nafcillin, neomycin, tobramycin, etc.
- **Antipyretics:** It helps to relieve against increased temperature. For example, paracetamol, Dolo, etc.
- **Analgesics:** It helps to relieve against bone pain. For example, voveran, tramadol, etc.

Surgical

- **Wound debridement:** To remove necrotic bone tissue and to replace it with healthy bone tissue.
- **Sequestrectomy:** It is a surgical procedure in which an opening is made in the involucrum and the sequestrum is removed.
- **Saucerization:** It is a surgical procedure in which the bone cavity is converted into a 'saucer' by removing its wall and this allows free drainage of the infected material.
- **Amputation:** Performed on patients who have massive infections that have not responded to one or more conventional treatments.
- **Myocutaneous flaps or skin and bone grafting:** If there is extensive destruction, grafting is performed.

Nursing

- Ask the patient to wash the hands frequently.
- Instruct the patient not to smoke.
- Encourage the patient to make healthy lifestyle practices.
- Make sure to clean the minor skin wound well and cover it with a clean, sterile bandages.
- Encourage the patient to eat a balanced diet as it boosts the immune system.
- Instruct the patient to participate in weight reduction program.

OSTEOPOROSIS

Definition

Osteoporosis or porous bone (fragile bone disease) is a chronic, progressive metabolic bone disease characterized by low bone mass and structural deterioration of bone tissue, leading to increased bone fragility.

Etiology

- Long-term use of heparin, oral corticosteroids and antiseizure medications
- Hyperthyroidism
- Stroke
- Rheumatoid arthritis
- Amenorrhea
- Chemotherapy

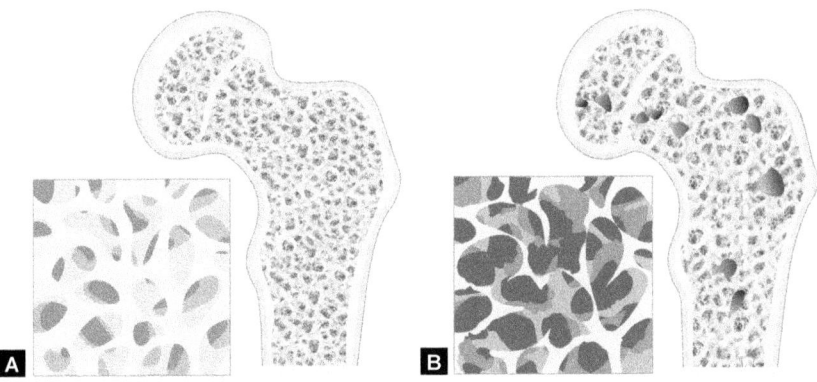

Figs. 12.12A and B: (A) Healthy bone; (B) Osteoporosis.

- Malabsorption
- Poor nutrition.

Risk Factors

Non-modifiable

- Advanced age (both men and women)
- Female sex
- Thin and small body frames
- Estrogen deficiency following menopause in women
- Decrease testosterone levels in men
- Family history of fracture
- Personal history of fracture as an adult
- European or Asian ancestry.

Modifiable

- Excessive alcohol
- Vitamin D deficiency
- Increased parathyroid hormone production
- Low body mass index
- Low dietary calcium intake
- Tobacco smoking
- Physical inactivity
- Weight bearing exercise
- Low-level exposure to heavy metals like cadmium
- Soft drinks as it contains phosphoric acid in it
- Having osteopenia, which is low bone mass.

Pathophysiology

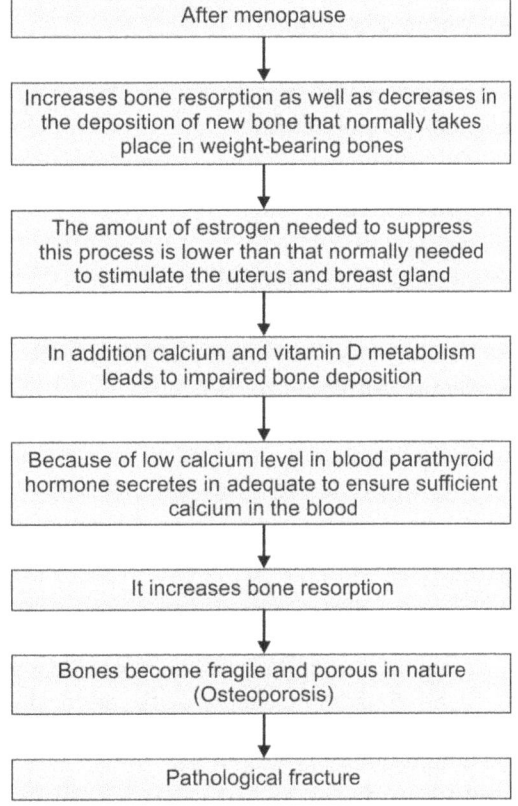

Clinical Features

- Fragile and porous bones
- Increased bone resorption

- Loss of bone mass
- Loss of bone strength
- Decreased estrogen level in blood
- Impairment in bone deposition
- Decreased calcium level in blood
- Weakness
- Dorsolumbar spine fracture
- Colle's fracture
- Fracture of the neck of the femur
- Loss of vertical height of a vertebra
- Cod fish appearance of the disk due to its biconvex shape
- Ground glass appearance of the bones.

Complications

- Fragility fracture
- Hip fracture
- Vertebral fracture
- Decreased quality of life
- Deep vein thrombosis
- Pulmonary embolism
- Pneumonia.

Diagnostic Tests

- History
- Physical examination
- X-ray examination
- Dual energy X-ray absorptiometry scan
- Blood examination
- Neutron activation analysis
- Bone biopsy
- Electromyography.

Management

Medical

- **Antiresorptive agents:** It inhibits bone removal, thus tipping the balance in favor of bone rebuilding and increased bone density. For example, alendronate, risedronate, ibandronate, calcitonin, etc.
- **Recombinant parathyroid hormone:** It acts like parathyroid hormone and stimulates osteoblasts. For example, teriparatide, etc.
- **Dual action bone agents (DABAs):** It stimulates the proliferation of osteoblasts as well as inhibiting the proliferation of osteoclasts. For example, strontium ranelate, etc.
- **Estrogen replacement therapy:** It helps to prevent osteoporosis by reducing bone resorption. For example, premarin, esterase, etc.
- **Selective estrogen receptor modulator (SERM):** It acts on the estrogen receptor throughout the body in a selective manner and it acts on the bone by slowing resorption by the osteoclasts. For example, raloxifene, etc.
- **Calcium supplements:** It supports bone growth, bone healing and maintains bone strength. For example, calcium.
- **Vitamin D supplements:** It reduces fracture in an elderly and also increases bone density. For example, vitamin D.

Surgical

- **Kyphoplasty:** It is the surgical procedure in which correction is made in the vertebral column due to slight loss of height and increased kyphosis due to compression of the anterior part of the spine.
- **Vertebroplasty:** It is the procedure in which surgical correction is made in the vertebral column as there is loss of vertical height in a vertebra due to a collapse.

Nursing

- Encourage to take high protein diet as it is helpful in the formation of the organic matrix of bone.
- Instruct them to avoid any falls or accidents in their routine day to day life.
- Encourage use of braces to prevent pathological fractures.
- Ensure a nutritious diet with adequate calcium intake.
- Instruct the patient to avoid second-hand smoking.
- Ensure the patient to maintain an adequate supply of vitamin D.
- Encourage the patient to participate in regular physical activity.
- Instruct the patient to avoid the intake of alcohol.

PAGET'S DISEASE

Definition

Paget's disease (osteitis deformans) is a chronic metabolic bone disorder in which increased bone loss results in enlarged and deformed bones throughout the body.

Etiology

- Slow virus infection (paramyxoviruses especially measles virus)
- Poor diet or bone injury early in life
- Genetic predisposition
- Idiopathic.

Risk Factors

- Being males
- Most common in older people
- Family history of Paget's disease
- It is more common in Europeans.
- It is more common in Australia and New Zealand.

Pathophysiology

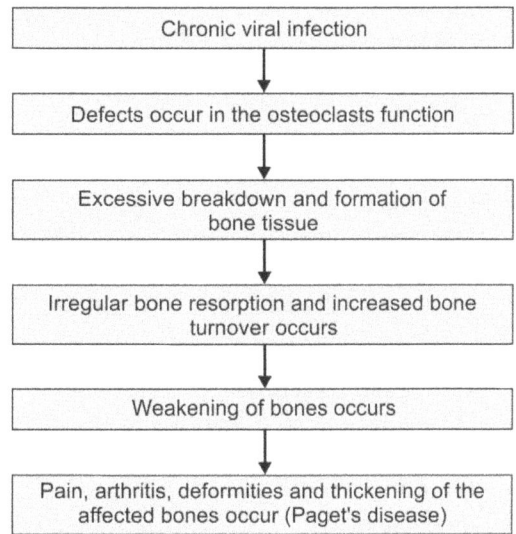

Clinical Features

- Localized bone pain adjacent to areas of the joints affected
- Headache

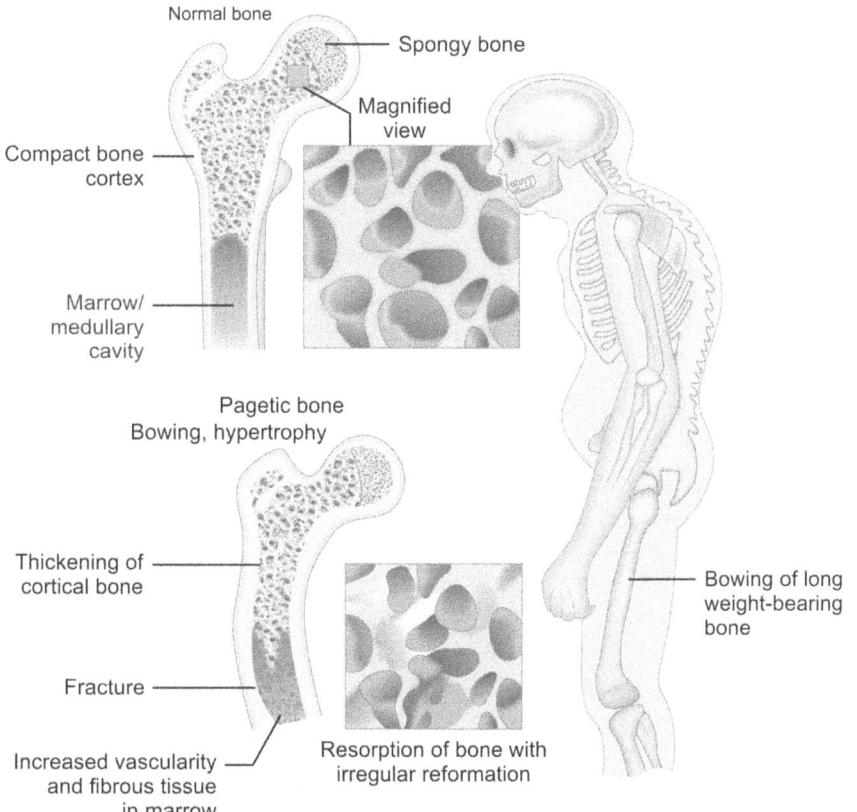

Fig. 12.13: Shows the comparison of normal bone with that of the pagetic bone (Paget's disease).

- Hearing loss
- Pressure on nerves
- Drowsiness
- Somnolence
- Paralysis
- Increased head size, bowing of limb or curvature of spine
- Hip pain
- Damaged joint cartilage
- Teeth may spread intraorally
- Chalkstick fractures.

Complications
- Pathological fracture
- Severe degenerative arthritis
- Bone deformity (bending)
- Bone enlargement
- Loss of hearing
- Heart disease
- Kidney stones
- Nerve system pressure
- Bone sarcoma
- Teeth loosening
- Disturbance in chewing
- Loss of vision.

Diagnostic Tests
- History
- Physical examination
- Blood examination
- X-ray examination
- Bone scan.

Management

Medical
- **Biphosphonates:** It helps to relieve bone pain and to reduce the progression of the disease. For example, pamidronate, zoledronate, risedronate, tiludronate, etidronate, etc.
- **Calcitonin:** It helps to prevent the progression of the disease. For example, miacalcin, etc.
- **Analgesics:** It helps in reducing pain caused by osteoarthritis and nerve compression. For example, paracetamol, ibuprofen, etc.

Nursing
- Encourage regular exercise to maintain joint mobility.
- Encourage to take protein and calcium-rich diet (except in case of renal stones).
- Reduce the activity of the patient to the level of pain-free functioning.
- Increase the activity of the patient in graduated fashion after several weeks of rest and improved symptoms.

RHEUMATOID ARTHRITIS

Definition
Rheumatoid arthritis is a chronic, progressive and disabling autoimmune disease that causes inflammation (swelling) and pain in the joints,

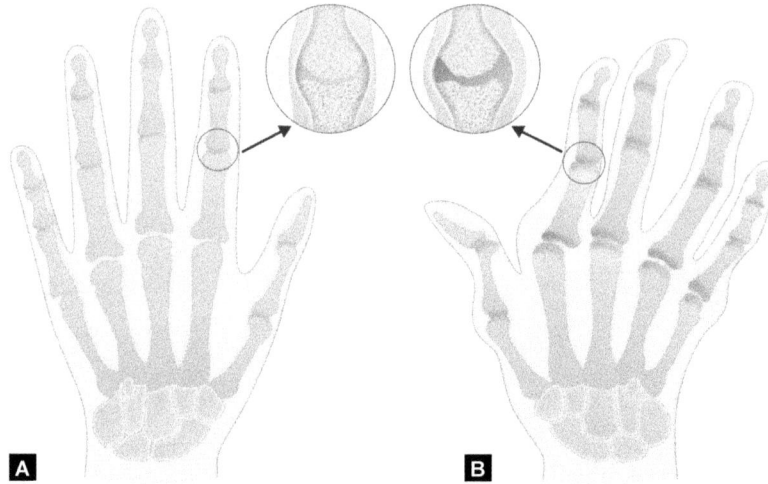

Figs. 12.14A and B: (A) Normal; (B) Rheumatoid.

the tissue around the joints and other organs in the human body.

Etiology

- Autoimmune disease
- Hormonal replacement therapy
- Use of oral contraceptives
- Intake of vitamin D.

Risk Factors

- Being females
- Family history of rheumatoid arthritis
- Those who are between the ages of 30 and 60 years
- Smoking
- Physical activity
- Early life exposure.

Pathophysiology

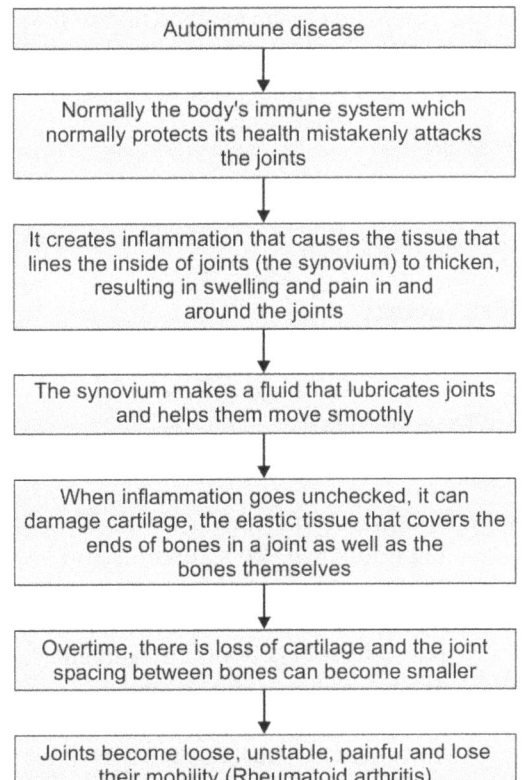

Clinical Features

- Joint pain, tenderness, swelling or stiffness for 6 weeks or longer
- Morning stiffness for 30 minutes or longer
- Redness or swelling in the joints
- More than one joint is affected
- The same joints on both sides of the body are affected
- Fatigue
- Loss of appetite
- Low-grade fever
- Malaise
- Depression
- Weight loss
- Anemia
- A feeling of warmth around the joint
- Deformities and contractures of the joint
- Nodules or lumps particularly around the elbow.

Complications

- Rheumatoid lung
- Hardening of the arteries
- Rheumatoid vasculitis
- Congestive cardiac failure
- Spinal cord injury.

Diagnostic Tests

- History
- Physical examination
- Blood examination
- X-ray examination
- Joint ultrasound
- Synovial fluid analysis
- Magnetic resonance imaging (MRI) scan
- Computed tomography (CT) scan
- Bone mineral density.

Management

Medical

- **Disease modifying antirheumatic drugs (DMARDs):** It helps in the treatment of rheumatoid arthritis. For example, methotrexate, leflunomide, etc.
- **Nonsteroidal antiinflammatory drugs (NSAIDs):** It helps to decrease swelling, pain and fever. For example, ibuprofen, naproxen, etc.
- **Anti-malarial agents:** It helps to relieve pain. For example, hydroxychloroquine, etc.

- **Corticosteroids:** It helps to reduce the joint swelling and inflammation. For example, prednisone, etc.
- **Selective COX-2 inhibitors:** It prevents the synthesis of a chemical called prostaglandin by inhibiting an enzyme called cyclooxygenase 2 (COX-2). Prostaglandins are important mediators of pain and inflammation in the body. For example, celecoxib, etoricoxib, etc.
- **Biologic agents:** It is used in the treatment of rheumatoid arthritis. For example, rituximab, abatacept, etc.

Surgical

- **Synovectomy:** It is the removal of diseased synovium and this reduces the pain and swelling of rheumatoid arthritis and prevents or slows down the destruction of joints.
- **Arthroscopy:** It is a surgical procedure in which the surgeon makes a small incision in the knee thereby irrigating and removing loose pieces of cartilage.
- **Partial knee replacement:** It is a surgical procedure in which the surgeon replaces only the part of the knee that is worn out.
- **Total knee replacement:** It involves resecting the ends of the bones of the knee and replacing them with a combination of metal and plastic.
- **Osteotomy:** It involves cutting the bone and reorienting the alignment of the knee.
- **Cartilage procedure:** It involves harvesting cartilage cells and transplanting them into the area of disease in the knee.

Nursing

- Ask the patient to maintain a healthy and active lifestyle.
- Encourage the patient to eat a balanced diet as it boosts the immune system.
- Instruct the patient to participate in weight reduction program.
- Instruct the patient to perform light to moderate exercise, interspersed with rest periods.
- Instruct the patient not to smoke.
- Encourage the patient to perform activities of daily living without muscle fatigue or intolerance.
- Encourage the patient and his family to verbalize their concerns and feelings and allow time for the patient and their family to process the information.
- Encourage the patient and family participation in care activities to promote feelings of self-esteem and control over the situation.

SPRAIN

Definition

A sprain is excessive stretching of one or more ligaments that usually result from twisting movements during a sports activity, exercise, or fall. Ligaments are tough bands of fibrous tissue that connect one bone to another. Common locations for sprains are ankles and knees.

Etiology

- Poor technique of using martial arts
- Sports injury
- Falls or trauma.

Risk Factors

- Poor conditioning of the muscles
- Improper warm-up exercise
- Tired muscles.

Types

- *First-degree (mild type)*
  - Ligament will be stretched and tear slightly.
  - The injured area will be somewhat painful, especially with movement.
  - The injured area will be tender.
  - Not much of swelling will be present.
  - The client can put weight on the joint.
- *Second-degree (moderate type)*
  - The fibers in the ligament will tear, but they don't rupture completely.
  - The joint is tender, painful and difficult to move.

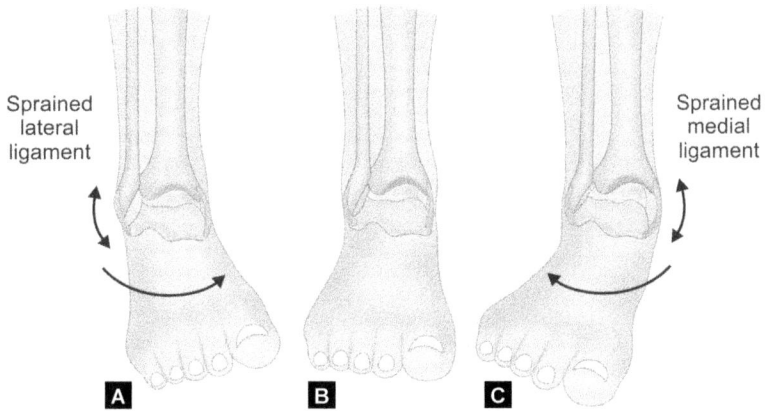

Figs. 12.15A to C: Ankle sprains: (A) Inversion; (B) Normal; (C) Eversion.

- The injured area will be swollen.
- The clients may feel unsteady when they try to bear weight on their joint.
- *Third-degree (severe type)*
  - One or more ligaments will tear completely.
  - The area will be painful.
  - The clients can't move their joint or put weight on it.
  - The joints will become swollen.
  - The injury may be difficult to distinguish from a fracture or dislocation, which requires medical care.

Pathophysiology

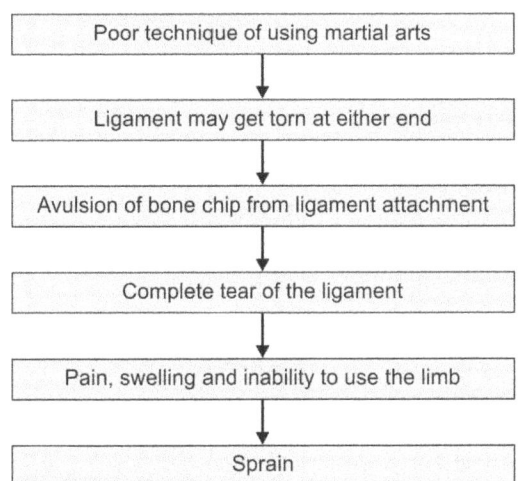

Clinical Features

- Swelling
- Localized tenderness
- Pain
- Limitations in using the limbs
- Tear of the ligaments
- Ecchymosis
- Bruising
- Muscle weakness
- Popping sounds
- Hemarthrosis
- Discomfort.

Complications

- Inability to use the limbs
- Long-term joint or tissue damage
- Inability to bear weight
- Stiffness of joint.

Diagnostic Tests

- History
- Physical examination
- Blood examination
- X-ray examination
- Magnetic resonance imaging (MRI) scan
- Arthrography
- Arthroscopy.

Management

Medical

- **Apply ice packs:** It helps to relieve against swelling of the joint muscles.
- **Physiotherapy:** It helps to provide maximal stability and strength to the injured joint.
- **Analgesics:** It helps to relieve pain. For example, ibuprofen, acetaminophen, etc.

Surgical

- **Immobilization:** It is practiced in second-degree sprain and the part is immobilized for 4–6 weeks.
- **Splints/Braces:** It helps in immobilizing the affected part either temporarily or during transportation.

Nursing

Till recovery continues with **P.R.I.C.E** treatment as follows:

- Instruct to immobilize the area and to protect it from further injury **(P-Protect)**.
- Instruct to avoid activities which cause pain, discomfort or swelling **(R-Rest)**.
- Encourage the use of ice to reduce swelling in the affected part **(I-Ice)**.
- Instruct to compress the area with an elastic bandage to reduce swelling **(C-Compress)**.
- Educate to elevate the injured area about the heart level to as gravity helps to reduce swelling **(E-Elevate).**

STRAIN

Definition

A strain is an injury to a muscle or a tendon (tissue that connects muscle to bone). In a strain, a muscle or tendon is stretched or torn.

Etiology

- Lifting heavy objects the wrong way
- A recent injury
- Overstressing the muscles.

Risk Factors

- Playing sports
- Sports such as soccer, football, hockey, boxing and wrestling
- Playing gymnastics, tennis, rowing and golf.

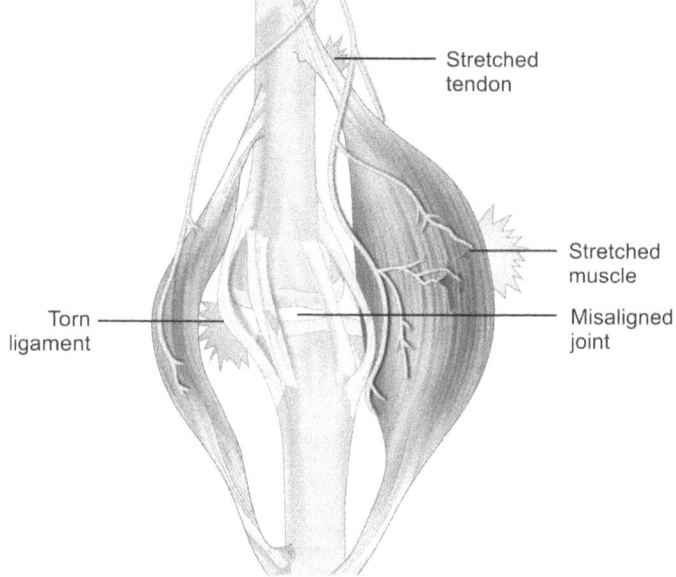

Fig. 12.16: Strain.

Pathophysiology

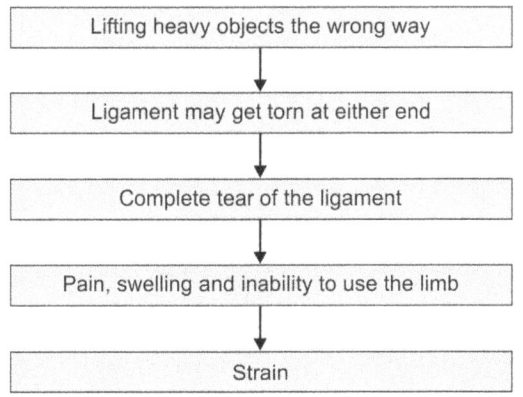

Clinical Features

- Pain
- Muscle spasms
- Muscle weakness
- Swelling
- Cramping
- Trouble in moving the muscle.

Complications

- Inability to use the limbs
- Long-term joint or tissue damage
- Inability to bear weight
- Stiffness of joint.

Diagnostic Tests

- History
- Physical examination
- Blood examination
- X-ray examination
- Magnetic resonance imaging (MRI) scan
- Arthrography
- Arthroscopy.

Management

Medical

- **Apply ice packs:** It helps to relieve against swelling of the joint muscles.
- **Physiotherapy:** It helps to provide maximal stability and strength to the injured joint.
- **Analgesics:** It helps to relieve pain. For example, ibuprofen, acetaminophen, etc.

Nursing

- Ask the patient to avoid exercising or playing sports when tired or in pain.
- Instruct the patient to avoid falling.
- Encourage the patient to eat a well-balanced diet to keep the muscles strong.
- Make sure the patient wear shoes that fit well.
- Encourage the patient to maintain a healthy weight.
- Ensure the patient performs exercise at regular intervals.
- Ask the patient to wear protective equipment when playing.

SYSTEMIC LUPUS ERYTHEMATOSUS

Definition

Systemic lupus erythematosus is a chronic autoimmune disorder that can affect virtually any organ of the body (skin, joints, kidneys, lungs, nervous system and other organs of the body). Most patients feel fatigue and have rashes, arthritis and fever.

Etiology

- Viral infection (Cytomegalovirus, Epstein-Barr virus, etc.)
- Exposure to chemicals
- Exposure to ultraviolet rays
- Genetic predisposition.

Risk Factors

- Being females
- More common in African-American and Asians
- Being black
- Those who are between the ages of 15 and 45 years
- Family history of systemic lupus erythematosus
- Smoking
- Being children
- Presence of other autoimmune disorders.

Disorders of Musculoskeletal System

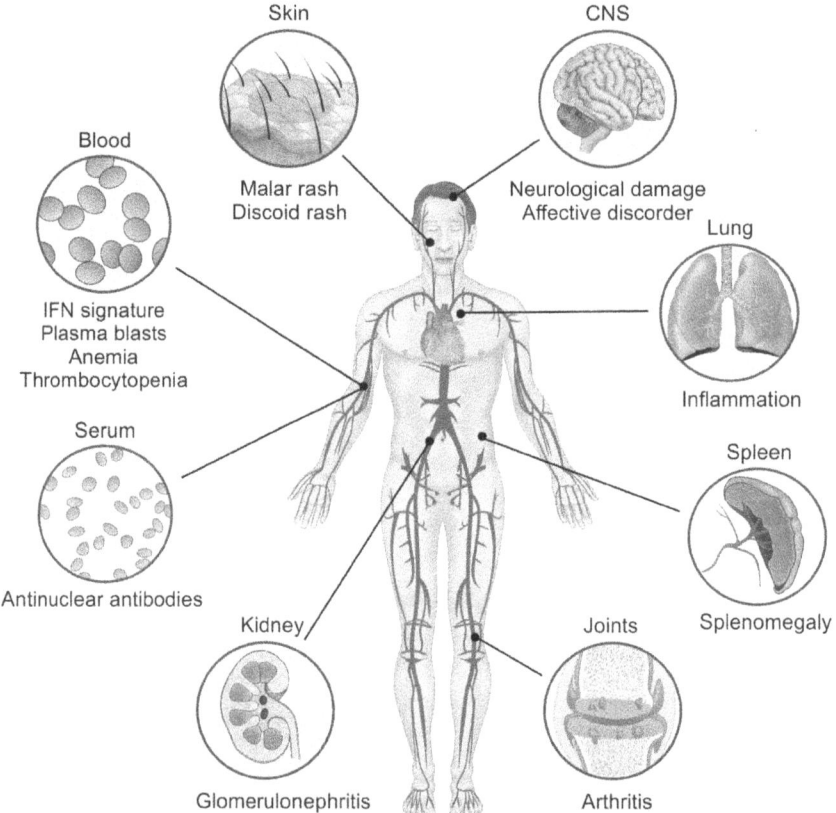

Fig. 12.17: Shows the cardinal features of systemic lupus erythematosus (SLE).

Pathophysiology

```
Viruses (Cytomegalovirus, Epstein-Barr virus, etc.)
                        ↓
When healthy, the immune system protects the
body by making antibodies (blood proteins) that
       attack foreign germs and cancers
                        ↓
With lupus, the immune system misfires and
instead of producing protective antibodies, an
autoimmune disease makes autoantibodies which
         attack the patient's own tissues
                        ↓
As the attack goes on, other immune cells join the
fight and this leads to inflammation and abnormal
              blood vessels (Vasculitis)
                        ↓
These antibodies then end up in cells in organs,
         where they damage those tissues
                        ↓
         Systemic lupus erythematosus
```

Clinical Features

- Achy joints (Arthralgia)
- Fever
- Swollen and painful joints
- Prolonged fatigue
- Skin rashes
- Anemia
- Swollen ankles
- Chest pain upon deep breathing (Pleurisy)
- Butterfly-shaped rash across cheeks and nose
- Sensitivity to sun
- Unusual hair loss
- Abnormal blood clotting problems
- Pale or purple fingers from cold or stress
- Seizures
- Mouth ulcers.

Complications

- Anemia
- Antiphospholipid syndrome

- Thrombocytopenia
- Neutropenia
- Acute lupus hemophagocyte syndrome
- Lymphomas
- Heart attack
- Stroke
- Lupus nephritis
- Pleurisy
- Lupus pneumonitis
- Osteoporosis.

Diagnostic Tests

- History
- Physical examination
- Blood examination
- X-ray examination
- Kidney biopsy
- Electroencephalogram
- Magnetic resonance imaging (MRI) scan
- Computed tomography (CT) scan
- Bone mineral density.

Management

Medical

- **Nonsteroidal anti-inflammatory drugs (NSAIDs):** It helps to decrease swelling, pain and fever. For example, ibuprofen, naproxen, etc.
- **Anti-malarial agents:** It helps to relieve some lupus symptoms such as fatigue, rashes, joint pain or mouth sores. For example, hydroxychloroquine, etc.
- **High-dose corticosteroids:** It helps to reduce the severity of the disease. For example, prednisone, etc.
- **Immune suppressants:** It helps to suppress the immune system. For example, azathioprine, cyclophosphamide, cyclosporine, etc.
- **Biologic agents:** It is used in the treatment of rheumatoid arthritis. For example, rituximab, abatacept, etc.

Nursing

- Ask the patient to maintain a healthy and active lifestyle.
- Instruct the patient to perform light to moderate exercise, interspersed with rest periods.
- Instruct the patients to minimize their exposure to crowds or people with contagious illnesses.
- Instruct the patient to maintain good personal hygiene.
- Ask the patient to avoid exposure to sunlight.
- Encourage the patient to take adequate rest of at least 8 hours.

13 CHAPTER

Communicable Diseases

CHAPTER OUTLINE

- Acquired immunodeficiency syndrome
- Chikungunya
- Chickenpox
- Chlamydia
- Cholera
- Dengue fever
- Diphtheria
- Ebola virus disease
- Filariasis
- Gonorrhea
- Influenza
- Japanese encephalitis
- Kala-azar
- Leprosy
- Leptospirosis
- Malaria
- Measles
- Mumps
- Pertussis
- Plague
- Poliomyelitis
- Rubella
- Severe acute respiratory syndrome
- Smallpox
- Swine flu
- Syphilis
- Tetanus
- Typhoid
- Yellow fever
- Zika virus disease

ACQUIRED IMMUNODEFICIENCY SYNDROME

Definition

Acquired immunodeficiency syndrome (AIDS) is a chronic, potentially life-threatening condition caused by the human immunodeficiency virus (HIV). By damaging your immune system, HIV interferes with your body's ability to fight the organisms that cause disease.

Etiology

- Viral infection (Human immunodeficiency virus)
- Multiple partners
- Blood transfusion without screening
- Sharing infected needles
- Injectable drug abuse
- From infected mother to child.

Risk Factors

- Having unprotected sex
- Infected with another STIs (sexually transmitted infections)
- Using intravenous drugs
- Uncircumcised man.

Stages

HIV infection passes through a series of steps or stages before it turns into AIDS. These are as follows:

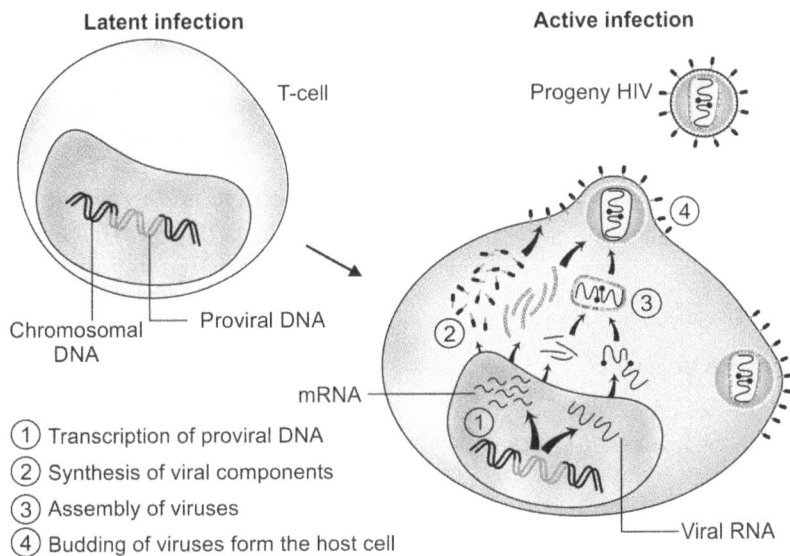

Fig. 13.1: Shows the pathogenesis of AIDS.

1. ***Seroconversion illness:*** This occurs in 1–6 weeks after acquiring the infection.
2. ***Asymptomatic infection:*** After seroconversion, virus levels are low and replication continues slowly. CD4 and CD8 lymphocyte levels are normal. This stage has no symptoms and may persist for years together.
3. ***Persistent generalized lymphadenopathy (PGL):*** The lymph nodes in these patients are swollen for three months or longer and not due to any other cause.
4. ***Symptomatic infection:*** This stage manifests with symptoms. In addition, there may be opportunistic infections. This collection of symptoms and signs is referred to as the AIDS-related complex (ARC) and is regarded as a prodrome or precursor to AIDS.
5. ***AIDS:*** This stage is characterized by severe immunodeficiency. There are signs of life-threatening infections and unusual tumors. This stage is characterized by CD4 T-cell count below 200 cells/mm^3.

Pathophysiology

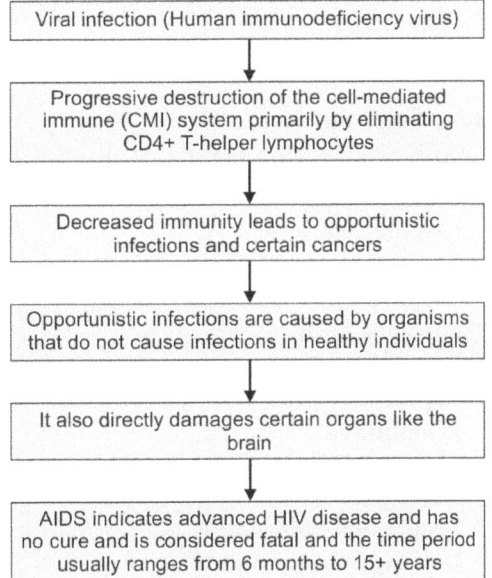

Clinical Features

Within First Few Weeks

- Fever
- Headache

- Sore throat
- Rashes
- Swollen lymph glands.

Few Years Later

- Diarrhea
- Weight loss
- Fever
- Cough
- Shortness of breath.

Progression of Disease to AIDS

- Soaking night sweats
- Shaking chills or fever higher than 100 °F for several weeks
- Cough and shortness of breath
- Chronic diarrhea
- Persistent white spots or unusual lesions on the tongue
- Headache
- Persistent, unexplained fatigue
- Blurred and distorted vision
- Weight loss
- Skin rashes.

Complications

- Tuberculosis
- Salmonellosis
- Cytomegalovirus
- Candidiasis
- Cryptococcal meningitis
- Toxoplasmosis
- Cryptosporidiosis
- Kaposi's sarcoma
- Lymphomas
- Liver or kidney damage
- Hepatitis
- Urinary tract infections
- Wasting syndrome
- Neurological complications.

Diagnostic Tests

- History
- Physical examination
- CD4 count
- ELISA test
- Western blot test
- Viral load test
- Drug resistance test.

Management

Medical

- **Non-nucleoside reverse transcriptase inhibitors (NNRTIs):** It disables a protein needed by HIV to make copies of it. For example, efavirenz, etravirine, nevirapine, etc.
- **Nucleoside reverse transcriptase inhibitors (NRTIs):** These are faulty versions of building blocks that HIV needs to make copies of itself. For example, abacavir, emtricitabine, tenofovir, lamivudine, zidovudine, etc.
- **Protease inhibitors (PIs):** It disables protease, another protein that HIV needs to make copies of it. For example, atazanavir, darunavir, fosamprenavir, ritonavir, etc.
- **Entry or fusion inhibitors:** These drugs block HIV's entry into CD4 cells. For example, enfuvirtide, maraviroc, etc.
- **Integrase inhibitors:** It works by disabling integrase, a protein that HIV uses to insert its genetic material into CD4 cells. For example, raltegravir, etc.

Nursing

- Use a clean and sterile needle for every individual patient.
- Encourage the individual use of a new condom every time whenever they have sex.
- Enforce medical treatment right away when they are pregnant to cut off the risk of their baby two-thirds.

CHIKUNGUNYA

Definition

Chikungunya disease is a viral disease transmitted in humans by the bite of infected mosquitoes. *Aedes aegypti* mosquito (also called yellow fever mosquito) is the primary transmission agent for chikungunya virus (CHIKV) which breeds in clean water stagnation in artificial containers.

Communicable Diseases

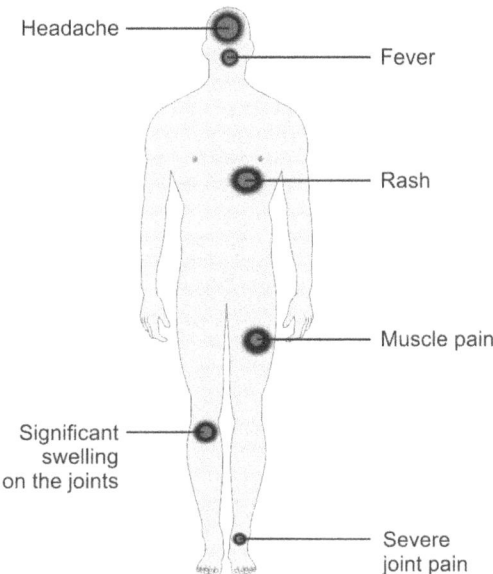

Fig. 13.2: Symptoms of chikungunya virus infection.

Clinical Features

- Initial symptoms include chills, fever, vomiting, nausea, headache and joint pain.
- Later fever up to 104° Celsius and severe joint pain
- Redness in eye and difficulty in looking at night
- Rashes may appear on limbs and trunks.

Complications

- Respiratory failure
- Cardiovascular decompensation
- Myocarditis
- Acute hepatitis
- Renal failure
- Meningoencephalitis
- Flaccid paralysis
- Guillain-Barr syndrome.

Etiology

Aedes aegypti mosquito (also known as yellow fever mosquito).

Risk Factors

- Stagnated clean water
- Travel to underdeveloped countries
- During daytime, particularly around sunrise and sunset
- Slums
- Elderly
- Homeless
- Diabetes
- Chemotherapy
- AIDS
- Weakened immunity
- Rainy season.

Diagnostic Tests

- History
- Physical examination
- Blood examination
- ELISA blood test
- Four-fold hemagglutination inhibition test
- Detection of virus nucleic acid in serum by RT-PCR.

Management

Medical

- **Analgesics and antipyretics combination:** It helps to relieve from severe joint pain. For example, paracetamol, etc.
- **Nonsteroidal anti-inflammatory agents:** It is a propionic acid derivative with analgesic, antipyretic and anti-inflammatory activity used for the treatment of chikungunya. For example, naproxen, chloroquine phosphate, etc.

Nursing

- Instruct the patient to avoid sources of standing water, such as stagnant ponds or even flower pots that have collected rain.
- Encourage patients to use screens, windows and doors to keep mosquitoes from coming into the home.

Pathophysiology

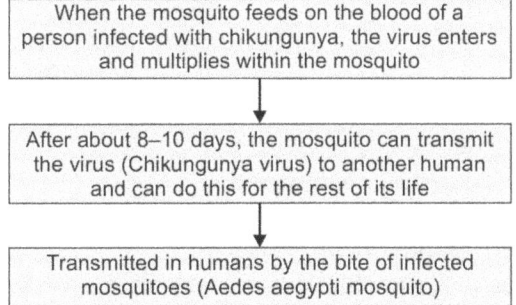

- Encourage sufficient rest to the patient.
- Encourage more fluids to the patient.
- Instruct to patient to take honey and lime mix at regular intervals as it gives a soothing effect.
- Instruct the patient to cover exposed skin by wearing long-sleeved shirts, long pants and hats.
- Instruct the patient to use an appropriate insect repellent as directed.

CHICKENPOX

Definition

Chickenpox is a viral infection a person develops extremely itchy blisters all over the body caused by varicella zoster virus, a member of the herpes virus family.

Etiology

Viral infection (Varicella-zoster virus).

Risk Factors

- Have not had chickenpox
- Have not been vaccinated for chickenpox
- Children under 10 years of age
- Pregnant women
- Late winter and early spring months
- Those who are in direct contact with open sores
- Living with children
- Weakened immune system
- People on chemotherapy
- Long-term use of steroids.

Pathophysiology

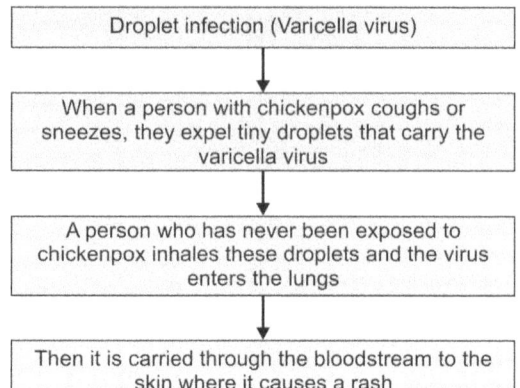

Droplet infection (Varicella virus)

↓

When a person with chickenpox coughs or sneezes, they expel tiny droplets that carry the varicella virus

↓

A person who has never been exposed to chickenpox inhales these droplets and the virus enters the lungs

↓

Then it is carried through the bloodstream to the skin where it causes a rash

Clinical Features

- A red, itchy rash, initially resembling insect bites, on your face, scalp, chest and back
- Small, liquid-filled blisters that break open and crust over
- Fever
- Abdominal pain
- Loss of appetite
- Mild headache
- Malaise
- Dry cough
- Raised papules
- Vesicles
- Crusts and scabs.

Complications

- Sepsis
- Pneumonia
- Encephalitis
- Toxic shock syndrome
- Reye syndrome
- Shingles.

Diagnostic Tests

- History
- Physical examination
- Virus culture
- Immunofluorescence assay
- Polymerase chain reaction (PCR).

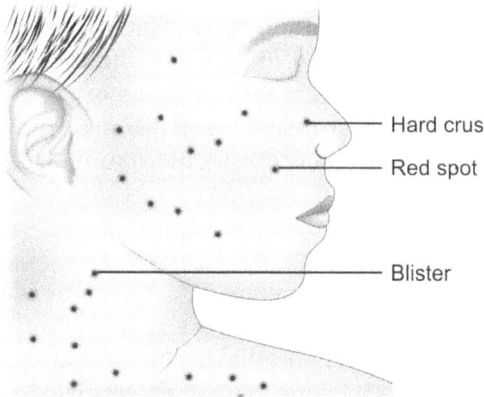

Fig. 13.3: Chickenpox.

Management

Medical

- **Antiviral agents:** It helps to minimize the symptoms of chickenpox, but it is only effective if it is started within the first 24 hours after exposure. For example, acyclovir, etc.
- **Antihistamines:** It focuses on relieving the annoying itch of chickenpox blisters and preventing broken blisters from getting infected from scratching. For example, diphenhydramine, etc.
- **Non-aspirin agents:** It helps to lower the temperature among the patients. For example, ibuprofen, acetaminophen, etc.

Nursing

- Encourage the patient to use cool wet compresses or give baths in cool or lukewarm water every 3-4 hours for the first few days.
- Instruct the patient not to rub the body dry.
- Encourage the patient to eat foods that are cold, soft and bland because chickenpox in the mouth can make drinking or eating difficult.
- Instruct the patient to wear gloves to prevent scratching that can lead to scarring.
- Restrict the patient from having salty or citrus foods.
- Provide information to patient regarding chickenpox vaccine.

CHLAMYDIA (SILENT INFECTION)

Definition

Chlamydia is a bacterial infection of the genital tract that spreads easily through sexual contact.

Etiology

- Bacterial infection (*Chlamydia trachomatis*)
- From mother to her child.

Risk Factors

- Age under 25
- Women using an intrauterine device (IUD)
- Being women

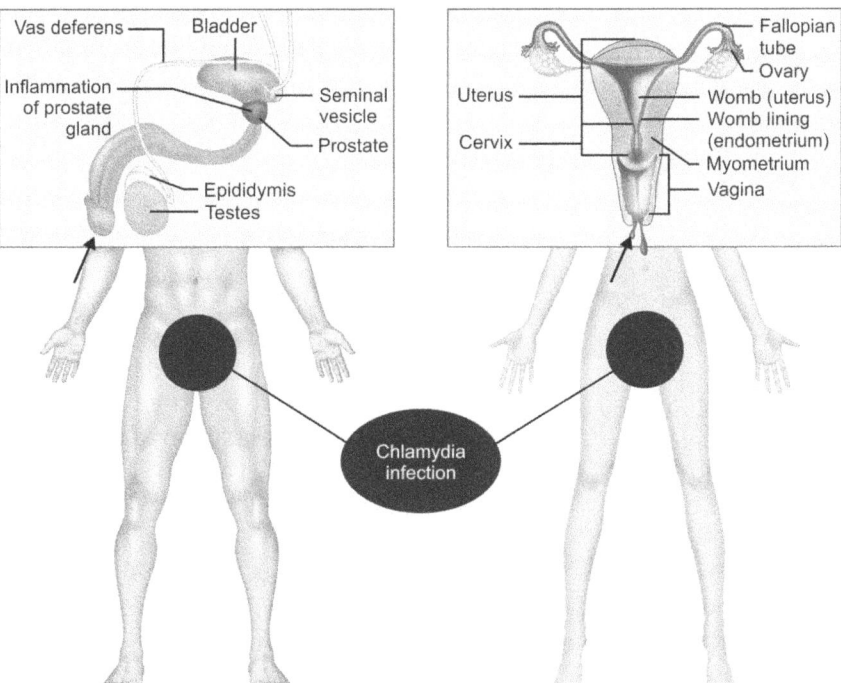

Fig. 13.4: Chlamydia infection.

- Multiple sex partners within the past year
- Not using a condom consistently
- History of prior sexually transmitted infection
- Douching among women
- Unprotected sex.

Pathophysiology

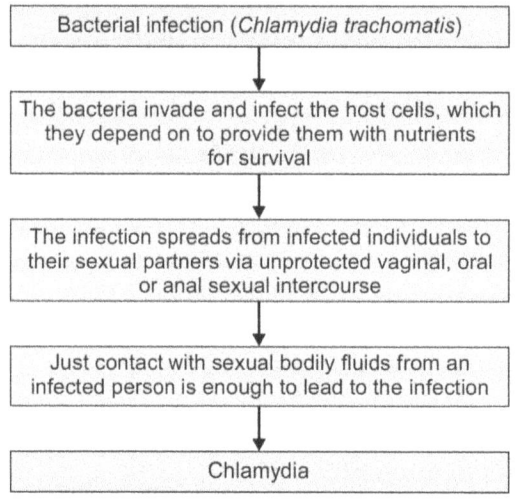

Clinical Features

In Women

- Unusual vaginal discharge
- Burning feeling when urinating
- Pain during sex
- Bleeding or spotting between periods or bleeding after sex
- Lower abdominal pain
- Nausea
- Fever.

In Men

- Discharge from the penis
- Discomfort when urinating
- Swelling of the testicles
- Burning or itching in opening of penis
- Testicular pain.

Complications

- Human immunodeficiency virus
- Sexually transmitted infections
- Pelvic inflammatory disease
- Chronic pelvic pain
- Infertility
- Epididymitis
- Prostatitis
- Rectal inflammation.
- Eye infections
- Infections in newborn.

Diagnostic Tests

- History
- Physical examination
- Pap smear test
- Cultural swab
- Urine test.

Management

Medical

Antibiotics: It helps to prevent secondary infections. For example, azithromycin, doxycycline, erythromycin, etc.

Nursing

- Instruct the patient to get regular screenings for sexually transmitted diseases.
- Educate the patient to avoid multiple sex partners.
- Instruct women to avoid using douche.
- Educate the patient to use condoms during every sexual encounter.
- Instruct the patients to undergo regular screenings.

CHOLERA

Definition

Cholera is an acute bacterial infection of the small intestine caused by *Vibrio cholerae* and characterized by extreme diarrhea with rapid and severe depletion of body fluids and salts. Bacterial disease usually spreads through contaminated water.

Etiology

- Contaminated water supply
- *Vibrio cholerae*
- Seafood

Communicable Diseases

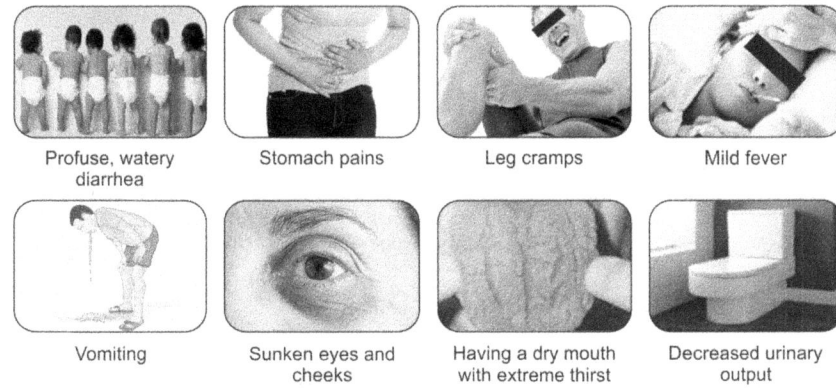

Fig. 13.5: Symptoms of cholera.

- Raw fruits and vegetables
- Grains.

Risk Factors

- Malnutrition
- Hypochlorhydria or Achlorhydria
- Household exposure
- Compromised immunity
- Type O blood
- Raw or undercook shellfish.

Pathophysiology

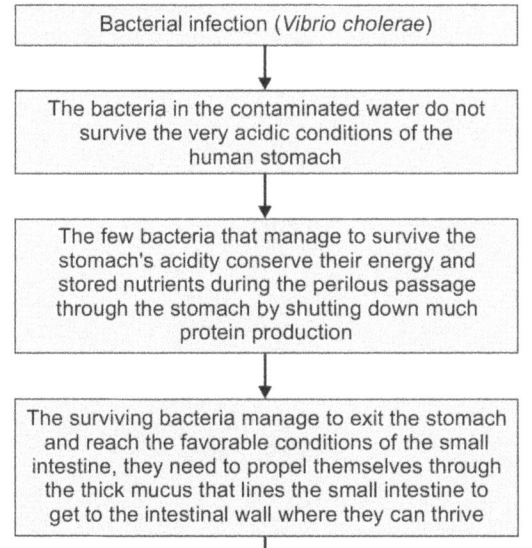

Clinical Features

- Severe, watery diarrhea
- Nausea
- Vomiting
- Muscle cramps
- Dehydration
- Sunken eyes and cheeks
- Stomach pain
- Dry mouth with extreme thirst
- Decreased urine output

- Hypovolemic shock
- Extreme drowsiness
- Mild fever
- Convulsions.

Complications
- Hypoglycemia
- Hypokalemia
- Renal failure.

Diagnostic Tests
- History
- Physical examination
- Stool sample test
- Dipstick test.

Management

Medical
- **Antibiotics:** It helps to shorten diarrhea duration. For example, azithromycin, etc.
- **Zinc supplements:** It decreases and shortens the duration of diarrhea.
- **Oral rehydration salts:** It replaces fluids and electrolytes lost through diarrhea. For example, ORS packets, etc.

Nursing
- Encourage the patient for frequent handwashing.
- Instruct the patient to avoid untreated water.
- Encourage patient to eat foods that is completely cooked and hot.
- Instruct the patient to avoid improperly cooked sea foods.

DENGUE FEVER

Definition
Dengue fever or dengue hemorrhagic fever (DHF) is an acute febrile disease found in the tropical region and caused by four closely related virus serotypes of the genus Flavivirus, family Flaviviridae. It is also known as breakbone fever or bonecrusher disease. It is an acute illness of sudden onset that usually follows a benign course with symptoms such as headache, fever, exhaustion, severe muscle and joint pain, swollen glands and rash.

Etiology
- *Aedes aegypti* mosquito
- Flavivirus.

Risk Factors
- Living or traveling in tropical areas
- Prior infection with a dengue fever virus
- Presence of water-holding containers in and around

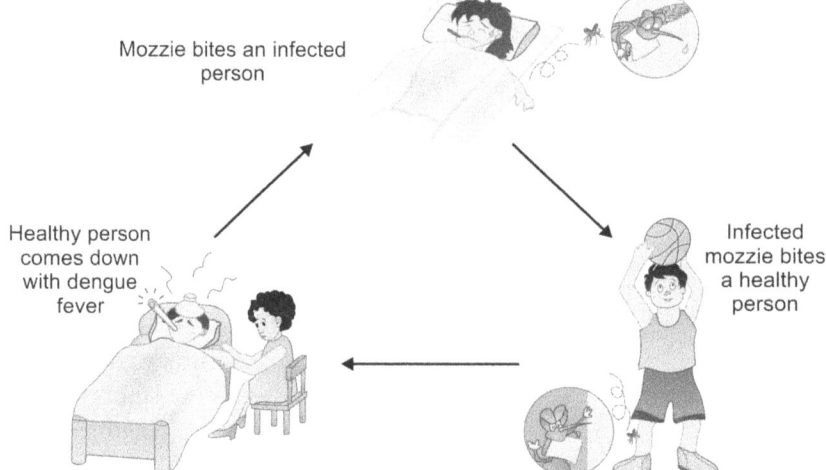

Fig. 13.6: Depicts pathogenesis of dengue fever.

- Being a neonate or young child
- Being females
- High body mass index
- Diabetes
- Asthma.

Pathophysiology

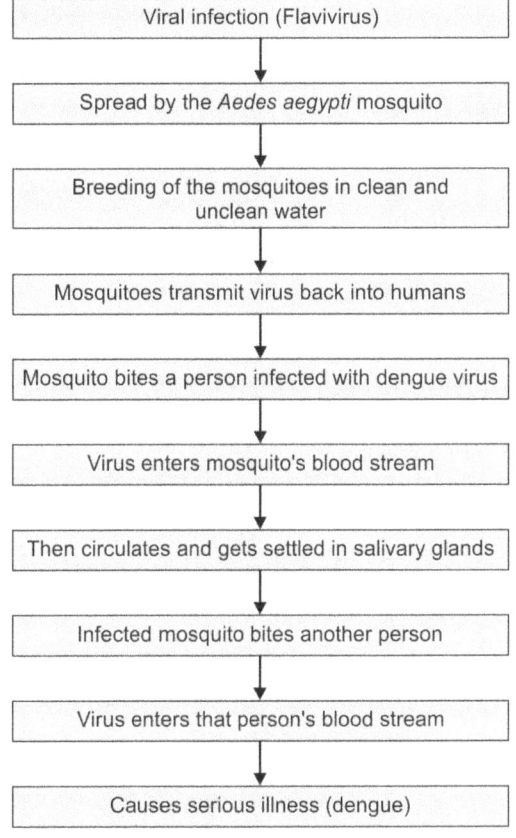

Clinical Features

- Sudden onset of severe headache
- Muscle and joint pains (Myalgia and arthralgia)
- Fever
- Appearance of bright red petechial rashes appearing first on the lower limbs and the chest and then they spread to cover most of the body.
- Bleeding gums
- Severe pain behind the eyes
- Red palms and soles
- Gastritis
- Severe abdominal pain
- Nausea
- Persistent vomiting
- Diarrhea
- Thrombocytopenia
- Sore throat
- Nasal stuffiness
- Cough
- Difficulty in breathing
- Swollen lymph nodes
- Fatigue.

Complications

- Dengue shock syndrome
- Liver damage
- Blood vessel damage
- Severe bleeding
- Sudden drop in blood pressure
- Brain damage
- Febrile convulsions
- Severe dehydration
- Death.

Diagnostic Tests

- History
- Physical examination
- Blood examination
- Antibody titer
- Polymerase chain reaction test
- Positive tourniquet test
- Liver function test.

Management

Medical

The mainstay of treatment is timely supportive therapy to tackle shock due to hemo-concentration and bleeding.

- **Supplementation with intravenous fluids:** It helps in preventing dehydration and significant concentration of the blood if the patient is unable to maintain the oral intake.
- **Platelet transfusion:** When the platelet level drops significantly below 20,000 or if there is significant bleeding.
- **Acetaminophen:** It helps to relieve from pain and fever. For example, tylenol, etc.

- **Paracetamol preparations:** It helps in relieving the patient from the symptoms of pain and fever. For example, Crocin, Dolo, etc.
- **Immunosuppressant agents:** It inhibits dengue replication. For example, mycophenolic acid, ribavirin, etc.

Nursing

- Recommend to the patient to take increased oral fluid intake to prevent dehydration.
- Instruct the patient to wear long-sleeved shirts, long pants, socks and shoes when they go into mosquito-infested areas.
- Encourage the patients to use mosquito repellants.
- Instruct the patient to travel during periods of minimal mosquito activity.

DIPHTHERIA

Definition

Diphtheria is an acute infectious disease of humans that affects the upper respiratory tract caused by the bacterium *Corynebacterium diphtheriae*. This disease primarily affects the mucous membranes of the respiratory tract (respiratory diphtheria), although it may also affect the skin (cutaneous diphtheria) and lining tissues in the ear, eye, and the genital areas.

Etiology

Bacterial infection (*Corynebacterium diphtheriae*).

Risk Factors

- Undernourished people
- People who have a compromised immune system
- People living in crowded or unsanitary conditions
- Children and adults who do not have up-to-date immunizations.
- Anyone who travels to an area where diphtheria is endemic.
- Being women
- Individuals addicted to alcohol and illicit drug users
- Homosexual men
- Old age.

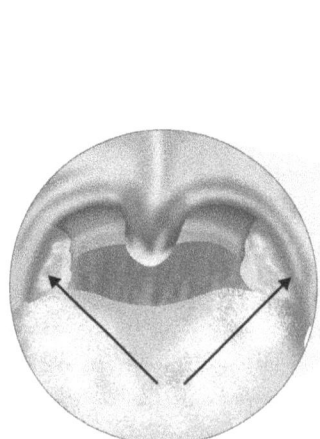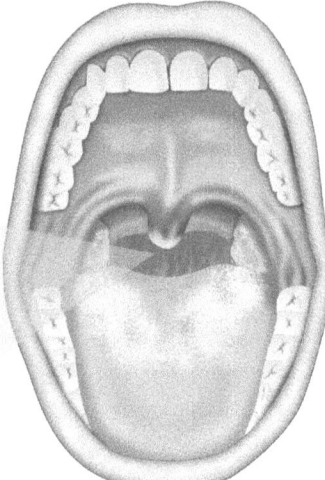

Fig. 13.7: Diphtheria.

Pathophysiology

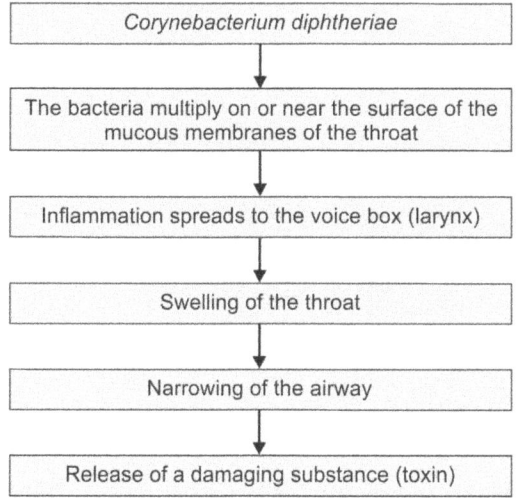

Clinical Features

- Sore throat
- Fever and chills
- Swollen glands in the neck
- Malaise
- Hoarseness
- Nasal discharge
- Painful swallowing
- Difficulty in breathing.

Complications

- Myocarditis
- Congestive cardiac failure
- Heart valve infection
- Heart rhythm disturbance
- Paralysis of the palate
- Vision problems
- Muscle weakness
- Nonhealing skin cancer
- Bone infection
- Localized infection
- Death.

Diagnostic Tests

- History
- Physical examination
- Throat culture
- Blood examination
- ECG.

Management

Medical

- **Antibiotics:** It helps to eradicate the bacteria, thereby stopping toxin production, and also it helps to prevent transmission of diphtheria to close contacts. For example, penicillin, erythromycin, etc.
- **Antitoxin:** It neutralizes the diphtheria toxin already circulating in the body. For example, diphtheria antitoxin, etc.

Nursing

- Instruct to the patient the importance of vaccination in prevention of diphtheria.
- Encourage the patient to take booster dose immunization when needed.
- Encourage the patient to practice strict hygienic techniques.

EBOLA VIRUS DISEASE

Definition

Ebola virus disease (EVD) is a viral hemorrhagic fever of humans and other primates caused by Ebola viruses.

Etiology

Viral infection (Ebola virus).

Risk Factors

- Travel to Africa
- Those who conduct animal research
- Attending burial ceremonies of someone who has died from Ebola
- Exposure to infected objects, such as needles
- Those who provide medical or personal care to family members
- Traveling to areas where a recent outbreak has occurred.

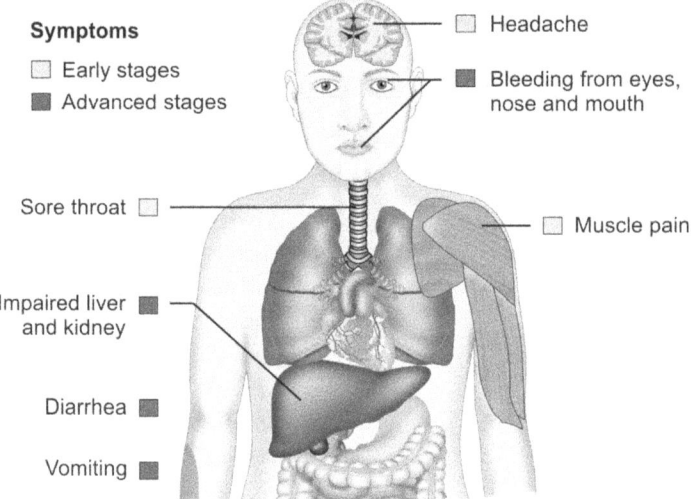

Fig. 13.8: Shows the cardinal features of Ebola virus disease.

Pathophysiology

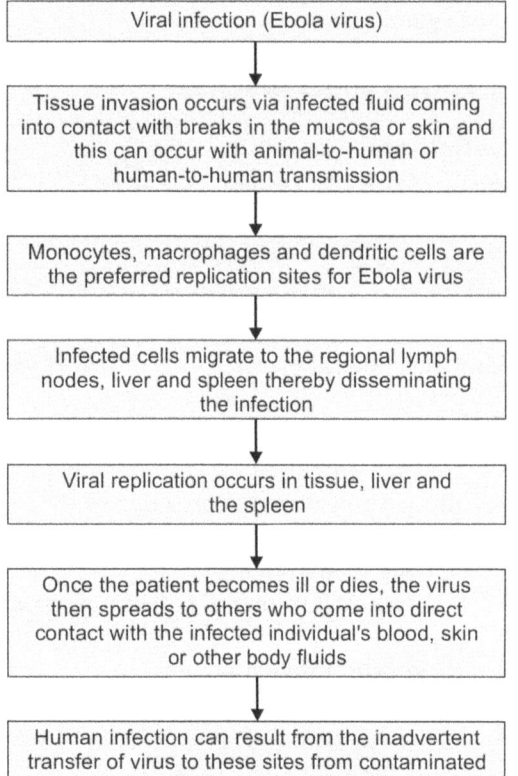

Clinical Features

Initial Symptoms are Flu-like and may Include

- Muscle aches and pains
- Sore throat
- Headaches.

Illness then Progresses with Symptoms such as

- Bleeding from eyes, nose and mouth
- Impaired liver and kidney
- Vomiting
- Diarrhea.

Other Features Include

- Sudden onset of fever
- Confusion
- Rash
- Cough
- Extreme tiredness and collapse.

Complications

- Multiple organ failure
- Severe bleeding
- Jaundice
- Delirium

- Seizures
- Coma
- Shock.

Diagnostic Tests

- History
- Physical examination
- ELISA test
- Blood examination
- Virus isolation
- Polymerase chain reaction test.

Management

Medical

The mainstay of treatment for Ebola virus disease involves supportive care to maintain adequate cardiovascular function while the immune system mobilizes an adaptive response to eliminate the infection.

- **Fluid and electrolyte replacement:** It can be administered orally or intravenously depending upon the stage of illness and the clinical presentation and may assist in guiding volume replacement in the absence of more accurate measures. For example, 0.9% sodium chloride solution, etc.
- **Respiratory support:** Invasive mechanical ventilation (intubation) is the best option for patients with progressive respiratory failure.
- **Antibiotics:** It covers against common respiratory pathogens as per guidelines for community-acquired or nososcomial pneumonia. For example, levofloxacin, quinolones, macrolides, etc.
- **Antiviral agents (Nucleoside analog agents):** It inhibits the coronaviral proteases, thus blocking the processing of the viral replicase polyprotein and preventing the replication of viral DNA. For example, ribavirin, oseltamivir phosphate, lopinavir, etc.
- **Antipyretic agents:** It decreases fever associated with Ebola virus disease. For example, paracetamol, acetaminophen, etc.
- **Antimotility agents:** It helps to control diarrhea and decreases fluid and electrolyte losses. For example, loperamide, etc.
- **Antiemetics:** It helps in controlling nausea and vomiting. For example, dramamine, bonine, etc.

Nursing

- Instruct them to avoid areas in which infections have been reported and suspected.
- Avoid direct contact with infected people.
- Instruct the patient to avoid wild-caught bushmeat.
- Isolate patients with Ebola from others.
- Teach proper infection control and sterilization techniques to everyone related to patients.
- Instruct them not to handle items that may have come in contact with an infected person's blood or body fluids.

FILARIASIS

Definition

Filariasis is a parasitic infection caused by thread-like nematodes (filariae) that belong to the roundworm superfamily filarioidea which results in an altered lymphatic system and the abnormal enlargement of body parts, causing pain, severe disability and social stigma.

Etiology

Parasitic infection (*Wuchereria bancrofti*).

Risk Factors

- Residence in tropical or subtropical areas where the disease is endemic
- Poor mosquito control and an infected population within an area
- Person on long-term work assignments like humanitarian workers, missionaries and military personnel.
- Presence of water-holding containers in and around.
- Poverty or cultural practices
- High body mass index.

Communicable Diseases

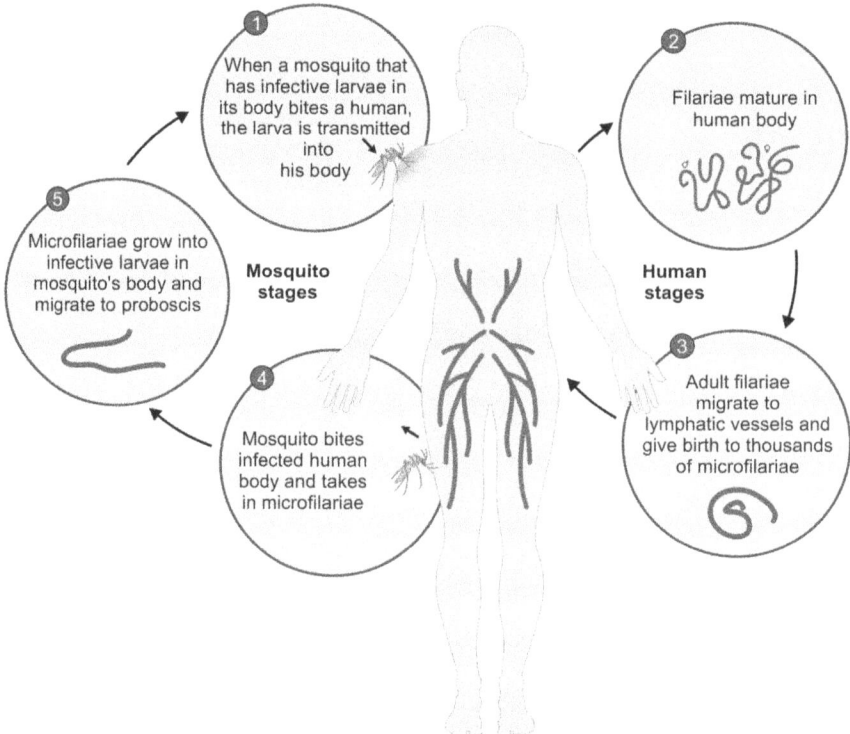

Fig. 13.9: Depicts pathogenesis of filariasis.

Pathophysiology

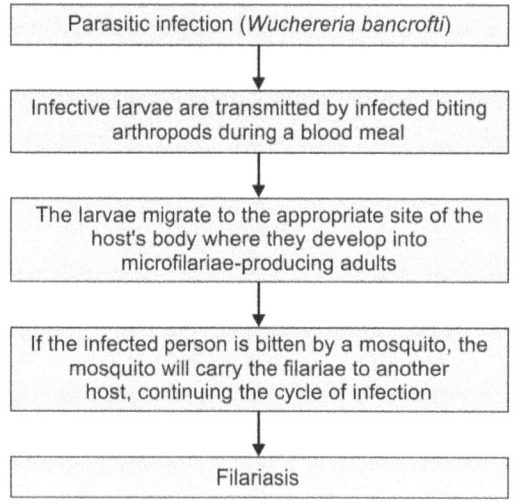

Clinical Features

- Fever with chills
- Enlargement of the lymph nodes
- Swelling in the area where the adult worms are present
- Muscle aches and pains
- Photophobia
- Headache
- Vertigo
- Fatigue
- Excessive sweating
- Nausea with or without vomiting.

Complications

- Elephantiasis
- Cellulitis
- Lymphangitis
- Fibrosis of the affected tissue
- Severe pain
- Kidney damage
- Gross disfigurement
- Sexual dysfunction
- Venous thrombosis.

Diagnostic Tests

- History
- Physical examination
- Finger prick test
- Blood examination
- Polymerase chain reaction (PCR)
- Magnetic resonance imaging (MRI)
- Computed tomography (CT) scan
- DEC provocation test.

Management

Medical

- **Antibiotics:** It helps to prevent secondary infections. For example, azithromycin, doxycycline, erythromycin, etc.
- **Anthelmintics:** It is used in the treatment of lymphatic filariasis by killing the circulating microfilariae in the blood. For example, diethylcarbamazine, etc.

Nursing

- Encourage the patient to sleep under a mosquito net.
- Encourage the patient to use insect repellant on exposed skin between dusk and dawn.
- Instruct the patient wear long sleeves, long trousers, closed footwear and socks.
- Instruct the patient to elevate and exercise the swollen arm or leg to move the fluid and improve the lymph flow.

GONORRHEA

Definition

Gonorrhea is a sexually transmitted bacterial infection caused by the organism *Neisseria gonorrhoeae* that is transmitted by sexual contact.

Etiology

Bacterial infection (*Neisseria gonorrhoeae*).

Risk Factors

- Younger age
- New sex partner
- Multiple sex partners
- Previous gonorrhea diagnosis
- Having other sexually transmitted infections
- Vaginal or anal sex with an infected partner
- Very close physical contact
- From mother to her baby at birth
- Inconsistent use of barrier methods.

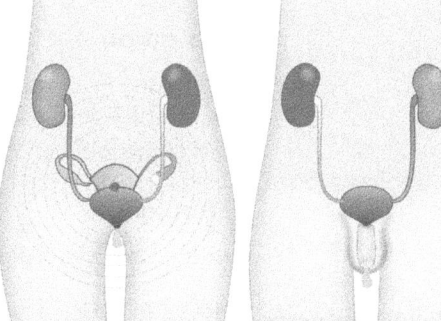

Fig. 13.10: Gonorrhea: Signs and symptoms.

Pathophysiology

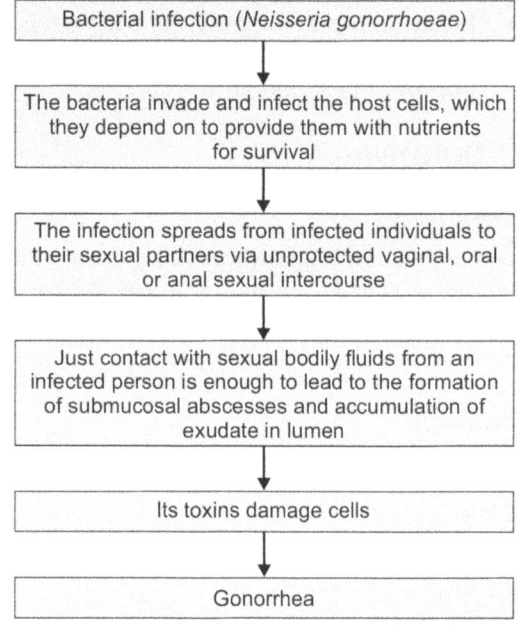

Clinical Features

In Women

- Yellowish vaginal discharge
- Abnormal vaginal bleeding
- Low abdominal or pelvic tenderness
- Burning or frequent urination
- Redness and swelling of the genitals
- Burning or itching of the vaginal area
- Inflammation of the fallopian tubes and ovaries
- Painful infection of the pelvis (fever, pelvic cramping, abdominal pain, and pain during intercourse).

In Men

- White, yellow or green thick discharge from the tip of the penis
- Inflammation of the testicles and prostate gland
- Irritation or discharge from the anus
- Urethral itch and pain or burning sensation when passing urine.

Complications

- Infertility in women
- Infertility in men
- Infection that spreads to the joints and other parts of the body
- Increased risk of HIV/AIDS
- Blindness may develop among babies.

Diagnostic Tests

- History
- Physical examination
- Urine testing
- Swab test of the affected area.

Management

Medical

Antibiotics: It helps to prevent secondary infections. For example, ciprofloxacin, levaquin, tequin, etc.

Nursing

- Educate the patient to abstain from sex in order to prevent the occurrence of gonorrhea and is the best possible way of prevention.
- Encourage the patient to use condom during sexual encounters.
- Instruct the patient partner also to have diagnostic tests.
- Instruct the patient to avoid having sex with someone who has unusual symptoms.
- Instruct the patient to have regular screening test for gonorrhea.

INFLUENZA

Definition

Influenza is a viral infection that attacks our respiratory system—the nose, throat and lungs. It is commonly known as flu.

Etiology

Influenza virus types A and B.

Risk Factors

- Young children
- Old adults
- Healthcare workers
- Weakened immune system
- Chronic illnesses
- Pregnancy.

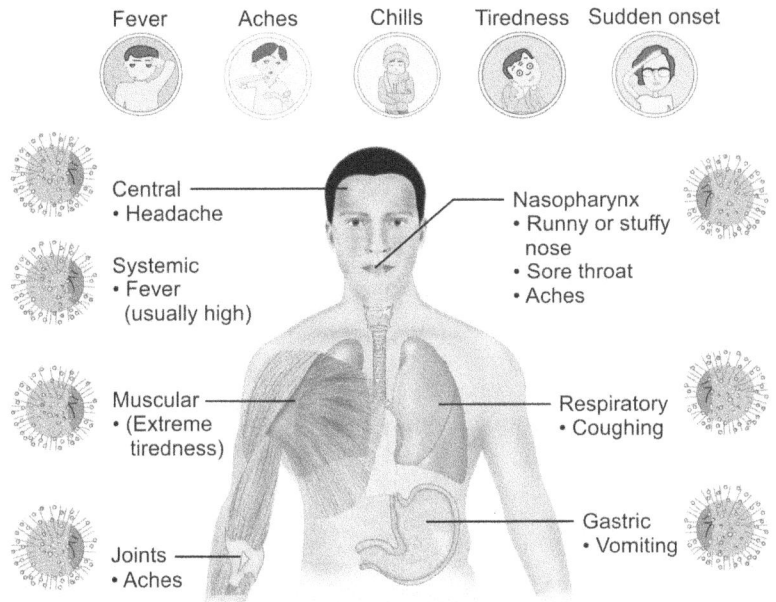

Fig. 13.11: Symptoms of influenza.

Pathophysiology

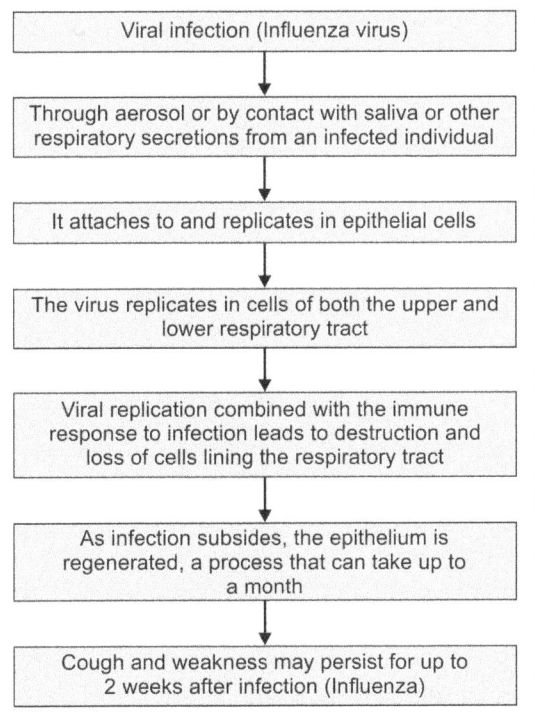

Clinical Features

- Common cold with a running nose
- Sore throat
- Sneezing
- Fever over 100° Fahrenheit
- Chill and sweat
- Headache
- Dry cough
- Muscle ache especially in back, arms and legs
- Fatigue
- Weakness
- Nasal congestion.

Complications

- Pneumonia
- Bronchitis
- Sinus infections
- Ear infections.

Diagnostic Tests

- History
- Physical examination

- Blood examination
- Viral tissue cell culture
- Rapid molecular assay test.

Management

Medical

- **Antiviral agents:** It helps in preventing the serious complications and also it shortens the illness by a day or so. For example, oseltamivir (tamiflu), zanamivir (relenza), amantadine, etc.
- **Acetaminophen:** It helps to combat the achiness associated with influenza. For example, tylenol, ibuprofen, etc.

Nursing

- Encourage the patient to drink plenty of fluids.
- Avoid sharing food, utensils, cups or bottles.
- Instruct the patient to take adequate rest to help their immune system fight infection.
- Encourage thorough and frequent hand-washing with alcohol based-hand sanitizers among patients to prevent infections.
- Ask them to cover their mouth with a tissue when coughing and throw it away after use.
- Instruct them to avoid touching their eyes, nose and mouth.

JAPANESE ENCEPHALITIS (JE)

Definition

Japanese encephalitis (JE) is a mosquito-borne zoonotic viral disease caused by arbovirus (flavivirus), involving the central nervous system.

Etiology

- *Aedes aegypti* mosquito
- Viral infection (Flavivirus).

Risk Factors

- Residence in tropical or subtropical areas where the disease is endemic
- Poor mosquito control and an infected population within an area
- Person on long-term work assignments like humanitarian workers, missionaries and military personnel

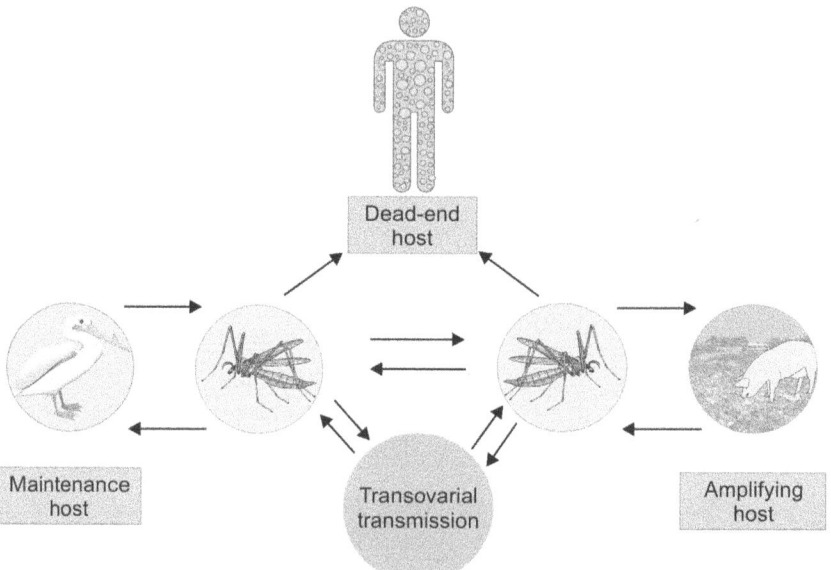

Fig. 13.12: Depicts pathogenesis of japanese encephalitis.

- Presence of water-holding containers in and around
- Poverty or cultural practices
- High body mass index.

Pathophysiology

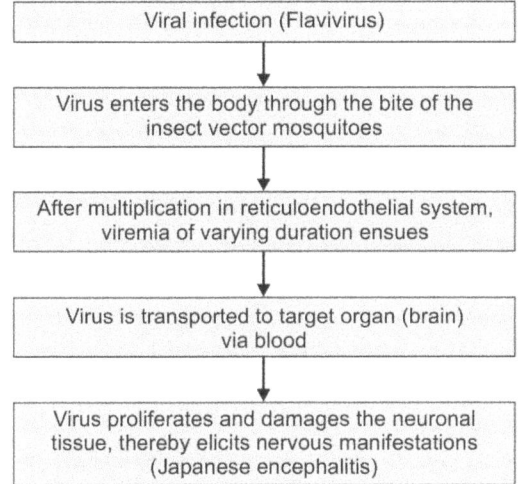

Clinical Features

- High fever with rigors
- Involuntary movements
- Altered sensorium
- Headache
- Sleepiness
- Lack of normal activity
- Neck stiffness
- Difference in movements on both sides of the body
- Vacant look (starring look)
- Wide-open eyes
- Convulsions
- Hyperventilation
- Marked loss of weight.

Complications

- Acute encephalitis
- Paralysis
- Seizures
- Coma
- Death.

Diagnostic Tests

- History
- Physical examination
- Cerebrospinal fluid (CSF) examination
- Blood examination
- Reverse transcription polymerase chain reaction (RT-PCR) test
- Routine viral culture.

Management

Medical

- **Immunization agent:** It works by exposing to a small dose of the virus that causes the body to develop immunity to the disease. For example, ixiaro, etc.
- **Osmotic diuretics:** It decreases intracranial pressure through reducing subarachnoid space pressure by creating an osmotic gradient between CSF in the arachnoid space and plasma. For example, mannitol, etc.
- **Acetaminophen (Paracetamol):** It helps to combat the achiness associated with influenza. For example, tylenol, ibuprofen, etc.
- **Antimalarial agents:** It inhibits the glutathione-dependent destruction of ferriprotoporphyrin IX in the malaria parasite resulting in the accumulation of this peptide which is toxic for the parasite. For example, quinine, artesunate, etc.

Nursing

- Encourage the patient to sleep under a mosquito net.
- Encourage the patient to use insect repellant on exposed skin between dusk and dawn.
- Instruct the patient wear long sleeves, long trousers, closed footwear and socks.
- Instruct the patient to elevate and exercise the swollen arm or leg to move the fluid and improve the lymph flow.

KALA-AZAR (VISCERAL LEISHMANIASIS)

Definition
Kala-azar is a group of parasitic diseases caused by protozoan flagellates of the genus *Leishmania*, transmitted through the infective bite of an insect vector, the phlebotomine sand fly.

Etiology
- Parasitic infection (*Leishmania donovani*)
- Female phlebotomine sandfly.

Risk Factors
- Poor housing and domestic sanitary conditions
- Sleeping outside or on the ground
- Malnutrition
- Population mobility
- Environmental and climate change
- Young children
- Travellers who are nonimmune
- Being male
- Immunodeficient persons.

Pathophysiology

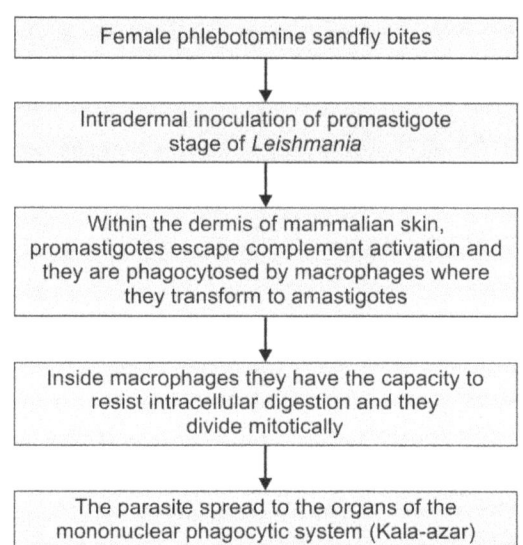

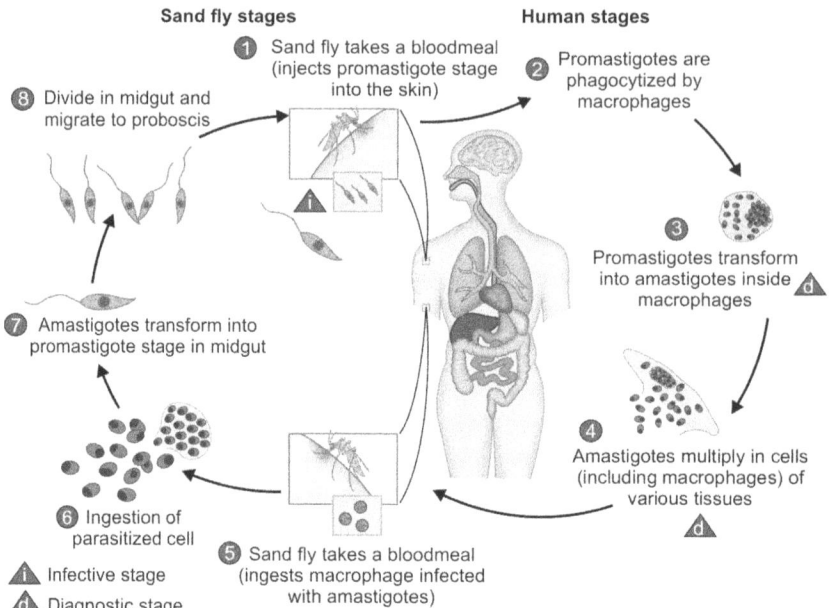

Fig. 13.13: Depicts pathogenesis of kala-azar.

Clinical Features

- Fatigue
- Weakness
- Cough
- Loss of appetite
- Fever that lasts for weeks
- Enlarged spleen
- Enlarged liver
- Decreased production of red blood cells (RBCs)
- Night sweating
- Vomiting
- Abdominal discomfort (Diarrhea)
- Thinning hair
- Scaly, grey, dark, ashen skin
- Weight loss.

Complications

- Bleeding (hemorrhage)
- Deadly infections due to immune system damage
- Disfigurement of the face.

Diagnostic Tests

- History
- Physical examination
- Dipstick test
- Blood examination
- Biopsy of the spleen and culture
- Bone marrow biopsy and culture
- Direct agglutination assay
- Indirect immunofluorescent antibody test
- *Leishmania*-specific PCR test
- Liver biopsy and culture
- Lymph node biopsy and culture.

Management

Medical

- **Pentavalent antimonials:** It directly inhibits DNA topoisomerase I leading to inhibition of both DNA replication and transcription of *Leishmania donovani*. For example, meglumine antimoniate, sodium stibogluconate, etc.
- **Antifungal agents:** It inhibits the growth of *Leishmania* donovani in a liquid medium. For example, amphotericin B, etc.
- **Alkylphospholipid derivatives:** It works by inhibiting in vitro activity against the promastigote and amastigote stages of *Leishmania* species. Miltefosine, etc.
- **Aminoglycoside antibiotics:** It works by stopping the growth of parasites in the intestines. For example, paromomycin, etc.
- **Azoles:** It results in inhibition of ergosterol synthesis and increased fungal cellular permeability. For example, ketoconazole, fluconazole, itraconazole, etc.
- **Aminoquinoline analog:** It inhibits heme polymerase activity and this results in accumulation of free heme, which is toxic to the parasites. For example, sitamaquine, etc.
- **Aromatic diamidine:** For example, pentamidine, etc. It interferes with nuclear metabolism producing inhibition of the synthesis of DNA, RNA, phospholipids, and proteins of *Leishmania* species.

Nursing

- Instruct the patient to wear clothes that cover the skin as much as possible.
- Encourage the patient to use insect repellant on exposed skin between dusk and dawn.
- Instruct the patient to put fine mesh netting around the bed.
- Ask the patient to screen the windows to prevent sandfly bites.

LEPROSY (HANSEN'S DISEASE)

Definition

Leprosy is a chronic infection caused by the bacteria *Mycobacterium leprae*, an acid fast, rod-shaped bacillus.

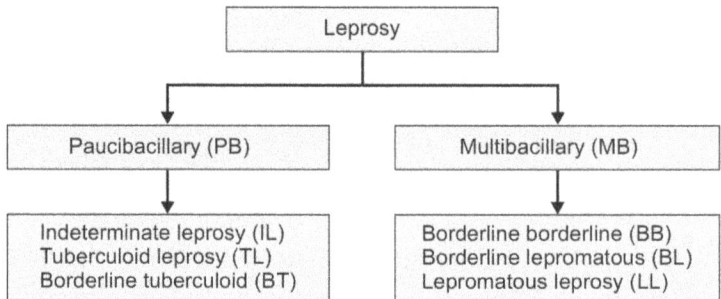

Etiology

Bacterial infection (*Mycobacterium leprae*).

Risk Factors

- Close contacts among patients with leprosy untreated
- Being children
- Persons living in countries with highly endemic disease
- It is more common among warm, wet areas in the tropics and subtropics.

Types

It has six classifications based on severity of symptoms. They are as follows:

1. ***Indeterminate***
   - It is the earliest and mildest form of the disease.
   - Few numbers of hypopigmented macules (cutaneous lesions) may occur.
   - Loss of sensation is rare.
   - Most cases progress into a later form, although patients with strong immunity may either clear the infection on their own or persist in this form without progressing.
2. ***Tuberculoid***
   - Can be either one large red patch with well-defined raised borders or a large hypopigmented asymmetrical spot
   - Lesions become dry and hairless
   - Loss of sensation may occur at site of some lesions
   - Tender, thickened nerves with subsequent loss of function are common.
   - Spontaneous resolution may occur in a few years or it may progress to borderline or rarely lepromatous types.
3. ***Borderline tuberculoid***
   - Similar to tuberculoid type except that lesions are smaller and more numerous.
   - Disease may stay in this stage or convert back to tuberculoid form, or progress.
4. ***Borderline borderline***
   - Numerous, red, irregularly shaped plaques
   - Sensory loss is moderate
   - Disease may stay in this stage, improve or worsen.
5. ***Borderline lepromatous***
   - Numerous lesions of all kinds, plaques, macules, papules and nodules. Lesions looking like inverted saucers are common.
   - Hair growth and sensation are usually not impaired over the lesions.
6. ***Lepromatous***
   - Early nerve involvement may go unnoticed.
   - Numerous lesions of all kinds, plaques, macules, papules and nodules
   - Early symptoms include nasal stuffiness, discharge and bleeding, and swelling of the legs and ankles.
   - If left untreated, the following problems may occur:
     - Skin thickens over forehead (leonine facies), eyebrows and eyelashes are lost, nose becomes misshapen or collapses, earlobes thicken, upper incisor teeth fall out.

- Eye involvement causing photophobia (light sensitivity), glaucoma and blindness.
- Skin on legs thickens and forms ulcers when nodules break down.
- Internal organ infection causing enlarged liver and lymph nodes.
- Slow scarring of peripheral nerves resulting in nerve thickening and sensory loss.
- Fingers and toes become deformed due to painless repeated trauma.

Pathophysiology

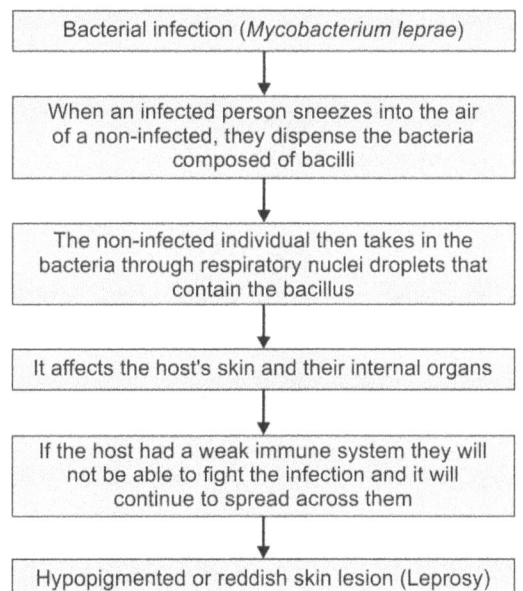

Clinical Features

- Appearance of white patches on the skin
- Loss of sensation in the affected areas
- Thick, stiffy or dry skin
- Severe pain
- Growths on the skin
- Muscle weakness or paralysis (especially in the hands and feet)
- Enlarged nerves
- A stuffy nose
- Nose bleeds
- Eye problems that may lead to blindness
- Ulcers on the soles of feet.

Complications

- Disfigurement
- Muscle weakness
- Permanent nerve damage in the arms and legs
- Sensory loss.

Diagnostic Tests

- History
- Physical examination
- Tissue biopsy or scraping
- Lepromin skin test.

Management

Medical

- **Dapsone:** It inhibits bacterial growth by preventing formation of folic acid. For example, avlosulfon, etc.
- **Rifampin:** It inhibits DNA-dependent bacterial RNA polymerase. For example, rifadin, rimactane, etc.
- **Clofazimine:** It inhibits mycobacterial growth, binds preferentially to mycobacterial DNA. For example, lamprene, etc.
- **Fluoroquinolones:** It exerts their antibacterial effect by preventing bacterial DNA from unwinding and duplicating. For example, ofloxacin, etc.
- **Macrolides:** It inhibits bacterial protein synthesis. For example, azithromycin, erythromycin, etc.
- **Minocycline:** It exerts antimicrobial effect by the inhibition of protein synthesis. For example, dynacin, minocin, etc.
- **Aspirin:** It helps to combat the achiness associated with leprosy. For example, tylenol, ibuprofen, etc.
- **Prednisone:** It helps to reduce the severity of the leprosy by suppressing the immune factor that mistakenly attacks its own tissues. For example, prednisone, etc.
- **Thalidomide:** It inhibits release of tumor necrosis factor alpha from monocytes,

and modulates other cytokine action. For example, thalomid, etc.

Nursing

- Instruct to avoid contacts with body fluids and the rashes of people who have leprosy.
- Encourage them to go for improvements in living conditions to assist in reducing the occurrence of leprosy.
- Teach and encourage early detection and treatment of leprosy and promote awareness among individuals.
- Encourage the individual to opt for specialized footwear.
- Tell patients and their families that leprosy is curable, and the drugs help stop the disease from spreading.

LEPTOSPIROSIS

(Also known as canicola fever, hemorrhagic jaundice, infectious jaundice, mud fever, spirochetal jaundice, swamp fever, Sewerman's flu).

Definition

Leptospirosis is an infectious disease of humans and animals that is caused by pathogenic spirochetes of the genus *Leptospira*.

Etiology

Bacterial infection (*Leptospira interrogans*).

Risk Factors

- Traveling abroad
- Sewage workers
- Farmers
- Veterinarians
- Slaughterhouse workers
- Rodent control workers
- Freshwater swimming
- Domesticated livestock
- Military personnel
- Pet dogs.

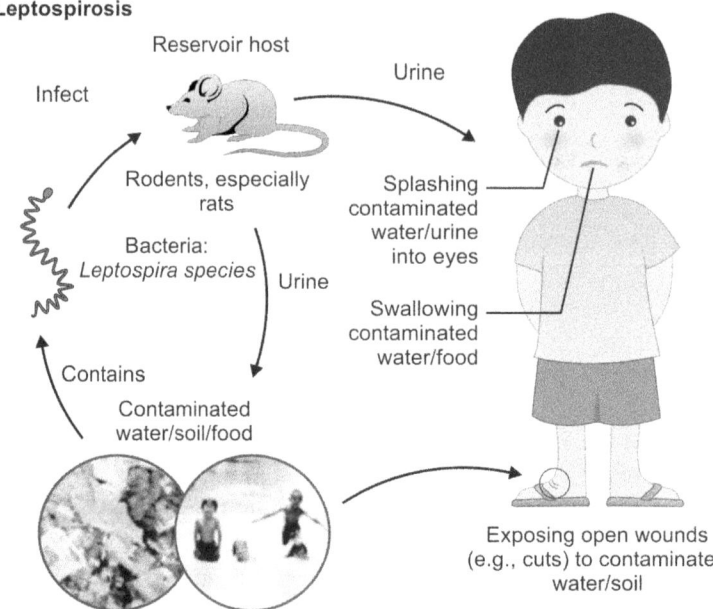

Fig. 13.14: Depicts pathogenesis of leptospirosis.

Pathophysiology

```
The bacteria enter a host via portals such as
damaged skin, certain mucus membranes,
the lungs and conjunctival membranes
            ↓
Once within the host tissues, pathogenic strains
can reproduce as they are optimized for
metabolism at body temperatures
            ↓
Their survival depends on the lack of an effective
host immune response
            ↓
The bacteria that survive entry and the immediate
innate response will rapidly migrate to the
bloodstream and lymphatic system and spread
throughout the host body within a very short time
            ↓
Virulent strains are rapidly removed by the
immune system, but the speed of spread is far
higher than in other bacterial infections and
a host can show leptospira within blood samples
in a matter of minutes from exposure
            ↓
Pathogenic bacteria reproduce by binary fission,
so the colony increases exponentially and the
typical doubling time is 8 hours
            ↓
The growth continues unchecked until the adaptive
immune response develops or the host dies
```

Clinical Features

- Headache
- Myalgia particularly associated with the calf muscles and lumbar region
- Fever (38–40° Celsius)
- Chills
- Arthralgia
- Conjunctival suffusion
- Meningeal irritation
- Anuria or oliguria
- Jaundice
- Hemorrhages (from the intestines and lungs)
- Cardiac arrhythmia or failure
- Skin rash
- Gastrointestinal symptoms such as nausea, vomiting, abdominal pain, diarrhea, etc.
- Dry cough.

Complications

- Jarisch-Herxheimer reaction when penicillin is given
- Meningitis
- Acute kidney injury
- Severe pulmonary hemorrhagic syndrome
- Hepatic dysfunction
- Thrombocytopenia.

Diagnostic Tests

- History
- Physical examination
- Cerebrospinal fluid examination
- Blood tests
- Kidney function test
- Enzyme-linked immunosorbent assay (ELISA) test
- Polymerase chain reaction (PCR)
- MAT (Microscopic agglutination test) serological test.

Management

Medical

- **Antibiotics:** It inhibits bacterial cell wall synthesis by binding and inactivating proteins present in the bacterial cell wall. For example, penicillin G, ampicillin, amoxicillin, doxycycline, cefotaxime, ceftriaxone, etc.
- **Oral corticosteroids:** It helps to reduce the severity of the leptospirosis by suppressing the immune factor that mistakenly attacks its own tissues. For example, prednisolone, dexamethasone, etc.

Nursing

- Instruct people to avoid rodent populations by preventing rodent access into the buildings.
- Educate people to wash hands after any contact with natural water or after handling any animals.

- Educate people that the risk of infection can be greatly reduced by not swimming or wading in water that might be contaminated with animal urine.
- Educate that there is no human vaccine available against leptospirosis.
- Instruct them to wear protective clothing (rubber boots, gloves, goggles) when exposure is unavoidable.

MALARIA

Definition

Malaria is a life-threatening disease caused by parasites (*Plasmodium*) that are transmitted to people through the bites of infected female Anopheles mosquitoes.

Etiology

- Parasitic infection (*Plasmodium vivax*)
- Female Anopheles mosquitoes.

Risk Factors

- Residence in tropical or subtropical areas where the disease is endemic
- Poor mosquito control and an infected population within an area
- Mobile populations
- Presence of water-holding containers in and around
- Nonimmune migrants
- Infants
- Children under 5 years of age
- Pregnant women
- Patients with HIV/AIDS
- Travellers.

Stages of Malaria

There are three stages in malaria. The two first stages take place exclusively into the human body, while the third one starts in the human body and is completed into the mosquito organism. They are as follows:

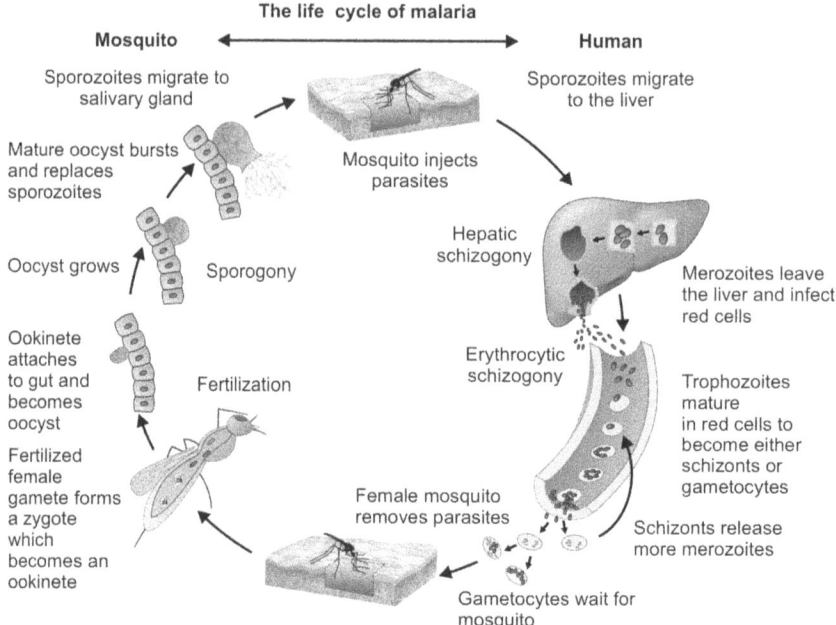

Fig. 13.15: Depicts pathogenesis of malaria.

1. ***Infectious phase (infection of a human with sporozoites):*** The human infection begins when an infected female Anopheles mosquito bites a person and injects infected with sporozoites saliva into the blood circulation. That is the first life stage of plasmodium (stage of infection).
2. ***Exo-erythrocytic and erythrocytic phase (asexual reproduction):*** The next stage in malaria life cycle is the one of asexual reproduction that is divided into different phases: the pre-erythrocytic (or better, exo-erythrocytic) and the erythrocytic phase. Within only 30-60 minutes after the parasites inoculation, sporozoites find their way through blood circulation to their first target, the liver. The sporozoites enter the liver cells and start dividing leading to schizonts creation in 6-7 days. Each schizont gives birth to thousands of merozoites (exo-erythrocytic schizogony) that are then released into the blood stream marking the end of the exo-erythrocytic phase of the asexual reproductive stage.
3. ***Sporogonic cycle (sexual reproduction):*** Merozoites released into the blood stream, are directed towards their second target, the red blood cells (RBCs). As they invade into the cells, they mark the beginning of the erythrocytic phase. The first stage after invasion is a ring stage that evolves into a trophozoite. The trophozoites are not able to digest the haem so they convert it in hemozoin and digest the globin that is used as a source of amino acids for their reproduction. The next cellular stage is the erythrocytic schizont (initially immature and then mature schizont). Each mature schizont gives birth to new generation merozoites (erythrocytic schizogony) that, after RBCs rupture, are released in the blood stream in order to invade other RBCs. This is when parasitemia occurs and clinical manifestations appear. The liver phase occurs only once while the erythrocytic phase undergoes multiple cycles; the merozoites release after each cycle creates the febrile waves. A second scenario into the RBCs is the parasite differentiation into male and female gametocytes that is a nonpathogenic form of parasite. When a female anopheles mosquito bites an infected person, it takes up these gametocytes with the bloodmeal (mosquitoes can be infected only if they have a meal during the period that gametocytes circulate in the human's blood). The gametocytes, then, mature and become microgametes (male) and macrogametes (female) during a process known as gametogenesis. The time needed for the gametocytes to mature differs for each plasmodium species: 3-4 days for *P. vivax* and *P. ovale*, 6-8 days for *P. malariae* and 8-10 days for *P. falciparum*. In the mosquito gut, the microgamete nucleus divides three times producing eight nuclei; each nucleus fertilizes a macrogamete forming a zygote. The zygote, after the fusion of nuclei and the fertilization, becomes the so-called ookinete. The ookinete, then penetrates the midgut wall of the mosquito, where it encysts into a formation called oocyst. Inside the oocyst, the ookinete nucleus divides to produce thousands of sporozoites (sporogony). That is the end of the third stage (stage of sexual reproduction/sporogony). Sporogony lasts 8-15 days. The oocyst ruptures and the sporozoites are released inside the mosquito cavity and find their way to its salivary glands but only few hundreds of sporozoites manage to enter. Thus, when the above-mentioned infected mosquito takes a bloodmeal, it injects its infected saliva into the next victim marking the beginning of a new cycle.

Pathophysiology

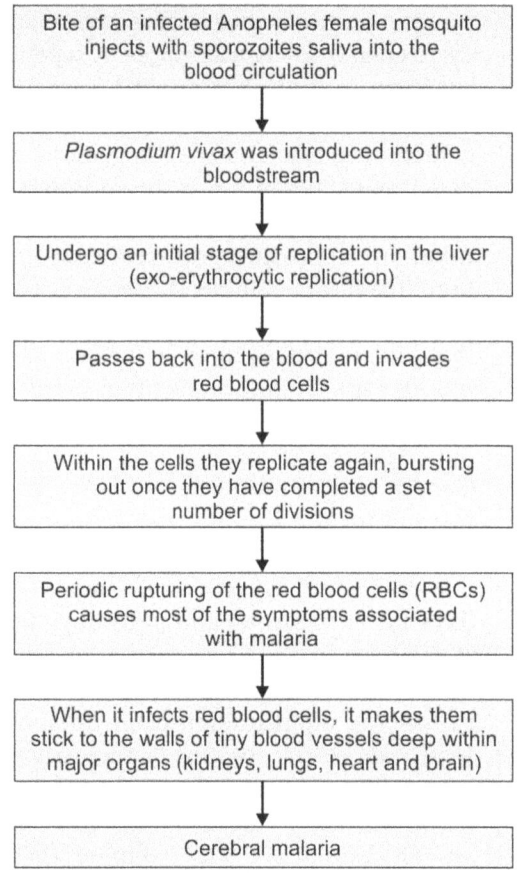

Clinical Features

- High fever with chills
- Profuse sweating
- Headache
- Nausea
- Vomiting
- Diarrhea
- Muscle pain
- Convulsions
- Coma
- Bloody stools.

Complications

- Respiratory distress
- Cerebral malaria
- Organ failure of kidneys, liver or spleen
- Anemia due to destruction of red blood cells (RBCs)
- Low blood sugar
- Shock.

Diagnostic Tests

- History
- Physical examination
- Microscopic examination
- Quantitative buffy coat (QBC) test
- Indirect fluorescent antibody test (IFAT)
- Enzyme-linked immunosorbent assay (ELISA)
- Rapid diagnostic test (RDT)
- Polymerase chain reaction (PCR).

Management

Medical

- **Antimalarial agents:** It acts as blood schizonticidal and weak gametocide against the malarial parasites and helps in treating malaria. For example, chloroquine, primaquine, quinine sulfate, artesunate, mefloquine, etc.
- **Antibiotics:** It helps to prevent secondary infections. For example, clindamycin, doxycycline, erythromycin, etc.
- **Analgesics and antipyretics combination:** It helps to relieve from high fever. For example, paracetamol, etc.

Nursing

- Encourage the patient to sleep under a mosquito net.
- Encourage the patient to use insect repellant on exposed skin between dusk and dawn.
- Instruct the patient to wear clothes that cover the skin as much as possible.
- Ask the patient to screen the windows to prevent malarial parasites.
- Instruct the patient to travel during periods of minimal mosquito activity.

MEASLES (RUBEOLA)

Definition

It is a highly contagious respiratory tract infection that is caused by the paramyxovirus.

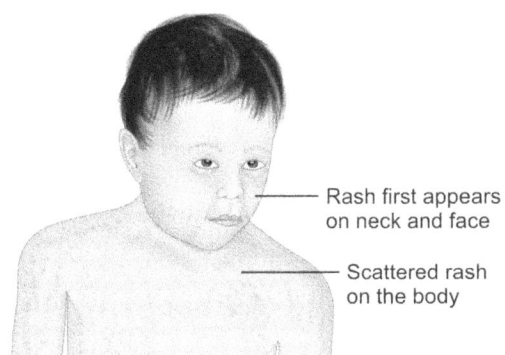

Fig. 13.16: Depicts cardinal features of measles.

Etiology

Viral infection (Paramyxovirus).

Risk Factors

- Being unvaccinated
- Having a vitamin A deficiency
- Traveling abroad
- Pregnant women
- Infants and children aged less than 5 years
- Adults aged more than 20 years
- People with compromised immune system (HIV infections, leukemia, etc).

Stages

The measles occurs in four stages as follows:
1. **Incubation stage:** It generally lasts from 10 to 14 days. During this stage, patients do not have any symptoms.
2. **Prodrome stage:** During this stage, symptoms appear. They usually begin 10-14 days after exposure. The common symptoms include: fever, fatigue, decreased appetite, red watery eyes, runny nose and cough. Other symptoms may include: vomiting, diarrhea, abdominal pain, sore throat, swollen glands and an enlarged spleen. It usually lasts 2-3 days. However, it can last up to eight days.
3. **Exanthem (rash) stage:** During this stage, a rash develops. The rash usually starts on the face and spreads to the neck, trunk, arms and legs. Often, patients will start to feel better about 48 hours after the rash appears. The rash starts to fade within 3-4 days after it appears. There may be some fine peeling of the skin after the rash fades. Patients are considered highly contagious from four days prior till four days after the onset of the rash.
4. **Recovery stage:** In this stage, cough may last for 1-2 weeks after the measles.

Pathophysiology

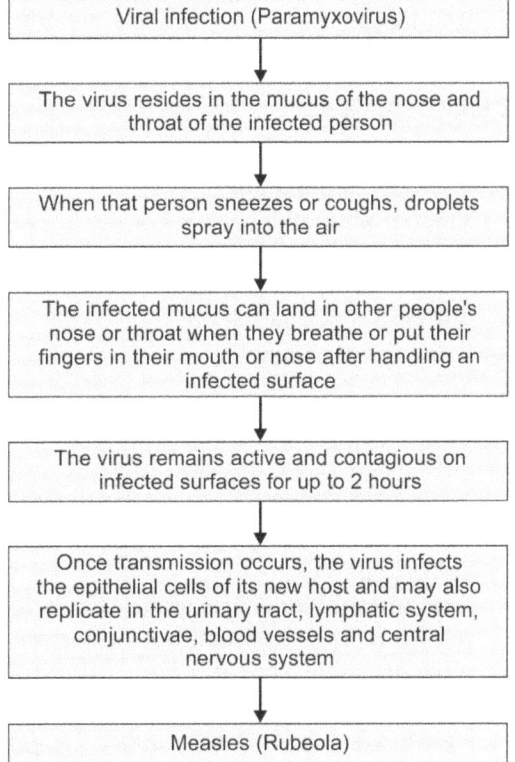

Clinical Features

- Full-body rashes (flat red spots on the forehead and slowly spread to the rest of the face, then down the neck and torso to the arms, legs and feet)
- Hacking cough
- Runny nose
- High fever (104° Fahrenheit)
- Red eyes
- Sore throat
- Muscle ache
- Koplik's spots (small red spots with blue-white centers that appear inside the mouth)
- Severe diarrhea.

Complications

- Ear infection
- Laryngitis
- Pneumonia
- Encephalitis
- Bronchitis
- Convulsions
- Thrombocytopenia
- Miscarriage or preterm labor
- Blindness
- Death.

Diagnostic Tests

- History
- Physical examination
- Blood examination
- Real-time polymerase chain reaction (RT-PCR)
- Throat swab examination
- Urine examination.

Management

Medical

- **Antibiotics:** It helps to prevent secondary infections. For example, ciprofloxacin, ceftriaxone, etc.
- **Acetaminophen (Paracetamol):** It helps to relieve fever and achiness associated with measles. For example, tylenol, ibuprofen, naproxen, etc.
- **Vitamin A supplements:** It helps to lessen the severity of the measles. For example, retinyl palmitate, retinol, etc.

Nursing

- Isolate them during and after the rash breaks out to prevent spreading to others as it is highly contagious.
- Ask them to get vaccinated for measles.
- Enforce measures to prevent resurgence of measles.
- Promote and preserve herd immunity among them.
- Ask the patient wear a mask or to cover the mouth and nose with a tissue when coughing or sneezing.
- Educate the patient not to share towels, bedding and eating utensils.
- Ask the patients to keep away from others as much as possible until the rashes come down.

MUMPS (EPIDEMIC PAROTITIS)

Definition

It is a contagious viral infection of the salivary glands that is caused by the paramyxovirus.

Etiology

Viral infection (Paramyxovirus).

Risk Factors

- Being unvaccinated
- Being infants
- Traveling abroad
- Pregnant women
- Children and teens
- Who never had mumps disease.

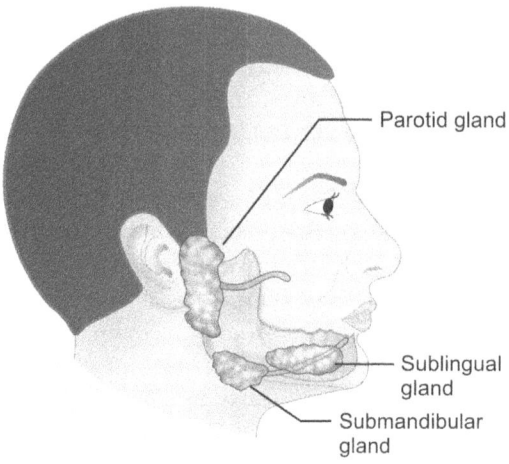

Fig. 13.17: Shows the infected salivary glands caused by paramyxovirus.

Pathophysiology

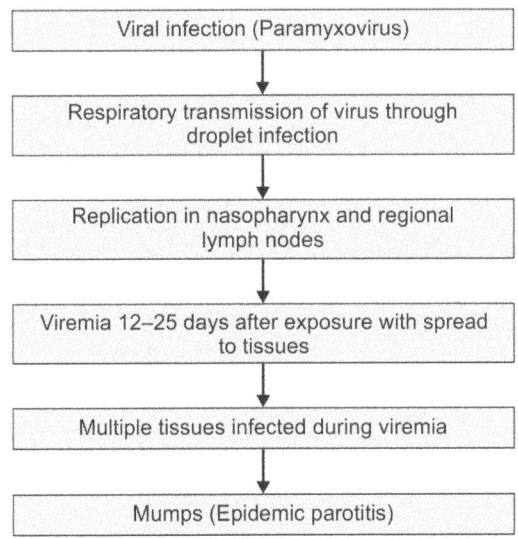

Clinical Features

- Swelling of the parotid glands
- Face pain
- Fever
- Headache
- Sore throat
- Swelling of the temples or jaw (temporo-mandibular area)
- Testicle lump (in males)
- Testicle pain (in males)
- Scrotal swelling (in males)
- Persistent vomiting or abdominal pain
- Persistent drowsiness
- Painful chewing and swallowing
- Eye redness.

Complications

- Orchitis
- Pancreatitis
- Unilateral deafness
- Death.

Diagnostic Tests

- History
- Physical examination
- Blood examination
- Polymerase chain reaction (PCR) test
- Urine examination
- Swab examination.

Management

Medical

Acetaminophen (Paracetamol): It helps to relieve achiness associated with mumps. For example, tylenol, ibuprofen, naproxen, etc.

Nursing

- Provide ice or heat packs to relieve pain.
- Isolate them to prevent spreading to others as it is highly contagious.
- Ask them to get vaccinated for mumps.
- Enforce measures to prevent resurgence of mumps.
- Ask the patient wear a mask or to cover the mouth and nose with a tissue when coughing or sneezing.
- Educate the patient not to share towels, bedding and eating utensils.
- Encourage them to take more fluids to stay hydrated.

▪ PERTUSSIS (WHOOPING COUGH)

Definition

Pertussis or whooping cough is an acute infectious disease caused by the bacteria *Bordetella pertussis*.

Etiology

Bacterial infection (*Bordetella pertussis*).

Risk Factors

- Being unvaccinated
- Having a weakened immune system
- Pregnant women
- Having sickle cell anemia
- Teens under long-term aspirin therapy
- Being renal patients

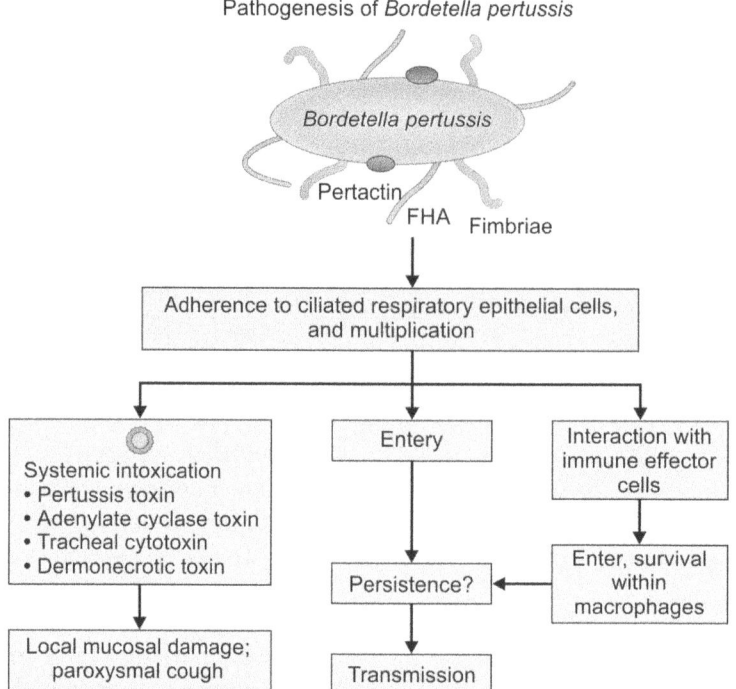

Fig. 13.18: Depicts pathogenesis of pertussis.

- Those receiving long-term treatment with steroids
- Being elderly
- Being under-five children.

Stages

The clinical course of the illness is divided into three stages as follows:

1. *Catarrhal stage (1–2 weeks):* It is characterized by the insidious onset of coryza (runny nose), sneezing, low-grade fever, and a mild, occasional cough, similar to the common cold. The cough gradually becomes more severe, and after 1–2 weeks, the second, or paroxysmal stage, begins. Fever is generally minimal throughout the course of the illness.
2. *Paroxysmal stage (1–6 weeks):* It is during this stage that the diagnosis of pertussis is usually suspected. Characteristically, the patient has bursts, or paroxysms, of numerous, rapid coughs, apparently due to difficulty in expelling thick mucus from the tracheobronchial tree. At the end of the paroxysm, a long inspiratory effort is usually accompanied by a characteristic high-pitched whoop. During such an attack, the patient may become cyanotic (turn blue). Vomiting and exhaustion commonly follow the episode. The person does not appear to be ill between attacks. Paroxysmal attacks occur more frequently at night, with an average of 15 attacks per 24 hours. During the first 1 or 2 weeks of this stage, the attacks increase in frequency, remain at the same level for 2–3 weeks, and then gradually decrease. It usually lasts 1–6 weeks but may persist for up to 10 weeks.
3. *Convalescent stage (weeks to months):* In this stage, recovery is gradual. The cough becomes less paroxysmal and disappears in 2–3 weeks. However, paroxysms often recur with subsequent respiratory infections for many months after the onset of pertussis.

Pathophysiology

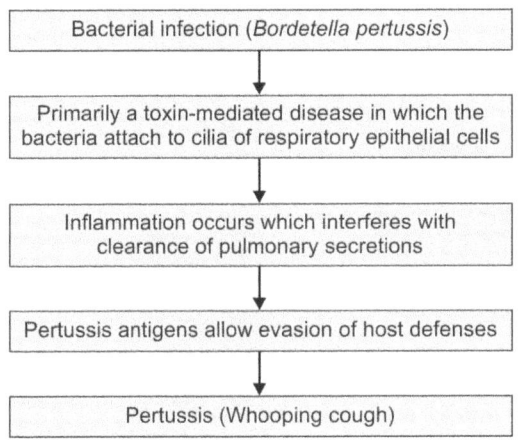

Clinical Features
- Runny nose
- Sore watery red eyes
- Sneezing
- Low-grade fever
- Malaise
- Mild conjunctival inflammation
- General unwellness
- Paroxysmal cough
- Coughing spells with inspiratory whoop
- Post-tussive vomiting.

Complications
- Difficulty in sleeping
- Urinary incontinence
- Pneumonia
- Rib fracture.

Diagnostic Tests
- History
- Physical examination
- Culture examination (Gold standard)
- Polymerase chain reaction (PCR) test
- Blood examination
- Direct fluorescent antibody test.

Management

Medical

Antibiotics: It eradicates the organism from secretions, thereby decreasing communicability and, if initiated early, may modify the course of the illness. For example, azithromycin, clarithromycin, erythromycin, trimethoprim sulfamethoxazole, etc.

Nursing

- Isolate them to prevent spreading to others as it is highly infectious.
- Ask them to get vaccinated for pertussis.
- Enforce measures to prevent resurgence of pertussis.
- Ask the patient wear a mask or to cover the mouth and nose with a tissue when coughing or sneezing.
- Educate the patient not to share towels, bedding and eating utensils.

■ PLAGUE

Definition
Plague is an infectious disease caused by *Yersinia pestis* that affects rodents, certain other animals (rats, rabbits, chipmunks, squirrels, etc.) and humans also.

Etiology
Bacterial infection (*Yersinia pestis*).

Risk Factors
- Recent flea bite
- Exposure to rodents
- Bites from infected domestic cats
- Touching the fluid draining from the swollen gland of an untreated, plague-infected person
- Touching the body of an animal that died from plague.

Types
There are three forms of plague as follows:
1. ***Bubonic plague (an infection of the lymph nodes):*** Patients develop sudden onset of fever, headache, chills, and weakness and one or more swollen, tender and painful lymph nodes (called buboes). This form is usually the result of an infected flea bite. The bacteria multiply in the lymph node closest to where the bacteria entered the human body. If the patient is not treated

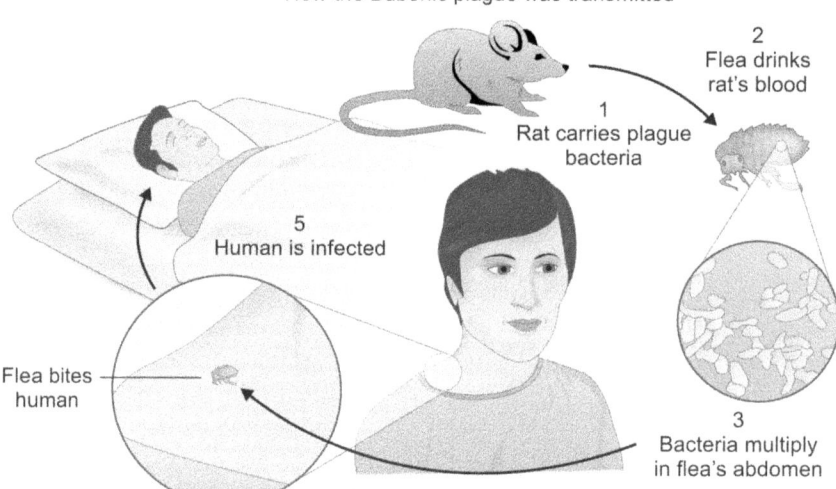

Fig. 13.19: Depicts pathogenesis of plague.

with appropriate antibiotics, the bacteria can spread to other parts of the body.

2. ***Septicemic plague (an infection of the blood):*** Patients develop fever, chills, extreme weakness, abdominal pain, shock, and possibly bleeding into the skin and other organs. Skin and other tissues may turn black and die, especially on fingers, toes, and the nose. Septicemic plague can occur as the first symptoms of plague, or may develop from untreated bubonic plague. This form results from bites of infected fleas or from handling an infected animal.

3. ***Pneumonic plague (an infection of the lungs):*** Patients develop fever, headache, weakness, and a rapidly developing pneumonia with shortness of breath, chest pain, cough, and sometimes bloody or watery mucus. Pneumonic plague may develop from inhaling infectious droplets or from untreated bubonic or septicemic plague that spreads to the lungs. The pneumonia may cause respiratory failure and shock. Pneumonic plague is the most serious form of the disease and is the only form of plague that can spread from person to person (by infectious droplets).

Pathophysiology

Bacterial infection (*Yersinia pestis*)

↓

Bitten by a flea that is infected with the plague bacteria (*Yersinia pestis*). Also can become infected from direct contact with infected tissues or fluids while handling an animal that is sick with or that has died from plague

↓

Finally people can become infected from inhaling respiratory droplets after close contact with cats and humans with pneumonic plague

↓

Chills, fever, cough, frothy, blood sputum and difficulty in breathing (Plague)

Clinical Features

The bubonic plague symptoms appear suddenly, usually after 2–5 days of exposure to the bacteria. Symptoms include:
- Chills
- Fever
- Malaise
- Headache
- Muscle pain
- Seizures
- Smooth, painful lymph gland swelling called a bubo.

Pneumonic plague symptoms appear suddenly, typically 2–3 days after exposure. They include:
- Fever
- Cough
- Difficulty in breathing
- Frothy, bloody sputum
- Pain in the chest when they breathe deeply
- Severe cough.

Septicemic plague may cause death even before its symptoms occur:
- Abdominal pain
- Bleeding due to blood clotting problems
- Diarrhea
- Fever
- Nausea
- Vomiting.

Complications
- Gangrene
- Meningitis
- Death.

Diagnostic Tests
- History
- Physical examination
- Blood examination
- Blood culture
- Sputum culture
- Culture of lymph node aspirate.

Management

Medical
- **Antibiotics:** It eradicates the organism from secretions, thereby decreasing communicability and if initiated early may modify the course of the illness. For example, penicillin, gentamycin, streptomycin, doxycycline, ciprofloxacin, levofloxacin, etc.

Nursing
- Instruct them to rodent-proof their home.
- Ask them to keep their pets free from fleas.
- Encourage them to use insect repellents.
- Ask the patient wear a mask or to cover the mouth and nose with a tissue when coughing or sneezing.
- Ask them not to handle sick or dead animal bodies without any protection.
- Ask them not to leave food sources outside as it may attract rodents.
- Instruct them to keep a minimum of 3 feet from those who have pneumonic form of plague.

POLIOMYELITIS

Definition
Poliomyelitis (polio) is a highly infectious viral disease caused by entero- virus, which mainly affects children under 5 years of age.

Etiology
Viral infection (Enterovirus).

Risk Factors
- Lack of immunization against polio
- Pregnancy
- Travel to an area that has had a recent polio outbreak
- Handling a laboratory specimen of the virus
- Taking care of or living with someone infected with polio
- Having the tonsils removed
- Extreme stress that compromises immune system function.

Types
There are three types of polio infections as follows:
1. **Subclinical:** Approximately 95 percent of polio cases are sub-clinical, and patients may not experience any symptoms. This form of polio does not affect the central nervous system (the brain and spinal cord).
2. **Non-paralytic:** This form does affect the central nervous system and produces only mild symptoms and does not result in paralysis.

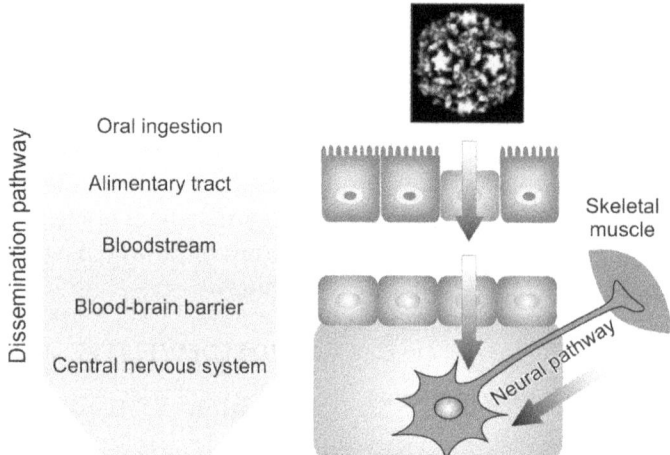

Fig. 13.20: Depicts pathogenesis of poliomyelitis.

3. ***Paralytic:*** This is the rarest and most serious form of polio, which produces full or partial paralysis in the patient. There are three types of paralytic polio: spinal polio (affects the spine), bulbar polio (affects the brainstem), and bulbospinal polio (affects the spine and brainstem).

Pathophysiology

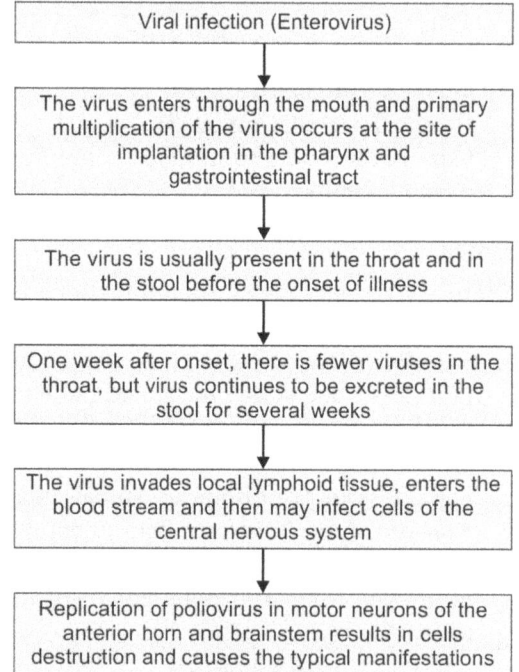

Clinical Features

If patients do have symptoms, they usually last for 72 hours or less and may include:
- Headache
- Sore throat
- Slight fever
- Vomiting
- General discomfort.

The symptoms of non-paralytic polio may last for a couple of days to a week or two and include:
- Fever
- Sore throat in the absence of upper respiratory infection
- Headache
- Vomiting
- Fatigue
- Abnormal reflexes
- Problems of swallowing and breathing
- Neck and back pain with stiffness, particularly neck stiffness with forward flexion of the neck.
- Arm and leg pain or stiffness
- Muscle tenderness and spasms.

People with paralytic polio experience the symptoms associated with paralytic-polio first. Soon after the following symptoms appear:
- Loss of reflexes
- Severe spasm and muscle pain
- Loose and floppy limbs

- Sudden paralysis
- Deformed limbs (especially the hips, ankles and feet due to prolonged weakness and the lack of appropriate orthopedic bracing.

Complications
- Post-polio syndrome
- Aspiration pneumonia
- Cor pulmonale
- Myocarditis
- Pulmonary edema
- Paralytic ileus
- Shock
- Death.

Diagnostic Tests
- History
- Physical examination
- Blood examination
- Blood culture
- Genome sequencing
- CSF examination
- Cultures of throat washings, stools or spinal fluid.

Management

Medical
- **Antibiotics:** It helps in relieving urinary infections and retention. For example, bethanechol, etc.
- **Analgesics:** It helps in relieving the symptoms of fever, headache, back and neck pain. For example, ibuprofen, diclofenac, acetaminophen, etc.

Nursing
- Instruct them to protect themselves through vaccination from polio virus infection.
- Enforce booster vaccinations for travellers to countries where polio occurs, health workers and laboratory workers handling specimens.
- Ask the patient wear a mask or to cover the mouth and nose with a tissue when coughing or sneezing.
- Instruct to avoid eating food prepared by someone who has polio.
- Instruct to avoid contact with nose and throat discharge of a person infected with the polio virus.

RUBELLA (GERMAN MEASLES OR THREE-DAY MEASLES)

Definition
Rubella, also known as German measles or three-day measles is an acute and contagious viral infection caused by rubella virus that causes a red rash on the body. Rashes may start a few weeks after the exposure and last for three days.

Etiology
Viral infection (Rubella virus).

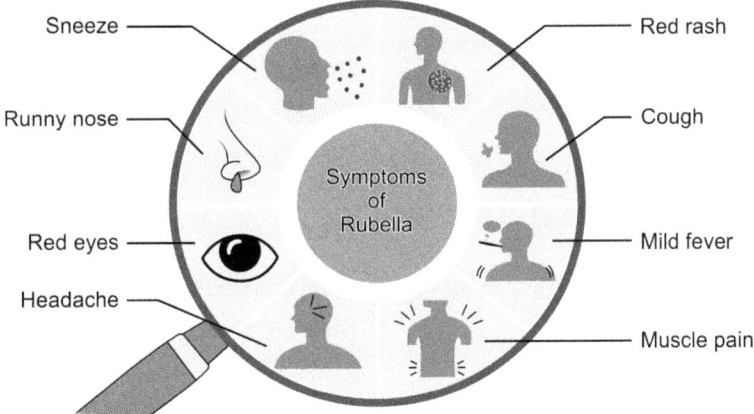

Fig. 13.21: Shows the cardinal features of rubella.

Risk Factors

- Being unvaccinated
- Having a weakened immune system
- Pregnant women
- Being infants and young toddlers
- Frequent travellers.

Pathophysiology

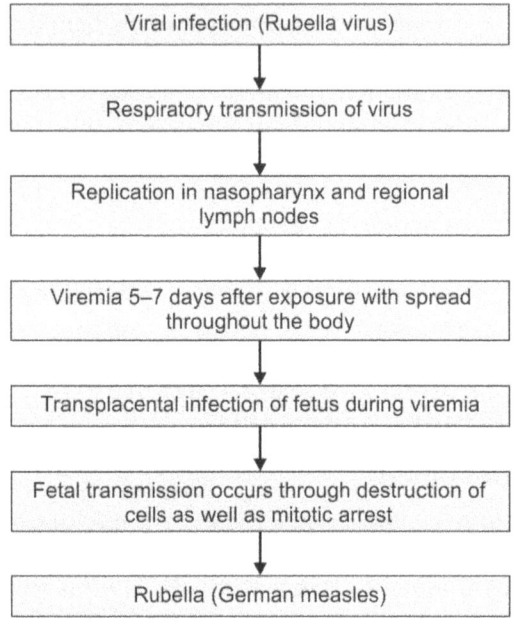

Clinical Features

- Pink or light red rashes that start on the face and spread to the rest of the body.
- Swollen and tender lymph nodes
- Fever
- Headache
- Malaise
- Loss of appetite
- Runny nose
- Bruising
- Inflammation of the eyes (bloodshot eyes)
- Maculopapular rash 14–17 days after exposure
- Muscle or joint pain.

Complications

- Arthralgia
- Arthritis
- Encephalitis
- Thrombocytopenic purpura
- Orchitis
- Neuritis
- Progressive panencephalitis.

Diagnostic Tests

- History
- Physical examination
- Blood examination
- Real-time polymerase chain reaction (RT-PCR)
- Throat swab examination
- Urine examination.

Management

Medical

Acetaminophen (Paracetamol): It helps to relieve achiness associated with rubella. For example, tylenol, ibuprofen, naproxen, etc.

Nursing

- Instruct them to take adequate bedrest.
- Ask them to get vaccinated for rubella.
- Enforce measures to prevent resurgence of rubella.
- Ask them to wear a mask or to cover the mouth and nose with a tissue when coughing or sneezing.
- Ask patients to keep away from others as much as possible until the rashes come down.

SEVERE ACUTE RESPIRATORY SYNDROME

Definition

Severe acute respiratory syndrome (SARS) is a viral respiratory illness caused by a virus called SARS-associated coronavirus (SARS-CoV).

Etiology

Viral infection (SARS-CoV).

Risk Factors

- People who had recently travelled to Asia.
- Healthcare workers who had cared for SARS patients.

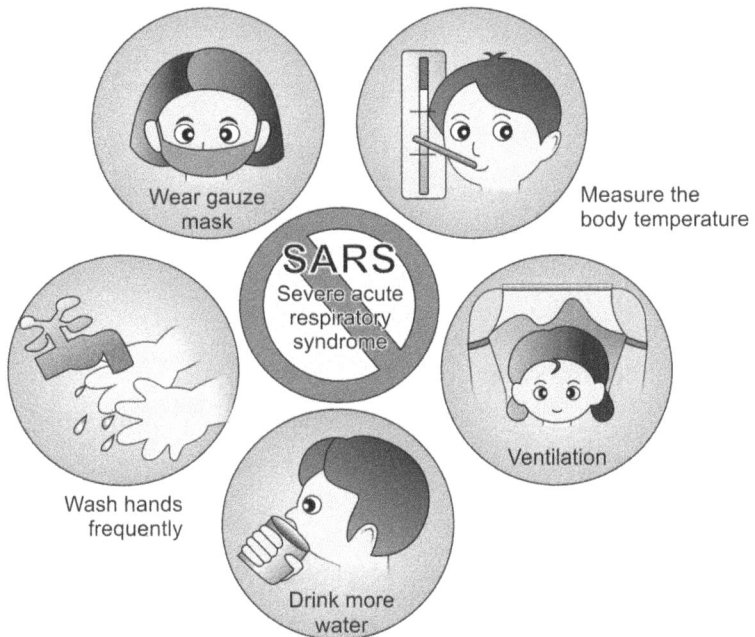

Fig. 13.22: Management of severe acute respiratory syndrome (SARS).

- Close family members of SARS patients.
- Sharing utensils for eating and drinking.
- Speaking to someone with SARS within 3 feet from them.
- Hugging and kissing someone with SARS.

Pathophysiology

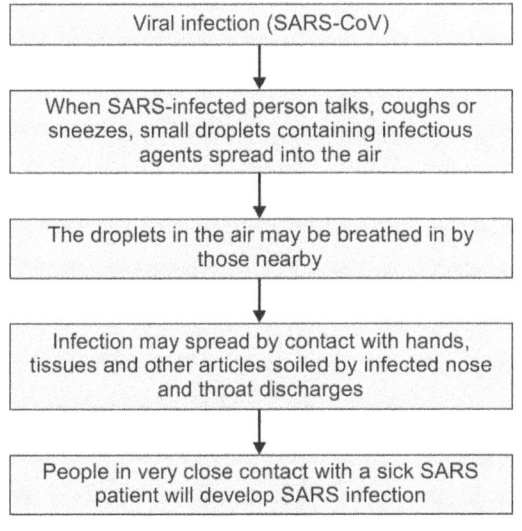

Clinical Features

The hallmark symptoms are:
- High fever (with a temperature exceeding 100.4° Fahrenheit)
- Difficulty in breathing
- Dry cough.

The most common symptoms are:
- Chills and shaking
- Muscle aches
- Headache.

Less common symptoms include:
- Cough that produces phlegm (sputum)
- Dizziness
- Poor appetite
- Nausea and vomiting
- Runny nose
- Sore throat
- Diarrhea.

Complications

- Respiratory failure
- Heart failure
- Liver failure.

Diagnostic Tests

- History
- Physical examination
- Arterial blood examination
- Blood clotting tests
- Blood chemistry tests
- Chest X-ray
- Chest CT scan
- Complete blood count (CBC)
- Antibody tests for SARS
- Direct isolation of the SARS virus
- Rapid polymerase chain reaction (PCR) test for SARS virus.

Management

Medical

- **Immunomodulators:** It helps to strike an optimal immune balance so that the patient can mount a sufficient adaptive response to eradicate the virus, but without the sequelae of irreversible lung damage from immune overreactivity. For example, methylprednisolone, thymosin alpha 1, etc.
- **Antibiotics:** It covers against common respiratory pathogens as per guidelines for community-acquired or nososcomial pneumonia. For example, levofloxacin, quinolones, macrolides, etc.
- **Antiviral agents (Nucleoside analog agents):** It inhibits the coronaviral proteases, thus blocking the processing of the viral replicase polyprotein and preventing the replication of viral DNA. For example, Ribavirin, oseltamivir phosphate, lopinavir, etc.

Nursing

- Instruct them to do frequent handwashing with an alcohol-based solution.
- Instruct to avoid touching the eyes, mouth or nose with unclean hands.
- Ask the patient wear a mask or to cover the mouth and nose with a tissue when coughing or sneezing.
- Educate the patient not to share towels, bedding and eating utensils.
- Ask the patients to keep away from others as much as possible until 10 days after the resolution of fever.

SMALLPOX

Definition

It is an acute contagious disease caused by the variola virus, a member of the orthopox virus family.

Etiology

Viral infection (Variola virus).

Risk Factors

- Physical contact with someone with smallpox
- Direct contact with infected bodily fluids
- Direct contact with contaminated surfaces
- Exposure to aerosolized particles from someone with smallpox
- Laboratory work with the virus
- Being military personnel
- Being unvaccinated
- Persons with weakened immune system
- Being pregnant women.

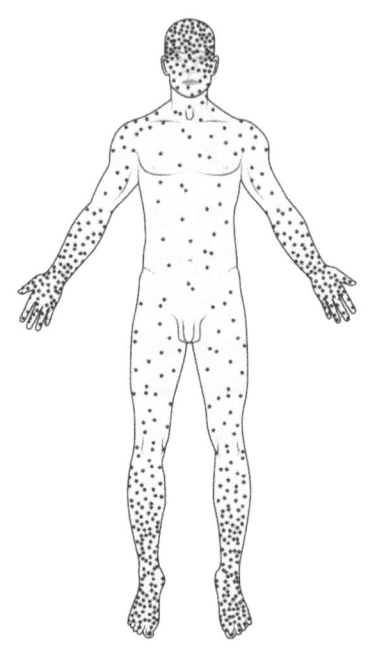

Fig. 13.23: Smallpox.

Stages

There are six stages of smallpox as follows:

- **Incubation not contagious stage:** It lasts for 7-17 days. Exposure to the virus is followed by an incubation period during which people do not have any symptoms and may feel fine. This incubation period averages about 12-14 days but can range from 7 to 17 days. During this time, people are not contagious.
- **Prodromal sometimes contagious stage:** It lasts for 2-4 days. The first symptoms of smallpox include fever, malaise, head and body aches, and sometimes vomiting. The fever is usually high, in the range of 101 to 104° Fahrenheit. At this time, people are usually too sick to carry on their normal activities. This is called the prodrome phase and may last for 2 to 4 days.
- **Early rash most contagious stage:** It lasts for about 4 days. A rash emerges first as small red spots on the tongue and in the mouth. These spots develop into sores that break open and spread large amounts of the virus into the mouth and throat. At this time, the person becomes most contagious. Around the time the sores in the mouth break down, a rash appears on the skin, starting on the face and spreading to the arms and legs and then to the hands and feet. Usually the rash spreads to all parts of the body within 24 hours. As the rash appears, the fever usually falls and the person may start to feel better. By the third day of the rash, the rash becomes raised bumps. By the fourth day, the bumps fill with a thick, opaque fluid and often have a depression in the center that looks like a bellybutton (hallmark feature of smallpox). Fever often will rise again at this time and remain high until scabs form over the bumps.
- **Pustular rash contagious stage:** It lasts for about 5 days. The bumps become pustules—sharply raised, usually round and firm to the touch as if there's a small round object under the skin. People often say the bumps feel like BB pellets embedded in the skin.
- **Pustules and scabs contagious stage:** It lasts for about 5 days. The pustules begin to form a crust and then scab. By the end of the second week after the rash appears, most of the sores have scabbed over.
- **Resolving scabs contagious stage:** It lasts for about 6 days. The scabs begin to fall off, leaving marks on the skin that eventually becomes pitted scars. Most scabs will have fallen off three weeks after the rash appears.

Pathophysiology

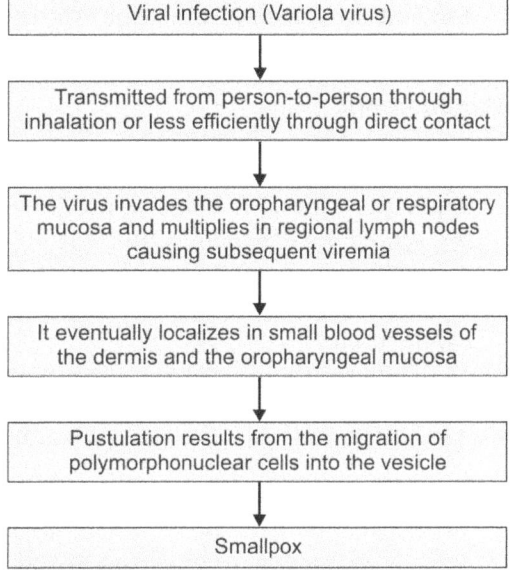

Clinical Features

- Backache
- Delirium
- Diarrhea
- Excessive bleeding
- Fatigue
- High fever
- Malaise
- Raised pink rash—turns into sores that become crusty on day 8 or 9
- Severe headache
- Vomiting.

Complications

- Arthritis
- Encephalitis
- Pneumonia
- Eye infections
- Scarring
- Severe bleeding
- Skin infection (from the sores)
- Death.

Diagnostic Tests

- History
- Physical examination
- Blood examination
- Polymerase chain reaction (PCR)
- Electron microscopy
- Enzyme-linked immunosorbent assay (ELISA) test.

Management

Medical

- **Antiviral agents:** It helps to minimize the symptoms of smallpox, but it is only effective if it is started within the first 24 hours after exposure. For example, cidofovir, etc.
- **Antibiotics:** It helps to prevent any secondary infections through bactericidal action in the body. For example, penicillin G, azithromycin, etc.
- **Nonaspirin agents:** It helps to lower the temperature among the patients. For example, ibuprofen, acetaminophen, etc.

Nursing

- Encourage the patient to use cool wet compresses or give baths in cool or lukewarm water every 3-4 hours for the first few days.
- Instruct the patient not to rub the body dry.
- Instruct the patient to wear gloves to prevent scratching that can lead to scarring.
- Restrict the patient from having salty or citrus foods.
- Provide information to patient regarding smallpox vaccine.

SWINE FLU

Definition

An acute and highly contagious form of human influenza caused by a filterable virus (orthomyxovirus) identical or related to a virus

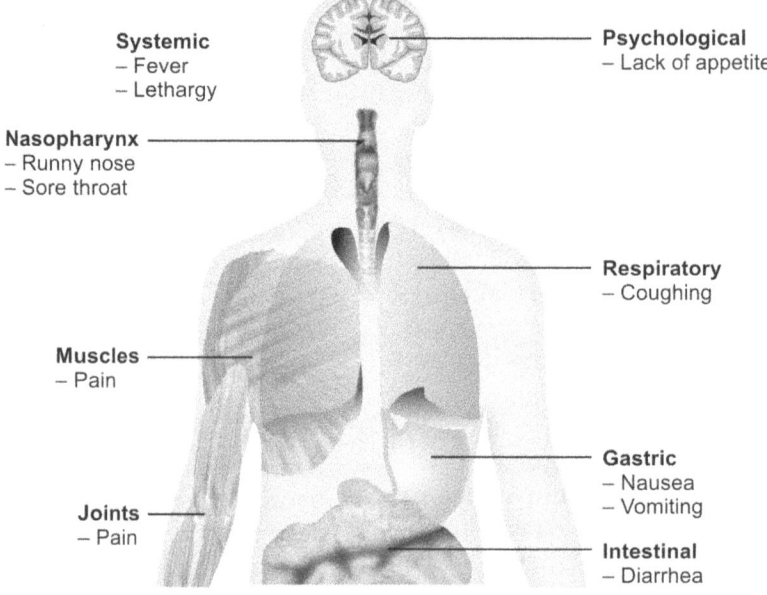

Fig. 13.24: Symptoms of swine flu.

formerly isolated from infected swine is known as swine flu.

Etiology

Viral infection (H1N1 or Orthomyxovirus).

Risk Factors

- Persons aged 65 years or older
- Children less than 5 years
- Pregnant women
- People with chronic illnesses (asthma, heart disease, diabetes, neuromuscular disease, etc.)
- People with compromised immune system (due to a disease such as AIDS)
- Adolescents who are receiving long-term aspirin therapy
- Residents of nursing homes and other chronic care facilities.

Pathophysiology

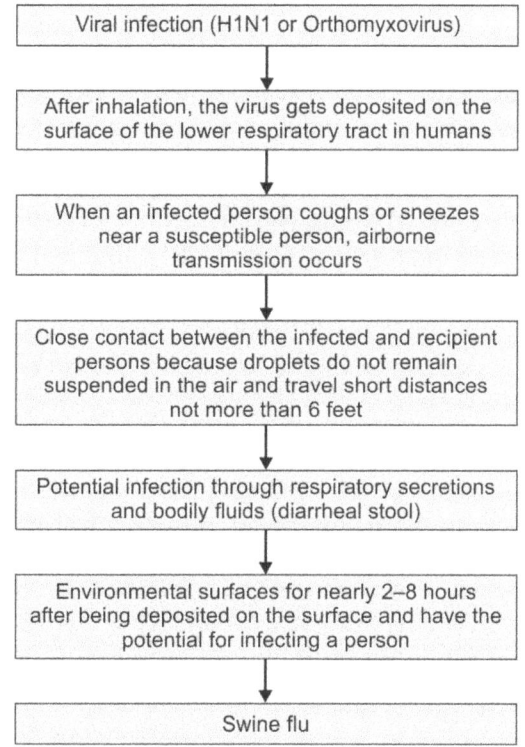

Clinical Features

- Fever
- Chills
- Headache
- Upper respiratory tract symptoms—cough, sore throat, rhinorrhea, shortness of breath
- Runny or stuffy nose
- Myalgia
- Arthralgia
- Fatigue
- Nausea
- Vomiting
- Diarrhea.

Complications

- Exacerbation of underlying chronic medical conditions
- Sinusitis
- Otitis media
- Pneumonia
- Status asthmaticus
- Post-infectious encephalopathy encephalitis
- Toxic shock syndrome.

Diagnostic Tests

- History
- Physical examination
- Blood examination
- Enzyme immune assays
- Routine viral culture
- Direct immune fluorescent assay
- Reverse transcription polymerase chain reaction (RT-PCR).

Management

Medical

- **Antiviral agents:** It inhibits the replication of influenza viruses by interfering with the uncoating of the virus inside the cell and helps in preventing the serious complications. For example, amantadine, oseltamivir (Tamiflu), zanamivir (Relenza), etc.
- **Acetaminophen:** It helps to combat the achiness associated with influenza. For example, tylenol, ibuprofen, etc.

Nursing

- Instruct the patient to keep away from others to prevent it spreading from others.

- Encourage to drink plenty of water and clear fluids to prevent dehydration.
- Ask them to cover mouth while coughing and sneezing and should not forget to wash their hands with soap and water or an alcohol-based hand wash after coughing or sneezing and after using tissues.
- Encourage them to wear a face mask if they are sharing common spaces with other family members to prevent spread of virus.
- Instruct them to avoid touching their eyes, nose or mouth to prevent spreading of germs.
- Ask them to keep a distance of minimum 6 feet from others especially when sneezing or coughing.

SYPHILIS

Definition

Syphilis is a sexually transmitted, infectious disease caused by the spirochete *Treponema pallidum*.

Etiology

Bacterial infection (*Treponema pallidum*).

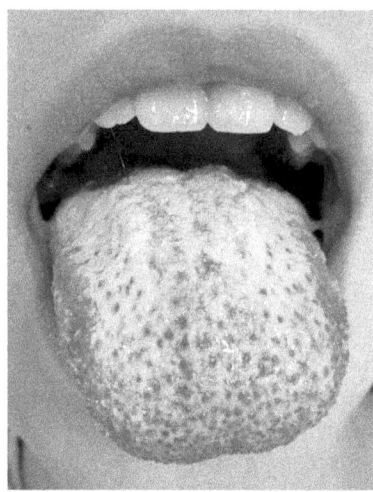

Fig. 13.25: Formation of chancre in syphilis.

Risk Factors

- Engaging in unsafe sex
- Having sex with more than one partner
- Homosexuals
- Not using a condom consistently
- Pregnant women
- Being HIV positive.

Stages of Syphilis

There are four stages of syphilis as follows:
1. **Primary stage:** It occurs about 3-4 weeks after they are infected with the bacteria. It begins with a small, round sore called a chancre. A chancre is painless, but it is highly infectious. This sore may appear wherever the bacteria entered the body, such as on or inside the mouth, genitals, or rectum. On an average, the sore shows up around three weeks after infection, but it can take between 10 and 90 days to appear. The sore remains for anywhere between 2 and 6 weeks. The syphilis is transmitted by direct contact with a sore. This usually occurs during sexual activity, including oral sex.
2. **Secondary syphilis:** During this stage, one may experience skin rashes and a sore throat. The rash will not itch and is usually found on the palms and soles, but it may occur anywhere on the body. Some people do not notice the rash before it goes away. These symptoms will go away whether or not one receives treatment. However, without treatment they will still be infected.
3. **Latent syphilis:** It is the third stage of syphilis. The primary and secondary symptoms disappear, and they will not have any noticeable symptoms at this stage. However, one will still be infected with syphilis. The secondary symptoms can reappear, or they could remain in this stage for years before progressing to tertiary syphilis.
4. **Tertiary syphilis:** It is the last stage of syphilis. Approximately, 15–30% of people

who do not receive treatment for syphilis will enter this stage. Tertiary syphilis can occur years or decades after they are initially infected. Tertiary syphilis can be life-threatening.

Pathophysiology

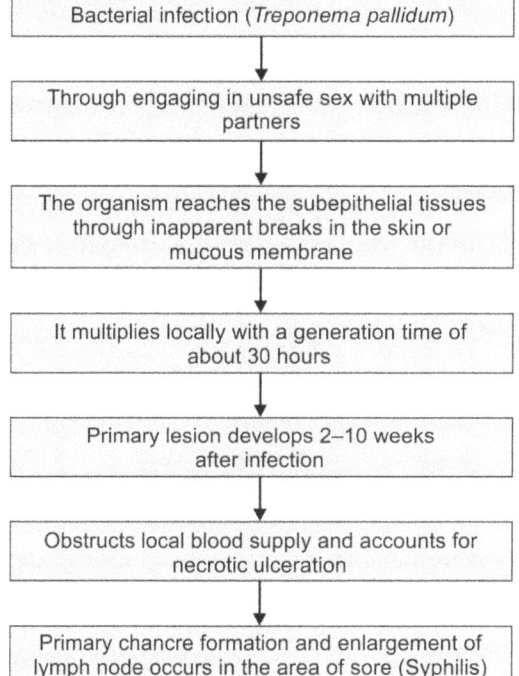

Clinical Features

Primary Features

- Small, painless open sore or ulcer (called a chancre) on the genitals, mouth, skin or rectum that heals by itself in 3–6 weeks
- Enlarged lymph nodes in the area of the sore.

Secondary Features

- Skin rashes, usually on the palms of the hands and soles in the feet
- Sores called mucous patches in or around the mouth, vagina or penis
- Moist, warty patches (called condylomata) in the genitals or skin folds
- Fever
- General ill-feeling
- Loss of appetite
- Muscle aches
- Joint pain
- Swollen lymph nodes
- Vision changes
- Hair loss.

Tertiary Features (the Late-phase of the Illness)

- Damage to the heart, causing aneurysm or valve disease
- Central nervous system disorders
- Tumors of skin, bones or liver.

Complications

- Aortitis and aneurysm
- Destructive sores of skin and bones (gummas)
- Neurosyphilis
- Syphilitic myelopathy
- Syphilitic meningitis
- Congenital syphilis.

Diagnostic Tests

- History
- Physical examination
- Examination of fluid from sore
- Echocardiogram
- Aortic angiogram
- Cardiac catheterization
- Blood examination
- Spinal fluid examination
- Rapid plasma reagin (RPR) blood test.

Management

Medical

Antibiotics: It helps to prevent any secondary infections through bactericidal action in the body. For example, penicillin G, benzathine penicillin, procaine penicillin, Bicillin C-R, etc.

Nursing

- Ask all pregnant women to screen for syphilis before pregnancy.

- Instruct the patient to get regular screenings for sexually transmitted diseases.
- Educate the patient to avoid multiple sex partners.
- Educate the patient to use condoms during every sexual encounter.

TETANUS (LOCKJAW)

Definition
Tetanus (lockjaw) is an infectious disease caused by contamination of wounds with the bacteria *Clostridium tetani*.

Etiology
Bacterial infection (*Clostridium tetani*).

Risk Factors
- Pregnancy
- Lack of immunization
- Contaminated wounds
- Tissue injury
- Deep penetrating wounds
- Infected umbilical stumps in newborn
- Surgical wounds
- Ear infections
- Summer or wet season
- Soil and intestines of animals and human.

Types
On the basis of clinical findings, three different forms of tetanus have been described:

1. ***Local tetanus:*** It is an uncommon form of the disease, in which patients have persistent contraction of muscles in the same anatomic area as the injury. These contractions may persist for many weeks before gradually subsiding. Local tetanus may precede the onset of generalized tetanus but is generally milder. Only about 1% of cases are fatal.
2. ***Cephalic tetanus:*** It is a rare form of the disease, occasionally occurring with otitis media (ear infections) in which *Clostridium tetani* is present in the flora of the middle ear, or following injuries to the head. There is involvement of the cranial nerves, especially in the facial area.
3. ***Generalized tetanus:*** It is the most common type (about 80%) of tetanus. The disease usually presents with a descending pattern. The first sign is trismus or lockjaw, followed by stiffness of the neck, difficulty in swallowing, and rigidity of abdominal muscles. Other symptoms include elevated temperature, sweating, elevated blood pressure, and episodic rapid heart rate. Spasms may occur frequently and last for several minutes. Spasms continue for 3–4 weeks. Complete recovery may take months.

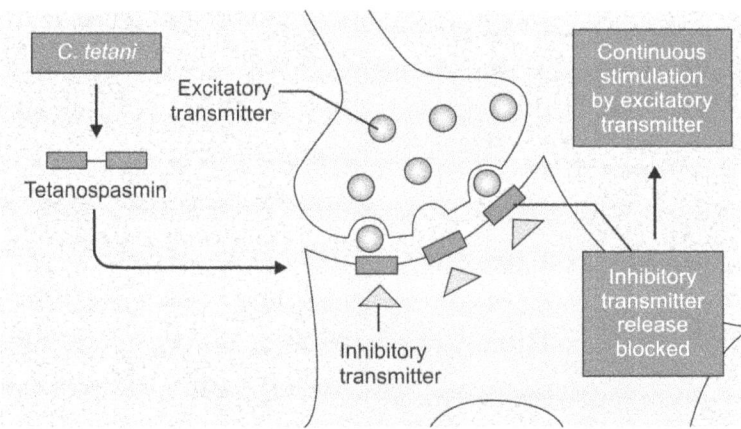

Fig. 13.26: Depicts pathogenesis of tetanus.

Pathophysiology

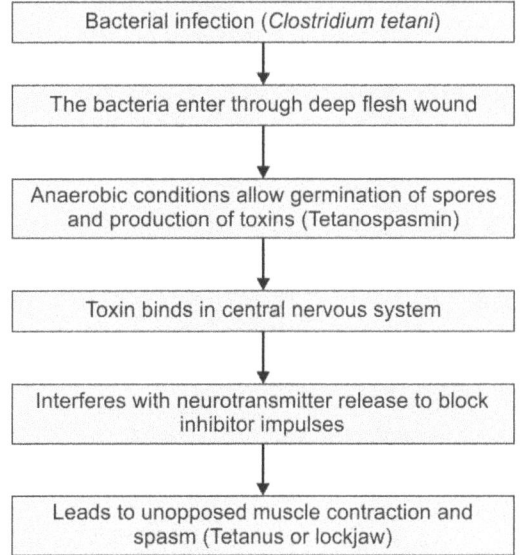

Clinical Features

- Mild spasm in the jaw muscles (Lockjaw)
- Spasm affecting the chest, neck, back and abdominal muscles
- Back muscle spasm cause arching (Opisthotonos) position
- Breathing problems
- Drooling
- Excessive sweating
- Fever
- Hand or foot spasm
- Irritability
- Swallowing difficulty
- Uncontrolled urination or defecation.

Complications

- Laryngospasm
- Fractures
- Hypertension
- Nosocomial infections
- Pulmonary embolism
- Aspiration pneumonia
- Death.

Diagnostic Tests

- History
- Physical examination
- Spatula test.

Management

Medical

- **Tetanus immune globulin (TIG):** It helps to remove unbound tetanus through neutralizing the toxins that the bacteria have created in the body. DTaP, Tdap, etc.
- **Antibiotics:** It helps to prevent any secondary infections through bactericidal action in the body. For example, penicillin, etc.
- **Muscle relaxants:** It helps in controlling the muscle spasm. For example, mephenesin, dicyclopropyl ketoxime, etc.

Nursing

- Encourage them to get vaccinated against tetanus.
- Instruct to keep the wound clean and sterile.
- Enforce thorough debridement of wounds.
- Provide facilitation to improve birth hygiene.
- Instruct to avoid traveling to remote areas.

■ TYPHOID (ENTERIC FEVER)

Definition

Typhoid fever is a bacterial infection caused by *Salmonella typhi*. It spreads through contaminated food, drink or water.

Etiology

Bacterial infection (*Salmonella typhi*).

Risk Factors

- Poor water sanitation
- Children
- Contaminated water
- Poverty
- Raw food
- Flies on food
- Developing nation
- International travel to typhoid-affected countries.

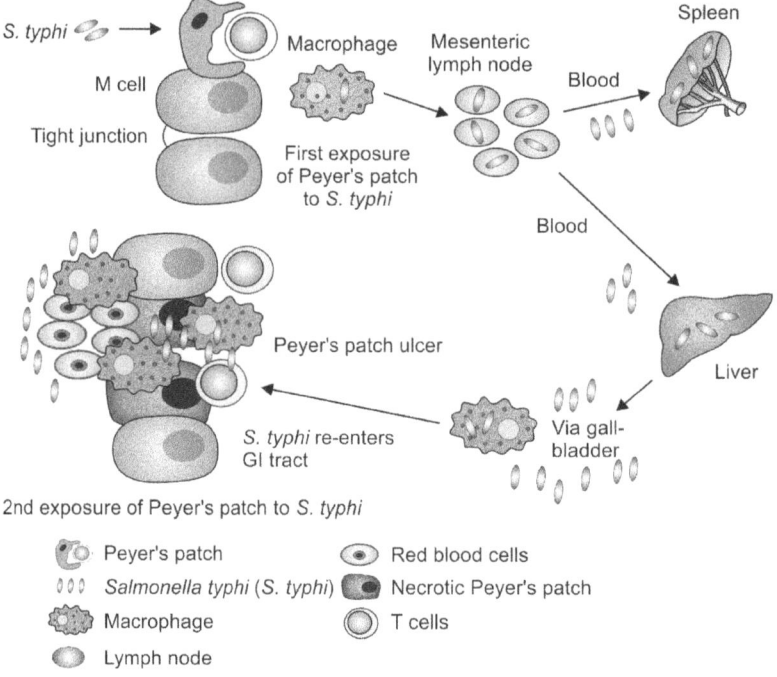

Fig. 13.27: Depicts pathogenesis of typhoid.

Pathophysiology

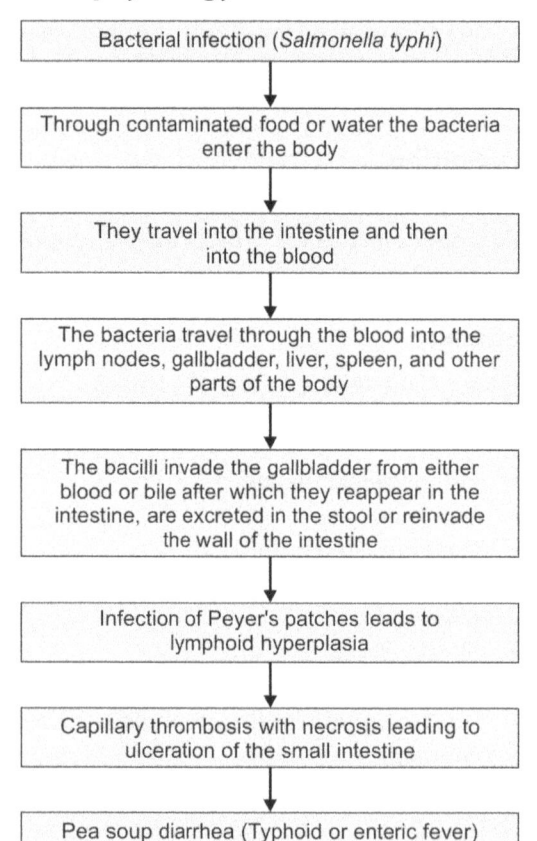

Clinical Features

- High fever (105° Fahrenheit)
- Severe diarrhea
- General ill-feeling
- Abdominal pain
- Develops small red spots (rose spots) on the abdomen and chest
- Abdominal tenderness
- Agitation
- Bloody stools
- Chills
- Confusion
- Difficulty in paying attention
- Delirium
- Fluctuating mood
- Hallucinations
- Nose bleeds
- Severe fatigue
- Slow, sluggish, lethargic feeling
- Weakness.

Complications

- Severe gastrointestinal bleeding
- Intestinal perforation
- Peritonitis
- Kidney failure.

Diagnostic Tests

- History
- Physical examination
- Blood examination
- Blood culture
- ELISA urine test
- Fluorescent antibody study
- Stool culture.

Management

Medical

- **Antibiotics:** It helps to prevent secondary infections. For example, ciprofloxacin, ceftriaxone, chloramphenicol, etc.
- **Acetaminophen (Paracetamol):** It helps to relieve fever as well as aches and pains associated with typhoid. For example, tylenol, etc.

Nursing

- Encourage to take single dose of vaccination at least one week before travel.
- Instruct to avoid drinking untreated water.
- Ask them to wash their hands after using the toilet.
- Ask them to ensure proper hygiene and sanitation.
- Encourage to consume hot and fresh foods as high temperature hinders the growth of bacteria.
- Encourage to keep all the household items properly clean and sanitized.
- Instruct to avoid eating raw veggies to keep the bacteria away.
- Encourage to drink more fluids to prevent dehydration.

YELLOW FEVER

Definition

Yellow fever is an acute viral hemorrhagic disease transmitted by infected *Aedes aegypti* mosquitoes.

Etiology

- *Aedes aegypti* mosquito
- Viral infection (Flavivirus).

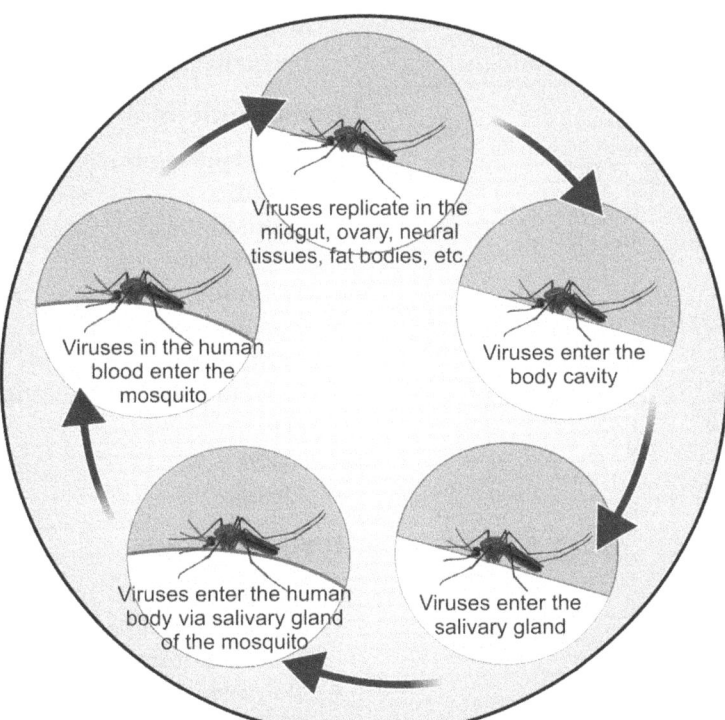

Fig. 13.28: Depicts pathogenesis of yellow fever.

Risk Factors

- Traveling to Africa or South America where the disease is known to be present
- Older adults
- Infants and neonates
- Unimmunized young men who are exposed to mosquito vectors through their work in forest areas
- Anyone exposed during the end of the rainy season and the beginning of the dry season.

Types

There are two types of yellow fever as follows:
1. **Urban yellow fever:** It is an epidemic viral disease of humans transmitted from infected to susceptible persons by *Aedes aegypti* mosquitoes, which breed in domestic and peri-domestic containers (e.g., water jars, barrels, drums, etc.) and thus in close association with humans.
2. **Jungle yellow fever:** It can most effectively be prevented by vaccination of human populations at risk for exposure.

Pathophysiology

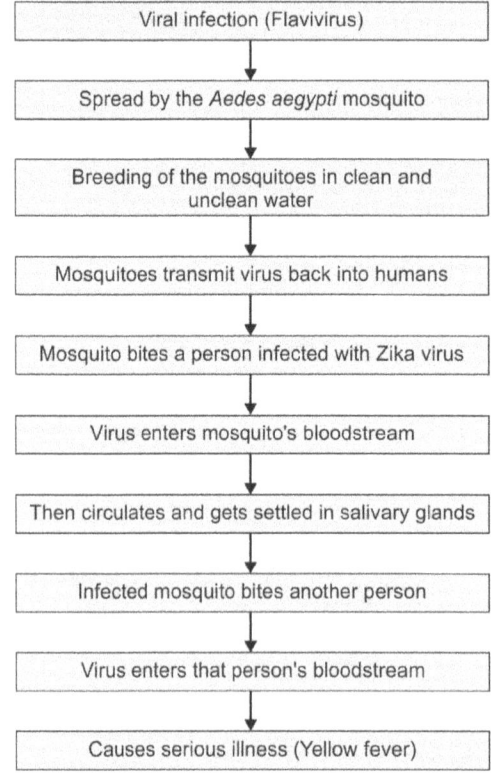

Clinical Features

The signs and symptoms will be experienced in three different phases as follows:
1. **Incubation phase**
   - During the first three to six days, there will not be any signs and symptoms experienced.
2. **Acute phase**
   - Fever
   - Headache
   - Muscle ache particularly at the back and knees
   - Nausea
   - Vomiting
   - Loss of appetite
   - Dizziness
   - Redness of eyes, face or tongue.
3. **Toxic phase**
   - Yellowness of the skin
   - Abdominal pain and vomiting something accompanied by blood vomiting
   - Decreased urination
   - Bleeding from the nose, mouth and eyes
   - Heart dysfunction
   - Brain dysfunction.

Complications

- Blood infection
- Jaundice
- Kidney failure
- Liver failure
- Delirium
- Pneumonia
- Parotitis
- Disseminated intravascular coagulation (DIC)
- Coma
- Death.

Diagnostic Tests

- History
- Physical examination
- Blood examination
- Polymerase chain reaction test
- ELISA test.

Management

Medical

Acetaminophen (Paracetamol): It helps to relieve fever as well as aches and pains associated with Zika virus disease as it reduces the production of prostaglandins in the brain. For example, tylenol, etc.

Nursing

- Ask them to take complete bedrest.
- Encourage to take single dose of vaccination to protect them for at least 10 years.
- Educate to reduce any exposure to mosquitoes.
- Encourage them to apply permethrin-containing mosquito repellants.
- Encourage them to sleep in screened housing.
- Ask the patient to wear clothing that fully covers their body.

ZIKA VIRUS DISEASE

Definition

Zika virus disease is a mild febrile viral illness caused by an arbovirus and transmitted by *Aedes aegypti* mosquitoes.

Etiology

- *Aedes aegypti* mosquito
- Viral infection (Flavivirus).

Risk Factors

- Anyone traveling to regions where Zika virus is circulating
- Pregnant women
- Fetuses in the first trimester
- Being a neonate.

Pathophysiology

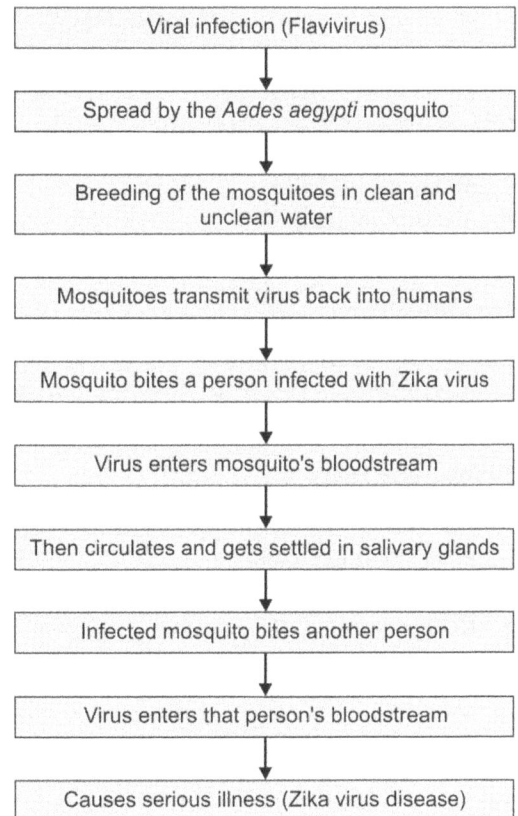

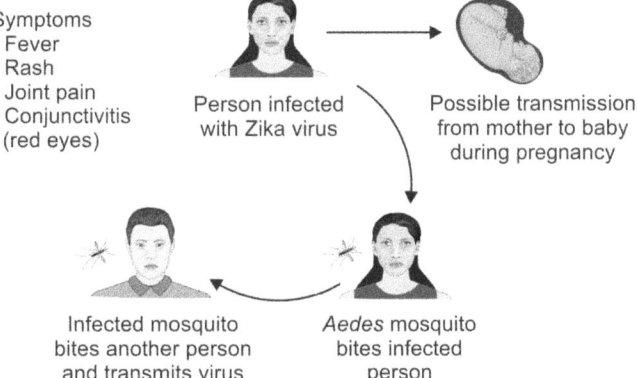

Fig. 13.29: Depicts pathogenesis of Zika virus disease.

Clinical Features

- Low-grade fever (between 37.8° Celsius to 38.5° Celsius)
- Chills
- Arthralgia (notably of small joints of hands and feet, with possible swollen joints)
- Myalgia
- Headache (retro-ocular headache)
- Conjunctivitis (red eyes)
- Pain behind the eyes
- Cutaneous maculopapular rash
- Fatigue
- Malaise
- Abdominal pain
- Vomiting.

Complications

- Guillain-Barre syndrome
- Birth defects (fetal microcephaly and intracranial calcifications).

Diagnostic Tests

- History
- Physical examination
- Blood examination
- Urine examination.

Management

Medical

Acetaminophen (Paracetamol): It helps to relieve fever as well as aches and pains associated with Zika virus disease as it reduces the production of prostaglandins in the brain. For example, tylenol, etc.

Nursing

- Ask the patient to get plenty of rest.
- Encourage the patient to drink more fluids to prevent dehydration.
- Ask the patient to cover exposed skin and to wear long-sleeved clothes
- Educate the patient to sleep under mosquito nets.
- Instruct the patients to unblock drains at home that could accumulate standing water.
- Instruct the patient to avoid accumulating garbage.
- Encourage the patient to use screens in windows and doors to reduce contact between mosquitoes and people.
- Ask the patient to cover domestic water tanks so that mosquitoes cannot get into it.

14 Oncology-related Disorders

CHAPTER OUTLINE

- Adrenal tumor
- Anal cancer
- Bile duct cancer
- Bladder tumor
- Bone tumor
- Brain tumor
- Breast cancer
- Cervical cancer
- Colon cancer
- Endometrial cancer
- Esophageal cancer
- Gallbladder cancer
- Head and neck cancer
- Kaposi's sarcoma
- Leukemia
- Liver cancer
- Lung cancer
- Lymphoma – Hodgkin's
- Lymphoma – Non-Hodgkin's
- Melanoma
- Multiple myeloma
- Nasopharyngeal cancer
- Ovarian cancer
- Pancreatic cancer
- Parathyroid tumor
- Penile cancer
- Pituitary gland tumor
- Prostate cancer
- Rectal cancer
- Renal cancer
- Skin cancer
- Spinal cord tumor
- Stomach cancer
- Testicular cancer
- Thyroid tumor
- Vaginal cancer
- Vulvar cancer

INTRODUCTION

Cancer is a genetic disease which occurs when changes in a group of normal cells within the body lead to uncontrolled growth causing a lump called a tumor; this is true of all cancers except leukemia (cancer of the blood). If left

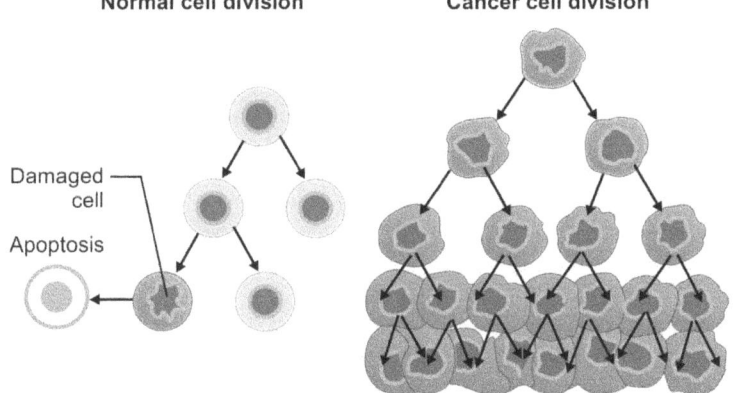

Fig. 14.1: Shows the normal cell division and cancer cell division.

untreated, tumors can grow and spread into the surrounding normal tissue, or to other parts of the body via the bloodstream and lymphatic systems.

ETIOLOGY

As with most illnesses, cancer is multifactorial and there is no single cause for any type of cancer. The various causes are as follows:
- Cancer-causing substances (carcinogens)
- Mobile phones
- Power lines
- Certain viruses (e.g., Epstein-Barr virus)
- Certain bacteria (e.g., *Helicobacter pylori*)
- Head injuries
- Excessive exposure to the ultraviolet rays of the sun
- Exposure to chemicals
- Physical inactivity
- Immunosuppression
- Exposure to radiations
- Dietary factors (e.g: Fat, alcohol, salt-cured or smoked meats, foods containing nitrates and nitrites).

RISK FACTORS

- More common in males than in females
- Hair dye
- Smoking
- Alcohol
- Being overweight
- Birth weight of more than 4 kg
- Hormone replacement therapy
- Previous history of cancer
- Genetic conditions (neurofibromatosis, tuberous sclerosis, Li-Fraumeni syndrome, Von Hippel-Lindau syndrome, Turner syndrome, Turcot syndrome, Gorlin syndrome and Cowden syndrome)
- Advanced age
- Family history of cancer.

PATHOPHYSIOLOGY

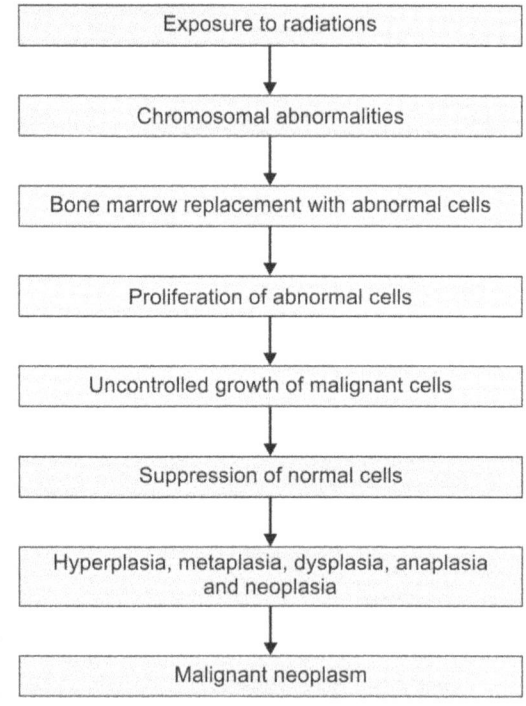

Steps Involved in Carcinogenesis

There are three steps involved as follows:
- ***Initiation:*** It involves carcinogens such as chemicals, physical factors and biologic

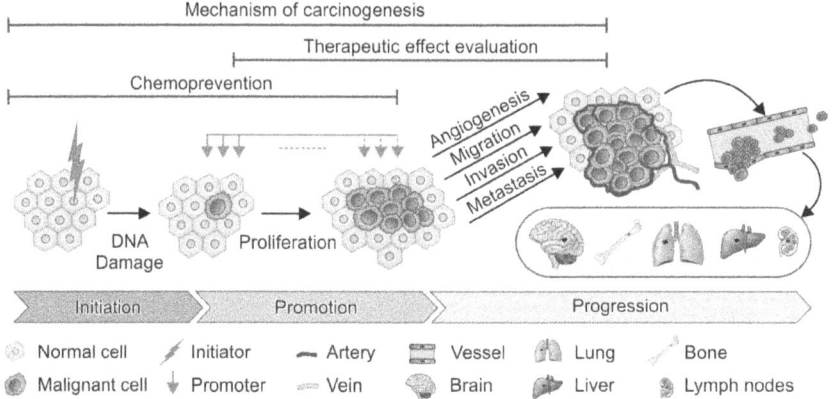

Fig. 14.2: Depicts the steps involved in carcinogenesis.

agents that alter the genetic structure of the cellular DNA.
- **Promotion:** It is the repeated exposure to promoting agents (co-carcinogens) that causes the expression of abnormal or mutant genetic information.
- **Progression:** It involves the cellular changes formed during initiation and promotion may now exhibit increased malignant behavior on the individuals.

TYPES OF CANCER

The major classification of cancer is as follows:
- **Carcinomas:** It arises from epithelial cells lining the internal surfaces of the various organs (e.g., mouth, esophagus, intestines, and uterus) and from the skin epithelium. The most common forms of cancer in this group are breast, prostate, lung and colon cancer.
- **Sarcomas:** It arises from mesodermal cells constituting the various connective tissues (e.g., fibrous tissue, fat and bone). The most common forms of cancer in this group are leiomyosarcoma, liposarcoma and osteosarcoma.
- **Lymphoma:** It arises from the cells of the bone marrow and immune systems. The most common forms of cancer in this group are Hodgkin's lymphoma and non-Hodgkin's lymphoma.
- **Leukemia:** It is a cancer of the white blood cells and bone marrow, the tissue that forms blood cells. The most common forms of cancer in this group are chronic myeloid leukemia and acute lymphocytic leukemia.

STAGES OF CANCER

TNM classification is used for staging of cancer as follows:

$T \rightarrow$ The extent of the primary tumor
$N \rightarrow$ The absence or presence and extent of regional lymph node metastasis
$M \rightarrow$ The absence or presence of distant metastasis.

Primary Tumor (T)

$Tx \rightarrow$ Primary tumor cannot be made
$T_0 \rightarrow$ No evidence of primary tumor
$T \rightarrow$ Carcinoma in site
$T_1, T_2, T_3, T_4 \rightarrow$ Increasing size and local extent of the primary tumor.

Regional Lymph Nodes (N)

$N_x \rightarrow$ Regional lymph nodes cannot be made out
$N_0 \rightarrow$ No regional lymph node metastasis.
$T \rightarrow$ Carcinoma in site
$N_1, N_2, N_3 \rightarrow$ Increasing size involvement of lymph nodes.

Distant Metastasis (M)

$M_x \rightarrow$ Distant Metastasis cannot be made out

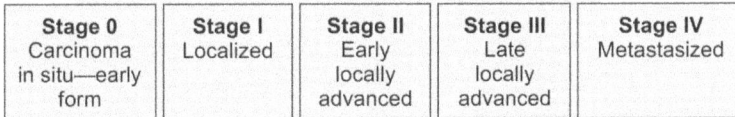

Fig. 14.3: Stages of cancer.

$M_0 \rightarrow$ No distant metastasis
$M1 \rightarrow$ Distant metastasis.

CLINICAL FEATURES

- Fatigue
- Alopecia
- Chronic pain
- Bleeding (or) Hemorrhage
- Low self-esteem
- Anorexia
- Cachexia
- Malabsorption
- Nausea
- Vomiting
- Stomatitis
- Impaired skin integrity
- Decreased immune response.

COMPLICATIONS

- Infection
- Sepsis
- Superior vena cava syndrome
- Spinal cord compression
- Hypocalcemia
- Pericardial effusion
- Dissemination intravascular coagulation
- Syndrome of inappropriate secretion of antidiuretic hormone (SIADH)
- Tumor lysis syndrome.

Types of cancer based on site of cancer including clinical features, complications, diagnostic test findings and management

Site of cancer	Clinical features	Complications	Diagnostic test findings	Management
Adrenal tumor	• Pain in the back or side (flank) • Feeling full with no appetite • Early puberty in children • Heart palpitations • Hypertension • Excessive hair growth • Unusual acne • Change in libido • Round, full face ("moon" face) • Easy bruising • Abdominal stretch marks • Fatigue • Muscle weakness • Weight gain and fluid retention • Diabetes • Osteoporosis • Headache • Insomnia • Hypokalemia • Tachycardia • Excessive perspiration • Mood changes	• Cushing's syndrome • Conn's syndrome • Neuroblastoma	• History • Physical examination • Blood tests • Urine tests • CT scan • MRI scan • PET scanners • Ultrasound scan • Angiography	• Surgery • Radiotherapy • Chemotherapy
Anal cancer	• Bleeding from the anus • Pain, discomfort and itching around the anus • Small lumps around the anus • Fecal incontinence • Discharge of mucus from the anus • Ulcers around the anus that can spread to the skin of the buttocks	• Perianal abscess • Intestinal obstruction • Gastrointestinal bleeding	• History • Physical examination • Digital rectal examination (DRE) • Anoscopy • Tissue biopsy • Ultrasound scan • PET scan • CT scan • Chest X-ray • MRI scan	• Surgery • Radiotherapy • Chemotherapy

Contd...

Contd...

Site of cancer	Clinical features	Complications	Diagnostic test findings	Management
Bile duct cancer	♦ Jaundice ♦ Itching ♦ Weight loss ♦ Loss of appetite ♦ Fever ♦ Abdominal pain	♦ Bleeding ♦ Infection ♦ Liver failure	♦ History ♦ Physical examination ♦ Blood tests ♦ Tumor marker tests ♦ Tissue biopsy ♦ Ultrasound scan ♦ CT scan ♦ Laparoscopy ♦ MRI scan	♦ Surgery ♦ Radiotherapy ♦ Chemotherapy
Bladder tumor	♦ Blood or blood clots in the urine ♦ Pain or burning sensation during urination ♦ Frequent urination ♦ Feeling the need to urinate many times throughout the night ♦ Feeling the need to urinate, but not being able to pass urine ♦ Lower back pain on one side of the body	♦ Anemia ♦ Hydronephrosis ♦ Urethral stricture ♦ Urinary incontinence	♦ History ♦ Physical examination ♦ Blood tests ♦ Urine tests ♦ Cystoscopy ♦ Tissue biopsy ♦ CT scan ♦ Laparoscopy ♦ MRI scan	♦ Surgery ♦ Chemotherapy ♦ Immunotherapy ♦ Radiotherapy
Bone tumor	♦ Pain where the tumor is located ♦ Joint swelling ♦ Tenderness ♦ Limping ♦ Fever ♦ General malaise ♦ Weight loss ♦ Anemia	♦ Phantom limb pain ♦ Pathological fracture ♦ Muscle wasting ♦ Reduced function	♦ History ♦ Physical examination ♦ Blood tests ♦ X-ray ♦ Bone scan ♦ Tissue biopsy ♦ CT scan ♦ PET scan ♦ MRI scan	♦ Surgery ♦ Chemotherapy ♦ Radiotherapy

Contd...

Contd...

Site of cancer	Clinical features	Complications	Diagnostic test findings	Management
Brain tumor	• Decerebrate posture • Decorticate posture • Decreased coordination • Decreased sensation of a body area • Diplopia • Emotional instability • Fever • Persistent headache which worsens when awakening • Hearing loss • Loss of memory • Impaired judgement • Personality and behavioral changes • Positive Babinski's reflex • Reduced alertness • Seizures • Speech difficulties • Lethargy • Weakness of the body area • Vomiting • Amenorrhea • Confusion • Breathing problem • Drooping of eyelids • Facial paralysis • Hand tremor • Hiccups • Impaired sense of smell • Obesity • Dysphagia • Uncontrollable movement	• Brain herniation • Vision changes • Personality changes • Seizures • Weakness • Loss of ability to function • Recurrent tumor growth • Permanent, progressive, profound neurologic losses	• History • Physical examination • Neurological examination • Positron emission tomography • CT scan of the head • Electroencephalogram • Histological examination • Examination of CSF • MRI scan of the head • Pneumoencephalography • Tissue biopsy	• Surgery • Radiotherapy • Chemotherapy • Targeted therapy • Electric field therapy

Contd...

Contd...

Site of cancer	Clinical features	Complications	Diagnostic test findings	Management
Breast cancer	• A lump in the breast • A change in the size or shape of the breast • Dimpling of the skin or thickening in the breast tissue • A nipple that's turned in (inverted) • A rash (like eczema) on the nipple • Discharge from the nipple • Swelling or a lump in the armpit	• Phantom breast pain • Lymphedema • Breast tenderness • Cachexia • Cerebral metastases • Opsoclonus • Loss of sexual interest • Depression • Lymphangitis carcinomatosa • Brachial plexus neuropathy • Mastalgia	• History • Physical examination • Mammography • Ultrasound scan • MRI scan • Tissue biopsy • Genomic tests • Blood tests • Tumor marker tests • X-ray • Bone scan • CT scan • PET scan	• Surgery • Radiotherapy • Chemotherapy • Hormonal therapy • Targeted therapy
Cervical cancer	• Abnormal vaginal bleeding • Persistent vaginal discharge • Postcoital pain and bleeding • Pelvic pain • Vaginal leakage of urine and stool from a fistula • Anorexia • Weight loss • Anemia • Periods become heavier and last longer than usual • Bleeding may present after menopause • Fatigue • Back pain • Leg pain • Single swollen leg	• Early menopause • Lymphedema • Hydronephrosis • Fistula • Emotional upset	• History • Physical examination • Blood tests • PET scan • CT scan • MRI scan • EUA (examination under anesthetic)	• Surgery • Radiotherapy • Chemotherapy

Contd...

Contd...

Site of cancer	Clinical features	Complications	Diagnostic test findings	Management
Colon cancer	• Blood in the stools which appears bright red or dark • Change in the normal bowel habit (diarrhea or constipation) that happens for no obvious reason and lasts longer than 3 weeks • Unexplained weight loss • Pain in the abdomen or back passage • Feeling of incomplete emptiness of the bowel • Unexplained tiredness • Obstruction in the bowel • Bloating	• Bowel obstruction • Constipation • Fecal impaction • Radiation enteritis	• History • Physical examination • Blood tests • PET scan • CT scan • MRI scan • Ultrasound scan • X-ray • Colonoscopy • Tissue biopsy • Molecular testing	• Surgery • Radiotherapy • Chemotherapy • Targeted therapy
Endometrial cancer	• Bulky uterus • Abnormal uterine bleeding • Abnormal menstrual bleeding • Lower abdominal pain or pelvic cramping • Thin white or clear vaginal discharge after menopause • Extremely long, heavy or frequent episodes of vaginal discharge after 40 years of age	• Anemia • Perforation of the uterus • Menorrhagia • Uterine enlargement	• History • Physical examination • Pelvic examination • Blood tests • Tumor marker tests • Hysteroscopic examination • PET scan • CT scan • MRI scan • Ultrasound scan • X-ray • Colonoscopy • Sonosalpingographic exam • Tissue biopsy • Pap smear tests	• Surgery • Radiotherapy • Chemotherapy

Contd...

Contd...

Site of cancer	Clinical features	Complications	Diagnostic test findings	Management
Esophageal cancer	• Difficulty and pain in swallowing • Pressure or burning in the chest • Indigestion or heartburn • Vomiting • Frequent choking on food • Unexplained weight loss • Cough • Hoarseness • Pain behind the breastbone or in the throat	• Tracheoesophageal fistula • Anemia • Pneumonia • Weight loss	• History • Physical examination • Esophagram or barium swallow • Upper endoscopy or esophagus-gastric-duodenoscopy (EGD) • Endoscopic ultrasound scan • Bronchoscopy • Tissue biopsy • Molecular tests • PET scan • CT scan • MRI scan	• Surgery • Endoscopic therapy • Radiotherapy • Chemotherapy • Targeted therapy
Gallbladder cancer	• Jaundice • Abdominal pain • Nausea • Vomiting • Bloating • A lump in the abdomen • Fever	• Cholestatic jaundice • Abdominal mass • Malignant transformation • Perforation of gallbladder	• History • Physical examination • X-ray • Endoscopic retrograde cholangiopancreatography (ERCP) • Percutaneous cholangiography • Laparoscopy • Blood tests • Endoscopic ultrasound scan • Tissue biopsy • PET scan • CT scan • MRI scan	• Surgery • Radiotherapy • Chemotherapy

Contd...

Contd...

Site of cancer	Clinical features	Complications	Diagnostic test findings	Management
Head and neck cancer	• Swelling or sore throat • Red or white patch in the mouth • Persistent sore throat • Lump or mass in the head or neck area, with or without painless • Hoarseness or change in voice • Nasal obstruction • Frequent nose bleeds • Dyspnea • Diplopia • Numbness or weakness of a body part in the head and neck region • Dysphagia • Ear or jaw pain • Blood in the saliva or phlegm • Loosening of teeth • Unexplained weight loss • Fatigue	• Oral mucositis • Infection • Xerostomia • Osteoradionecrosis	• History • Physical examination • Blood tests • Urine tests • HPV testing • Endoscopy • Tissue biopsy • Molecular testing • X-ray • Barium swallow • Panorex • PET scan • CT scan • MRI scan • Ultrasound scan • Bone scan	• Surgery • Radiotherapy • Chemotherapy • Targeted therapy
Kaposi sarcoma	• Slightly elevated purple, red or brown spots (lesions) on the skin • Lesions in the mouth or throat • Lymphedema • Unexplained cough or chest painless • Unexplained stomach or intestinal pain • Breathlessness • Cough • Nausea and vomiting • Diarrhea • Anemia	• Internal bleeding • Gastrointestinal bleeding • Anemia • Pleural effusion • Hemangioma	• History • Physical examination • Endoscopy • Tissue biopsy • X-ray • Bronchoscopy • CT scan	• Antiviral treatment • Surgery • Photodynamic therapy • Radiotherapy • Chemotherapy • Immunotherapy

Contd...

Contd...

Site of cancer	Clinical features	Complications	Diagnostic test findings	Management
Leukemia	• Fatigue • Weakness • Easy bruising • Bleeding that does not stop easily • Pale skin • Red pinhead-sized spots on the skin • Weight loss • Fever • Bone or abdominal pain • Dyspnea • Recurrent infections • Swollen lymph nodes • Enlarged liver or spleen • In women, menstruation that lasts longer than usual • Dizziness • Headache • Blurred vision • Nausea • Vomiting	• Splenomegaly • Anemia • Tumor lysis syndrome • Richter transformation • Death	• History • Physical examination • Blood tests • Bone marrow aspiration and tissue biopsy • Immunophenotyping or flow cytometry • Karyotyping or cytogenetics • Genetic testing • Lumbar puncture tests • CT scan • MRI scan	• Chemotherapy • Targeted therapy • Radiotherapy • Stem cell/bone marrow transplantation
Liver cancer	• Pain in the upper abdomen on the right side • A lump or a feeling of heaviness in the upper abdomen • Swollen abdomen (bloating) • Loss of appetite • Feeling of fullness • Weight loss • Nausea • Vomiting • Fever	• Ascites • Jaundice • Fatigue • Liver metastases • Bile obstruction • Liver failure	• History • Physical examination • Blood tests • CT scan • MRI scan • Ultrasound test • Tissue biopsy	• Liver transplant • Ablation • Embolization • Targeted therapy • Radiation therapy • Chemotherapy

Contd...

Contd...

Site of cancer	Clinical features	Complications	Diagnostic test findings	Management
Lung cancer	• A cough that lasts for 3 weeks or more • Repeated chest infections • Feeling breathless for no reason • A hoarse voice that lasts for 3 weeks or more • Pain in the chest or shoulder that doesn't get better • Feeling more tired than usual for some time	• Pleural effusion • Hemoptysis • Neuropathy • Pain • Lymphedema • Chemodrain	• History • Physical examination • CT scan • MRI scan • PET scan • Tissue biopsy • Bone scan • Molecular testing • Bronchoscopy • Thoracentesis • Thoracoscopy • Mediastinoscopy • Thoracotomy	• Surgery • Radiotherapy • Chemotherapy • Targeted therapy • Immunotherapy
Lymphoma – Hodgkin	• Painless swelling of lymph nodes in the neck, underarm or groin area that does not go away within a few weeks • Fatigue • Unexplained weight loss • Night sweats, usually drenching • Unexplained fever that does not go away • Pruritus, a generalized itching that may be severe • Pain in the lymph nodes triggered by drinking alcohol	• Weakened immune system • Infertility • Leukemia • Heart disease • Thyroid problems • Lung problems	• History • Physical examination • Bone marrow aspiration • Tissue biopsy (Reed-Sternberg cells) • Blood tests • Liver function tests • Kidney function tests • CT scan • PET scan • MRI scan • Pulmonary function tests • Echocardiogram • Multigated acquisition (MUGA) scan	• Chemotherapy • Radiotherapy • Stem cell/bone marrow transplantation

Contd...

Contd...

Site of cancer	Clinical features	Complications	Diagnostic test findings	Management
Lymphoma – Non-Hodgkin	• Enlarged lymph nodes in the abdomen, groin, neck or underarms • Hepatomegaly • Splenomegaly • Unexplained fever • Unexplained weight loss • Sweating • Chills • Fatigue	• Bone marrow infiltration • Disseminated intravascular coagulation • Pleural effusion • Superior vena cava obstruction • Spinal cord compression • Tumor lysis syndrome	• History • Physical examination • Bone marrow aspiration • Tissue biopsy • CT scan • PET scan • MRI scan • Molecular testing	• Watchful waiting • Chemotherapy • Radiotherapy • Immunotherapy • Stem cell/bone marrow transplantation
Melanoma	• Asymmetrical moles (A) – Irregular in shape • Border of a mole (B) – Blurred, uneven or has ragged edges • Color of a mole (C) – Mole has more than one color like black, brown, tan, etc. • Diameter (D) – Irregular moles are usually larger than 7 mm • Evolving (E) – Moles often change in size, shape, color or appearance • Any of the above-mentioned ABCDE features • A mole that tingles or itches • Crusting or bleeding of a mole • Any unusual marks on the skin that lasts more than a few weeks • Something growing under a nail	• Recurring melanomas • Hypopigmentation • Lymph adenopathy • Cutaneous nodules • Blue nails • Acanthosis nigricans	• History • Physical examination • Tissue biopsy • CT scan • PET scan • MRI scan • Ultrasound scan	• Surgery • Radiotherapy • Immunotherapy • Targeted therapy • Intralesional therapy • Chemotherapy • Isolated limb infusion therapy

Contd...

Contd...

Site of cancer	Clinical features	Complications	Diagnostic test findings	Management
Multiple myeloma	• Bone pain • Anemia • Fatigue • Hypercalcemia • Kidney damage or failure • Paraproteins in the blood or urine • Weight loss • Nausea • Fever • Lowered immunity	• Renal insufficiency • Bone marrow failure • Infection • Spinal cord compression • Pathologic fracture • Thrombocytopenia • Petechiae	• History • Physical examination • Blood tests • Urine tests • (M-proteins) • X-ray • Bone marrow aspiration • Tissue biopsy • CT scan • PET scan • MRI scan • Molecular testing	• Targeted therapy • Chemotherapy • Stem cell/bone marrow transplantation • Radiotherapy • Surgery
Naso-pharyngeal cancer	• A lump in the neck • Nasal obstruction or stuffiness • Troubles hearing • A sense of fullness or pain in the ear • Tinnitus • Sore throat • Breathlessness • Epistaxis • Pain, numbness or paralysis in the face • Frequent headaches • Difficulty opening the mouth • Blurred vision • Fatigue • Unexplained weight loss	• Paraneoplastic syndrome • Hypernasal speech • Middle ear effusion • Dysphagia	• History • Physical examination • Blood tests • Endoscopy • X-ray • Bone scan • Tissue biopsy • CT scan • PET scan • MRI scan • Ultrasound scan	• Radiotherapy • Chemotherapy • Surgery

Contd...

Contd...

Site of cancer	Clinical features	Complications	Diagnostic test findings	Management
Ovarian cancer	• Sense of pelvic heaviness • Abnormal ovarian mass • Discomfort in the lower abdomen • Pain during sex • Vaginal bleeding • Weight gain or loss • Abnormal menstrual cycles • Unexplained back pain that worsens over time • Increased abdominal girth • Indigestion • Anorexia • Nausea • Vomiting • Inability to ingest usual intake of food • Bloating • Increased urinary frequency or urgency • Excessive hair growth • Unexplained or extreme tiredness • Changes in bowel habits • Ascites	• Torsion of an ovarian cyst • Hemorrhage • Rupture of an ovarian cyst • Infection • Infertility	• History • Physical examination • Blood tests • Ultrasound scan • Laparoscopy • Laparotomy • X-ray • Tissue biopsy • CT scan • PET scan • MRI scan	• Surgery • Chemotherapy • Radiotherapy
Pancreatic cancer	• Pain or discomfort often begins in the upper abdomen and spreads to the back • Weight loss • Jaundice • Loss of appetite • Indigestion • Nausea • Vomiting • Depression • Feeling bloated after meals • Feeling extremely tired • Change in bowel habits	• Bowel obstruction • Liver failure • Problems with glucose metabolism • Malnutrition	• History • Physical examination • Blood tests • Tissue biopsy • MRI scan • PET scan • CT scan • Endoscopic retrograde cholangiopancreatography (ERCP) • Endoscopic ultrasound (EUS) • Percutaneous transhepatic cholangiography (PTC) • Molecular testing	• Surgery • Radiotherapy • Chemotherapy • Targeted therapy

Contd...

Contd...

Oncology-related Disorders

Contd...

Site of cancer	Clinical features	Complications	Diagnostic test findings	Management
Parathyroid tumor	♦ Feeling thirsty and passing a lot of urine ♦ Muscle weakness ♦ Nausea ♦ Vomiting ♦ Indigestion ♦ Loss of appetite ♦ Constipation ♦ Difficulty in speaking ♦ A lump in the neck ♦ Confusion ♦ Insomnia ♦ General malaise	♦ Hypercalcemia ♦ Bleeding in the neck ♦ Recurrent laryngeal nerve injury ♦ Wound infection	♦ History ♦ Physical examination ♦ Blood tests ♦ Urine tests ♦ Tissue biopsy ♦ MRI scan ♦ SPECT scan ♦ CT scan ♦ Ultrasound scan	♦ Surgery ♦ Radiotherapy ♦ Chemotherapy
Penile cancer	♦ Thickening or change in color of the skin ♦ Genital lesions on the penis ♦ Painless sore on penis ♦ Pain and bleeding from the penis ♦ Swollen lymph nodes in the groin ♦ Reddish, velvety rash beneath the foreskin ♦ Irregular swelling at the end of the penis	♦ Lymphedema ♦ Urethral stricture ♦ Wound infections ♦ Seroma ♦ Skin flap necrosis ♦ Phlebitis	♦ History ♦ Physical examination ♦ Tissue biopsy ♦ X-ray ♦ CT scan ♦ MRI scan	♦ Surgery ♦ Laser therapy ♦ Radiotherapy ♦ Chemotherapy
Pituitary gland tumor	♦ Headache ♦ Vision problems ♦ Unexplained tiredness ♦ Mood changes ♦ Irritability ♦ Acromegaly ♦ Infertility ♦ Changes in menstruation (in women)	♦ Diabetes insipidus ♦ Permanent hormone deficiency ♦ Pituitary apoplexy	♦ History ♦ Physical examination ♦ Blood tests ♦ Urine tests ♦ Tissue biopsy ♦ Lumbar puncture ♦ Visual field exam ♦ CT scan ♦ MRI scan	♦ Surgery ♦ Radiotherapy ♦ Hormonal therapy ♦ Chemotherapy

Contd...

Site of cancer	Clinical features	Complications	Diagnostic test findings	Management
Prostate cancer	• Pain in the back, hips or legs • Frequent urination • Difficulty in passing urine • Urge to urinate frequently at night • Feeling of incomplete emptying of bladder • Blood in the urine or semen • New onset of erectile dysfunction • Pain when passing urine or ejaculating • Unexplained weight loss • Fatigue • Change in bowel habits • Swelling or edema in the legs or feet	• Erectile dysfunction • Urinary incontinence • Acute kidney injury • Loss of libido	• History • Physical examination • Blood tests • Urine tests • PSA test • DRE test • Gene-based test • Transrectal ultrasound (TRUS) • Tissue biopsy • MRI fusion biopsy • Bone scan • CT scan • MRI scan	• Watchful waiting • Surgery • Radiotherapy • Androgen deprivation therapy • Chemotherapy • Immunotherapy
Rectal cancer	• Blood in the stools and it may be bright red or dark in color • Change in bowel habits • Unexplained weight loss • Unexplained tiredness • Pain in the abdomen or back passage • Feeling of incomplete emptying of bowel	• Bowel obstruction • Constipation • Fecal impaction • Radiation enteritis	• History • Physical examination • Blood tests • PET scan • X-ray • Tissue biopsy • Molecular testing • Virtual colonoscopy • Sigmoidoscopy	• Surgery • Chemotherapy • Radiotherapy • Targeted therapy
Renal cancer	• Blood in the urine • A dull pain in the side between the upper abdomen and back • High fever • Night sweats • Feeling very tired • Losing weight for no obvious reason • A lump in the tummy area, side or back	• Polycythemia • Hypercalcemia • Congestive heart failure • Death	• History • Physical examination • Blood tests • CT scan • MRI scan • Ultrasound test • Tissue biopsy	• Surgery • Targeted therapy • Radiotherapy

Contd...

Contd...

Site of cancer	Clinical features	Complications	Diagnostic test findings	Management
Skin cancer	• Flat, red spot which is scaly and crusty • Develops a crust or scab • Itching • Formation of painless ulcer • Bleed sometimes • Begin to heal but never completely heal • Waxy, smooth, pearly, red lump • Feel tender to touch	• Recurring melanomas • Hypopigmentation • Lymph adenopathy • Cutaneous nodules • Blue nails • Acanthosis nigricans	• History • Physical examination • CT scan • MRI scan • PET scan • Tissue biopsy	• Surgery • Radiotherapy • Chemotherapy
Spinal cord tumor	• Back and neck pain • Numbness • Tingling • Weakness in the arms or legs or both • Clumsiness • Difficulty in walking • Loss of bowel and bladder control (incontinence)	• Paralysis to varying degrees • Life-threatening spinal cord compression • Permanent damage to nerves	• History • Physical examination • Blood tests • Urine tests • CT scan • MRI scan • Tissue biopsy	• Surgery • Radiotherapy • Chemotherapy
Stomach cancer	• Heartburn or indigestion that doesn't go away • Burping a lot • Loss of appetite • Feeling full after eating only a small amount • Pain in the upper tummy area • Weight loss • Being sick • Dysphagia • Blood in the stools • Feeling tired • Breathlessness due to anemia	• Esophageal stricture • Cachexia • Gastric ulcer • Dysphagia • Bowel obstruction • Pyloric stenosis	• History • Physical examination • Endoscopic ultrasound • CT scan • PET scan • Laparoscopy • Ultrasound scan	• Surgery • Radiotherapy • Chemotherapy • Targeted therapy
Testicular cancer	• Pain or discomfort in the testicle • Feeling of heaviness in the scrotum • Dull ache in the back or lower abdomen • Lump or swelling in either testicle • Enlargement of a testicle • Gynecomastia	• Infertility • Pulmonary fibrosis • Peripheral neuropathy • Raynaud's phenomenon • Tinnitus • Hearing loss	• History • Physical examination • Blood tests • X-ray • Tissue biopsy • CT scan • PET scan • Ultrasound scan	• Surgery • Chemotherapy • Radiotherapy

Contd...

Contd...

Site of cancer	Clinical features	Complications	Diagnostic test findings	Management
Thyroid tumor	• A lump in the front of the neck (near the Adam's apple) • Hoarseness of voice • Swollen glands in the neck • Difficulty in swallowing • Pain in the throat or neck • Shortness of breath • Persistent cough	• Injury to the voice box • Hypocalcemia • Laryngeal nerve palsy	• History • Physical examination • Blood tests • X-ray • Tissue biopsy • PET scan • Ultrasound scan • Radionuclide scan • Molecular testing	• Surgery • Hormonal therapy • Radioactive iodine therapy • Radiotherapy • Chemotherapy • Targeted therapy
Vaginal cancer	• Pain in the pelvic area • Pain when passing urine • Urgency to pass urine often • Blood in the urine • Tenesmus • Swollen legs • Bleeding after the menopause, between periods or after sex	• Early menopause • Lymphedema • Hydronephrosis • Fistula • Emotional upset	• History • Physical examination • Blood tests • Pap smear test • Colposcopy • Tissue biopsy • X-ray • Endoscopy • CT scan • PET scan • MRI scan	• Radiotherapy • Surgery • Chemotherapy
Vulvar cancer	• Itching, burning or soreness in the vulva that doesn't go away • A lump, swelling or wart-like growth on the vulva • Thickened, raised, red, white or dark patches on the skin of the vulva • Bleeding or a blood-stained vaginal discharge not related to menstruation • Burning pain when passing urine • Tenderness or pain in the area of the vulva • A sore or ulcerated area on the vulva • A mole on the vulva that changes shape or color	• Lymphedema • Depression • Loss of interest	• History • Physical examination • Blood tests • PET scan • CT scan • MRI scan • EUA (examination under anesthetic)	• Surgery • Radiotherapy • Chemotherapy

PREVENTION OF CANCER

There are two levels of cancer prevention as follows:
1. **Primary prevention**
   - Avoiding known carcinogens
   - Adopting proper dietary pattern
   - Promoting healthful lifestyles
   - Educating the community regarding risk involved in cancer.
2. **Secondary prevention**
   - Early detection and screening to achieve early diagnosis and prompt intervention to halt the cancer process.

MANAGEMENT

Medical

- **Radiotherapy:** It is a procedure in which high-energy ionizing rays or particles are used to destroy a cancer cell's ability to grow and multiply. It can be given both externally and internally. External radiotherapy (*Teletherapy*) aims high energy X-rays at the affected area using a large machine. Internal radiotherapy (*Brachytherapy*) involves having radioactive material placed inside the body. It works by destroying cancer and certain amount of normal cells in the area that's being treated. Cancer cells cannot repair themselves after radiotherapy, but normal cells usually can.
- **Chemotherapy:** It is a procedure in which antineoplastic agents are used in an attempt to destroy tumor cells by interfering with cellular functions and reproduction.
  - *Alkylating agents:* It helps to alter the DNA structure by misreading DNA code and initiating breaks in the DNA molecule. For example, bisulfan, chlorambucil, cisplatin, cyclophosphamide, etc.
  - *Antimetabolites:* It interferes with the biosynthesis of metabolites or nucleic acids necessary for RNA and DNA synthesis. For example, 5-Fluorouracil, hydroxyurea, methotrexate, 6-mercaptopurine, etc.
  - *Antibiotics:* It interferes with DNA synthesis by binding to DNA. For example, bleomycin, dactinomycin, daunorubicin, doxorubicin, mitomycin, etc.
  - *Plant alkaloids:* It arrests metaphase by inhibiting mitotic tubular formation. For example, vincristine, vinblastine, etc.
  - *Taxanes:* It arrests metaphase by inhibiting tubulin depolymerization. For example, paclitaxel, docetaxel, etc.
  - *Nitrosoureas:* It crosses the blood-brain barrier, alters DNA structure by misreading DNA code and initiating breaks in the DNA molecule. For example, carmustine, lomustine, etc.
  - *Topoisomerase inhibitors:* It includes break in the DNA strand by binding to enzyme topoisomerase, preventing cells from dividing further. For example, irinotecan, topotecan, etc.
  - *Hormonal agents:* It binds to hormone receptor sites that alter cellular growth. For example, estrogens, antiprogestins, luteinizing hormone, etc.
  - **Immunotherapy:** It is the treatment modality which produces anti-tumor effects primarily through the action of natural host defense mechanism. It is capable of altering the immune system with either stimulatory or suppressive effects.
  - **Targeted therapy:** It is a treatment that targets the cancer's specific genes, proteins, or the tissue environment that contributes to cancer growth and survival. This type of treatment blocks the growth and spread of cancer cells while limiting damage to normal cells.
  - **Electric field therapy:** It uses low-intensity electrical fields to suppress cancer cell proliferation in the body.
  - **Hormonal therapy:** It delays the growth of cancer and helps reduce the risk of it coming back.

- **Gene therapy:** It is the approach that corrects genetic defects or manipulates genes to induce tumor cell destruction.
- **Thermal therapy:** It is a procedure in which temperature is generated greater than 106.7°F to destroy tumors in human cancers as the malignant cells are more sensitive than normal cells to the harmful effects of high temperature.
- **Endoscopic therapy:** It is a therapy used for mucosal cancers, whereas palliation is used for patients unwilling or unable to undergo surgery, chemotherapy or radiation.
- **Ablation therapy:** The main goal of ablation therapy is complete tumor destruction. With this form of treatment, individual tumors are destroyed using heat (radiofrequency ablation), cold (cryoablation) or chemical agents (percutaneous ethanol instillation). Ablative therapy is most often performed for tumors involving the liver, kidney, lung and painful tumors of bone.
- **Radioactive iodine therapy:** It is a nuclear medicine treatment used to treat thyroid cancer. When a small dose of radioactive iodine I-131 or I-123 (an isotope of iodine that emits radiation) is swallowed, it is absorbed into the bloodstream and concentrated by the thyroid gland, where it begins destroying the gland's cells.
- **Androgen deprivation therapy (ADT):** It is the mainstay of treatment for metastatic prostate cancer. It suppresses the disease for many years. It is also used as an adjunct to radiotherapy, but is not by itself a curative treatment for prostate cancer.
- **Isolated limb infusion (ILI) therapy:** It is a minimally invasive technique for delivering regional chemotherapy in patients with advanced and metastatic melanoma confined to a limb. It is essentially a low-flow isolated limb perfusion (ILP) performed via percutaneous catheters without oxygenation.

Surgical

- **Biopsy:** It is a surgical procedure in which a tissue sample is obtained for analysis of cells suspected to be malignant.
- **Surgery as primary treatment:** It is a surgical procedure in which malignant tumor and a margin of adjacent normal tissue is removed.
- **Debulking:** It is the surgical removal of the bulk of the tumor before starting chemotherapy.
- **Salvage surgery:** It is the surgical procedure which involves the use of an extensive surgical approach to treat a local recurrence after implementing a less extensive primary approach, for example, A mastectomy to treat recurrent breast cancer after primary lumpectomy and radiation.
- **Electrosurgery:** It is the surgical procedure in which electrical current is used to destroy the tumor cells.
- **Cryosurgery:** It is the surgical procedure in which liquid nitrogen is used to freeze the tissues that cause cell destruction.
- **Palliative surgery:** It is a surgery that attempts to relieve the complications of cancer such as hemorrhage, pain, obstruction, etc. when cure is not possible.
- **Chemosurgery:** It is the surgical procedure which uses combined chemotherapy and layer-by-layer surgical removal of abnormal tissue.
- **Photodynamic surgery:** It is the surgical procedure which makes use of light and energy aimed at an exact tissue location and depth to vaporize cancer cells.
- **Stereotactic radiosurgery:** It is a surgical procedure in which single and highly precise administration of high-dose radiation therapy used in some types of brain, head, and neck cancers.
- **Prophylactic surgery:** It is a surgical procedure in which nonvital tissues or organs that are likely to develop cancer are removed.

- **Reconstructive surgery:** It is a surgical procedure which follows curative or radical surgery in order to carry out an attempt to improve function or to obtain a more desirable cosmetic effort.
- **Bone marrow transplantation (Also known as stem cell transplantation):** Blood cells are produced in the bone marrow. The bone marrow is a tissue that is found in the center of bones, such as the back of the hips (the iliac crests) and the breastbone (the sternum). There are two categories of bone marrow transplantation as follows: autograft (the patient's own bone marrow or stem cells are used) and allograft (the bone marrow or stem cells from a donor are used). There are different types of donors like siblings (a brother or sister), MUD (a matched unrelated donor), alternative family donor (a parent, cousin or child) or syngeneic (an identical twin). A bone marrow or cord blood transplant is a medical procedure performed to replace unhealthy blood-forming cells with healthy ones.
- **Intralesional therapy:** It is a procedure involving the injection of medications (methotrexate, interferon, 5-fluorouracil, bleomycin, etc) into the skin for treating cutaneous neoplasms, with the aim of reducing the symptoms of cutaneous neoplasms. The injections were given as follows: using a 27-gauge needle, 0.3–2.0 cc of medications in a concentration of either 12.5 mg/mL or 25 mg/mL is injected each time.

Nursing

- Encourage the patient to increase the consumption of fresh vegetables in the diet.
- Educate the patient to maintain a healthy weight.
- Instruct the patient to reduce the intake of dietary fat and alcohol intake.
- Ask the patient to avoid excess consumption of salt-cured, smoked or nitrate-cured foods.
- Ask them to wear protective clothing.
- Instruct them to avoid overexposure to the sun.
- Encourage them to take vitamin-A, vitamin-C and fiber-rich diet.
- Ask them to safeguard against harmful radiations.

Index

Page numbers followed by *f* refer to figure.

A

Ablation therapy 498
Abortion 352
  complete 351
  elective 351
  habitual 351
  incomplete 351
  induced 351
  inevitable 351
  missed 351
  recurrent 351
  septic 351
    spontaneous 351
    therapeutic 351
    threatened 351
Abscess
  formation 6*f*
  retropharyngeal 133
Acetaminophen 433, 442, 443, 467, 476
Acetylcholinesterase inhibitors 3, 17, 73, 264, 267
Acetylsalicylic acid, topical 387
Achlorhydria 431
Achondroplasia 22
Acidosis 315
  metabolic 312
Acne vulgaris 371
  cardinal features of 371*f*
Acoustic reflectometry 151
Acquired immunodeficiency syndrome 424, 425
  pathogenesis of 425*f*
Acromegaly 91, 408
Activated partial thromboplastin time test 300
Acute respiratory distress syndrome 84, 258, 400
Acyclovir 160
Addison's disease 75, 96, 98
  signs of 75*f*
  symptoms of 75*f*
Adefovir dipivoxil 189
Adenoid glands, enlarged 134
Adenoidectomy 151
Adenomas, benign pituitary 91
Adenomyosis 354
Adenovirus 132, 159, 207, 333
  infection 112
Adrenal crisis 76

Adrenal enzyme inhibitors 78
Adrenal vein sampling test 87
Adrenalectomy 78, 87
  bilateral 78, 87
Adrenergic
  agents 292
  inhibitors 275
  receptor antagonists 328
Adrenocorticotropic hormone stimulation test 76, 100
Advancement rectal flap 165
Aedes aegypti mosquito 427, 432, 442, 473, 475
Age-related macular degeneration 105
Aggressive fluid resuscitation 368
Agitation 245
Airway
  injury, diffuse 215
  obstruction 154
Albuminuria 315
Albuterol 214
Alcohol 188
Alcoholism 193, 195
Aldosterone antagonists 264, 267, 274, 315, 319, 321, 325, 330
Algodystrophy 400
Alkalinizing agents 48
Alkalosis, metabolic 96, 330
Alkylphospholipid derivatives 445
Allen test 304
Allergen immunotherapy 156
Allergy shots 156
Alopecia 480
Alpha-antitrypsin deficiency 216
Alpha-blockers 275, 339, 348
Alpha glucosidase inhibitors 82, 85, 89
Alpha reductase inhibitors 339
Alveolar hypoxia 222
Alzheimer's disease 1, 16, 17, 343
  mild 2
  moderate 2
  severe 2
American Spinal Injury Association 57
Aminoglycoside 337
  antibiotics 445
Aminoquinoline analog 445
Aminosalicylates 175, 209
Amlodipine 184
Amoebae 202
Amoebiasis 161
Amoxicillin 160

Amphotericin B 229
Ampicillin 35, 41, 172
Amputation 412
Amsler grid test 106
Amyloid deposit inhibitors 17
Amyloidosis 263, 318, 322, 395, 412
Analgesics 6, 9, 27, 61, 70, 133, 135, 136, 143, 144, 151, 154, 158, 160, 170, 172, 201, 205, 219, 279, 283, 300, 342, 354, 391, 393, 395, 404, 405, 412, 416, 427
  simple 409
Anaphylaxis 311
Androgen deprivation therapy 498
Anemia 293, 293*f*
  aplastic 294, 295*f*
  pernicious 76, 98, 296, 296*f*
  severe 250
Aneurysm 59, 290, 469
  aortic 252, 253*f*, 255, 285
  ventricular 257
Anger control issues 25
Angina
  microvascular 251
  pectoris 250, 250*f*
  stable 251
  unstable 251
  variant 251
Angiogram
  coronary 267, 269
  pulmonary 241
Angiography 304
  pulmonary 239
Angioplasty 252
  extended 305
Angiotensin
  converting enzyme inhibitors 61, 71, 258, 274, 279, 281, 315, 319, 321, 323, 325, 330
  receptor blockers 61, 70, 264, 274, 315, 319, 321, 323, 325, 330
Angle-closure glaucoma 121
Anistreplase 279, 308
Ankle sprains 419*f*
Ankylosing spondylitis 282, 392, 394, 394*f*
Anorectal manometry 173
Anorexia 209, 480
Anovulatory menstrual cycles 359
Anoxic brain injury 10
Antacids 182, 184, 197, 201, 205, 315

Anti-androgen agents 372
Antibiotics 35, 39, 41, 76, 78, 80, 108,
    111, 125, 135, 146, 149, 158,
    163, 175, 181, 187, 197, 199,
    201, 203, 205, 209, 218, 219,
    225, 231, 272, 281, 283, 292,
    315, 320, 323, 326, 328, 330,
    333, 337, 342, 348, 354, 369,
    378, 412, 437, 464, 497
    oral 372, 382, 384
    topical 124, 372, 384
Antibody blood tests 76
Anticholinergics 170, 195
    agents 54, 214, 218, 221
Anticholinesterase 47
    agents 23, 52
Anticoagulants 68, 223, 239, 241, 252,
    255, 261, 264
Anticoagulation therapy 59
Anticonvulsant 4, 19, 21, 27, 36, 41, 56,
    285, 391
    drugs 89
Antidepressants 30, 33, 54, 317
    drugs 17
Antidiarrheal agents 181, 210
Anti-diuretic hormone 78, 100
    action of 102
    replacement 80
Antiemetics 170, 195, 197, 201, 203,
    205, 437
Antiepileptic 7, 33
    drugs 30
Antifibrinolytics 300, 310
    drugs 138
Antifungal agents 19, 41, 108, 272, 445
    topical 374, 385, 388
Anti-glutamates 4
Antigout agents 283, 402
Antihistamines 54, 113, 136, 149, 156,
    158, 317, 382, 389, 391
    agents 143, 186
    agonist 113
Antihypertensive agents 9, 37, 65
Antihypotensive 277
Anti-inflammatory agents 197, 199,
    281
Antimalarials 385
    agents 50, 203, 417, 423, 443
Antimetabolites 497
    agents 352
Antimicrobial
    agents 133, 156, 160
    therapy 7
Antineoplastic agents 45
Antioxidants 3, 18, 74
    vitamins 106
Anti-Parkinsonian agents 54
Antiphospholipid syndrome 359, 422
Antipsychotics 33, 56
    drugs 17
Antipyretics 272, 412
    agents 437
Antireflux surgery 184
Antiresorptive agents 414
Anti-seizure agents 45, 52

Anti-spasm agents 335, 337
Anti-spastic agent 4
Anti-thyroid drugs 94
Anti-vascular endothelial growth
    factor 106
    therapy 118
Antiviral
    agents 19, 41, 54, 125, 160, 391,
    437, 442, 464
    drugs 189
Antrectomy 183
Antrochoanal nasal polyps 148
Anxiety 54, 367
Anxiolytic agents 17
Aortic
    aneurysm, abdominal 253
    dissection 253, 320
    root dissection 286
Aortitis 469
Appendectomy, laparoscopic 167
Arbovirus 18
Arginine stimulation test 99
Aromatic diamidine 445
Arrhythmias 94, 227, 241, 251,
    265
Arterial blood gas analysis 84, 88, 217,
    221, 225, 245
Arterial gas embolism 13f
Arterial ligation 139
Arterial oxygen, pressure of 244
Arteriography 68
    coronary 252, 255
Arteriosclerosis 338
Arteritis, aortic 253
Artery thrombosis, large 69
Arthralgia 467
Arthritis 466
    chronic gouty 402
    inflammatory 401
    post-infectious 168
    psoriatic 386
    rheumatic 282
    septic 235, 412
    severe degenerative 416
Arthrography 419, 421
Arthropathy 299
Arthroscopy 409, 418, 419, 421
Artificial disc surgery 32
Ascaris lumbricoides 201, 202
Ascending reticular activating system
    9
Asexual reproduction 451
Aspergillus 228, 280
Aspiration pneumonia 154, 234, 461,
    471
Aspirin 252, 255, 269, 278, 304, 447
Asthma
    allergic 213
    bronchial 213, 213f, 222
    mixed 213
    nonallergic 213
Astigmatism 114
Atelectasis 211, 217
    acute 212
    chronic 212

Atherectomy 256, 270
Atheroembolic disease 255
Atherosclerosis 252, 254, 254f, 268,
    285, 302
    coronary 250
Atherosclerotic coronary arteries 250
Athlete's foot 373, 373f
Atrial ectopic beat 260
Atrial fibrillation 259f, 260, 285, 288
Atrial natriuretic peptide 313
Atropine 48
Attention deficit hyperactivity disorder
    25
Autoimmune
    disease 18, 24, 26, 188, 417
    disorder 5, 301, 303, 307, 317,
    320, 359
    dysfunction 1
Automated lamellar keratoplasty 116
Autonomic system testing 54
Azathioprine 63
Azithromycin 457
Azoles 445

B

Bacillary dysentery 167
Bacitracin zinc 124
Back pain
    acute 392
    chronic 31
Bacteremia 168, 235, 326, 348
Bactericidal agents 243
Bacteriuria 326
Balanitis xerotica obliterans 331
Balloon
    angioplasty 256
    sinuplasty 159
Barbiturates 22
Barotrauma 245
Bartholin's abscess 352, 353f
Bartholin's duct cyst, chronic 353
Bartholin's glands 353f
Basal ganglia of brain 32f
Basal polyps, allergic 148
Beclomethasone 212, 217
Bell's palsy 5
    cardinal features of 5f
Benzathine penicillin G 160
Benzodiazepines 22, 26, 45
Benzoyl peroxide 372
Benzyl penicillin 35, 41
Beta-3 adrenergic receptor 335
Beta-adrenergic
    agents 214
    agonists 218, 221
    blockers 45
Beta-blockers 30, 61, 71, 94, 122, 252,
    254, 258, 261, 269, 274, 323,
    369, 385
Beta-interferons 45
Bevacizumab 118
Biguanides 82, 85, 88
Bile acid
    disorders 197
    sequestrants 256, 269, 278

Bile duct cancer 482
Biliary tract infections 171
Billroth procedure 205
Biologic agents 210, 418, 423
Biologic therapies 175
Biopsy 498
   myocardial 267, 269
   pericardial 283
   pleural 236
   renal 315
   tonsil 56
Biphosphonates 416
Bipolar diathermy 186
Birth control pills 365, 367
Bismuth subsalicylate 172, 181
Bisphosphonates 90
Bladder
   diverticula 339
   protectants 317
   slings 335
   stress test 335
   tumor 482
Bleeding, rectal 209
Blepharitis 107, 123
   anterior 107
   chronic 110
   posterior 107
Blepharospasm 54
Blindness 129, 129f, 391
Blood
   acidosis 222
   borne infections 310
   cells, types of 295f
   chemistry tests 464
   clots 241
   dyscrasias 138
   infections of 458
   loss, acute 291
   plasma transfusion 292
   pressure
      high 78, 106, 251
      pulmonary arteries, raised 240f
   stream 198f
   tests 3, 449
   thinners 223, 239, 241
   thinning agents 9, 61, 70, 279, 281, 308
   transfusions 297
   urea nitrogen 319
Bone 412
   Bone biopsy 414
   Bone density test 410
   Bone disorder 315
   Bone healing, stages of 398f
   Bone marrow 411f
   Bone marrow transplantation 297, 499
   Bone mineral density test 90
   Bone scintigraphy 400
   Bone tumor 482
   Bone, normal 4f, 410f, 415f
Bordetella pertussis 216, 455
Brachytherapy 256, 497
Bradycardia 37
Brain 2f, 7f, 40f, 62f
   abscess 6, 6f
   biopsy 56
   infection 142
   injury, traumatic 71, 72, 98, 128, 140
   stimulation, seep 26, 54
   surgery 79, 98
   temporal lobe of 18f
   tumor 483
Brainstem
   auditory evoked response 142, 146
   test 227
   herniation 103
Breast cancer 484
Brimonidine 122
Bronchial dilation test 217
Bronchial tube 217f
Bronchiectasis 215, 215f, 222, 231, 233, 249
Bronchiole 211f
Bronchitis 216, 217f, 441, 454
   acute 216
   chronic 216, 220, 220f, 240, 369
Bronchodilators 212, 216, 217, 219, 223, 225, 227, 231, 235, 241, 245
Bronchospasm 184
Brown pigment stones 171
Bubonic plague 457
Budesonide 148, 212
Buerger's disease 302, 303, 304f
Bullous impetigo 383, 383f
Burns 374
   chemical 119
   classification of 375f
Burst appendix 205

C

Cachexia 52, 480
Caecostomy 193
Caffeine, intake of 145
Calcimimetics 90
Calcineurin inhibitors 382
Calcipotriene 387
Calcitonin 416
Calcitriol 98
Calcium
   channel blockers 9, 30, 37, 61, 70, 184, 252, 256, 258, 261, 264, 267, 270, 274, 279, 313, 315, 323, 330
   stones 327
   supplements 414
Cancer
   anal 481
   cell division 477f
   drugs 409
   endometrial 485
   esophageal 486
   nasopharyngeal 491
   pancreatic 492
   parathyroid 89
   rectal 494
   renal 494
   stages of 479f
   types of 479
   vaginal 496
   vulvar 496
Candida 280
   albicans 132, 378
Candidal onychomycosis 385
Candidiasis 378, 378f, 426
   esophageal 378
Captopril suppression test 87
Carbimazole 94
Carbonic anhydrase inhibitors 122, 201
Carcinogenesis 478f
Carcinoma 479
   hepatocellular 196, 299
   pituitary 91
Cardiac arrest 257, 257f
   sudden 94, 290
Cardiac computed tomography scan 264
Cardiac enzyme test 258
Cardiac failure, congestive 260, 265, 265f, 299, 417, 435
Cardiac magnetic resonance imaging 264
   scan 283
Cardiac muscle 262f
   hypertrophy of 260
Cardiac resynchronization therapy 268
Cardiac system, disorders of 250
Cardiomyopathy 63, 222, 262, 262f, 265, 281, 285, 405
   dilated 263
   hypertrophic 263
   hypertrophic obstructive 251
   restrictive 263
Cardiovascular collapse 237
Cardiovascular disease 64, 106
Carditis 285
   chronic rheumatic 285
Carotid
   angioplasty 9
   artery
      angiography 60, 70
      disease 255
      Doppler examination 60
      endarterectomy 9, 61, 71
Carpal pedal spasms 410
Carpal tunnel
   release 397
   syndrome 92, 302, 395, 396f
Cataract 108
   congenital 109, 130
   eye 109f
   secondary 109
   traumatic 109
Catechol-O-methyl transferase inhibitors 54
Cathartics 187
Cauda equina syndrome 31, 395, 404
Cell
   division, normal 477f
   myocardial 277f, 280f
Cellulitis 379, 379f, 383, 385, 438
   pre-orbital 123
Central nervous system disorders 228

Cephalosporin 35, 41, 160, 167, 337
Cephalothin 172
Cerebellar degeneration 51
Cerebral
   aneurysm 28
   angiography 61, 73
   decompression sickness 14
   infarction 7, 7f
      atherosclerotic 8
      hemorrhagic 8
   neurons 20f
palsy 22, 128, 22
   venous thrombosis 36
Cerebrospinal fluid 34, 36, 65
   examination 56, 443
Cerebrovascular accident 59
Cerebrovascular disease 274
Cerumen impaction 134, 134f
Cerumenolytic agents 135
Cervical
   adenoiditis 208
   cancer 484
   stenosis 354
Cervicitis 358
Cestodes 202
Chalazion 110, 111f
Chancre, formation of 468f
Charcot joints 66
Chemical peel 373
Chemodiol 172
Chemosurgery 498
Chemotherapy 98, 401, 497
Chest
   pain, anterior 238
   physiotherapy 212, 229, 232, 235, 245
   radiography 65
   trauma 218, 218f
   blunt 218
      penetrating 236
   tube insertion 219
   X-ray 103
Cheyne-Stokes respiration 70
Chickenpox 428, 428f
Chikungunya 426
   virus 426
      infection, symptoms of 427f
Chills 230, 243
Chlamydia 342, 356, 358, 362, 429
   infection 352, 429f
   pneumonia 132
   trachomatis 332, 429
Chloramphenicol 113
Chloride channel activator 174
Chlorpropamide 88
Cholangitis 172
Cholecystectomy 170, 172
Cholecystitis 168, 172
Cholecystostomy 170, 172
Choledochojejunostomy 201
Choledocholithiasis 172
Choledochostomy 170
Cholelithiasis 170
Cholera 430
   symptoms of 431f
Cholesteatoma 151

Cholesterol
   high 78
   stones 171
Cholinergic agents 122
Cholinesterase inhibitor 193
Chondrocalcinosis 408
Chronic obstructive pulmonary
      disease 50, 212, 216, 220, 222
Churg-Strauss syndrome 148
Ciprofloxacin 167, 342, 459
Cirrhosis
   alcoholic 196
   biliary 196
   cardiac 196
   post-necrotic 196
   primary biliary 326
Citalopram 3, 74
Clarithromycin 457
Clofazimine 447
Clonidine 26
   stimulation test 100
Clopidogrel 252
Clostridium
   sordellii 367
   tetani 470
Clotrimazole 388
Clotting disorders 359
Coagulation
   mesh 138
   tests 323
Coblation turbinoplasty 157
Cocaine 48
Coccidioides 280
Coccydynia 392
Cochlear implant 141, 153
Cochlear otosclerosis 152
Cold 233
Colectomy
   subtotal 176
   total abdominal 176
Colitis 164
   ulcerative 208, 209f
Collagen vascular disease 231
Coloboma 130
Colon cancer 485
Colonic transit study 173
Colonoscopy 173
Colostomy 193
Colposuspension 335
Coma 9, 10f
Communicable diseases 424
Compartment syndrome 48, 399
Complete blood count 276, 464
Computed tomography scan 12, 31, 35, 37, 41, 44, 47, 52, 56, 58, 60, 65, 68, 70, 76, 78, 80, 87, 90, 92, 98, 100, 103, 136, 138, 141, 144, 146, 148, 153, 154, 156, 158, 160, 165, 172, 175, 187, 191, 194, 197, 198, 200, 203, 206, 219, 227, 229, 231, 232, 235, 237, 241, 247, 254, 255, 267, 269, 292, 299, 315, 317, 319, 321, 325, 326, 328, 330, 337, 357, 358, 363, 370, 393, 395, 402, 404, 407, 417, 423, 439

Conjunctiva 112f
Conjunctivitis 112, 112f
   allergic 112
   bacterial 112
   recurrent 107
   toxic 113
   viral 112
Connective tissue
   diseases 240
   disorder 138, 286, 302
Constipation 162, 172
Contact dissolution therapy 172
Contact lenses 128
Continuous renal replacement therapy 313, 315, 330
Contusions 72
Cor pulmonale 222, 222f, 247, 461
Cornea, curvature of 114
Corneal abrasion 119
Corneal inflammation, chronic 125
Corneal transplantation 131
Coronary artery
   bypass
      grafting 256, 259, 267, 270, 279
      surgery 252
   disease 63, 255, 257, 268, 268f, 274, 285
   spasm 250
   stenting 256
Coronavirus 132
   SARS-associated 462
Corpus callosotomy 22
Correctable refractive errors 114
   types of 114f
Cortical visual impairment 130
Corticosteroids 6, 7, 19, 27, 35, 41, 45, 47, 48, 50, 52, 100, 101, 113, 125, 133, 143, 144, 146, 154, 156, 160, 175, 199, 209, 212, 214, 217, 221, 223, 225, 227, 245, 247, 281, 283, 285, 300, 310, 320, 323, 326, 378, 397, 402, 404, 405, 418
   high dose 31, 58, 423,
   nasal spray 148
   oral 148, 389, 391, 449
   topical 163, 165, 382
   use of 124, 132
Corticotropin releasing hormone
      stimulation test 78
Corynebacterium diphtheriae 434
Cosmetic deformity 123
Cottle's test 136
Cover test 128
Cowden syndrome 478
Coxsackie virus 231
Cranial nerve palsies 128
Craniectomy, decompressive 37, 74
Craniotomy 37, 74
Creatine kinase 39
Cretinism 101
Creutzfeldt-Jakob disease 56
   iatrogenic 56
Cricothyroidotomy 249
Crohn's disease 163, 164, 174, 174f, 192, 197, 205, 394

Cromolyn sodium 113, 214
Crush
  injuries 218, 311
  syndrome 400
Cryoglobulinemia 189, 318
Cryopexy 127
Cryoprecipitate 301, 310
Cryosurgery 498
Cryotherapy 157
Cryptococcus neoformans 39
Cryptorchidism 340
Cryptosporidiosis 426
Crystalloids, intravenous 293
Cushing's syndrome 77, 77*f*, 81, 87
Cyanosis 245, 249, 266
  central 212
Cyclophosphamide 63
Cyst
  arachnoid 34
  aspiration 365
Cystic fibrosis 147, 215, 222, 224, 224*f*, 225, 228, 233
Cystine stones 328
Cystinosis 409
Cystitis 316, 316*f*
Cystolithiasis 339
Cystoscopy 317, 335, 337, 339
Cystourethrogram 337
  anterograde 332
Cystourethroscopy 332
Cytokines 210
Cytomegalovirus 159, 426

D

Dandy-Walker syndrome 34
Dapsone 447
D-dimer test 239, 308
DEC provocation test 439
Decompression
  posterior fossa 66
  sickness 12, 13*f*
    cutaneous 12
    neurological 13
Deep internal bleeding 310
Deep vein thrombosis 58, 307*f*, 414
Defecography 173
Defibrillation 259, 262
Deformity, external 136
Degenerative disease 43
Dehydrating hyperosmolar agents 9, 35, 37
Dehydration, chronic 80
Delirium 15, 15*f*, 16, 16*f*, 54, 88, 474
  hyperactive 15
  hypoactive 15
  mixed 15
Dementia
  cortical 16
  primary 17
  progressive 16
  secondary 17
  subcortical 16
Dengue
  fever 432
    pathogenesis of 432*f*
  shock syndrome 433

Depression 54
Dermatitis 381
  adult seborrheic 381
  allergic contact 367
  asteatotic 382
  atopic 381
  contact 381
  herpatiformis 76
  infantile seborrheic 381
  pompholyx 381
  varicose 382
Dermoplasty, septal 139
Desmopressin 300, 310
Dexamethasone 35, 78, 113, 118, 160
Diabetes insipidus 78
  central 79
  dipsogenic 79
  gestational 79
  nephrogenic 79
  pathophysiological aspects of 79*f*
Diabetes mellitus 8, 36, 59, 80, 92, 132, 154, 164, 269, 312, 314, 378
  pathophysiological aspects of 81*f*
Diabetic ketoacidosis 82, 83
  pathophysiological aspects of 83*f*
Diaphoresis 21, 214, 227, 251
Diarrhea 180, 180*f*
  acute
    bloody 180
    watery 180
  chronic 164
  persistent 180
Diathermy, submucous 157
Diethylstilbestrol 359
DiGeorge syndrome 96
Digital rectal examination 326, 339
Dihydrotestosterone, high levels of 338
Diltiazem 184, 252
Dimercaptosuccinic acid scintigraphy 326
Diphtheria 434, 434*f*
Dipstick test 432, 445
Disc arthroplasty 32
Discectomy 31
Discoid dermatitis 381
Disease-modifying antirheumatic drugs 395, 417
Dissecting aortic aneurysm 282
Disseminated intravascular coagulation 474
Distal intestinal obstruction syndrome 225
Distal limb amputation 305
Diuretics 36, 146, 223, 241, 245, 258, 264, 267, 281, 283, 397
Diverticulitis 192, 205
Diverticulosis 324
Dizziness 72, 86, 251
Dopamine
  agonists 54, 92
  blockers 16
Doppler echocardiography 223
Dorzolamide 122
Double crush syndrome 395
Down's syndrome 1, 22, 128

Doxycycline 342, 459
Drug resistance test 426
Dual action bone agents 414
Duraplasty 66
Durkan test 397
Dyschezia 172
Dysentery, amoebic 161
Dysmenorrhea 354, 355*f*
  primary 354
  secondary 355
Dyspepsia, flatulent 196
Dysphagia 184
Dyspnea 224, 230, 237, 243, 245, 269
  exertional 286
  paroxysmal nocturnal 286
Dysreflexia, autonomic 58
Dysrhythmias 217, 221, 245, 267, 275
  cardiac 259

E

Ear
  disorders of 132
  infections 441
    recurrent 142
  wax 134*f*
Ebola virus disease 435
  cardinal features of 436*f*
Ecchymosis 119, 419
Echocardiogram 50, 60, 70, 247, 254, 269, 276, 283, 285, 292, 321
Echocardiography 286, 290, 304
Eclampsia 311
Eczema 381
Edema 323*f*
  pulmonary 319
Ehlers-Danlos syndrome 252
Ejaculation problems 345*f*
Ejaculatory disorders 345
Ejection fraction testing 258
Electric field therapy 497
Electrocardiogram 3, 50, 60, 65, 70, 237, 247, 252, 255, 269, 276, 281, 285, 292
Electrocardiography 223
Electrocochleogram 141, 153
Electrocochleography 142, 146
Electroencephalogram 21, 23, 187, 227, 423
Electroencephalography 12, 56, 61, 73
Electromyogram 27, 31, 405
Electromyography 6, 23, 391, 397, 404, 414
Electron microscopy 466
Electronystagmography 141, 146, 153
Electrooculogram 130
Electrophysiology study 261
Electroretinogram 130
Electrosurgery 498
Elephantiasis 438
Emphysema 222, 236, 240
  pulmonary 220, 221
Empyema 231
Encephalitis 18, 28, 79, 391, 428, 454, 466
  acute 443
    disseminated 18

arboviral 18
limbic 51
primary 18
secondary 18
Encephalopathy
  hepatic 186, 189, 196
  hypertensive 319
  toxic metabolic 10
  uremic 329, 329f
Endarteritis 303
Endocarditis 235, 271, 271f, 286
  bacterial 6
  infective 285
  rheumatic 285
Endocervical culture 358
Endocrine, disorders of 75
Endolymphatic hydrops 145
Endometrial biopsy 358, 360, 362, 363
Endometrial polyps 354
Endometriosis 354, 356
Endometritis 352, 357
Endometrium 358f
Endophlebitis 303
Endoscopic retrograde
    cholangiopancreatography
    172, 486
Endoscopic sinus surgery 149
Endoscopic therapy 498
Endothelial cells 62f
Endothelin receptor antagonist 241, 304
Endotracheal intubation 249
Endovascular repair 254
Entamoeba histolytica 161, 193, 201, 202, 228
Enteritis, regional 164
Enterocolitis, necrotizing 206
Enteroscopy 175
Enterovirus 39, 132, 159, 459
Enthesitis 395
Envenomation 138
Enzyme-linked immunosorbent assay
    test 426, 427, 437, 449, 452,
    466, 473, 474
Eosinophilia 203
Epididymis, inflamed 342f
Epididymitis 341, 348
Epilepsy 19
  phases of 21
Epistaxis 137, 285
Epstein-Barr virus 132, 159, 478
Erectile dysfunction 92, 343, 343f
Erection problems 345f
Erysipelas 380
Erythema nodosum 175
Erythrocytosis 222
Erythromycin 48, 124, 160, 457
Erythropoiesis-stimulating agents 297
Erythropoietin agents 315
Escharotomy 377
Escherichia coli 39, 193, 325, 336, 347, 352, 411
Esophageal immune function 228
Esophageal sphincter, lower 183
Esophagitis 183

Esophagogastroduodenoscopy 205
Estrogen
  receptor modulators 90
  replacement therapy 370, 414
Ethmoidal nasal polyps 148
Eustachian tube dysfunction 156
Evoked response test 44
Ewing's sarcoma 398
Exacerbation, acute 412
Exercise stress testing 255
Extra-capsular cataract extraction 110
Extracorporeal membrane oxygen 239
Extracorporeal shock wave lithotripsy
    170, 328
Extracranial-intracranial arterial
    bypass 9, 61, 71
Extraskeletal bone, deposition of 406f
Extraventricular drain 37
Eye
  disorders of 105
  glasses 128
  normal 109f
  tests 50
  trauma 119
    penetrating 119f
Eyelid lacerations 120
Ezetimibe 256, 270, 279

F

Facet joint osteoarthritis 392
Facial
  cellulitis 380
  nerve palsy 151
  swelling, unilateral 133
Fainting, sudden 63
Fallopian tube 363f
Fanconi syndrome 409
Farsightedness 115
Fasciitis, necrotizing 154, 380
Fasciotomy 377
Fatigue 86, 251, 298, 467
Fatty liver disease, nonalcoholic 195
Febrile convulsions 433
Fecal occult blood test 297
Fertility
  agents 365
  promoting agents 360
Fever
  acute rheumatic 160
  dengue hemorrhagic 432
  enteric 471
  scarlet 383
Fibrates 256, 270, 279
Fibric acid derivatives 256, 270, 279
Fibrin sealants 300, 310
Fibrinogen test 300
Fibroids
  hysteroscopic resection of 362
  uterus 354, 361, 361f
Fibromuscular dysplasia 8
Fibromyalgia 392
Fibrosis
  pulmonary 245, 247
  retroperitoneal 312

Filariasis 222, 437
  pathogenesis of 438f
Finger prick test 439
Fissure, anal 162, 173, 164
Fissurectomy 163, 165
Fistula
  extrasphincteric 165
  intersphincteric 164
  suprasphincteric 164
Fistulotomy 165
Fitz-Hugh-Curtis syndrome 363
Flaccid
  paralysis 427
  penis 343f
Flagellates 202
Flail chest trauma 218
Flaring nostrils 249
Flavivirus 432, 442, 473, 475
Flavoxate 337
Floppy infant syndrome 22, 23f
Fluconazole 229
Fluid
  and electrolyte
    imbalance 203
    replacement 437
  deprivation test 80
  intravenous 433
  replacement therapy 326, 328,
      333, 337
  restriction 103
Flunisolide 148
Fluorescein angiography 106, 118
Fluoride therapy 153
Fluorometholones acetate 113
Fluoroquinolones 337, 447
Fluoxetine 3, 74
Fluticasone 148, 217
Fluvoxamine 3, 74
Four-fold hemagglutination inhibition
    test 427
Fracture 397
  pathological 412, 416
Fresh frozen plasma 301, 310
Friedreich's ataxia 57
Functional endoscopic sinus surgery
    157, 159
Fungal
  infection 39, 132, 228, 233, 271,
      280, 281, 373, 384, 385,
      387, 387f
  contagious 373f
  keratitis 125
  nail infection 384
Fusidic acid 113
Fusion inhibitors 426

G

Gallbladder 169f, 171f
  cancer 486
  radionuclide scan 172
Gallstones 171f
Gamete intrafallopian transfer 360
Gamma-aminobutyric acid 26
Gangrene 380

Gas exchange 244*f*
Gastrectomy 183
Gastric 54
   decompression 193
   mucosa, inflamed 182*f*
   ulcer 204
Gastritis 181, 182*f*
Gastroesophageal reflux 213
   disease 132, 150, 158, 183
Gastrointestinal surgery, postoperative 199
Gastrointestinal system, disorders of 161
Gastroparesis 82
Gene therapy 498
Genetic
   diseases 129
   testing 299, 405
Genital candidiasis 378
Gentamicin 167, 459
German measles 461
Giardia lamblia 197
Gigantism 91
Gilles De La Tourette syndrome 24
Glaucoma 120, 121*f*
   congenital 121
   open-angle 121
   post-traumatic 120
   secondary 121
Gliclazide 88
Glipizide 88
Glomerular
   capillaries 318*f*
   disease 323*f*
   filtration 329*f*
Glomerulonephritis 189, 318
   acute 133, 318
   chronic 314, 319, 321
Glomerulopathy 322
Glucagonoma 81
Glucocorticoids 76, 276
Glycerol 35
Glycoprotein receptor inhibitors 256, 270, 279
Glycosides, cardiac 258, 261, 264, 267
Goldflam disease 45
Gonadotropin-releasing
   analogs 341
   hormone agonists 360
Goniotomy 122
Gonorrhea 342, 356, 358, 362, 439
   signs 439*f*
   symptoms 439*f*
Goodpasture's syndrome 318
Gorlin syndrome 478
Gout 401
   cardinal features of 401*f*
Granulomas 49*f*
Grave's disease 46, 76, 92, 93
Growth hormone
   receptor antagonist 92
   releasing hormone test 99
Guanfacine 26
Guanylate cyclase C-agonist 174
Guillain-Barr syndrome 26, 26*f*, 102, 128, 244, 427, 476

Guttate 386
   psoriasis 383, 385

H

H1N1 467
H2-receptor antagonists 183, 184, 201, 205
Haemophilus influenzae 141, 144, 411
Hallucinations 330
Haloperidol 17, 74
Hand cellulitis 380
Hansen's disease 445
Hashimoto's thyroiditis 100
Hay fever 156
Head
   and neck cancer 487
   injury, severe 36
Headache 28, 28*f*, 39
   cervicogenic 28
   cluster 29
   inflammatory 29
   muscular 28
   myogenic 28
Hearing aids 141
Hearing loss 139
   central 140
   conductive 140
   mixed 140
Heart
   disease 416
      congenital 228, 257, 260, 265
      coronary 265
      ischemic 268
      rheumatic 265, 271
      valvular 285, 286*f*, 290
   failure 230, 274
      congestive 275
      hypertensive 273*f*
      hypotensive 275*f*
   muscle 277*f*
      biopsy 281
   pumps 268
   rate, accelerated 80
   transplantation 259, 268
   valves 286*f*
Heat 186
Helicobacter pylori 181, 203, 478
Helminthes 202
Hemarthrosis 399, 419
Hematuria 339
Hemicraniectomy, decompressive 9
Hemilaminectomy 32, 59
Hemispherectomy 22
Hemochromatosis 98, 263, 298, 298*f*
Hemodialysis 313, 315, 320, 321, 325, 330, 369
Hemoglobin, glycated 82, 84, 88
Hemolytic anemia 295, 295*f*
Hemolytic uremia syndrome 168
Hemophilia 299, 299*f*
   A 300
   acquired 300
   B 300
   C 300
Hemoptysis 215, 241, 243, 247

Hemorrhage 60, 72, 399
   external 291*f*
   internal 291*f*
   intraventricular 34
   vitreous 120
Hemorrhoidectomy 186
   cryosurgical 186
Hemorrhoids 173, 185, 185*f*, 370
   external 185
   internal 185
Hepatic dysfunction 449
Hepatic failure 48
Hepatitis 186, 188, 322, 426
   A 188
   acute 427
   B virus 188
   C 188
   D 188
   E virus 188
   viral 26
Hepatobiliary iminodiacetic scan scan 170
Hepatomegaly 196, 203, 298
Hepatorenal syndrome 196
Hernia 189
   epigastric 190
   femoral 190
   incisional 190
   inguinal 191, 341
   repair, open 191
   types of 190*f*
   umbilical 191
Hernioplasty 191
Herniorrhaphy 191
Heroin 48
Herpes simplex 26
   encephalitis 18
   virus 18, 39, 132, 159, 333
Heterotopic ossification 58, 73, 406
Hiccups 230
High dose dexamethasone suppression test 78
Histamine analog agents 146
Histoplasma 280
Histoplasmosis 76
Hodgkin's disease 26
Hodgkin's lymphoma 489
Holter monitoring 65
   ambulatory 252
Hordeolum 123
   external 123
   internal 123
Hormonal therapy 362, 497
Hormone
   replacement therapy 76, 78, 101, 171, 237, 344, 346, 360, 417
   test 258
Horner syndrome 66
Human B-type natriuretic peptide 264
Human chorionic gonadotropin 341
   stimulation test 341, 350, 357
Human immunodeficiency virus 424, 430
   infection 193, 195
Human metapneumovirus 233
Huntington's disease 16, 32, 32*f*

Hydantoin 22
Hydration, intravenous 48
Hydrocele testis 341
Hydrocephalus 34, 34f, 60, 73
    non-obstructive 35
Hydrocortisone 100
Hydrogen breath test 198
Hydronephrosis 339
Hydrotherapy 377
Hyperaldosteronism 85
    pathophysiological aspects of 86f
Hyperbaric oxygen chamber 14
Hypercalcemia 52, 199, 247
Hypercalciuria 327
Hypercapnia 245
Hypercholesterolemia 8, 36
Hyperglycemia 377
Hyperkalemia 312, 315
Hyperlipidemia 251, 266, 322, 323f
Hyperlipoproteinemia 8
Hypermature senile cataract 109
Hypermetropia 115
Hyperopia 123
Hyperosmolar hyperglycemic
    nonketotic syndrome 82, 87
    pathophysiological aspects of 87f
Hyperoxaluria 327
Hyperparathyroidism 89, 173, 199
    pathophysiological aspects of 89f
Hyperphosphatemia 312
Hyperpituitarism 91, 91f
Hyperplasia, benign prostatic 338f
Hypertension 59, 70, 82, 92, 94, 138, 260, 266, 269, 273, 285, 312, 314, 326, 343, 386
    chronic thromboembolic pulmonary 240
    portal 240
    pulmonary 239, 240, 288, 302
        arterial 240, 247
        venous 240
Hyperthyroidism 46, 92
    etiological aspects of 93f
Hypertonic saline infusion test 80
Hypertrophy
    benign prostatic 312
    left ventricular 274
Hyperuricemia 312
Hyperuricosuria 327
Hyperventilation 37, 443
Hypervolemia 266
Hyphema 119, 120
Hypoalbuminemia 322, 323f
Hypocalcemia 48, 209, 312, 330, 410
Hypochlorhydria 431
Hypoglycemia 76, 94, 99, 366, 432
    cycle of 95f
    mild 95
    moderate 95
    severe 95
Hypogonadism 299, 343
Hypokalemia 86, 432
Hypolipidemic agent 80
Hypometabolism 99
Hyponatremia 312, 330
Hypoparathyroidism 76, 96
    congenital 96, 97
    idiopathic 97
    pathophysiological aspects of 97f
Hypoperfusion, renal 311
Hypophosphatasia 409
Hypophosphatemia 409, 410
Hypophysectomy, pranssphenoidal 78, 92
Hypophysitis, lymphocytic 98
Hypopituitarism 76, 98
Hypospadias surgery 331
Hypotension 58, 76, 94, 99, 200, 238, 275
    neurally mediated 276
    orthostatic 54, 276
    postprandial 276
    postural 84, 276
Hypothalamic disorders 91
Hypothalamus, malfunctioning 79
Hypothermia 377
Hypothyroidism 99, 100, 100f, 101, 158, 266, 282, 395
    post-operative 97
Hypotonia 22, 23f
    congenital 22
Hypoventilation 211
Hypovolemia 377
    signs of 84
Hypoxemia 238, 245, 377
Hypoxia 224, 225, 240, 260, 275
    acute 226f
    anemic 226
    chronic 226f
    histotoxic 226
    hypoxic 226
    stagnant 226
Hysterectomy 352, 362, 365
    vaginal 370
Hysterosalpingography 360, 362
Hysteroscopy 358, 362

I

Ibuprofen 68, 135, 342
Ileal pouch anal anastomosis 210
Ileostomy 176, 193, 210
Iminostilbenes 22
Immune
    disorders 151
    suppressants 423
    system, abnormal 51f
Immunoglobulin 24, 27
    intravenous 39, 52, 63
Immunomodulators 50, 175, 209, 464
Immunoreactive trypsinogen test 225
Immunosuppressant 47, 50, 52, 382
    agents 45, 320, 434
    topical 382
Immunotherapy 497
Impetigo 382
    large blisters 383
    nonbullous 383, 383f
Implantable cardioverter defibrillator 259, 262, 264, 267, 281
In vitro fertilization 360
Incontinence
    functional 334
    mixed 334
    transient 334
    urge 334
Indirect fluorescent antibody test 452
Infarction
    migrainosus 29
    myocardial 251, 260, 265, 275, 277, 277f
    post-myocardial 282
Infection
    amoebic 202f
    bacterial 1, 39, 81, 107f, 112, 123, 125, 132, 143, 153, 159, 167, 193, 203, 216, 228, 231, 233, 242, 271, 280, 281, 325, 332, 336, 347, 352, 367, 371, 379, 383, 385, 394, 411, 429, 434, 439, 446, 448, 455, 457, 468, 470, 471
    gonorrheal 352
    maternal 350
    nosocomial 471
    parasitic 39, 161, 193, 197, 228, 333, 437, 444, 450
    pulmonary 6, 215
    symptomatic 425
Inferior vena cava 239
Infertility 348, 350
    causes of 359f
    female 359, 359f
    male 345
Inflammatory bowel disease 208, 307
Influenza 132, 233, 440
    symptoms of 441f
Injury
    depth of 375f
    traumatic 253
    tubular 311
Inotropic agent 292
Insomnia 341, 402
Insulin 82, 89
    induced hypoglycemia test 76
    secretion inhibitors 96
    therapy 85
        inadequate 84
    tolerance test 100
Integrase inhibitors 426
Intermittent anti-vertigo agents 146
International Spinal Cord Injury Classification System 57
Interstitial lung disease 236, 240
Intestine
    failure of 198f
    infections of 161f
    large 166f, 192f
Intra-capsular cataract extraction 110
Intracorneal rings 117
Intracranial pressure 36, 36f
Intracytoplasmic sperm injection 360
Intralesional therapy 499
Intraocular implants 116
Intraocular lens 110
Intraocular steroid agents 118
Intraurethral therapy 344, 346
Intrauterine device 429
Intrauterine insemination 360

Invasive candidiasis 378
Ipratropium bromide 158
Iridectomy 122
Iridodialysis 120
Iridotomy 122
Iron
   chelation therapy 297
   deficiency anemia 138, 293, 294*f*
   supplements 362
Irrigation 120
Irritants 112
Ischemia 275
   mesenteric 192
   silent 251
   visceral 255
Isolated limb infusion therapy 498
Isopropyl alcohol poisoning 22
Itchy eyelids 108

J

Japanese encephalitis 442
   pathogenesis of 442*f*
Jarisch-Herxheimer reaction 449
Joint and limb pain decompression
   sickness 12

K

Kala-azar 444
   pathogenesis of 444*f*
Kaposi's sarcoma 426, 487
Kartagener's syndrome 158
Kawasaki disease 144
Kennedy's disease 38, 38*f*
Keratectomy, photorefractive 115
Keratitis 124, 124*f*
   amoebic 124
   bacterial 125
   exposure 125
   nonulcerative sterile 125
   onchocercal 125
   ulcerative 125
   viral 125
Keratoplasty, conductive 116
Keratotomy, astigmatic 116
Ketoconazole 229, 388
Kidney
   biopsy 321
   disease 79, 98
      chronic 89, 314, 401
      cystic 327
   function
      impaired 87
      test 292, 315, 321, 323, 325,
         326, 328, 330, 368, 449
   hypoperfusion of 311
   injury, acute 311, 311*f*, 329, 449
   interstitial tissue of 325*f*
   stones 327
   ultrasonogram 321
Klinefelter's syndrome 341
Knee
   joint 408*f*
   replacement, partial 418
Kuru Creutzfeldt-Jakob disease 56
Kyphoplasty 414

Kyphoscoliosis 222
Kyphosis 92

L

Labyrinthectomy 147
Labyrinthitis 141, 145, 151
Lacunar cerebral infarction 8
Lambert-Eaton myasthenic syndrome
   50
Laminectomy 31, 58, 66, 393, 404
Laminotomy 31, 58
Lamivudine 189
Laparoscopic laser cholecystectomy
   170, 172
Laparoscopy 191, 357, 358, 363
Laparotomy 207
Laryngitis 233, 454
Laser
   angioplasty 256
   epithelial keratomileusis 116
   in situ keratomileusis 116
   photocoagulation 106, 118
   therapy 139, 186, 306
   thermal keratoplasty 116
   trabeculoplasty 122
Latanoprost 122
Latex agglutination test 41, 208
Laxatives 165
Leg cellulitis 380
Leishmania
   donovani 444, 445
   specific PCR test 445
   trypanosomea 201, 202
Leishmaniasis, visceral 444
Leprosy 445
Leptospira 448
   interrogans 448
Leptospirosis 448
   pathogenesis of 448*f*
Leukemia 479, 488
   chronic lymphocytic 154, 159
Leukocytosis 229, 326
Leukotriene inhibitors 214
Levofloxacin 342, 459
Levothyroxine, synthetic 101
Li-Fraumeni syndrome 478
Lightheadedness 72
Limb perfusion, isolated 498
Lipase supplements 199
Lipid profile test 101, 323, 372
Lipoprotein, low-density 323, 325
Liquid challenge test 103
Lithium 385
Lithotripsy 328
Liver
   abscess 193
      amoebic 193
   biopsy 194, 196
   cancer 488
   cells 194*f*
   cirrhosis 86, 195, 195*f*, 206, 230,
      233, 299, 311
   disease 225, 298
   dysfunction 197
   failure of 187*f*

   function test 84, 88, 172, 187, 194,
      196, 292, 299, 372, 433
   tissue, inflamed 188*f*
Lobectomy 216, 229, 235
Lodoxamide tromethamine 113
Loeys-Dietz syndrome 252
Long-term lithium therapy 89
Lopidine 122
Lou Gehrig's disease 3
Low dose dexamethasone suppression
   test 78
Loxapine 74
Lumbar disk herniation 402, 403*f*
Lumigan 122
Luminal amoebicides 162
Lump, formation of 111*f*
Lung
   abscess 228, 228*f*
      primary 228
      secondary 228
   biopsy 223
   cancer 489
   cystic 224
   disease 230
      acute 222
      chronic 233, 236, 265
      diffuse infiltrative 222
   disorders 63
   failure 405
   infections of 458
   sonography 237
   transplantation 223, 235, 241
Lupron 360
Lupus
   hemophagocyte syndrome, acute
      423
   nephritis 423
   pneumonitis 423
Luteinizing hormone urine test 360
Lyme disease 16
Lymph nodes, infections of 457
Lymphadenitis 374
Lymphadenopathy, persistent
   generalized 425
Lymphangitis 374, 438
Lymphomas 423, 426, 479

M

Macrolides 447
Macular degeneration
   dry age-related 106
   wet age-related 106
Maculopathy 106
Magnetic resonance
   angiography 61, 70
   cholangiopancreatography 201
   imaging scan 6, 12, 19, 21, 25, 35,
      41, 50, 58, 61, 68, 70, 78, 80,
      92, 100, 141, 144, 148, 154,
      156, 160, 165, 175, 187, 194,
      197, 203, 206, 223, 239, 254,
      255, 267, 285, 292, 315, 325,
      337, 363, 370, 391, 393, 402,
      407, 417, 421, 439
Malabsorption syndrome 197, 409

Malaria 450
  pathogenesis of 450f
Malignancy, hematological 138
Malnutrition 243
Mannitol 35
Marfan's syndrome 236, 252, 271
Marsupialization 354
Mast cell
  inhibitors 214
  stabilizer 113
Mastoid cells, inflammation of 143f
Mastoidectomy 145
Mastoiditis 143, 143f, 151, 208
Maternal systemic diseases 350
McArdle's disease 48
Measles 452
  cardinal features of 453f
Mechanical ventilation 219, 245
Medrysone 113
Meglitinide analogs 82, 85, 88
Meibomian cyst 123
Meibomian gland dysfunction 123
Melanoma 490
Meniere's disease 145, 145f
Meniere's syndrome 140
Meninges 40f
Meningitis 8, 28, 39, 65, 79, 98, 134,
    151, 208, 235, 247, 449
  aseptic 40
  bacterial 40
  cryptococcal 426
  viral 40
Meningoencephalitis 427
Meningomyelocele 57
Menstrual cycles, irregular 92
Menstruation, painful 355f
Meperidine 172
Metabolic disorders 63, 151, 263, 395,
    408
  inherited 8
Metabolic syndrome 251, 386
Metformin 88
Methenamine 337
Methyldopa 26
Methylprednisolone 160, 217
Methylxanthines 214, 221
Miconazole 388
Microdiscectomy 31, 58, 393, 404
Microscopic agglutination test 449
Middle ear infections 136
Migraine 28, 29, 39
Mineral 106
  disorder 315
Mineralocorticoid 76
  receptor antagonists 87
Minimal invasive surgical treatments
    340
Minocycline 447
Miotics agents 122
Miscarriage 351
Mitral valve prolapse 287
Moccasin 373
Moebius syndrome 42
  cardinal features of 42f
Molecular test 225

Monoamine
  depletors 33
  oxidase inhibitors 54
Mononucleosis 26, 144
  infectious 154, 159
Mood stabilizers 16, 33
Moraxella catarrhalis 141, 144
Morphine 172
Multiorgan dysfunction syndrome 258
Multiple endocrine neoplasia
    syndrome 77, 89
Multiple myeloma 16, 43, 43f, 57, 173,
    322, 343, 398, 491
Multiple system atrophy 276
Mumps 454
Muscarinic receptor antagonists 125
Muscle
  atrophy 404
  biopsy 23, 405
  integrity test 115
  relaxants 27, 31, 45, 58, 393, 404
  strain 406f
  tone 23f
Muscular dystrophy 22, 404, 405f
Musculoskeletal system, disorders
    of 392
Myalgia 224, 467
Myasthenia gravis 45, 45f, 51, 76, 128
  congenital 46
  generalized 46
  ocular 46
  transient neonatal 46
Mycobacterium
  leprae 445, 446
  tuberculi 231, 242
Mycoplasma 233
  genitalium 332
  pneumoniae 233
Myectomy, septal 264
Myelin 43f
Myelogram 31, 393, 404
Myelography 66
Myelomeningocele 34
Myocardial infarction, acute 282
Myocardial perfusion scintigraphy 252
Myocarditis 279, 280f, 427, 435, 461
Myoclonus 330
Myoglobinuria 47
Myomectomy 360, 362
Myopia 114
Myositis 52
  ossificans 400, 406, 406f
Myringoplasty 151
Myringotomy 144, 151
Myxedema 100, 101, 282
Myxomatous degeneration 285, 286

N

Naegleria fowleri 39
Naproxen 135
Narcotic 393
Narcotic analgesics 233
Nasal
  cavity 155f
  corticosteroid

  spray 137
  topical 158
  decongestant 136, 156, 158
  endoscope 136, 138, 148, 156
  polyps 147, 147f, 156, 225
    nonallergic 148
  septum 135f
Nateglinide 88
Nausea 467
Nearsightedness 114
Necrosis
  avascular 400
  papillary 312
Nedocromil sodium 113, 214
Needle aspiration 160
  test 160
Neisseria gonorrhoeae 132, 332, 439
Nematodes 202
Neomycin 187
Neoplasm 338
Nephritic syndrome 230
Nephritis 208
  heredity 318
Nephropathy
  diabetic 82
  membranous 322
Nephrosclerosis 274, 320, 320f
  benign 320
Nephrostolithotomy, percutaneous
    328
Nephrotic syndrome 86, 311, 319,
    322, 323f
Nephrotoxic
  agents 311
  drugs 314
  medication 312
Nerve
  compression of 67f
  conduction
    study 4
    tests 404
    velocity 23, 27, 391
  transfer 59
Nervous system, disorders of 1
Neural transplantation 54
Neuralgia, postherpetic 391
Neurectomy, selective vestibular 147
Neuritis 462
Neuroendocrine dysfunction 73
Neurofibromatosis 478
Neurogenic thoracic outlet syndrome
    67
Neuroleptic 3, 25, 74
  malignant syndrome 48
Neurological tests 50, 247, 344
Neurons, degeneration of 32f
Neuropathy
  diabetic 82, 343
  peripheral 52, 168, 247
  sensory 1
Neuropsychological testing 3, 17
Neurosarcoidosis 49, 49f
Neurotomy, selective peripheral 59
Neurotoxin 26
  agents 335

Neutron activation analysis 414
Neutropenia 423
Niacin 256, 270, 279
Nicardipine 252
Nissen fundoplication 184
Nitrates 252, 255, 258, 269, 278
Nitrofurantoin 337
Nitrosoureas 497
N-methyl D-aspartate
    receptor antagonist 3, 73
    blockers 18
Nometasone 148
Non-Hodgkin lymphoma 490
Non-nucleoside reverse transcriptase
    inhibitors 426
Nonspecific-type thoracic outlet
    syndrome 68
Nonsteroidal anti-androgen agents
    365
Nonsteroidal anti-inflammatory
    agents 285, 427
    drugs 30, 31, 45, 50, 58, 65, 68, 133,
        135, 136, 143, 144, 154, 158,
        160, 232, 247, 314, 348, 356,
        362, 367, 397, 402, 404, 409,
        417, 423
Nose, disorders of 132
Nucleoside
    analog agents 437, 464
    reverse transcriptase inhibitors
        426
Nutritional deficiencies 15
    correction of 199

O

Obstruction
    aqueductal 34
    intestinal 192
    tracheal 248
Obstructive sleep apnea 160
Ocular coherence tomography scan
    118
Odynophagia 154, 184
Olanzapine 17, 74
Olfactory system testing 54
Omega 3 fatty acids 108
Onchocerciasis 129
Onychomycosis 379, 384, 384f
    lateral subungual 384
    proximal subungual 384
    total dystrophic 385
Oophorectomy 365
Open-heart surgery 239
Opioids 393
    weak 409
Opsoclonus-myoclonus syndrome 51
Optic
    nerve hypoplasia 130
    neuritis 129
Optical coherence tomography 106
Oral dissolution therapy 172
Oral glucose tolerance test 82, 96
Oral hypoglycemic agents 365
Oral iron supplements 297
Oral rehydration salts 432
Oral salt loading test 86
Oral thrush, appearance of 378f
Orbital cellulitis 380
Orchidopexy 341
    two-stage 341
Orchitis 455, 462
Oropharyngeal airway insertion 249
Oropharyngeal candidiasis 378
Orthomyxovirus 467
Orthopnea 286
Osmodiuretics 19, 41
Osmotic diuretics 48, 61, 70, 443
Osteoarthritis 400, 403, 408
Osteomalacia 398, 409, 400, 410f, 411,
    411f
Osteonecrosis 408
Osteo-odonto-keratoprosthesis,
    modified 131
Osteopenia 92
Osteoporosis 76, 92, 94, 225, 398, 412,
    413f, 423
Osteotomy 409, 418
Otitic hydrocephalus 151
Otitis media 149, 149f, 150, 156, 160,
    208, 467
    acute suppurative 150
    chronic suppurative 150
    recurrent 150
Otosclerosis 151
    diffuse active 152
    early focal 152
    quiescent 152
Otoscope, pneumatic 151
Ovarian cancer 492
Ovary, normal 364f
Oxazolidinediones 22
Oxiconazole 388
Oxygen therapy 14, 212, 219, 223, 225,
    227, 229, 231, 232, 235, 237,
    241, 245, 247, 368, 412
Oxygenation 84
Oxymetazoline 158

P

Pacemaker, cardiac 262
Paget's disease 266, 398, 415, 415f
Pain
    acute scrotal 342
    chronic 410, 480
    pleural 212
    pleuritic 238
    severe chronic 66
Palliative surgery 498
Pallidotomy 54
Pan retinal photocoagulation 118
Pancreatic function test 198
Pancreaticoduodenectomy 201
Pancreaticojejunostomy 201
Pancreatitis 81, 84, 172, 199, 200f,
    205, 455
    acute 199, 282
    chronic 199
    familial 199
Panencephalitis, progressive 462
Papillary muscles, rupture of 265
Papilledema 37
Paracentesis 197
Paracetamol 342, 443, 476
    preparations 434
Paralysis 443
    intermittent 86
Paralytic ileus 192, 461
Paramyxovirus 454f
Paraneoplastic syndromes 50
Parathyroid hormone 89, 102
    recombinant 98, 414
    secretion of 99f
Parathyroidectomy
    partial 90
    total 90
Parkinson's disease 53, 53f, 98, 173,
    343, 386
    advanced 16
Parotitis 474
    epidemic 454
Pelvic
    bone fractures 331
    cavity 369f
    congestion syndrome 354
    infections 358
    inflammatory disease 206, 354,
        359, 362, 363f, 430
    laparoscopy 362
    malignancy 312
    pain, chronic 363, 430
    peritonitis 358
Penicillin 160, 337, 459
Penile
    cancer 493
    implants 344, 347
    ultrasound 344
Peptic ulcer disease 91, 199, 203, 204f
Percutaneous needle aspiration 195
Percutaneous tibial nerve stimulation
    335
Percutaneous transhepatic
    cholangiography 172
Percutaneous transluminous coronary
    angioplasty 256, 279
Percutaneous transthoracic tube
    drainage 229
Perfusion lung scan 239
Pericardiectomy 283
Pericardiocentesis 283
Pericarditis 235, 281, 282f
    chronic 282
    constrictive 282, 283
Periodontal disease 154, 228
Periorbital cellulitis 380
Peripheral artery disease 255, 290, 312
Peritoneal dialysis 206, 313, 316, 330
Peritonitis 205
    primary 206
    secondary 206
Peritonsillar abscess 153, 160
Pertussis 455
    pathogenesis of 456f
Petrosal sinus 78
Petrositis 151
Peyronie's disease 343

Phalen's test 397
Pharyngitis 207, 207f
    acute 132, 132f
    previous episodes of 132
Phenazopyridine 337
Phenformin 88
Phenylephrine 158
Phenytoin 36, 409
Phimosis 347
Phlebectomy
    ambulatory 306
    transilluminated powered 306
Phlebitis 306
Phlebotomy 223, 299
Phosphodiesterase inhibitors 241, 339, 344, 346
Photocoagulation
    infrared 186
    laser surgery 127
Photodynamic therapy 107, 372
Photokeratitis 125
Phototherapy 382
Physical therapy 52, 68, 405
Pick's disease 16
Pilocarpine 122
Pink-to-red annular patches 387f
Piperacillin 35, 41
Piriformis syndrome 392
Plague 457
    pathogenesis of 458f
    pneumonic 458
    septicemic 458
Plant alkaloids 497
Plaque 386
Plasma exchange 45, 52
Plasmapheresis 24, 27, 45, 52, 297
Plasminogen activator 308
Plasmodium
    toxoplasma 201, 202
    vivax 450
Platelet
    aggregation test 310
    inhibiting agents 9, 61, 70
    transfusion 293, 433
Pleural effusion 154, 230, 244
Pleurectomy 231
Pleurisy 231, 232f, 423
Pleuritic chest pain 230, 237
Pleuritis 231
Pleurodesis 229, 237
Pleurodynia 231
Pneumonectomy 216
Pneumonia 27, 60, 208, 217, 230, 233, 233f, 243, 391, 400, 414, 428, 441, 454, 466, 467, 474
    community-acquired 234
    hospital-acquired 234
    necrotizing 228
    opportunistic 234
Pneumothorax 221, 231, 235, 236f, 244
    simple 236
    traumatic 236
Poliomyelitis 459
    pathogenesis of 460f
Polyarteritis nodosa 318

Polycystic kidney 324f
    disease 314, 324, 329
Polycystic ovary 364f
    disease 364, 364f
    syndrome 81, 365
Polymerase chain reaction 428, 439, 449, 452, 466
    test 133, 433, 437, 455, 457, 474
Polymyositis 48
Polymyxin B sulphate 124
Polyp biopsy 148
Polypectomy 149
Pontine myelinolysis, central 103
Porphyria 26
Positive tourniquet test 433
Positron emission tomography 73
    scan 52, 255, 269
Postphlebitic syndrome 308
Post-polio syndrome 461
Post-streptococcal glomerulonephritis 160, 383, 385
Post-thrombotic syndrome 239
Post-void residual volume test 339
Potassium
    permanganate 164
    sensitivity test 317
    sparing diuretics 197, 365
Prasugrel 252
Prednisolone 35
Prednisone 63, 118, 212, 447
Pregnancy
    ectopic 356, 357f
    termination of 350f
Premature ventricular contraction 261
Prematurity, retinopathy of 130
Premenstrual syndrome 366, 366f
Presbyopia 115
Pressure hydrocephalus, normal 35
Prinzmetal's angina 251
Proctocolectomy, total 210
Propionibacterium acnes 371
Propylthiouracil 94
Prostaglandin 352, 357
    analogs 122, 205
    inhibitors 80
    renal 313
Prostate
    biopsy 339
    cancer 494
    enlarged 338f
    inflamed 347f
    normal 347f
    specific antigen test 339, 348
    transurethral
        incision of 339
        resection of 339, 348
Prostatectomy, open 339
Prostatic stents 340
Prostatitis 347, 347f
    bacterial 348
    non-bacterial 348
Protease inhibitors 426
Protein, abnormal accumulation of 55f
Proteinuria 321, 322, 323f
Prothrombin time test 300

Proton pump inhibitors 183, 184, 205
Protozoa 202
Pruritus 315
Pseudohypertrophy 405
Pseudohypoparathyroidism 97
Pseudomonas aeruginosa 411
Psoriasis 378, 385, 386f
Psychiatric disorders 63
Pulmonary embolism 230, 237, 414, 471
Pulmonary function test 212, 214, 216, 223, 225, 405
Pulse oximetric examination 212, 235
Pulsed light therapy 306
Punch excision 373
Pyelogram, intravenous 319, 328, 330
Pyelonephritis 317, 325, 328, 336
    acute 326
    chronic 326
Pyemia 412
Pyloroplasty 183
Pyoderma gangrenosum 175
Pyogenic arthritis, acute 412
Pyogenic liver abscess 193
Pyuria 326

Q

Quantitative buffy coat test 452
Quetiapine 17

R

Radial keratotomy 116
Radiation
    fibrosis 312
    infrared 186
    therapy 96, 230, 353
Radioactive iodine therapy 94, 498
Radiofrequency catheter ablation 259, 262, 265
Radiofrequency occlusion 306
Radioiodine uptake test 94
Radioisotope liver scan 200
Radionuclide scan 337
Radiotherapy 497
Ramsay Hunt syndrome 391
Ranibizumab 118
Rapid antigen tests 133
Rapid diagnostic test 452
Rapid molecular assay test 442
Rapid plasma reagin blood test 469
Rapid polymerase chain reaction 464
Raynaud's phenomenon 301, 301f
Real-time polymerase chain reaction 454
Red blood cells 293f, 294f, 452
    decreased production of 445
Refraction test 115
Regurgitation
    aortic 286
    mitral 288
    pulmonic 288
    tricuspid 289
Reiter's syndrome 168
Renal artery 86
    stenosis 86, 329

Renal calculi 327
Renal disease 320
　　end-stage 314, 319
Renal duplex echography 323
Renal failure 245, 427, 432
　　acute 311
　　chronic 314f, 409
Renal function test 229
Renal system, disorders of 311
Renal transplantation 313, 316, 320, 325, 331
Renin inhibitors 275, 315, 330
Repaglinide 88
Reproductive system
　　disorders of 338
　　female 350
　　male 338
Respiratory disease, family history of 244
Respiratory failure 46, 58, 66, 239, 244, 427
　　acute 237, 244
　　chronic 244
Respiratory infection, childhood 216
Respiratory muscles, paralysis of 27
Respiratory system, disorders of 211
Respiratory tract infections, viral 213
Restlessness 245
Retina 62f
　　normal 117f
Retinal detachment 126, 126f
　　rhegmatogenous 126
　　secondary 126
Retinitis pigmentosa 129, 130
Retinoids 372, 387
Retinopathy
　　diabetic 82, 117, 117f, 126, 129
　　mild nonproliferative 117
　　moderate nonproliferative 117
　　proliferative 117
　　severe nonproliferative 117
Retinopexy, pneumatic 127
Retrolental fibroplasias 129
Reverse transcription polymerase chain reaction 467
　　test 443
Reye syndrome 428
Rhabdomyolysis 48, 84
Rheumatic fever 208, 282, 283, 285, 286
　　cardinal features of 284f
Rheumatoid 416f
　　arthritis 46, 101, 230, 280, 301, 395, 408, 416
　　lung 417
　　vasculitis 417
Rheumatologic disorders 286
Rhinitis 155
　　allergic 132, 156
　　infectious 156
　　nonallergic 156
Rhinoplasty 137
Rhinovirus 132
Rib fracture fixation 219
Rifampin 447

Rifaximin 187
Rimantadine 160
Ring worm 387f
Rinne test 135
Risperidone 17, 74
Royal disease 299
Rubber band ligation 186
Rubella 461
　　cardinal features of 461f
　　virus 461
Rubeola 452

S

Sacral
　　colpopexy 370
　　neuromodulation 335
Sacroiliac joint disease 392
Salbutamol 217
Saline suppression test 86
Salivary glands 454f
Salmeterol 214
Salmonella typhi 471
Salmonellosis 426
Salpingitis 358
Salvage surgery 498
Sarcoidosis 98, 100, 246, 263, 280
Sarcomas 479
Sarcoptes scabiei 388
Scabicidal agents, topical 389
Scabies 388, 389f
Scalene muscle hypertrophy 67
Scar tissue 111f
Schistosoma fasciola 201, 202
Schistosomiasis 222, 240
Scleral buckling 127
Scleroderma 301
Sclerosis
　　amyotrophic lateral 3, 4f
　　tuberous 324, 478
Sclerostomy 122
Sclerotherapy 186, 306
Scoliosis 66, 405, 406
Scrotal fistula, cutaneous 342
Scrotum 349f
Sedatives 16
Seizure 19, 29, 60, 73, 168, 443
　　absence 20
　　atonic 20
　　complex partial 21
　　myoclonic 20
　　partial 21
　　simple partial 21
　　tonic clonic 20
Selective COX-2 inhibitors 409, 418
Selective estrogen receptor modulator 414
Selective serotonin reuptake inhibitors 3, 56, 74, 367
Senile cataract
　　immature 109
　　mature 109
Sensorineural hearing loss 140
Sepsis 311, 317, 336, 428
Septal ablation 265

Septicemia 154, 235, 358, 383, 412
Septoplasty 137, 139, 157
Septostomy, atrial 223
Sequestrectomy 412
Seroconversion illness 425
Serological test 449
Sertraline 3, 74
Seton placement 165
Severe acute respiratory syndrome 462
　　management of 463f
Severe pulmonary hemorrhagic syndrome 449
Sexual dysfunction 66
Sexual reproduction 451
Sexually transmitted infections 362, 430, 342, 356, 358
Sheehan's syndrome 98
Shigella dysenteriae 167
Shigellosis 167
Shingles 390, 390f
Shy-Drager syndrome 276
Sickle cell
　　anemia 240, 295, 296f
　　disease 222, 411
Sickness, pulmonary 14
Sigmoidoscopy 173, 175
Simmond's disease 98
Simultaneous red reflex test 128
Single photon emission computed tomography 21, 54
Sinus
　　arrhythmia 260
　　bradycardia 260
　　cavity, inflamed 157f
　　headache 29
　　infections 441
　　　chronic 147
　　　frequent 136
　　surgery, Open 159
　　tachycardia 260
　　tract malignancy 412
Sinusitis 28, 156, 157, 208, 213, 217, 367, 467
　　acute 158
　　chronic 158
　　recurrent 158
　　subacute 158
Sitz bath 164
Skeletal muscle dysfunction 221
Skeletal traction 400
Skin
　　allergy test 158
　　cancer 495
　　disorders of 371
　　inflamed 386f
　　normal 386f
　　rash 390f
　　traction 400
Slit-lamp test 106, 108, 115, 124
Small bowel movements 173f
Small incision cataract surgery 110
Smallpox 464, 464f
Snellen test 130
Sodium valproate 36

Soft tissue
  biopsy 412
  fillers 372
  resulting 406f
Somatostatin analogues 92
Sonohysterography 362
Sore throat 132
Spasticity 58, 73
Sphincterectomy, lateral internal 163
Sphincterotomy, endoscopic 170, 197
Spina bifida 65, 341
Spinal arachnoiditis 65
Spinal bulbar muscular atrophy 38
Spinal cord
  compression 480
  cystic enlargement of 65f
  injury 57, 58f, 65, 173, 320, 343, 345, 417
  stimulation 59
  tumor 65, 495
Spinal fusion 32, 58, 406
Spinocerebellar ataxia 57
Spondylolisthesis, isthmic 392
Sporozoa 202
Sports injuries 398
Sprain 418
Spurs 136
Sputum culture examination 212
Squamous cell carcinoma 412
Squint eyes 127, 128f
Stapedectomy 151
  partial 153
  total 153
Staphylococcal infection 112
Staphylococcus aureus 123, 141, 228, 367, 383, 411
  methicillin-resistant 383
Staphylococcus pyogenes 383
Statins 48, 323
Status migrainosus 29
Steatohepatitis, nonalcoholic 195
Steatorrhea 169
Stein-Leventhal syndrome 364
Stem cell transplantation 297
Stenosis
  aortic 287
  mitral 288
  pulmonic 289
  renal 320
  tricuspid 290
Stereotactic radiosurgery 92, 498
Steroids
  topical 387
  weak topical 108, 111
Stiff person syndrome 51
Stimulants 174
Stomach 183f
  cancer 495
  defective lining of 204f
  ulcer 205, 291
Stomatitis 480
Stool
  sample test 432
  softeners 163, 174
Strabismus 127, 128f, 129
Strain 420, 420f

Streptococcal tonsillitis 385
Streptococcus
  milleri 193
  organisms 379
  pneumoniae 141, 143
  pyogenes 141, 143, 159, 367
Streptokinase 239, 279, 308
Streptomycin 459
Stress
  emotional 63
  incontinence 334
  test 276
Striated muscle, breakdown of 47f
Stroke 59
  hemorrhagic 60
  ischemic 60
  types of 59f
Struvite stones 327
Subinguinal varicocele ligation 346, 350
Substance abuse disorder 367
Substantia nigra 53f
Succinimides 22
Sulfamethoxazole 457
Sulfonylureas 82, 85, 88
Superficial white onychomycosis 384
Superior vena cava syndrome 480
Surgery
  abdominal 206
  endoscopic 397
Susac's syndrome 62, 62f
Swab test 363
Sweat chloride test 225
Swine flu 466
  symptoms of 466f
Swollen
  gastrointestinal tract 174f
  lymphoid follicles 207
  tonsils 159f
Sympathectomy 303
  lumbar 305
  periarterial 305
Sympathomimetic 122
  catecholamine 292
Synarel 360
Syncope 63, 64f
Syndrome of inappropriate
    antidiuretic hormone secretion 102, 480
  pathophysiological aspects of 102f
Synovectomy 418
Synovial fluid analysis 417
Syphilis 163, 285, 468, 468f
Syringobulbia 66
Syringomyelia 65
  congenital 65
  idiopathic 66
  traumatic 65
Systemic lupus erythematosus 8, 26, 39, 46, 230, 301, 318, 322, 421
  cardinal features of 422f

T

Tachycardia 21, 84, 133, 214, 223, 227, 229, 230, 235, 238, 285

atrial 260
junctional 261
Tachypnea 212, 227, 229, 235, 237, 238
Taenia echinococcus 201, 202
Tarsorrhaphy 43
Taxanes 497
Tay-Sachs disease 22
Teletherapy 497
Tenesmus 168
Tenofovir 189
Tension pneumothorax 236
Terbinafine 388
Testes, undescended 340, 345
Testicular
  atrophy 350
  cancer 341, 495
  dysfunction 76
  infarction 342
  injury 341
Tetanus 470
  immune globulin 471
  pathogenesis of 470f
Tetany 98
Tetracycline 172, 337
  antibiotics 103
Thalamotomy 54
Thalassemia 293, 294f
Thalidomide 447
Thecoperitoneal shunting 66
Theophylline 217
Thermal therapy 498
Thiamine hydrochloride 16
Thiazide diuretics 80, 275, 315, 320, 330
Thiazolidinediones 82, 85, 89
Thoracentesis 213, 231, 233, 236
Thoracic
  aortic aneurysm 253
  myelopathy 14
  outlet syndrome 67
  ultrasonogram 237
Thoracotomy 231, 233, 235, 237
Throat, disorders of 132
Thrombectomy 239
  venous 308
Thromboangiitis obliterans 303, 304f
Thrombocytopenia 52, 423, 449, 454
Thrombocytopenic purpura 462
Thrombocytosis 52
Thromboembolism 288
Thromboendarterectomy, pulmonary 241
Thrombolytic 68, 256, 279, 308
  agents 239
Thrombosis, venous 307
Thymectomy 47
Thyroid
  agenesis, congenital 100
  disease 343
  dysfunction 260
  eye disease 127
  function test 3, 94, 101
  hormone 102
  tumor 496
Thyroidectomy 94
  subtotal 94

Thyroiditis, chronic 76
Thyrotoxicosis 265
Ticagrelor 252
Tilt table test 276
Timolol 122
Tinea
    corporis 379, 387, 387f
    mentagrophytes 384
    pedis 373, 379
Tinel's test 397
Tinnitus 142
Tissue
    amoebicides 162
    freezing 157
    plasminogen activator 239, 279
Toenails, infections of 384f
Tolbutamide 88
Tongue wasting 66
Tonometric test 130
Tonsillectomy 151, 155, 160
Tonsillitis 132, 159
Topoisomerase inhibitors 497
Total knee replacement 418
Tourette syndrome, complex clinical spectrum of 24f
Toxic shock syndrome 138, 367, 367f, 428
Toxoplasmosis 426
Trabeculectomy 122
Tracheitis 367
Tracheostomy 249
Traction 400
    headache 29
Tractional retinal detachment 126
Tranquilizers 33
Transaxillary approach 68
Transcranial Doppler ultrasound 73
Transient ischemic attack 59, 69, 69f
Transmyocardial revascularization 270
Transoral incisionless fundoplication 184
Transsphincteric fistula 164
Transurethral microwave therapy 340
Transurethral needle ablation 340
Travatan 122
Trematodes 202
Treponema pallidum 468
Triamcinolone 118, 148
Trichiasis 107
Trichomonas vaginalis 333
Trichophyton rubrum 373, 384, 385, 387
Tricyclic antidepressants 391
Triglycerides 78
Trimethoprim 457
    sulfamethoxazole 337
Tube thoracostomy 231
Tuberculin skin test 76, 243
Tuberculosis 79, 98, 215, 228, 281, 358, 426
    miliary 243
    pulmonary 222, 242, 242f
Tube-shunt surgery 122
Tumor
    adrenal 481
    cancerous 51f
    necrosis factor 210
    noncancerous 361f
    parathyroid 493
    pituitary gland 493
    resection 22
Tumorlysis syndrome 480
Turbinectomy 157
Turcot syndrome 478
Turner syndrome 252, 478
Tympanocentesis 151
Tympanoplasty 151
Typhoid 471
    pathogenesis of 472f

U

Ulcer, duodenal 204
Ultrasonogram 315, 341, 400
    vaginal 358
Ultrasonography 317, 363, 397
Uncover test 128
Upper endoscopy 486
Upper respiratory tract infection 5, 216, 410
Urea 35
Ureteroscopy 328
Ureterovesical reflux 325
Urethral dilation 332
Urethral stent placement 332
Urethral strictures 312, 331, 331f
Urethritis 332, 332f, 347
Urethrostomy 332
Uric acid stones 327
Urinalysis 80, 84, 88, 328, 330, 335, 336
Urinary analgesics 317, 325, 326, 328, 333, 337
Urinary flow test 339
Urinary incontinence 73, 334
Urinary retention 54
    acute 339
Urinary tract
    infection 27, 314, 317, 328, 331, 335, 336, 336f, 342, 370, 426
    frequent 347, 370
    microbial invasion of 336f
    obstruction 314
Urination, frequency of 326
Urine analysis 342, 344, 348
Urokinase 279, 308
Ursodiol 172
Uterine
    artery embolization 362
    prolapse 369, 369f
Uterus
    inflamed 363f
    irritated lining of 358f
    pregnancy outside of 357f
Uveitis 395

V

Vacuum erection devices 344, 347
Vaginal canal 369f
Vaginal pessary 370
Vaginitis 379
Vagotomy 183
Valproates 22
Valsalva maneuver test 276
Valve
    regurgitation 285
    stenosis 285
Valvular disorders 265
Valvular dysfunction, severe 257
Vancomycin 35, 41
Vaporization 340
Varicella zoster virus 390, 428
Varicocele 349, 349f
    embolization 346, 350
    ligation, laparoscopic 346, 350
Varicocelectomy 346, 350
Vas deferens 342f
Vascular disease
    ischemic 199
    peripheral 274, 411
Vascular disorders 138, 152
Vascular system, disorders of 291
Vascular thoracic outlet syndrome 68
Vasculitis 39, 253, 311
Vasoconstrictive agents 138
Vasodilators 241, 264, 267, 275, 303
Vasopressin
    receptor antagonists 103
    test 80
Vasopressor 277
Vasospasm 60
    coronary 268
Veins
    dilated abdominal 196
    distended jugular 238
    enlarged 349f
    ligation 306
    normal 349f
    stripping 307
    varicose 305, 305f
Venography 68
Ventilation 84, 239
Ventriculostomy 36
Verapamil 184, 252
Vernal keratitis 125
Vertebroplasty 414
Vertigo 72
Vibrio cholerae 430
Violent coughing spells 63
Viral infection 26, 39, 81, 132, 145, 151, 159, 188, 199, 216, 231, 233, 281, 333, 385, 428, 442, 459, 461, 467, 473, 475
Viral load test 426
Viral respiratory infection 233
Virus infection 112
Viscocanalostomy 122
Vision
    blurred 72
    therapy 129
Visual acuity test 99, 106, 108, 110, 113, 115, 122, 124, 128
Visual field test 122, 130
Visual impairment 129, 129f
Vitamin 197
    B absorption, failure of 296f
    D supplements 414
    replacements 297
    supplements 243

Vitiligo 76
Vitrectomy 118, 127
Voiding cystourethrogram 326
Vomiting 184, 480
von Hippel-Lindau syndrome 324, 478
von Willebrand's disease 138, 308, 309*f*
von Willebrand's factor
    activity test 310
    antigen test 310
Vulvovaginal candidiasis 378

W

Wasting syndrome 426
Water pills 241
Weber test 135
Wegener's granulomatosis 318
Western blot test 426
Whipple's disease 197
Whipple's procedure 201
Whooping cough 455
Wilson's disease 96, 409
Wuchereria bancrofti 437

X

Xathine oxidase inhibitors 313
X-ray 6, 73
Xylose absorption test 198

Y

YAG laser 186
Yeast infection 378
Yellow fever 473
    jungle 474
    pathogenesis of 473*f*
    urban 474
Yersinia pestis 457

Z

Zidovudine 160
Zika virus disease 475, 476
    pathogenesis of 475*f*
Zinc supplements 432
Zoladex 360
Zollinger-Ellison syndrome 197, 204
Zygote intrafallopian transfer 360

www.ingramcontent.com/pod-product-compliance
Ingram Content Group UK Ltd.
Pitfield, Milton Keynes, MK11 3LW, UK
UKHW050319210425
457661UK00008B/362